Exam Preparatory Manual for Undergraduates

Oral Medicine and Radiology

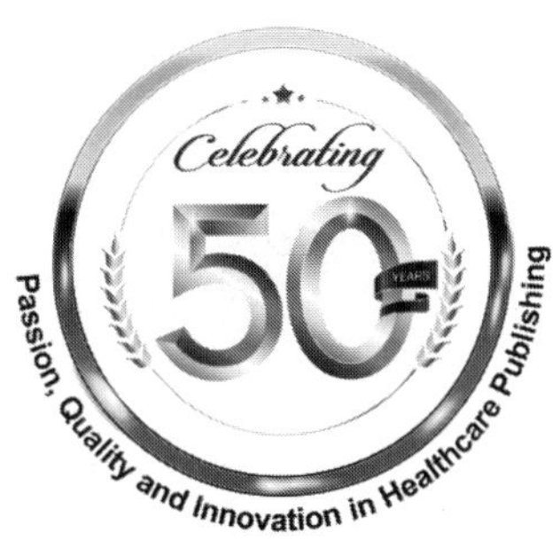

Exam Preparatory Manual for Undergraduates
Oral Medicine and Radiology

K Anbarasi MDS PhD
Associate Professor
Faculty of Dental Sciences
Department of Oral Medicine and Radiology
Sri Ramachandra Dental College
Sri Ramachandra Institute of Higher Education and Research (DU)
Chennai, Tamil Nadu, India

Foreword
N Gnanasundaram

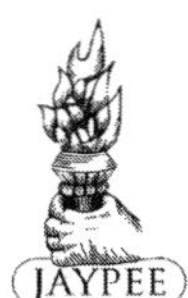

JAYPEE BROTHERS MEDICAL PUBLISHERS
The Health Sciences Publisher
New Delhi | London

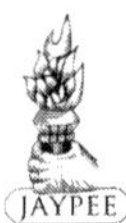

Jaypee Brothers Medical Publishers (P) Ltd

Headquarters
Jaypee Brothers Medical Publishers (P) Ltd
4838/24, Ansari Road, Daryaganj
New Delhi 110 002, India
Phone: +91-11-43574357
Fax: +91-11-43574314
Email: jaypee@jaypeebrothers.com

Overseas Office
J.P. Medical Ltd
83 Victoria Street, London
SW1H 0HW (UK)
Phone: +44 20 3170 8910
Fax: +44 (0)20 3008 6180
Email: info@jpmedpub.com

Website: www.jaypeebrothers.com
Website: www.jaypeedigital.com

Inquiries for bulk sales may be solicited at: jaypee@jaypeebrothers.com

Exam Preparatory Manual for Undergraduates: Oral Medicine and Radiology

First Edition: **2020**

ISBN 978-93-5270-602-0

Printed at Sanat Printers

Contributors

Chapter Contributor (Radiology)

TN Uma Maheswari MDS PhD
Professor
Saveetha Dental College and Hospitals
Chennai, Tamil Nadu, India

Appendix

1. **Aarthi Mu**
2. **Abbyraamy N**
3. **Abinaya R**
4. **Abitha V**
5. **Ahamed Anwer**

Alumni (2010–15 Batch)
Faculty of Dental Science
Sri Ramachandra Dental College
Sri Ramachandra Institute of Higher Education and Research (DU)
Chennai, Tamil Nadu, India

Art Work

MC Pandi Meena MDS
Alumni (2015–2018)
Department of Oral Medicine and Radiology
Sri Ramachandra Dental College
Sri Ramachandra Institute of Higher Education and Research (DU)
Chennai, Tamil Nadu, India

Foreword

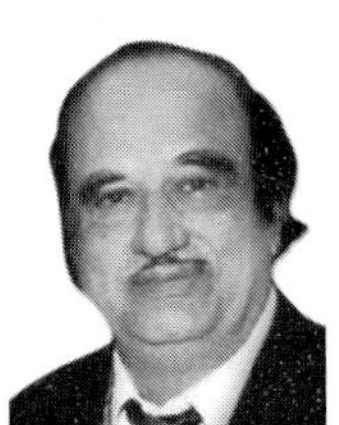

The art of teaching in a specialty subject is rewarded by the student's excellence in the particular domain. The author of this manual is my student and I am happy about her merits.

When students are studying, they need to gain knowledge and write exam to prove their learning level. Mere teaching will not help the students to crack the exams easily. Exam preparatory guides always solve the issue in a placid approach.

Dr Anbarasi, MDS in Oral Medicine and Radiology has 13 years of experience in the subject and she is one of the best teachers in her institution. She has done PhD in dental education and familiar about the students needs and she has written this guide on the exam point of view of a student. She has given model questions and answers for essays, short notes, MCQs and sample viva voce questions for each chapter. This guide will really help the students for exam preparation in a better way as it reduces the burden of studying voluminous material in the textbook.

I recommend students to read the textbooks for the better understanding of the subject and gain knowledge from your teachers to sustain in the field with good credits. Students can use this exam preparatory manual as a key to open the doors of examination and walk out with good marks.

I am sure that this preparatory manual will make students preparation much easier and also motivate the students to prepare the exam syllabus with a complete understanding. Students should use this manual to appear for the examination with more confidence and clarity. I appreciate the work by Dr Anbarasi to help the students and her efforts in satisfying the students' needs.

N Gnanasundaram
Professor
Visiting Faculty
Department of Oral Medicine and Radiology
Faculty of Dental Sciences
Sri Ramachandra Institute of Higher Education and Research
Former Principal and Professor
Government Dental College
Chennai, Tamil Nadu, India

Preface

Textbook are the ultimate source of providing knowledge. The students need to progress with consistent learning goals and dynamic academic strategies throughout their course period. The hardest and most challenging part in this period is facing examination. The exam preparation requires systematic planning of time management, appropriate course materials, ability to keep up with the materials, hard work, reading, and memorizing. The amount of information need to be understood and memorize is huge in oral medicine and radiology. Many students experience difficulty in understanding the concepts and proper application of the understanding to analytically and interpretively tackle the questions. All these factors lead to increased "anxiety" and "burn out" feeling during the exam time which ultimately reduce their potential and performance.

This preparatory manual was started with the interest of overcoming these concerns and providing a fruitful solution for the exam preparation. Great care was taken to consolidate and integrate the topics in a relevant manner. Each topic is provided with an introduction, headings and subheadings for clarity and meaningful connections. In addition, flowcharts and tables were used to explain the concepts and line diagrams to encourage the art work in the answer sheets. The whole idea is to set the task of studying for the exams and helping the undergraduate dental students to apply the theoretical information to solve the exam puzzle.

The topics are intellectually compiled by carefully reviewing the standard works of pioneers in the field as well as the recent advances added by experts in journal articles. Maximum effort was taken to cover all the relevant topics dictated by Dental Council of India and the exam requirement of different institutions at national as well as Pan Asian level.

This radiology annexure aims to create an interest and basic idea on dental radiology. The work focuses on normal anatomy and interpretation of most common dental diseases associated with pulp, periapical and periodontal structures in everyday practice. It is exclusively a practical guidance for undergraduates on many things that may be missed out.

This annexure was prepared by a team of interns under my guidance. The interns have put in lots of effort in compiling radiographs from patients that walk in Department of Oral Medicine and Radiology, Sri Ramachandra Institute of Higher Education and Research (SRIHER). With all our hard work behind the process, we thought of sharing our experience in the journey of learning radiology with beginners of dentistry. The visual representations were made for the better perceptive which will raise beginner's curiosity in examination of radiograph and diagnosis. Hence, this annexure is an, ***"Introduction to dental radiology to dental students by dental students".***

This manual will help the students to prepare the contents well in advance the class schedule and utilize the lecture hours for discussion. The faculty members can also extend the scope of their classes beyond exam point of view.

In this fine moment, I like to sincerely register my acknowledgment for the support and encouragement of my institution, SRIHER central library staff members, postgraduate trainees of my department, and all my beloved students.

The reviewer commends, critical suggestions, and publishers support are the great boon to complete this task in a successful way.

I hope the good intention and sincere effort taken to prepare this book will be recognized by the faculty members and students. I wish a very happy and hazel free learning experience for all students.

Best wishes and good luck for all students

K Anbarasi

Contents

PART 3

APPENDIX

1

PART

Part 1 Outline

1. Red, White and Mixed Red and White Lesions
2. Vesiculobullous and Ulcerative Diseases
3. Orofacial Pain
4. Pigmented Lesions of Oral Mucosa
5. Salivary Gland Diseases
6. Dental Consideration for Patients with Systemic Diseases/Disorders
7. Bleeding Disorders
8. Cervicofacial Lymphadenopathy
9. Oral Cancer —Investigation and Treatment Procedures
10. Focal Sepsis
11. Acquired Immune Deficiency Syndrome
12. Infectious Disease of Oral Cavity
13. Discoloration of Teeth
14. Odontogenic and Nonodontogenic Cysts
15. Odontogenic and Nonodontogenic Tumors
16. Temporomandibular Joint Disorders
17. Oral Manifestations of Endocrine Disorders
18. Immunological Diseases
19. Bone Disorders
20. Oral Manifestations of Nutritional Disorders
21. Dental Caries
22. Drugs Used in Dentistry
23. Developmental Disorders of Teeth and Orofacial Structures
24. Infection Control in Dental Clinics
25. Miscellaneous Topics

CHAPTER 1

Red, White and Mixed Red and White Lesions

HIGHLIGHTS

Lesions that involve the epithelium and superficial connective tissue of oral mucosa are known as surface lesions. Surface lesions are divided into three categories based on their clinical appearance: White, red and white and red. They may be due to a range of causes from hereditary to potentially malignant disorders.

Learners are expected to know about:

- Classification of mucosal lesions.
- Description of the characteristic or unique clinical features of the lesions.
- Potentially malignant disorders.
- Differential diagnosis and medical management of various lesions.

ESSAY QUESTIONS

1. Define submucous fibrosis. Write about etiopathogenesis, clinical features, investigation, and medical management of oral submucous fibrosis.

Definition (Pindborg in 1966)

Oral submucous fibrosis is an insidious, chronic disease affecting any part of the oral cavity and pharynx. Occasionally it is preceded by vesicle formation but always associated with a juxtaepithelial inflammatory reaction. Inflammation is progressed to fibroelastic changes of the lamina propria, and submucosal myofibrils causing stiffness of the oral mucosa. The resultant symptoms include decreased mouth opening and tongue protrusion.

Etiopathogenesis

- The etiologic factors are divided into *initiators and promoters* of oral submucous fibrosis.
- The initiators include—habitual chewing of areca nut and tobacco, chilies.
- The promoters include—iron deficiency anemia, deficiencies of B complex and folate vitamins, protein malnutrition, and immunologic disorders.
- Defect in collagen metabolism due to the imbalance in collagen production and breakdown is considered as a significant pathogenic part.
- The various components of areca nut play different role in the pathogenesis. (Flowchart 1)
- Autoimmune condition: The increased frequency of HLA, A10/DR3, B8/DR3 and A10/B8 suggests the immunological cause for this condition.

Clinical Features

Stage 1: *Stomatitis*: Mucosa appears erythematous. Oral ulcers, pigmentation, and petechia are the frequent findings. Vesicles are rare.

Stage 2: *Fibrosis*: The hallmark of oral submucous fibrosis. Thick, fibrous bands are formed in the posterior buccal mucosa, running in a vertical direction, and palpable fibrous bands encircle the lips. Fibrosis results in a pale, marble-like mucosa and a restricted mouth opening.

The progressive changes include:

- Blanched mucosa.

Flowchart 1: Sescribing the pathogenesis of oral submucous fibrosis.

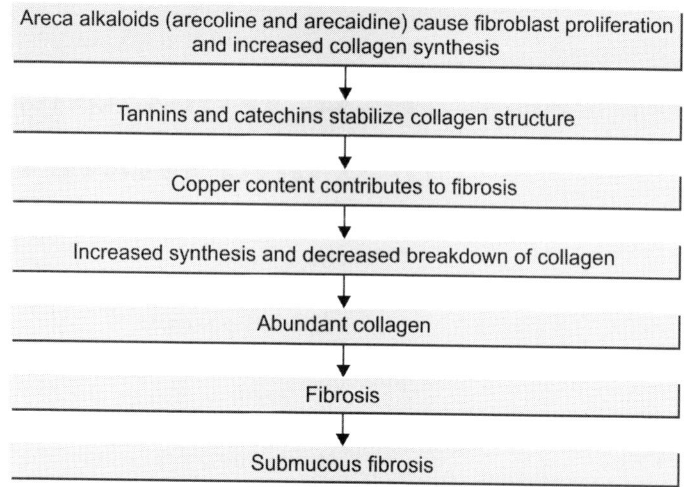

- Decreased mouth opening (trismus)
- Difficulty in tongue protrusion
- Pale gingiva
- Decreased pliability soft palate
- Blanched and atrophied uvula (or) bud shaped (or) hockey stick appearance of uvula: The thickness of fibrous band differs between a whitish coat on the soft palate causing no symptoms and a dense fibrosis that shorten and deviation the uvula.
- Sinking of the cheeks, disproportionate to age or nutritional status.

Classification of Oral Submucous Fibrosis based on Clinical Findings

- Lai Dr (1995) grouped oral submucous fibrosis into four categories based on inter-incisal distance:
  - Group A: >35 mm
  - Group B: Between 35–30 mm
  - Group C: Between 20–30 mm
  - Group D: <20 mm
- Rajendran R (2003) classified OSMF into two stages:
  1. Early oral submucous fibrosis: Burning sensation, recurrent oral inflammation or ulceration, excessive salivation, reduced taste perception, and dry mouth.
  2. Advanced oral submucous fibrosis: Blanched, pale, and firm mucosa, fibrous bands in palate, faucial pillars and buccal mucosa. Tongue movement is gradually restricted, and mouth opening becomes difficult.

Differential Diagnosis

- Oral manifestations in scleroderma
- Oral manifestations in Plummer-Vinson syndrome.

Investigations

- Complete hemogram
- Toludine blue test
- Incisional biopsy.

General Management

Supportive Care

- Elimination of the habit is the first step to be considered to prevent further progress especially in early stage and improve the response to treatment.
- Minimizing chillies and spicy foods.
- Proper oral hygiene.
- ***Nutritional support:*** Supplementation of iron, vitamins, and minerals with antioxidant potential (vitamin A, C, E, zinc, selenium) for 6–8 weeks, and high protein diet.
- Topical vitamin A application 50,000 IU/day.

- Ferrous fumarate tablets 200 mg once daily.
- Lycopene therapy: Lycopene is a carotene, carotenoid pigment and photochemical present in tomatoes, carrots, watermelons, and papayas. Lycopene has both anticancer and antioxidant properties. It has therapeutic benefits in potentially malignant disorders at the dose of 16 g/day.

Medical Management

Steroids

- Steroids are immunosuppressive drugs and inhibit the release of inflammatory cytokines and thereby reduce the proliferation of fibroblasts and collagen deposition. Relapse is common following treatment. Steroids also prevent or suppress the inflammatory reactions and hence reduce the symptoms.

Topical Steroids

- Topical application of steroids reduces the symptoms.
- Triamcinolone acetonide 0.1% 2–3 times/day. It heals inflammatory mucosal lesions.

Intralesional Injections

- Triamcinolone acetonide (10 mg/mL) and hyaluronidase (1,500 IU) combination for 22 weeks at 15 days interval.
  - Hyaluronidase facilitates the action of triamcinolone acetonide by dissolving the rigid connective tissue matrix hyaluronic acid.
  - Triamcinolone acetonide increases vascularity due to the fibrinolytic, anti-allergic and anti-inflammatory action.
- ***Placental extracts:*** Around 2 mL twice weekly for 4–6 weeks increases physiological function. The actions include anti-inflammatory and analgesic effect, improves blood circulation and tissue vascularity, and lowers immune response factors.
- Hyaluronidase and chymotrypsin are the two enzymes used in the treatment of OSMF. Hyaluronidase (1,500 IU submucosal injections) exhibit rapid and effective action in reducing the burning sensation and painful ulceration. It improves mouth opening by decreasing collagen formation. But recurrence is common.
- Methylxanthine derivative (pentoxifylline) is a vasodilator. The use of pentoxifylline increases the mucosal vascularity. It also suppresses the leukocyte function and stimulates fibrinolysis. This drug also stimulates the neutrophil degranulation and release of peroxides, promoting natural killer cell activity and inhibiting the production of tumor necrosis factor.

Oral Physiotherapy to Improve Mouth Opening

Muscle stretching exercises using wooden spatula and Hister's jaw exercise will improve the mouth opening and prevent relapse when complemented with medical management..

Complication

Submucous fibrosis is a potentially malignant condition with 7–13% of patients developing oral cancer.

2. Define leukoplakia. Write in detail about the various clinical types, etiology, malignant risk, and management.

Definition

Oral leukoplakia is a nonscrapable white patch or plaque that cannot be categorized as any other disease by clinical and histological examinations. Habit of tobacco consumption is the only causative factor.

World Health Organization Definitions For Leukoplakia

- A white plaque not related to physical or chemical agents excluding tobacco products.
- A white patch or plaque that cannot be defined clinically or histopathologically as any other disease and has the potential for malignant transformation.

Etiology

- Tobacco consumption is the well-recognized causative agent. Smokers are affected more than nonsmokers.
- Alcohol plays an additive effect along with tobacco.
- Human papillomavirus (HPV) also plays a recognized role in etiology.

Types of Leukoplakia

- *Homogeneous lesions* are uniformly flat and thin and usually asymptomatic. Clinical appearance may be focal and smooth or homogeneous with an associated low-risk of malignant transformation.
- Other lesions may be *heterogeneous or nonhomogeneous* (speckled, erosive, ulcerative) which may be interspersed with red or atrophic areas but retaining the predominant white color, and has the probability for dysplastic and malignant changes.
- *Exophytic type* (verrucous leukoplakia and proliferative verrucous leukoplakia). Proliferative verrucous leukoplakia is an aggressive type of leukoplakia that carries high-risk for cancerous changes. This type occurs as a diffused lesion and is resistant to treatment. Gingiva, buccal mucosa and alveolar ridge are the commonly involved sites.
- Leukoplakia has the tendency for transitions from one clinical form to another. The location of the leukoplakia is recognized in eight sites: Tongue, the floor of mouth, buccal and lower labial mucosa, hard palate, upper and lower alveolar ridges, and gingiva.

Malignant Transformation

- Around 1–2% of leukoplakia tends to become malignant in 5 years. Leukoplakia occurring at the floor of the oral cavity, tongue, and ventral surface has a high-risk for malignant transformation.
- Risk factors that initiate malignant transformation in leukoplakia:
  - Female gender
  - Long-standing leukoplakia
  - Leukoplakia in nontobacco users (idiopathic leukoplakia)
  - Leukoplakia involving tongue and floor of the mouth
  - Size >200 mm^2
  - Nonhomogeneous variety
  - Presence of invasive *C. albicans*
  - Epithelial dysplasia
  - History of head-and-neck carcinoma.

Investigations

- Biopsy and histopathological diagnosis is the confirmatory method to differentiate between dysplastic and nondysplastic lesions.
- A brush biopsy is a noninvasive method to collect the basal layer of cells for pathological examination.
- Toluidine blue vital staining is used to identify the presence of dysplastic changes in the lesion and select the appropriate site for biopsy.
- Chemiluminescence (ViziLite system) is based on the fluorescence property of the healthy and leukoplakia tissue to specific light wavelength.

Treatment

- The treatment goal for leukoplakia is to prevent the malignant transformation.
- In the absence of histologically demonstrated dysplastic changes, routine follow-up observation is appropriate in conjunction with the elimination of any tobacco habit and medical management.

Chemoprevention: It is aimed for scavenging the free radicals, destroying the caricinogenic byproducts of tobacco, and inhibiting mutation.

- Retinoids
- Vitamins (A, C, E)

- Carotenoids
- Topical retinoic acid (vitamin A) — prevents keratin production, inflammatory response and carcinogenesis.
- Candida-associated leukoplakias respond to topical antifungal therapy (clotrimazole 1% cream 4 times/day for 2 weeks).

If dysplastic changes present:

- Topical bleomycin 1% (cytotoxic antibiotic) can be used for 2 weeks.
- Surgical treatment is also recommended (conventional surgery, electrocauterization, laser ablation, or cryosurgery).

3. Classify oral candidiasis. Explain the clinical features, investigations, and management of acute candidal infections.

Classification

Primary oral candidiasis (group 1)

- Acute types:
  - Primary pseudomembranous candidiasis (thrush)
  - Erythematous.
- Chronic types:
  - Pseudomembranous (occurs in HIV infected individuals and in patients using steroid inhaler for long period)
  - Erythematous
  - Hyperplastic
  - Nodular
  - Plaque-like.
- Candida associated:
  - Angular cheilitis
  - Denture stomatitis
  - Median rhomboid glossitis.
- Keratinized primary lesions superimposed with candida:
  - Leukoplakia
  - Lichen planus
  - Lupus erythematosus.

Secondary oral candidiasis (group 2)

- Candidiasis endocrinopathy syndrome
- Mucocutaneous candidiasis.

Causative Agent

- *Candida albicans* is the frequently associated organism in 70–95% of reported patients. *Candida tropicalis, Candida krusei*, and *Candida glabrata* are also associated in oral infection.

Predisposing Factors

- Chronic local irritants like removable dentures.
- Altered oral biology or changes in the oral flora caused by long time medications (antibiotics and corticosteroid).
- Dry mouth
- Deficiencies of iron and vitamins.
- Immunological and endocrine disorders
- Malignant and chronic diseases
- Radiotherapy and chemotherapy
- Extremities of age
- Hospitalization
- Epithelial alterations
- Heavy smoking.

Acute Oral Candidiasis

Acute pseudomembranous candidiasis (oral thrush)

- It manifests as pseudomembranous white patches on the oral mucosa, palate, and tongue composed of desquamated cells, fibrin, and fungal hyphae. The surface appears white or whitish yellow confluent plaque resembling curd or cheese. When swiping with a swab, the membrane is scraped off and leaves a red base.
- Commonly affects newborn babies (due to immature immune system), older individuals (immune decline), individuals using steroid inhaler (inhibits local immunity) or an underlying disease.
- The patient may present with the mild symptom of altered taste or slight tingling sensation in acute disease, whereas the chronic form may cause dysphagia.

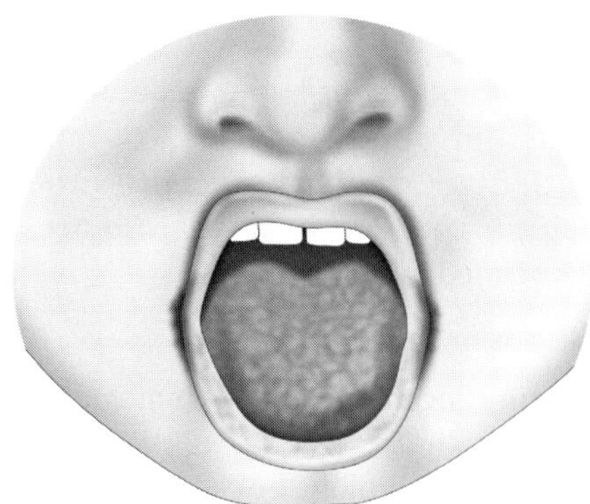

Fig. 1: Angular stomatitis.

Erythematous (or) acute atrophic candidiasis

It is a rare form. The occurrence is associated with prolonged use of corticosteroids and broad-spectrum antibiotics administration or HIV infection. It may also a squeal of persistent acute pseudomembranous candidiasis, when the pseudomembranes shed, the acute form changes to atrophic form. It appears as red, depapillated surfaces on the dorsum of the tongue, erythematous patches on the palate, or buccal mucosa. Pain and discomfort are frequently associated symptoms.

Angular stomatitis (perleche, angular cheilitis)

Fissuring and cracking at the commissural areas of the mouth (Fig. 1). It is commonly associated with denture stomatitis, iron deficiency anemia, vitamin deficiencies, and HIV infection. It is either asymptomatic or associated with pain, and irritation at one or both commissars.

Investigations

- *Smears detection:* Smear should be collected from the active lesion site using a wooden spatula and fixed immediately on two slides, one for Gram staining and other for periodic-acid Schiff (PAS) technique. Direct microscopic examination of smears reveals yeast cells appearing dark blue in Gram staining and red or purple in PAS preparations.
- *Swabs:* The lesion site is swabbed and seeded on Sabouraud agar growth medium. Incubation at 25°C will encourage the growth.
- *Imprint culture technique:* A sterile, square, plastic foam pad (2.5 × 2.5 cm) dipped in peptone water is placed over the mucosal lesion for 30–60 seconds. Then the plastic foam is incubated on sabouraud's agar at 37°C for 48 hours. Candida density is expressed as colony-forming units per mm^2. More than 30 colony-forming units (CFU) per cm^2 of mucosa in the dentulous patients and 49 CFU per cm^2 in denture wearers suggest candidal infection.
- *Salivary culture technique:* This is done by collecting 2 mL of mixed, unstimulated saliva in a sterile, container and incubated in sabouraud's agar medium. The number of candida in salivary sample is expressed as CFU.
- *Oral rinse technique:* The patient should rinse the mouth for 60 seconds with 10 mL of sterile saline or sterile water and then returns the oral rinse to the sterile container. The collected oral rinse is centrifuged and inoculated on appropriate media to assess CFU per mL of the sample.
- *Serological tests for invasive candidiasis:* Useful to detect candida antibodies by-
  - Slide agglutination
  - Latex agglutination
  - Immunodiffusion
  - Phytohemagglutination.

Management

Oral candidiasis in immunocompetent individuals are treated with topical antifungals, and in immunocompromised individuals, both topical and systemic antifungals are used.

- Eliminating the predisposing factors
- Proper oral hygiene home practices
- Using anticandidal mouthwashes like:
  - Triclosan
  - Chlorhexidine gluconate (0.12%) 15 mL mouth rinse 3 times per day.

- Essential oil formulations: Plant derivatives like thymol, eucalyptol and bioflavonoids have an anticandidal property by fungal cell membrane disruption and enzyme inhibition.

- Antifungal agents:
  - *Topical azoles*
    - Clotrimazole 1% cream 4 times/day for 2 weeks.
    - Clotrimazole 10 mg/mL suspension, swab 1–2 mL over the lesion 3 times/day for 2 weeks.
  - *Transmucosal drugs:* It should be used until 2 days after symptoms subsides
    - Miconazole buccal tablet 50 mg-1 tab/day for 2 weeks; applied in gum region.
    - Nystatin suspension 4,00,000–6,00,000 units, 4–6 mL/day, swish and swallow.
  - *Systemic medication:*
    - Fluconazole (400 mg as starting dose followed by 200 mg/day for 15 days).
    - Ketoconazole 200 mg tab/day for 7–10 days.
  - *For angular cheilitis:*
    - A mixture of topical antifungal and antibacterial ointment (e.g. nystatin and mupirocin) is preferred 3 times/day for 2 weeks.
    - Miconazole is an antifungal drug with effective antistaphylococcal effect. Hence, miconazole oral gel can be used for angular cheilitis.

4. Define lichen planus. Describe its clinical features, diagnosis, and management briefly.

Lichen planus is a chronic inflammatory disease of skin and mucosa. The occurrence of oral lichen planus (OLP) is more common than the cutaneous form. Oral lesions are long-lasting and resistant to treatment.

Etiology

- Lichen planus is an autoimmune disorder characterized by abnormal T-cell-mediated immune response. The basal epithelial cells are recognized as antigens due to their cell surface changes.
- Activation of mast cells (associated with vascular and neuronal supply of oral mucosa) directs inflammatory cells in the bloodstream towards mucosa and facilitates OLP.

Predisposing Factors

- Cell-mediated hypersensitivity reactions.
- Stress induces a significant change in immune response.

Clinical Features

Lichen planus has the preference for middle-aged women. Men and children are occasionally affected.

Clinical Types (Fig. 2)

Reticular Oral Lichen Planus

It is the most prevalent type. Lesions manifests as a multiple radiating keratotic striae with an elevated white dot at the point of intersection of these line known as Wickham's striae. The white striae are present bilaterally on the buccal mucosa, vestibule, gingiva, tongue, palate and rarely lips. Usually asymptomatic but may associate with burning sensation on taking spicy foods.

Erosive Oral Lichen Planus (Atrophic form)

The erosive form is the second common type of OLP. It presents as a combination of red and ulcerated surface surrounded by faint radiating white striae at the periphery. It is commonly present in gingiva and erosive lichen planus involvement of the gingiva is called as *desquamative gingivitis.* Involvement of buccal mucosa, vestibule, and floor of the mouth also occurs. The lesions may become widespread and patient's complaints range from intermittent pain to severe discomfort that interferes with chewing.

Plaque-like Oral Lichen Planus

Plaque-like form clinically resembles homogeneous leukoplakia. These plaque-like lesions are smooth and flat or irregular and

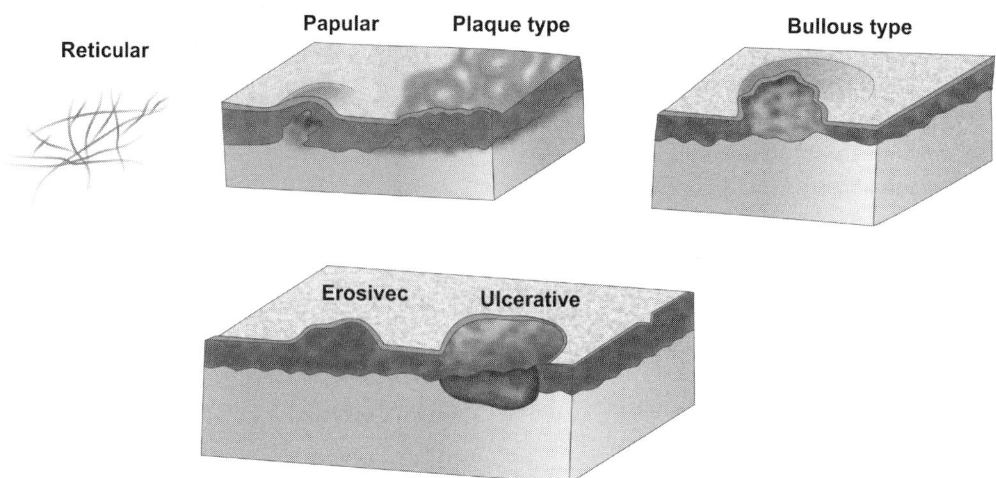

Fig. 2: Types of lichen planus.

elevated in appearance. This type involves the dorsum of the tongue and buccal mucosa. This is a variant form of the reticular lesion, usually asymptomatic but may associate with burning sensation on taking spicy foods.

Bullous Lichen Planus

The bullous form is a rare variety and affects the buccal mucosa and the lateral borders of the tongue. The bullae rupture immediately and lead to an ulcerative form of lichen planus. Nikolsky's sign is positive in bullous form.

Papular

The papular form is sporadic and is the transient form of other types of OLP. Multiple white spots are present with faint radiating white lines at the periphery.

Differential Diagnosis

- *Reticular type:* Lichenoid reaction, candidiasis, discoid lupus erythematosus, frictional keratosis.
- *Plaque type:* Leukoplakia.
- *Erythematous and bullous type:* Pemphigus, pemphigoid.

Investigations

- Incisional biopsy and histopathological examination.
- Immunohistochemical reactions.

Management

- The primary care should involve good oral hygiene with the elimination of all local irritants and superadded candidal infection using 0.12% chlorhexidine gluconate rinse.
- *Corticosteroid:* The drug of choice to revise the immune reaction.
  - Topical corticosteroid is used in mild to moderately symptomatic lesions.
  - The following preparations are used in terms of increasing potency:
    - 0.1% triamcinolone acetonide ointment 3 times/day
    - 0.05% clobetasol propionate gel
    - 0.1% or 0.05% betamethasone valerate gel
    - 0.05% fluocinonide gel
    - 0.05% clobetasone butyrate ointment or cream.
    - For widespread lesions, 1.0 mg/mL aqueous triamcinolone acetonide or 0.1 mg/mL dexamethasone elixir is effective. Patients should use 5 mL of this solution for 2 minutes after every meal and at night time.

Advantage of topical steroid application:

- Side effects are minimal than the systemic preparations.
- Direct release of the drug at the lesion site.

Adverse Effects

- Secondary candidal infection and mucosal atrophy.
- High potent topical corticosteroids can cause adrenal suppression when for long periods.

Intralesional injection of corticosteroid: Administered for recalcitrant lesions. Around 0.2–0.4 mL of a 10 mg/mL solution of triamcinolone acetonide is used.

Systemic steroid therapy: It should be reserved for patients in whom topical steroid are ineffective. Prednisone tablet 10–20 mg/day for moderately severe conditions and up to 35 mg/per day for severe conditions.

Other preferred medications:

- 0.1% tacrolimus ointment
- Topical retinoids and vitamin A
- Antioxidants.

Clinical Significance

Oral lichen planus is a potential malignant disorder especially erosive and atrophic forms. This necessitates appropriate management with regular follow-up care.

5. Briefly mention the reason for oral white lesions and Classify white lesions of oral mucosa.

The whitish appearance of mucosa is due to:

- Increase in thickness of one or more epithelial layers
- Abnormal thick keratin layer
- Reduced vascularity of underlying mucosa.
- Increase in the amount of edema in epithelium (leukodema).

They are classified by keratotic or nonkeratotic nature.

Classification Based on Keratinization

- *Keratotic white lesions: Nonscrapable white lesions.*
  - Frictional keratosis
  - White sponge nevus
  - Reticular lichen planus
  - Leukoplakia
  - Hairy leukoplakia.
- *Nonkeratotic white lesions: Scrapable white lesions.*
  - Candidiasis
  - Chemical burns.

Classification Based on Origin and Pathogenesis

- *Hereditary or developmental white lesions*
  - Leukoedema
  - White spongy nevus
  - Hereditary benign intraepithelial dyskeratosis
  - Pachyonychia congenita
  - Dyskeratosis congenita
- *Reactive white lesions*
  - Frictional keratosis
  - Morsicatio buccarum
  - Nicotine stomatitis
  - Tobacco pouch keratosis
  - Chemical burn
- *Immunologic white lesions*
  - Lichen planus
  - Lichenoid mucositis
  - Discoid lupus erythematosus
  - Graft-versus-host disease
- *Bacterial or viral or fungal white lesions*
  - Candidiasis
  - Mucous patches of secondary syphilis
  - Oral hairy leukoplakia
- *Systemic disease—causing oral white lesions*
  - Uremic stomatitis
- *Potentially malignant disorders*
  - Leukoplakia
  - Actinic cheilitis.

SHORT NOTES

1. Actinic keratosis (or) actinic cheilitis.

- Chronic exposure to sunlight may cause keratotic changes in the lip. It has the tendency for malignant transformation.
- Usually, patients are asymptomatic. In atrophic form, ulceration, pain, and bleeding are common.

There are 4 types:
1. Hyperkeratotic form
2. Pigmented form
3. Lichenoid form
4. Atrophic form.

Treatment

- A strict advice to be given to the patient to avoid sun exposure as much as possible.
  - Diclofenac sodium 3% gel, topical application for 60–90 days.
  - Cryosurgery with liquid nitrogen for *freezing off* the actinic keratosis.
  - 5-fluorouracil—a cytotoxic topical cream that causes the lesion to become red and inflamed before they fall off.
  - Photodynamic therapy.
  - CO_2 or Er:YAG laser therapy. Laser resurfacing technique is used to treat diffuse form.
  - Electrocautery.

2. Denture stomatitis (or) denture sore mouth (or) chronic atrophic candidiasis.

- The characteristic features of denture-induced stomatitis include the erythematous and edematous changes of the mucosa that contacts the fitting maxillary denture base (palate and gingiva).
- The involvement of mucosa contacting lower denture base is infrequent. The patients are asymptomatic but occasionally complaint about soreness. The associated angular stomatitis may cause difficulty in mouth opening.
- Etiology includes local and systemic factors.
  - Local factors:
    - Poor oral and denture hygiene
    - Microbial colonization
    - Old dentures
    - Hypersensitivity for denture base materials and residual monomer
    - Dryness of mouth.
  - Systemic factors include:
    - Diabetes mellitus
    - Immunodeficiency
    - Nutritional disorders.
- Newton classification of denture stomatitis:
  - Type I—a localized simple inflammation or a pinpoint hyperemia.
  - Type II—erythematous type: more diffuse erythema involving a part of or the entire denture-covering mucosa.
  - Type III—granular type (inflammatory papillary hyperplasia) frequently affecting the middle of the hard palate and the alveolar ridge (Fig. 3).

The causative factorcandida. The yeast form of candida colonizes the oral mucosa beneath denture along with bacterial colonization. The attachment is facilitated by mucous and serum and decreased by the presence of salivary pellicle. The use of soft liners in dentures adds hazard by providing mechanical locking for plaque and yeasts to the denture base.

Management

- Disinfection of the denture with:
  - 10% solution of household bleach.
  - Socking in boric acid.
  - Applying nystatin cream before inserting the denture.
  - Denture adhesives should be removed on daily basis.
  - Overnight storage of dentures in water.
  - An antifungal treatment will resolve the bright red appearance of the mucosa.
  - The papillomatous appearance of mucosa requires surgical excision following antifungal therapy and discontinuing the denture wearing.

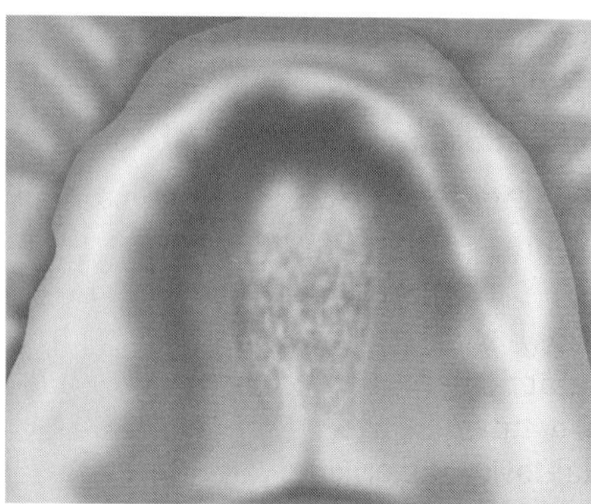

Fig. 3: Denture stomatitis.

3. Discuss hairy tongue (or) black hairy tongue.

Hairy tongue is a term for the abnormal acquired coating on the dorsal surface of the tongue. It is a temporary condition that gives the tongue a furry, carpet-like appearance. There is defective desquamation and sheading of the papilla that leads to accumulation of keratinized layers. The filiform papillae are approximately 1 mm in length, and become elongated and hypertrophic due to keratinization and can reach 12–18 mm length, with a width of 2 mm, giving a hair-like appearance. The over-retention of papillae cause food and bacteria, to accumulate in the hair-like mesh and various colors like brown, white, green, and pink to the surface of the tongue. Secondary bacterial and fungal infections can even a black appearance, referred to as *black hairy tongue*.

Etiology

Multifactorial: It can occur from poor oral hygiene, prolonged or excessive use of antibiotics, radiotherapy for head and neck region, food habits like coffee or tea drinking, or tobacco usage. It may also develop in edentulous persons because of their soft food diet that will not aid in the stimulation of normal shedding of the papillae. Regular use of mouthwashes containing oxidizing agents, such as peroxide, or astringent agents, such as menthol also causes this condition. Decreased consumption of coarse food and restricted tongue movement also leads to poor desquamation of the papilla.

Clinical Features

- Asymptomatic but occasionally associated with burning sensation.
- Gagging or a tickling sensation in the soft palate due to the contact of elongated structures.
- Halitosis and unusual taste due to the taste buds holding onto debris in the mouth.

Treatment

- Maintenance of improved oral hygiene and eliminating the contributing factors will resolve black hairy tongue.
- Use of tongue scraper and rinsing with dilute hydrogen peroxide mouth rinse will promote desquamation. Increased consumption of raw fruits and vegetables is helpful.
- Topical use of 30% urea solution and trichloroacetic acid can be used. It may cause mild local irritation.

4. Lichenoid reactions (or) oral lichenoid lesions.

- Oral lichenoid reactions (or) lesions represent a similar clinical manifestation to a reticular pattern of oral lichen planus but are often unilateral. It is a response to external agents (drugs, dental restorative materials, allergens) or altered self-antigens and can be cured if the inciting factor is identified and eliminated. Oral lichenoid reactions may also result from systemic drug exposure [oral lichenoid drug reaction; (OLDR)] or local allergic contact hypersensitivity (OLCR).
- Dental amalgam restoration is the most common etiological factors. The amalgam reacts with oral fluid and releases degradation products which initiate the lichenoid reaction.

Lichenoid Drug Reactions

- It may involve the skin, oral mucosa, or both. The duration between drug administration and development of OLDR is variable, with an average of 2–3 months. Based on the causative drug, the lesions appear either as white reticular papules or as erosions and sometimes associated with pain. These lesions are associated with the use of nonsteroidal anti-inflammatory drugs (aspirin, ibuprofen, indomethacin), antihypertensives (atenolol, enalapril,

hydrochlorothiazide, methyldopa, metoprolol), and HIV antiretrovirals (zidovudine).
- There are no universal criteria for the diagnosis. Proposed diagnostic criteria include a history of systemic medication intake, clinical and histological features of lichenoid mucositis, and resolution of lesions with drug discontinuation.

Treatment

Discontinuation of the suspect medication and substitution with an alternate medication will resolve the lesion within few weeks to months, but delayed responses may also occur. If the causative medication cannot be discontinued or if residual lesions persist after drug elimination, topical corticosteroid can be used.

5. Allergic contact stomatitis.

- It is an immune-mediated (T-cell-mediated) inflammatory reaction to an exogenous allergen that has direct contact with oral mucosa. Pain, burning sensation, and itching sensation are the associated symptoms.
- Lesions are located in apposition or near proximity (within 1 cm) to the offending allergen, and lesions are restricted to the sites of contact. Typical sites include the lateral borders of the tongue and buccal mucosa. Dental restorative materials, cinnamon and other spices, chewing gums, impression materials, and orthodontic appliances may induce the hypersensitivity reactions. Erythema, vesicles, ulcers, and hyperkeratotic patches are the various clinical forms.

Differential Diagnosis

Plasma cell gingivitis, anemic stomatitis, lichen planus.

Diagnosis

It is confirmed based on examination finding and by the disappearance of the lesion following the elimination of the causative factor.

Treatment

Elimination of causative agent.

6. Oral hairy leukoplakia.

- Oral hairy leukoplakia is a vertically radiating white lesion of the lateral border of the tongue with slightly elevated, ill-defined, and corrugated *hairy* surface. Lesions cannot be rubbed off and are symptomless. It is caused by Epstein-Barr virus (EBV) and is a sign of immunosuppression.
  - Present in patients with acquired immunodeficiency syndrome (AIDS) and less often seen in drug abusers, hemophilic, blood transfusion recipients and organ transplant patients.
- The lesions are bilateral and asymptomatic but rarely cause burning sensation.

Treatment is not essential as they would not cause any serious symptoms. For people with widespread lesions and who is experiencing discomfort or altered taste are treated with topical application of podophyllin resin.

7. Describe graft-versus-host disease.

Graft-versus-host disease (GVHD) is a complication of allogeneic hematopoietic stem cell transplantation (HSCT). GVHD occurs in two forms: Acute and chronic.

1. *Acute graft-versus-host disease:* It occurs within 100-days following transplantation, whereas chronic form manifests at a later period is more than 100 days, and reveals some of the features of autoimmune diseases. Chronic form may develop either de novo or following resolution of/or as an extension of acute GVHD.

   The acute form is precipitated by many conditions like radiotherapy, chemotherapy, neutropenia, herpes infection and treatment with cytokines. Oral findings include mucosal erythema, ulcerations, and painful desquamative lesions.
2. *Chronic graft-versus-host disease:* Involves the skin, oral, vaginal and conjunctival mucosa, salivary and lacrimal glands and

liver. Around 40–70% of engrafted patients develop cGVHD which can persist for months to years and require long-term management from multiple disciplines.

- The oral presentation is variable and includes lichen planus-like changes of mucosa, hyperkeratotic plaques, mucosal atrophy and ulcers, and secondary Sjogren's syndrome.

Management

Topical corticosteroid or tacrolimus can be used to reduce pain and discomfort.

8. Describe erythroplakia.

Definition

Erythroplakia is a red-patch that cannot be diagnosed as any other lesion by clinical or pathological findings.

Predisposing Factors

Tobacco and alcohol.

Clinical Features

Erythroplakia appears as fiery-red, flat or depressed lesion with a smooth or granular surface. In many cases, the lesion appears as a mixed form with predominant red and some white spots and is called as *erythroleukoplakia*.

Differential Diagnosis

Erythematous lichen planus and atrophic candidiasis—these lesions have multifocal involvement.

Symptoms

Pain and burning sensation.

Histopathology

Erythroplakia shows some degree of dysplastic features or features of carcinoma in situ or invasive carcinoma.

Treatment

Cold knife or laser surgery is the recommended treatment modality.

9. What is frictional keratosis?

- Frictional or traumatic keratosis appears as a white patch with rough and ragged mucosal surface adjacent to a source of mechanical irritation.
- Sharp cusps, broken teeth, rough denture borders, clasps, and irregular edges of orthodontic appliances are the potential source and usually resolve.
- Asymptomatic.
- Keratotic patches disappear gradually within 2 weeks following the removal of irritants.
- Differential diagnosis: Leukoplakia, lichenoid reactions.
- Biopsy should be considered in nonhealing lesions that persist after the removal of irritation.

10. Median rhomboid glossitis.

- Median rhomboid glossitis (Fig. 4) is a central papillary atrophy of the tongue and is located around the midline of the dorsum of the tongue. It appears as a well-defined, symmetrical depapillation, anterior to the circumvallate papillae. The surface of the lesion is smooth or lobulated and demarcated from the surrounding sites. Usually asymptomatic, but occasionally associated with pain, irritation, or pruritus.

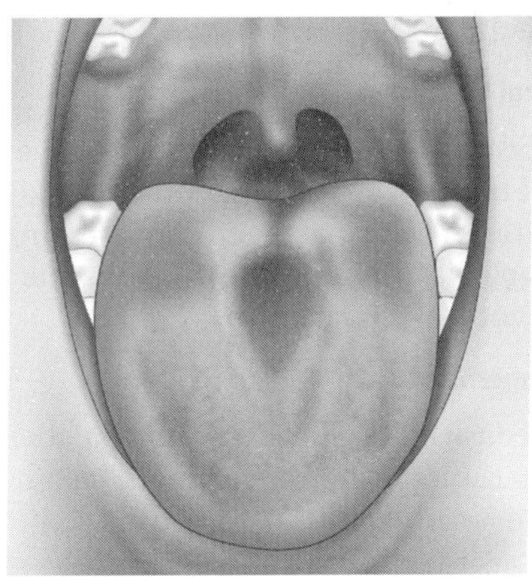

Fig. 4: Median rhomboid glossitis.

- When median rhomboid glossitis is associated with a palatal inflammation, it is called as *kissing lesion*. It is frequently seen in HIV infected individuals and hence when present, necessary investigations should be carried out to rule out AIDS.
- Predisposing factors associated are smoking, diabetes mellitus, a prolonged course of antibiotic treatment and candidal infection. It is asymptomatic. Topical anticandidal medication is the treatment of choice.

11. Candidal leukoplakia.

Candidal leukoplakia is a nonscrapable, chronic candid infection that resembles leukoplakia in appearance. The terms *chronic hyperplastic candidiasis* and *candidal leukoplakia* are used synonymously.

Clinical Presentation

- White plaque that cannot be rubbed off and presenting at the following oral sites in decreasing order of frequency: Oral commissars, cheek mucosa, palate, and the tongue.
- Candidal hyphae invade the superficial layers of the epithelium and cause epithelial atrophy, hyperplasia, and dysplasia. Systemic conditions like diabetes, poor immunological conditions and deficiencies of vitamins A, B_1, B_2, folic acid and iron predisposes this condition.

Clinical Features

It appears as a distinct, elevated lesion either small transparent or large opaque plaques which are nonscrapable and hence resembling leukoplakia. Some areas of the plaque may have nodular characteristics.

Management

- Medical management: Antifungal therapy, topical application of retinoids, bleomycin, and β-carotene.
- Surgical excision.

12. Proliferative verrucous leukoplakia.

- Proliferative verrucous leukoplakia is a severe form of oral leukoplakia. It preferably occurs in women (female-to-male ratio of 4:1) not having the habit of tobacco. It presents as a multifocal white patch or plaque with rough surface projections. These lesions tend to spread slowly and involve other oral mucosal regions. More frequently occurs on the gingival but other sites may also be affected.
- It tends to recur after surgical excision and has the risk for transformation into *squamous cell carcinoma* usually within 8 years of initial diagnosis.
- Five major and four minor criteria were proposed to allow for a definitive diagnosis of PVL.

Major Criteria

- Leukoplakia presenting at more than two different oral sites preferably in the gingiva, alveolar processes, and palate.
- The existence of a verrucous surface.
- The lesions should be widespread.
- There has been a recurrence in a previously treated area.
- Histopathologically leukoplakia should present as simple epithelial hyperkeratosis or verrucous hyperplasia or verrucous carcinoma or oral squamous cell carcinoma or in situ or infiltrating.

Minor Criteria

- Oral leukoplakia measuring a minimum of 3 cm size.
- Female patient.
- The patient must be free of tobacco habit.
- More than 5 year duration.

To confirm the diagnosis of PVL, the following guideline if followed:

- Three major criteria (with histopathological criteria, as one in 3).
- Two major criteria (histopathological change as one criteria) + two minor criteria.

Management

- There is no definitive treatment.
- Surgical excision, CO_2 laser evaporation, laser surgery, chemo, and radiotherapy

are the different modalities preferred for management.

13. Chemical burn (or) scrapable white lesions of oral mucosa (or) nonkeratotic white lesions of oral mucosa.

- Chemicals with *caustic potential* like aspirin, silver nitrate, formocresol, sodium hypochlorite, hydrogen peroxide, and cavity varnish and acid-etching materials, when retained in the mouth for a long period leads to the formation of *whitish pseudomembrane* with necrotic surface and exudates.
  - *Aspirin burn:* When aspirin is held in the mucobuccal fold adjacent to the painful tooth for relief, it causes focal superficial necrosis with white pseudomembrane that can be easily scraped off leaving an underlying erythematous mucosa.
  - *Silver nitrate:* This chemical is sometimes used in the treatment of aphthous ulcer as a cautery agent. It gives immediate pain relief by burning the nerve ends at the ulcer site. At the same time, it causes severe necrosis at the application site with pseudomembrane formation.
  - *Hydrogen peroxide:* Concentration of hydrogen peroxide is greater than 3% as an oral rinse for periodontal problems may lead to epithelial necrosis.
  - *Sodium hypochlorite:* It is used as an intracanal irrigant in endodontic procedures and when accidental contact with the oral mucosa or gingiva causes severe ulceration with superficial necrosis.
  - *Dentifrices and mouth rinse:* Cinnamon-flavored dentifrices often cause sensitivity or allergic reaction on the oral mucosa resulting in necrosis and sloughing of the epithelium.
  - Mouthrinses containing chlorhexidine and alcohol also occasionally causes caustic burns in some individuals.

Clinical Features of Chemical Burn

- It is commonly seen on mucobuccal fold and gingiva as an irregularly shaped area with white pseudomembrane.
- When the tissue involvement is extensive, severe damage with sloughing of necrotic mucosa will cause pain.
- In case of mild contact of the agent with mucosa, superficial white and wrinkled appearance without necrosis is present.

Management

- A protective emollient agent like methylcellulose can be used for milder cases and heals within 1–2 weeks.
- For deep tissue necrosis, debridement of the surface followed by systemic antibiotic and anti-inflammatory coverage is essential.

14. Snuff dipper's lesion (or) Pouch keratosis (or) smokeless tobacco keratosis.

- The habit of keeping tobacco quid in the buccal or labial vestibule causes white patch or plaque lesions on the vestibule. These lesions may involve the adjoining tissues like gingiva and buccal mucosa.
- Early lesions may show slight wrinkling that disappears when the tissues are stretched. Older lesions appear as hyperkeratotic, granular patches. Long-standing lesions, with persistent habit exhibit grayish-white mucosa with well-developed folds and fissures. There will be no associated pain or burning sensation.
- Smokeless tobacco keratosis takes about 5 years to develop but breaking the habit leads to a normal mucosa within 2–6 weeks. For lesions that remain more than 6 weeks, a biopsy should be considered.

15. Nicotina stomatitis (or) smokers palate.

- Nicotine stomatitis develops as a response to cigar smoking or from cigarette smoking. The hot smoke released strikes the palate and cause hyperkeratotic alteration of the palatal mucosa.

- The palatal mucosa becomes thickened and whitish in appearance with a fissured surface. Papular elevations with red centers also a common feature which represents the partial occlusion of the duct orifice with keratotic plugging and inflamed orifice of the minor salivary gland ducts. The changes are more localized to the glandular zone of hard palate alone.
- Though nicotine stomatitis is a tobacco-related condition, it has no malignant transformation potential. Discontinuation of the smoking habit reverse the condition.

16. Viadent leukoplakia (or) sanguinaria-associated keratosis (or) sanguinaria leukoplakia.

- Sanguinaria canadensis (a type of flower) has been found to be effective against plaque build-up and gingivitis. Sanguinaria-associated leukoplakia is a unique form of oral leukoplakia attributed to the chronic use of oral rinses and toothpaste containing the extract of the sanguinaria plant. It is usually located on the attached gingiva and the alveolar mucosa of the maxillary vestibule.
- The duration of usage of the product and development lesion may vary between 6 months to 12 years.
- The lesion appears as a white, velvety, wrinkled or corrugated patch in the maxillary vestibule involving both attached gingiva and vestibular mucosa. Involvement of mandibular anterior vestibule is also common. The site specificity is due to prolonged retention of the product in vestibule due to their greater distance from major salivary gland ducts. The lesion is well demarcated from the surrounding mucosa.

Management

Discontinue the use of sanguinaria containing products and careful follow-up.

17. Describe parulis (or) gumboil.

- Parulis is an oral lesion characterized by a soft erythematous papule (or red spot) that develops on the alveolar process or attached gingiva of a tooth in association with periapical abscess or with a periodontal abscess. It represents the drainage tract of pus with an inflamed orifice, and is made up of granulation tissue.
- The lesion appears as a red or normal mucosal colored gingival swelling surrounded by erythema. It is fluctuant on palpation and is less than 5 mm in size. On examination with a periodontal probe, a small orifice adjacent to the fistulous tract can be identified. Pus discharge may present at the orifice.
- The parulis presents with variable symptoms. It may be painless or produces a noticeable pain. The pain persists until pus drains out through the surface opening.

Diagnosis

A sterile gutta-percha (GP) point can be inserted into orifice of the fistulous tract and a periapical radiograph should be taken with the GP point. The proximity of the gutta-percha point to the apex of the nonvital tooth can be evaluated on the radiograph.

Treatment

Endodontic procedures or extraction is indicated if the affected tooth is nonvital. If the tooth is associated with a deep periodontal pocket, periodontal therapy is indicated. Once the underlying cause is treated, the parulis resolves and does not recur.

18. Discoid lupus erythematosus.

- Discoid lupus erythematosus (DLE) is an autoimmune, connective tissue disorder affecting the skin and oral mucosa. The oral discoid lesions present with a characteristic central erythematous zone and a periphery of white radiating lines or hyperkeratotic plaques and striae. The distribution of discoid lupus erythematosus is usually asymmetric. Peripheral striae are faint. The oral lesions occur along skin lesions or before the onset of skin lesions and rarely oral lesions alone may be present without skin involvement.

- The labial mucosa, the vermilion border of the lip and the buccal mucosa are the commonly involved sites. Burning sensation, tenderness, dryness and pain are the associated symptoms.
- The diagnosis is based on the coexistence of skin lesions, histopathology, and immunofluorescent studies.

Differential diagnosis of lichen planus:

- Topical steroid (triamcinolone acetonide 0.1% is effective in treating the skin and oral lesions).
- Intralesional steroids are helpful for treating chronic conditions.
- In resistant cases, antimalarial drugs like chloroquine, hydroxychloroquine, and mepacrine are used.

Other topical agents:

- 0.1% tacrolimus ointment twice daily
- 0.05% clobetasol propionate ointment twice daily

Failure of early treatment may lead to permanent scar and pigmentation.

19. Uremic stomatitis.

- Uremic stomatitis is a complication of advanced renal failure. The onset is abrupt, with white plaques present predominantly on the buccal mucosa, tongue, and floor of the mouth. The odor of ammonia or urine may be smelled on the patient's breath. The principal cause is the elevated levels of ammonia. Uremia-induced hemorrhagic disorders to cause a decrease in the resistance of mucosal tissues to infection resulting in ulceration and pseudomembrane formation.
- Four forms of uremic stomatitis are recognized:
  1. Ulcerative form
  2. Hemorrhagic form
  3. Pseudomembranous form
  4. Hyperkeratotic form.

Pseudomembranous form and hyperkeratotic form appears white.

Management

- In some conditions, uremic crystals may clear within 2–3 weeks following dialysis.
- In persistent conditions, acidic mouth rinses like hydrogen peroxide may clear the uremic deposits.
- Palliative therapy with ice cubes is also advisable.

20. What is the classification and staging of leukoplakia?

LSCP classification and staging of leukoplakia:

L—extent of the lesion
S—site of the lesion
C—clinical aspects
P—histopathological features.

Classification

Extent of the lesion:

L_0 = No evidence of lesion
L_1 = Lesion ≤2 cm
L_2 = Lesion 2–4 cm
L_3 = Lesion ≥4 cm
L_X = Not specified

Site of the lesion:

S_1 = All oral site except floor of mouth and tongue.
S_2 = Floor of mouth and/or tongue.
S_X = Not specified

Clinical aspects:

C_1 = Homogeneous
C_2 = Nonhomogeneous
C_X = Not specified

Histopathological features

P_1 = No dysplasia
P_2 = Mild dysplasia
P_3 = Moderate dysplasia
P_4 = Severe dysplasia
P_X = Not specified

Staging

Stage 1: Any L, S_1, C_1, P_1, or P_2
Stage 2: Any L, S_1 C_2, P_1, or P_2
Any L, S_2 C1, P_1, or P_2
Stage 3: Any L, S_2 C_2, P_1, or P_2
Stage 4: Any L, any S, any C, P_3, or P_4

In case of widespread lesion, the highest L and the highest S should be considered.

MULTIPLE CHOICE QUESTIONS

1. Gallenkamp colony counter is used to assess ***candida density***.
   a. Candida density
   b. Viral load
   c. Lactobacillus count
   d. Oral flora
2. One of the following *genetic (hereditary) disorder* cause *white lesions on mucosa is* ***dyskeratosis congenita.***
   a. Cowden's syndrome
   b. Digeorge's syndrome
   c. Dyskeratosis congenita
   d. Peutz-Jeghers syndrome
   (**Note:** Genetic (hereditary) disorder cause *white lesions on mucosa* are *white sponge nevus, hereditary benign intraepithelial dyskeratosis and dyskeratosis congenita*).
3. Morsicatio buccarum denotes ***chronic chewing of buccal mucosa***.
   a. Ulcer caused by natal teeth
   b. Chronic chewing of buccal mucosa
   c. Traumatic ulcer of buccal mucosa
   d. Dryness of buccal mucosa
   (**Note:** Buccal mucosa—*morsicatio buccarum;* Labial mucosa—*morsicatio labiorum*
   Lateral border of tongue—*morsicatio linguarum*).
4. *Mucous patches* are associated with ***secondary syphills.***
   a. NOMA
   b. Canker sores
   c. Secondary syphilis
   d. HIV infection
   (**Note:** Mucous patches are mucosal necrosis appearing as grayish white patches and seen in secondary syphilis).
5. *Bowens's disease* is the result of ***arsenic ingestion.***
   a. Lead ingestion
   b. Mercury ingestion
   c. Bismuth ingestion
   d. Arsenic ingestion
   (**Note:** *Bowens's disease is the result of arsenic ingestion* and characterized by localized *intraepidermal squamous carcinoma of the skin* that may progress to invasive carcinoma).
6. *Kobner's phenomenon* is associated with *appearance of new lesion* ***along the line of trauma.***
   a. After a relapse
   b. Along the line of trauma
   c. After complete healing
   d. Along the midline
7. *Witkop's disease* manifestation in oral cavity is ***white plaques.***
   a. White plaques
   b. Erythematous patches
   c. Bullous lesions
   d. Mucosal nodules
   (**Note:** *Witkop's disease* is hereditary benign intraepithelial dyskeratosis and associated with oral white plaques and bilateral limbal conjunctival plaques).

VIVA VOCE

1. What is quid?

Quid is a mixture of substances containing tobacco and areca nut in either raw or manufactured form placed in the mouth, chewed and kept in contact with oral mucosa.

2. What are potentially malignant disorders?

World Health Organization defines potentially malignant disorders (PMDs) of oral cavity as an inherent cancerous nature of a lesion or condition in which the probability for malignant transformation at the lesion site or any part of the orodigestive tract is higher in the succeeding phases.

- Precancerous lesion — a benign lesion with morphologically altered tissue which has a greater than normal risk of transforming into malignancy.

- Precancerous condition—a generalized disease state that may or may not alter the clinical appearance of tissues but prone to develop a cancerous state than normal tissues.

3. Give examples for premalignant lesions and disorders.

- Premalignant lesions:
  - Leukoplakia, erythroplakia, proliferative verrucous leukoplakia, palatal lesions in reverse smokers, submucous fibrosis, actinic cheilitis, and dyskeratosis congenita.
- Premalignant conditions:
  - Lichen planus, discoid lupus erythematosus, and xeroderma pigmentosum, Plummer-Vinson syndrome, immunosuppressive diseases (AIDS).

4. What is field mapping? (or) What is field effect in cancer? What is field cancerization?

Morphologically normal epithelium present in close proximity to the tumor, may have precancerous cells and genetic potential to develop into multiple primary tumor. Multiple biopsies in the clinically suspecious area is recommended to diagnose the multiple primary or recurrent tumor.

5. What is orabase?

Orabase is a oral adhesive paste composed of gelatin, pectin, and sodium carboxymethylcellulose used to facilitate the adhesion of intraoral gel or ointment. The prescribed medication can be mixed with equal parts of orabase and applied to the mucosal tissues for better retention.

6. Discuss leukoedema.

It is a *normal variant of the oral mucosa*. It manifests as diffuse, faint, white and filmy-wrinkling appearance of mucosa bilaterally. Common in buccal mucosa but involves labial mucosa, soft palate, and floor of mouth occasionally. *No treatment* is required.

7. What is white sponge nevus?

- It is an autosomal dominant disorder affecting oral mucosa and sometimes mucous membrane of nose, esophagus, genitalia, and rectum.
- Bilateral symmetrical, white, soft, spongy and velvety thick plaques appear on buccal and labial mucosa, ventral tongue, floor of the mouth and soft palate. It is asymptomatic and requires no treatment.

8. What is linea alba?

Linea alba is a bilateral horizontal white streak extending from commissure to posterior teeth. The causative factors include friction or irritation from buccal cusps of teeth and reduced overjet of posterior teeth. No treatment is required.

9. What is morsicatio buccarum or labiorum or linguarum?

- Chronic irritation caused by self-chewing, nibbling or sucking results in a localized area of thickened, scared and pale area of the oral mucosa. Patient experiences roughness or felling of delicate tissues. Sometimes erythema or ulceration also present with the white patch.
- Stress or psychological disorder is considered as an underlying disorder.
- To stop the predisposing habits, occlusal night guard or splint is advised. Antidepressants may be helpful for some patients.

10. What is thrush?

Thrush is the superficial candidal infection of the outer layer of epithelium causing white plaques or flecks on the mucosal surface resembling the white belly of the singing bird *thrush*. The white plaques are easily scrapable.

11. What are the predisposing factors for oral candidiasis?

- Altered oral microflora due to routine use of antibacterial mouth rinse or prolonged use of antibiotics.

- Administration of steroid inhalants and topical steroids.
- Poor oral hygiene.
- Diabetes mellitus.
- Chronic local irritation due to dental appliances.
- Pregnancy
- Immunological deficiency like HIV infection, cancer chemotherapy, head and neck radiation, leukemia and lymphomas, bone marrow transplantation.
- Malabsorption and malnutrition.

12. Why antioxidants are used in the management of submucous fibrosis?

The components of commercial betel nut products release free radicals that damage the cell structures, and biological molecules. Also the associated nutritional deficient status delays the routine repair mechanism of the inflamed mucosa leading to an atrophic condition. Antioxidants stabilize and deactivate the free radicals before they attack cells. Vitamins A, B complex, C, D, E and minerals like iron, copper, and magnesium are used as a standard or adjunct supplement in controlling the signs and symptoms of OSMF.

13. What are Fordyce's granules?

Fordyce's granules are ectopic sebaceous glands within the oral mucosa. They are normal tissue in an abnormal location. They present as a group of multiple-yellowish orange papules on buccal mucosa and vermilion borders of the lip. They are asymptomatic and require no treatment.

14. Enumerate the six *P*'s of Lichen Planus.

Pruritic, purple, polygonal, planar, papules, and plaques—these are the six patterns of lichen planus manifestation.

BIBLIOGRAPHY

1. Awan KH, Morgan PR, Warnakulasuriya S. Utility of chemiluminescence (ViziLite™) in the detection of oral potentially malignant disorders and benign keratoses. J Oral Pathol Med. 2011;40(7):541-4.
2. Borle RM, Borle SR. Management of oral submucous fibrosis: a conservative approach. J Oral Maxillofac Surg. 1991; 49(8):788-91.
3. Brouns ER, Baart JA, Bloemena E, et al. The relevance of uniform reporting in oral leukoplakia: definition, certainty factor and staging based on experience with 275 patients. Med Oral Patol Oral Cir Bucal. 2013;18(1):e19-26.
4. Cerero-Lapiedra R, Baladé-Martínez D, Moreno-López LA, et al. Proliferative verrucous leukoplakia: a proposal for diagnostic criteria. Med Oral Patol Oral Cir Bucal. 2010;15(6):e839-45.
5. Farah CS, Lynch N, McCullough MJ. Oral fungal infections: an update for the general practitioner. Aust Dent J. 2010;55(Suppl 1):48-54.
6. Feller L, Wood NH, Khammisa RA, Lemmer J. allergic contact stomatitis. Oral surgery, oral medicine, oral pathology and oral radiology. 2017 May 1;123(5):559-65.
7. Gandolfo S, Scully C, Carrozzo M. Oral medicine. Elsevier Health Sciences; 2006.
8. Gendreau L, Loewy ZG. Epidemiology and etiology of denture stomatitis. J Prosthodont. 2011;20(4):251-60.
9. Kramer IR, Lucas RB, Pindborg JJ, et al. World Health Organization Collaborating Centre for Oral Precancerous Lesions. Definition of leukoplakia and related lesions: an aid to studies on oral precancer. Oral Surg Oral Med Oral Pathol. 1978;46(4):518-39.
10. Krinsky NI. Mechanism of action of biological antioxidants. Proc Soc Exp Biol Med. 1992;200(2):248-54.
11. Kumar V, Abbas AK, Aster JC. Robbins Basic Pathology E-Book. Elsevier Health Sciences; 2017.
12. McCullough MJ, Ross BC, Reade PC. Candida albicans: a review of its history, taxonomy, epidemiology, virulence

attributes, and methods of strain differentiation. Int J Oral Maxillofac Surg. 1996; 25(2):136-44.

13. Mollaoglu N. Oral lichen planus: a review. British Journal of Oral and Maxillofacial Surgery. 2000;38(4):370-7.
14. Nisa L, Giger R. Black hairy tongue. Am J Med. 2011;124(9):816-7.
15. Pappas PG, Kauffman CA, Andes D, et al. Clinical practice guidelines for the management of candidiasis: 2009 update by the Infectious Diseases Society of America. Clin Infect Dis. 2009;48(5):503-35.
16. Parihar S. Oral candidiasis-A review.
17. Pindborg JJ, Sirsat SM. Oral submucous fibrosis. Oral Surg Oral Med Oral Pathol. 1966;22(6):764-79.
18. Rajendran R. Oral submucous fibrosis: etiology, pathogenesis, and future research. Bulletin of the World Health Organization. 1994;72(6):985-96.
19. Ranganathan K, Mishra G. An overview of classification schemes for oral submucous fibrosis. J Oral Maxillofac Pathol. 2006; 10(2):55-9.
20. Samaranayake LP, Cheung LK, Samaranayake YH. Candidiasis and other fungal diseases of the mouth. Dermatol Therapy. 2002;15(3):251-69.
21. Samlaska CP, Winfield EA. Pentoxifylline. J Am Acad Dermatol. 1994;30(4):603-21.
22. Schepman KP, van der Waal I. A proposal for a classification and staging system for oral leukoplakia: a preliminary study. Eur J Cancer B Oral Oncol. 1995;31B(6):396-8.
23. van der Waal I, Reichart PA. Oral proliferative verrucous leukoplakia revisited. Oral oncology. 2008;44(8):719-21.
24. Warnakulasuriya S, Johnson N, van der Waal I. Nomenclature and classification of potentially malignant disorders of the oral mucosa. J Oral pathol Med. 2007;36(10): 575-80.
25. Williams D, Lewis M. Pathogenesis and treatment of oral candidosis. J Oral Microbiol. 2011;3(1):5771.

CHAPTER 2

Vesiculobullous and Ulcerative Diseases

HIGHLIGHTS

Oral lesions often manifest as vesicle and bulla but pathologically differ from each other. These vesicle and bulla rupture immediately after their manifestation because of their fragile nature and forces associated with mastication, movements of tongue and lips. Many of these lesions involve cutaneous surface. The oral lesions precede the onset of skin lesions, occur simultaneously or develop at the later stage. This chapter enlightens about different types of vesiculobullous lesions, their etiology, pathogenesis, clinical course, necessary investigations, and drugs for management.

Learners are expected to know about:

1. Classification of vesiculobullous lesions
2. Description of the etiopathogenesis of each lesion
3. Clinical features of the lesions
4. Differential diagnosis and medical management of individual lesions.

ESSAY QUESTIONS

1. Describe the etiopathogenesis, clinical features, investigations, and management of recurrent herpes simplex virus infection.

(or)

Write in detail about recurrent herpes labialis.

Herpes simplex virus (HSV) is a DNA group of virus and has the pathognomonic features of latency and reactivation following primary infection.

It has two subtypes: (1) HSV-1 causes a nongenital lesion (i.e. lesions occur above the waist) and is usually transmitted between 6 months and 14 years of age, preferably, before 5 years; (2) HSV-2 causes genital lesions.

The primary form of HSV-1 gingivostomatitis infection affects preschool children. After the primary infection, the virus travel and reach the sensory ganglion and remains in a dormant state. The inactive period begins a *latent* form infection in the V, VII, and X nerve ganglia. Sometime the primary infection will be subclinical and does not cause any clinical presentation.

Pathogenesis

The HSV travels from the primary site of oral or skin lesions and reach the dorsal root ganglion, and multiplies in the neurons, dermal, and epidermal cells. The dormant state persists for a variable period.

The reactivation of HSV-1 at trigeminal ganglia affects the facial, oral, labial, oropharyngeal, and ocular mucosa.

Reactivation of the latent virus requires *triggering factors* like exposure to sunlight, stress, menstrual periods, illness, and injury. The lesion appears 24–36 hours after a trigger. Recurrence of oral infection differs between one to six times in a 12 month period.

Clinical Features

Many patients experience a *"prodrome"* of fever followed by burning, prickling, or itching sensation at the potential sites where the lesion develops. Submandibular lymphadenopathy is also common.

Cold sores appear as clusters of vesicles on the lips, at the junction of the labial mucosa and the vermilion border of the lips or in the nasal mucosa. The vesicles soon rupture and form ulcers and crustation. Healing begins at 3rd or 4th day, and complete re-epithelialization may take 7 or 8 days.

Differential Diagnosis

- Aphthous ulcers
- Behçet's syndrome.

Diagnosis

The various laboratory investigations to diagnose HSV-1 include:

- Tzanck test
- Culture test
- Polymerase chain reaction (PCR)
- Serological examination
- Fluorescent antibody test.

Swab Preparation

Fresh vesicles (those formed <48 hours) are essential for obtaining viral culture. A sterile scalpel or needle should be used to unroof the new vesicle and to scrape the base. The vesicular content is absorbed in a swab. The swab should be sent to the laboratory in a suitable viral transport media and should be protected from heat.

Direct Fluorescent Assay

The swabs so prepared are rolled on the microscopic slides in multiple areas (up to five sites), each measuring 5–10 mm in diameter and air dried. The slide is stained with fluorescein-labeled antibody. The examination of the slide under the fluorescent microscope will reveal the apple green fluorescent spots in the nucleus and cytoplasm if the individual is positive for HSV infection.

Indirect Serological Test

From the suspected individual, 8–10 mL of blood is collected in a test tube in the absence of anticoagulant. The tube is centrifuged to separate the serum. The serum is subjected to serological testing. Both acute and convalescent phase sera need to be examined. If HSV-1 is not isolated from acute sera but isolated from convalescent sera, it indicates the infection is a primary type (primary HSV-1). If the HSV isolation is present in both acute and convalescent sera, it means recurrent HSV infection.

Polymerase Chain Reaction

Polymerase chain reaction is a more sensitive test to HSV infection and is particularly helpful for the detection of asymptomatic viral infection.

Tzanck Test

This test is done by scrapping the floor of the herpetic vesicle; spread the content over the microscopic slide. The slide should be stained with Giemsa stain or Papanicolaou stain and examined under light microscope. The positive condition reveals multinucleated giant cells. However, the results do not specify the type of herpes infection.

Treatment

For patients manifesting 3–5 episodes yearly—preventive therapy should be initiated with sunblock agents and a topical antiviral drug. *For patients presenting with 6 or more recurrence lesions in a year,* those in whom recurrence triggers erythema multiforme (EM) and for patients in an immunocompromised state should be treated with a specific protocol.

Topical Therapy

Acyclovir cream 5%, five times/day or penciclovir 1% cream every 2 hours.

Systemic Therapy

- Acyclovir 400 mg, five times/day for 5 days
  or
- Valacyclovir 2 g two dose for 1 day
  or
- Famciclovir 1,500 mg single dose for 1 day.

Suppressive Therapy

- Acyclovir 400 mg twice a day.

Antiviral therapy is helpful in relieving the symptoms earlier and shortens the healing time.

2. Discuss in detail about the etiology, clinical features, and management of postherpetic neuralgia.

Herpes zoster (shingles) is an acute, self-limiting infection caused by varicella-zoster virus (VZV), a DNA group of virus. Chickenpox is the primary infection, whereas herpes zoster is the reactivated form of the VZV.

Herpes zoster occurs as painful vesicular rash involving single dermatome and resolves within few weeks.

Herpetic neuralgia: Pain associated with the occurrence of rashes that may continue up to 4 weeks is called as acute herpetic neuralgia. Pain present between the 2nd and 4th months (30–120 days) is the subacute herpetic neuralgia and persisting pain after 4 months (>120) of the onset of herpes zoster rash is the postherpetic neuralgia (PHN).

Postherpetic neuralgia: PHN is a recurrent type of shooting pain that lasts for short duration, and remains after the healing of mucocutaneous rashes.

For the PHN, the risk of occurrence increases after 6th decade of life probably due to the decreased immune level.

The reason for postherpetic pain is unclear. The suggested reasons include atrophy of the posterior horn of the spinal cord, fibrosis of the dorsal root ganglion, and degeneration of axonal or cell bodies of primary afferent neurons may give rise to pain.

The pain may be either spontaneous or evoked after a stimulus. Some patients may report abnormal sensations like numbness, itching, and paresthesias in the affected dermatome. Shooting pain exacerbated response to mild touch, and loss of sensory function are also common in the affected dermatome.

There are three subtypes in PHN which are as follows:

1. Sensitized nociceptor burning pain (spontaneous experience of pain and mechanical allodynia in the affected dermatome)
2. Partially deafferented burning pain (experience extreme pain to light touch)
3. Deafferented burning pain (severe sensory loss and deafferentation pain).

Etiopathogenesis

After primary varicella (chickenpox) is subsided, the zoster virus remains in a dormant form (viable but do not replicate) either at the dorsal ganglia of spinal nerves or extramedullary ganglia of cranial nerves (Fig. 1). Varicella-zoster virus *becomes reactivated* with increasing age or immunosuppression. Conditions like human immunodeficiency virus (HIV), cancer chemotherapy, immunosuppressive drugs, and hematological malignancy increase the risk of a chance of severe and fatal form of zoster infection.

Clinical Features

Herpes zoster infection develops as vesicles on the skin and mucosa innervated by the affected nerve. The skin supplied by the thoracic (45%), cervical (23%) and trigeminal (15%) regions is the frequently affected dermatome. The frequently affected nerves are C3, T5, L1, L2, and the ophthalmic division of cranial nerve V (Fig. 2).

There are three stages in the clinical course:

1. Prodromal stage
2. Active or acute stage
3. Chronic stage (PHN and develops in 10% of affected individuals).

Antiviral therapy for herpes zoster:

- 800 mg acyclovir five times/day for 1 week (or)
- 800 mg famciclovir three times/day for 1 week (or)

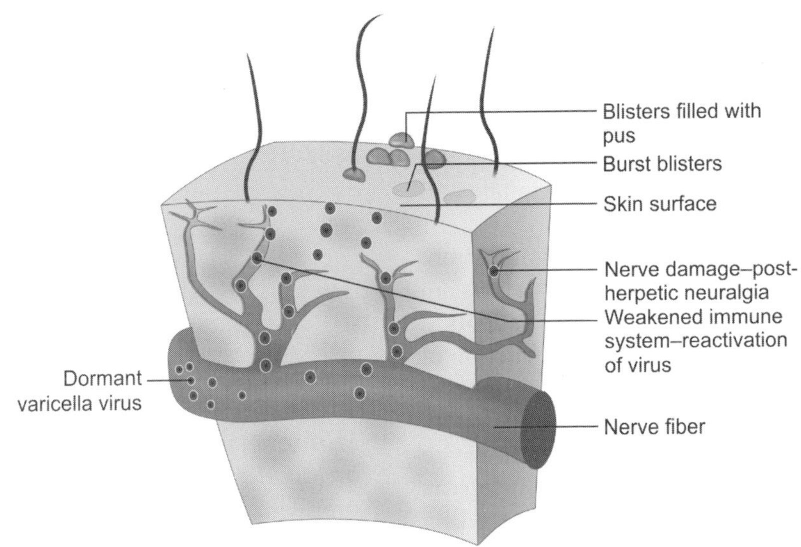

Fig. 1: Postherpetic neuralgia.

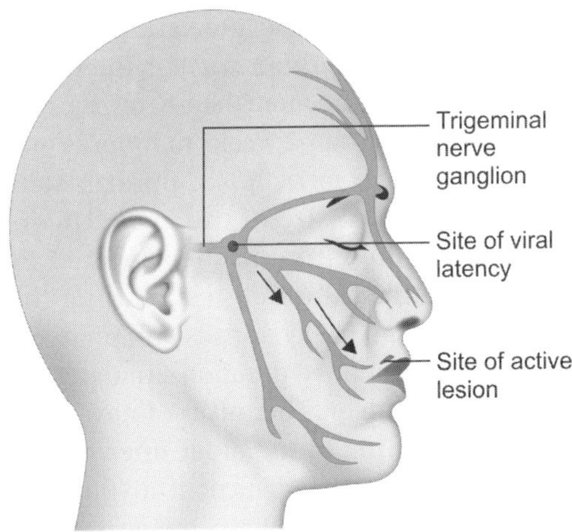

Fig. 2: Course of herpes zoster infection.

- 1,000 mg valacyclovir three times/day for 1 week.

Investigations

- Viral isolation in tissue culture.
- Polymerase chain reaction.

Treatment

- Topical lignocaine 5%.
- Topical application of 8% capsaicin—an extraction of hot chili pepper.
- Tricyclic antidepressants such, as amitriptyline, nortriptyline, and desipramine.
    - Anticonvulsants—gabapentin up to 3,600 mg/day in divided dose for 1–2 weeks. Effective in pain management and enhancing the quality of daily activities.

Response to therapy shows significant inhomogeneity probably due to damage to various neurological pathways.

3. Define recurrent aphthous stomatitis and explain about its etiology, clinical presentation, investigations, and management.

Recurrent aphthous stomatitis (RAS) is a clinical presentation of frequent ulcers that affects only oral mucosa of individuals who are otherwise healthy.

Etiology

There are many hypotheses for the etiology of RAS.

Host Factors

- *Genetics*: There is a genetic predisposition for RAS. The chance for developing RAS is 90% for an individual if both parents are affected with RAS, but only 20% if parents are not affected. The human leukocyte antigen

(HLA) subtypes are associated with RAS. Positive family history will favor the onset at the young age and severe symptoms.

- *Food allergies*: Foods, such as cheese, tomatoes, chocolate, coffee, peanuts and gluten-containing wheat flour may precipitate RAS in some patients.
- *Hematological deficiency*: Hematinic (iron, folic acid, vitamins B_6 and B_{12}) defects are commonly associated with RAS patients.
- *Immune reaction*: The cytotoxic action of lymphocytes and monocytes in the oral epithelium is likely to cause the ulceration. The preulcerative and healing phases are prevailing with T-helper cells, whereas the ulcerative phase is dominated by T-suppressor cells.
- *Psychological stress*: Stress may play a trigger or a modifying role in the manifestation of RAS.
- *Hypersensitivity reaction*: *Streptococcus sanguis* L-form has been suggested to cause autoimmunity to the oral mucosal homogenate and produces oral ulcers.

Environmental factors include microtrauma, local tissue injury, and chemical contact.

Clinical Presentation

- *Site of occurrence*: The ulcers are typically seen on the nonkeratinized structures like labial and buccal mucosa, soft palate, floor of the oral cavity, and tongue (Fig. 3). Involvement of palate and gingiva are extremely infrequent except in diffused presentation in severely immunocompromised patients.
- *Prodromal features*: Localized burning sensation or pain for 24–48 hours usually precedes the ulcers.
- *Signs and symptoms*: Ulcers are ovoid or round in shape with a well-defined erythematous periphery and shallow central necrosis. All ulcers have a yellow-grayish membrane at the base. The lesions are painful, and the pain gets aggravated by chewing, swallowing and talking. The duration of the pain is typically 3–4 days.

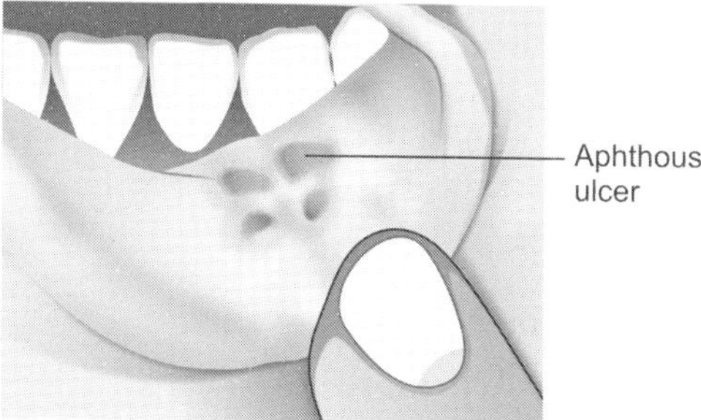

Fig. 3: Aphthous ulcer.

Three types of clinical presentations of RAS:

1. *Minor recurrent aphthous stomatitis or Mikulicz's diseases*: This is the most prevalent type of RAS comprising 75–85% of all cases of RAS. They typically measure 5–10 mm in size, last for 10–14 days and heal without scarring. After healing, there is a variable ulcer-free interval.
2. *Major RAS or Sutton's disease*: The ulcers typically measure more than 10 mm in size, last for more than 2 weeks to months and *heal with scar formation*. Approximately 10–15% of RAS are of this type. Ulcers occur on the multiple sites covered by nonkeratinized mucosa including the posterior oral cavity, tonsils and pharynx. The more extended duration simulates the malignant ulcer. The onset of new ulcer before healing of the older ones causes almost one persistent ulcer at anytime.
3. *Herpetiform ulcers*: They occur as multiple crops of several ulcers. Each crop measures less than 5 mm and unites to form a larger ulcer with a surrounding erythematous border. They persist for 10–14 days and are painful than other forms. Approximately 5–10% of RAS occur as a herpetiform type. The ulcers often look like of primary type of herpes simplex infection (HSV), but the duration of recurrence is variable.

Investigations

- The recurring nature and examination findings help in the diagnosis. The medical history of a celiac disease, Crohn's disease, neutropenia, HIV, and Behçet's syndrome should be ruled out.

- Complete blood cell count, hematinic estimation to rule out vitamin and iron deficiencies and malabsorption syndrome.
- The possibility of an autoimmune disorder is ruled out by performing antiendomysial antibody test.

Differential Diagnosis

- Recurrent herpes viral infection
- Recurrent EM
- Cyclic neutropenia.

Syndromes associated with RAS

- Behçet's disease (syndrome) is a blood vessel inflammatory disorder, manifesting a triad of recurring oral, ocular and genital ulcers. Oral ulcers resemble both major and minor forms of aphthous.
- PFAPA syndrome comprises periodic fever, aphthous stomatitis, pharyngitis and cervical adenitis.
- *Mouth and genital ulcers with inflamed cartilage (MAGIC) syndrome*: Ulcers in the oral cavity and genital organs with cartilage inflammation.
- Celiac disease is a gluten hypersensitivity disorder of the small intestines. Recurring oral aphthae is a common manifestation.

Management of Aphthous Stomatitis

As the etiology is unknown, the treatment plan should be developed individually for each patient. The management should be aimed for:

- Eliminating the discomforts
- Decreasing the number and size of ulcers
- Extending the ulcer-free period.

Topical Treatments

- The antiseptics and anti-inflammatory drugs are the first-line treatment. 0.2% chlorhexidine rinse or gel, three times a day and 3% topical diclofenac are efficient in pain relief.
- Amlexanox is also widely prescribed for RAS. It antiallergic action inhibits leukotrienes and histamines and thereby accelerates complete healing. Its anti-inflammatory property reduces the pain. Dosage: 5% amlexanox, two to four times/day.
- 0.1% triamcinolone acetonide is applied three to ten times/day. It is effective for minor aphthous associated with less pain and discomfort.
- Clobetasol ointment 0.05% in orabase or fluocinonide ointment 0.05% in orabase is indicated in larger ulcers and/or ulcers with severe pain.

Oral Rinse

- Elixir forms of corticosteroids, such as dexamethasone can be used as an oral rinse for patients with multiple ulcerations.
- Tetracycline or doxycycline or minocycline in oral rinse preparation will lessen the pain and frequency of RAS. 100 mg capsule should be dissolved in 10 mL of water and used as rinse for 2–3 minutes/time and four times every day for 3 days will be beneficial.

Systemic Therapy

- Corticosteroid—prescribed only for RAS patients with frequent episodes and severe symptoms.
  - Oral prednisone 25 mg/day for 2 weeks is the regular course. The dose should be progressively reduced to 12.5 mg/day on the subsequent 2 weeks and then 6.25 mg/day for 2 more weeks. The tapering is maintained by 6.25 mg on alternate days for 2 weeks. This is the stepwise dose reduction for 2 months. The benefit of this therapy is effective pain relief and healing by surface epithelialization.
  - Copper, iron, zinc, folate, vitamin B_{12}, and iron supplementation.

Miscellaneous

Pentoxifylline, colchicine, dapsone, and thalidomide may be used, but their adverse effects should be considered before starting the therapy.

4. Write about the etiopathogenesis, clinical features, and management of erythema multiforme.

Erythema multiforme is an acute, inflammatory, mucocutaneous disorder. It is self-limiting and is characterized by the symmetrical distribution of skin lesions primarily on the extremities. It tends to recur and is occasionally chronic. Erosions or bullae occur in the mucosa of the genital tract, eye, or oral cavity. EM involving mucosal surfaces is known as major type, and without mucosal involvement is minor type.

Erythema multiforme that repeatedly occurs for many years is called as recurrent EM. Herpes infection is the common precipitating factor for recurrent EM; however, the cause is still unclear. EM has preference for young adults, and females.

Etiopathogenesis

The suspected causes include infection, medication, neoplasm, autoimmune disease, radiation exposure, immunization, and menstruation. Underlying infection corresponds for 90% of cases, and the widely reported pathogen is HSV followed by *Mycoplasma pneumoniae.*

Isolatwed Type of Erythema Multiforme

- Infections—HSV, mycoplasma pneumonia.
- Drugs—nonsteroidal anti-inflammatory drugs (NSAIDs), sulfonamides, antiepileptics, antibiotics.

Recurrent (>6 Episodes of EM/Year)

- Infections—HSV (both type 1 and 2), mycoplasma pneumonia, hepatitis C.
- Others—benzoic acid consumption.

Persistent

- Infections—HSV, hepatitis C, Epstein-Barr virus.

Others—inflammatory bowel disease, malignancy.

Pathogenesis

Herpes simplex virus-induced EM is a delayed hypersensitivity reaction. It is a T cell mediated type IV reaction viral antigens. There is a possible genetic predisposition with HLA-DQB1 has been reported.

Clinical Features

- The disease tends to occur with an episode of 1–4 weeks. It usually affects young individuals and rare after 50 years.
- It has an acute and explosive onset with general symptoms like fever and malaise for less than 24 hours before the beginning of skin and mucosal lesions. The oral mucosa alone is affected in many cases.
- The specific target (iris) lesion of EM is clearly demarcated circular skin lesions with three concentric zones:
  1. Center is dusky with a blister or crust
  2. Next zone is pale pink and raised due to edema
  3. The periphery is bright red.

The iris is the initial lesion manifesting two zones: (1) dusky central and (2) outer red.

The lesions present in varying forms (multiforme). During an episode, in a given period, lesions at different development phases may present.

Oral lesions involve the nonkeratinized surfaces and are extensive in the lips and anterior part of the oral cavity (Fig. 4). Intraoral lesions appear as widespread blisters that immediately break down and form ill-defined ulcers which coalesce to form larger ulcers. Ulcers bleed profusely and the surface is covered by crustation and necrotic tissue tags.

- In severe cases, oral epithelium is denuded in larger area and the patient experiences difficulty during eating or drinking.
- A severe form of this disease is Stevens-Johnson syndrome with a generalized occurrence of bulla and vesicles involving the skin, oral mucosa, eyes, and genitals.

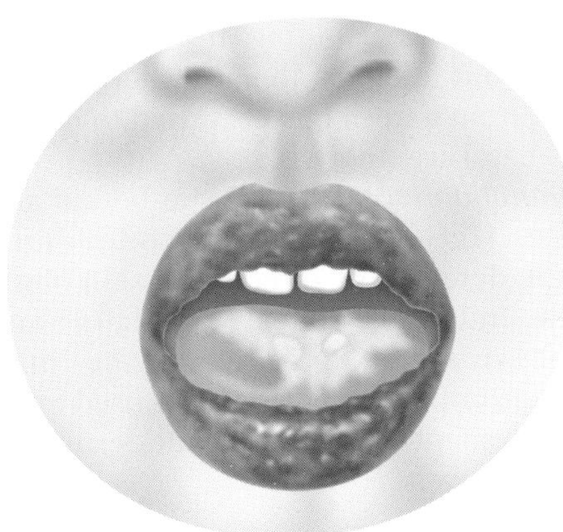

Fig. 4: Erythema multiforme involving the labial mucosa and tongue.

The most severe form is toxic epidermal neurolysis (TEN), with sloughing of larger areas of skin and mucosa.

Differential Diagnosis

- Urticaria
- Bullous pemphigoid
- Paraneoplastic pemphigus
- Fixed drug eruption
- Sweet's syndrome (acute febrile neutrophilic dermatosis).

Investigations

Since EM is frequently associated with HSV infection, patients should be subjected to HSV-specific investigations like Tzanck smear and PCR studies. Serologic tests for *M. pneumoniae* should be advised when the patient manifests respiratory symptoms. The investigation should include chest X-ray and PCR testing of throat swabs.

Management

Erythema multiforme is a self-limiting disease and resolves within weeks. The treatment is directed according to the causative agent.

- In drug-induced cases, the suspected drug should be stopped.
- In HSV-induced recurrent EM, antiviral prophylaxis should be initiated. One of the following drugs can be prescribed:
  - Acyclovir 400 mg twice daily (or)
  - Valacyclovir 500 mg twice daily (or)
  - Famciclovir 250 mg twice daily.

The drug should be continued until 4 months the patient becomes free of recurrence episodes. Gradual dose reduction is essential before withdrawal. If antiviral therapy is ineffective, cytotoxic drugs like azathioprine, dapsone, cyclosporine, or mycophenolate mofetil should be considered.

- Topical corticosteroid and oral antihistamines are considered for treating milder cases, whereas systemic steroids are indicated for severe cases with starting dose of 30–50 mg prednisone/day.
- The use of 0.05% chlorhexidine helps to prevent superinfection.

5. Classify chronic multiple oral ulcers of autoimmune etiology. Briefly describe the pathogenesis, clinical presentation, investigations, and management of pemphigus. (or) Describe the intraepithelial group of mucocutaneous diseases that cause multiple chronic oral ulcers.

Pemphigus is an *intraepithelial blistering* type of disease. Pemphigus vulgaris and pemphigus foliaceus are the two common entities.

Pemphigus Vulgaris

Greek word "pemphig" means bubble, and hence the name pemphigus for this blistering disease. It occurs at the 5th or 6th decade of life and involves skin and mucous membranes. The oral lesions occur as an isolated variety and cause severe morbidity but not life-threatening. Pemphigus vulgaris is sudden in onset and unpredictable in progression. Remission is a common feature, and apparent cure for the disease is possible.

Pathogenesis

Pemphigus vulgaris is an autoimmune disorder in which immunoglobulin G (IgG) serum antibodies are directed against adhesion molecules desmoglein 3 (Dsg3) present on the keratinocytes cell membrane. The antibody—desmoglein complex separates epithelial layers and leads to blisters formation. The result is the attachment loss of cells with each at the superficial epithelium, but the basal cells remain attached to the basement membrane of connective tissue, as they do not contain Dsg3.

The oral mucosa has only Dsg3, whereas skin has Dsg3 and Dsg1. The presence of antibodies against Dsg3 leads to mucosal pemphigus, whereas the presence of antibodies against Dsg1 and Dsg3 causes both cutaneous and oral lesions.

Clinical Features

Pemphigus has preference for Mediterranean origin and Jews and hence a genetic background. Oral lesions precede the skin lesions and remain the sole presentation for 2–6 months. Multiple blisters develop and immediately ruptured and result in painful bleeding ulcers. Sloughing is common. The lesion affects any part of the oral cavity but is common in the labial, buccal, and palatal mucosa. Pain and burning sensation are the associated symptoms. Profuse salivation and halitosis are also common in the advanced stage.

Multiple erosions localized on the gingiva, especially on the free gingival region may progress to desquamative or erosive gingivitis.

Investigations

Diagnosis is made by correlating the clinical features, histopathological results, and direct immunofluorescence (IF) findings.

Nikolsky's sign: It is demonstrated as a chairside test done by applying oblique pressure on the mucosa with the finger. The occurrence of a fresh bulla is the positive Nikolsky's sign. The technique is a highly specific and very useful in the preliminary diagnosis.

Histopathological finding: The Tzanck test is carried out to detect the acantholytic cells; smear from a fresh blister is used to identify suprabasal acantholysis.

Immunofluorescent test: Tissue-bound antibodies (IgG and IgA) and complement can be detected by direct IF of skin biopsy tissue. Indirect IF detects circulating antibodies in serum. Specific enzyme-linked immunosorbent assay (ELISA) is used for the measurement of individual antidesmoglein antibody levels.

Treatment

- Corticosteroid is the drug of choice. Mild localized lesions of the oral mucous membrane are treated with topical corticosteroid creams, 0.1% triamcinolone acetonide or 0.05% clobetasol propionate. Intralesional triamcinolone acetonide may be used for resistant lesions at a weekly interval till the symptoms subside.
- Patients with widespread disease or severe localized form are treated with systemic corticosteroids. Prednisone 60–80 mg/day with low maintenance dose on alternative days is given for years.
- Adjunctive therapy to reduce corticosteroid side effects includes azathioprine or cyclophosphamide. Other drugs to be considered include deflazacort, mycophenolate mofetil, gold and immunoglobulin.

Pemphigus Vegetans

Pemphigus vegetans is a variant of pemphigus vulgaris. It presents as "heaped up" vegetating lesions in the flexures. In the oral cavity, vegetations occur on the mucous membrane as soft dark granulations. The vegetant form is a rare presentation in oral cavity and seen in partially treated pemphigus. The occurrence is due to the exaggerated healing response of the eroded skin by forming hyperplastic granulation tissue, called as "Neumann type" in which early lesions are larger bullae. Verrucous hyperkeratotic vegetation formation during healing of milder pustular lesion is known as "Hallopeau type". The oral lesions are common in both and manifest as ulcers with a purulent surface.

Corticosteroids are the drug of choice.

Paraneoplastic Pemphigus

Paraneoplastic pemphigus is due to the interference of tumor-released products on the innate immune system and not because of tumor infiltration or metastasis.

It causes blisters and ulcers on the skin and mucous membranes. Oral lesions are sudden in onset and very painful. The oral ulcers are multiple, shallow, and irregular. They often spread to vermilion border and present as blisters, erosions, and blood crusts.

Occurrence of paraneoplastic pemphigus is a poor sign of prognosis.

Diagnosis is based on three major and three minor criteria.

Three major criteria:

1. Mucocutaneous eruptions
2. Internal malignancy
3. Serum antibodies.

Three minor criteria:

1. Acantholysis
2. Direct IF revealing IgG and complement at the intercellular region and basement membrane.
3. Indirect IF with rat bladder epithelium showing circulating autoantibodies.

Presence of three major or two major and two minor criteria confirms a definitive diagnosis.

Treatment

Systemic corticosteroid (prednisone) with other immunosuppressive drug like azathioprine, cyclophosphamide, or methotrexate.

6. Briefly describe the subepithelial mucocutaneous bullous disorders that cause multiple persistent ulcers of the oral cavity.

Subepithelial bullous disorders include bullous pemphigoid, mucous membrane pemphigoid (MMP), linear IgA diseases, paraneoplastic pemphigoid and erosive lichen planus. They are characterized by involvement of the basement membrane epithelium.

Bullous Pemphigoid

Bullous pemphigoid is an autoimmune disease characterized by subepidermal blistering affecting the elderly individuals and rarely young people.

Pathogenesis

Bulla will appear in the subepithelial region (in the lamina lucida region of basement membrane).

Clinical Features

The age of onset is typically between 60 years and 80 years. It is a self-limiting condition and lasts for few months to 5 years. It may present with other diseases like multiple sclerosis and malignancies due to aging and mortality rate is high.

Treatment

Tetracycline and nicotinamide.

Mucous Membrane Pemphigoid or Cicatricial Pemphigoid

It is a type of autoimmune, mucocutaneous disease which is characterized by the separation of epithelium from connective tissue, due to alteration in the anchoring proteins. MMP is also known as "*benign* MMP", "*cicatricial pemphigoid*" and "ocular or oral gingival pemphigoid". The disease has preference for middle aged and older women. Fluid-filled or sometimes blood-filled blisters develop following a mild to moderate trauma that ruptures and leads to ulcers. Patient experiences pain and difficulty on chewing and brushing.

The disease severity is variable ranging from occasional blisters to continuous severe blistering and ulceration. Scarring is uncommon in gingival lesions but occurs in other oral areas.

Investigations

Nikolsky's sign: Rubbing the margin of ulcer with a blunt instrument will lead to expansion of the ulcer in unaffected adjacent mucosal site.

Histopathological studies: Specimen will reveal the separation of epithelium and basement membrane with infiltration of acute and chronic inflammatory cells.

Direct IF: Reveals continuous straight band deposition of immunoglobulins (IgG and IgA) and complements (C3) at the basement membrane.

Indirect IF: Demonstrates the circulating autoantibodies (IgG and IgA) in patient's serum.

Treatment

Patients who exhibit only mild oral lesions may require no treatment. Many patients develop a tolerance to the oral lesions and stop complaining of oral discomfort despite the persistence of disease.

The treatment for oral lesions is the use of topical corticosteroid, such as fluocinonide. Systemic corticosteroid like prednisone may be used for severe cases. Cyclophosphamide, azathioprine, and methotrexate are used in combination with systemic corticosteroid. Intravenous immunoglobulin (IVIG) can also be used.

Erosive and Bullous Lichen Planus

In the erosive and bullous type of lichen planus, the epithelium is separated from connective tissue due to degeneration of basal cell layer of epithelium. If the lesion manifests directly as ulcer, it is known as erosive type, whereas the initial appearance of a vesicle or bulla that subsequently breaks into ulcer is known as bullous type of lichen planus.

Etiopathogenesis

An alteration in cell-mediated immunity is responsible for the onset of the disease. The immune system is triggered by an endogenous or exogenous factor resulting in apoptosis of keratinocytes in the basal layer and determines disease activity.

In erosive type, the triggering factors are exogenous and include:

- Drugs—NSAIDs, penicillamine, angiotensin-converting enzyme inhibitors.
- Underlying disease—hepatitis C.
- Lichenoid reaction—dental restoration.

Clinical Features

In the erosive form, bright red, well-demarcated erosions surrounded by faint white lines are present. In bullous type, vesicles, bullae and asymmetrical shallow ulcers are seen. Pain is severe and affects the regular functions.

Complication

Erosive lichen planus has a potential for malignant transformation.

Diagnosis

Histopathological features:

- Absence of epithelium
- Liquefaction of the basal layer
- Cytoid bodies, apoptotic bodies or civatte bodies.

Direct IF: IgM deposits are frequently seen in the subepithelial layer. IgA and C3 are also seen in the subepithelial layer sometimes.

Differential Diagnosis

Lupus erythematosus, pemphigus, pemphigoid.

Treatment

- Topical corticosteroids—0.1% triamcinolone acetonide two to three times/day.
- 0.1% tacrolimus ointment.
- For indolent lesion—intralesional steroids.
- For cases with severe exacerbation—systemic steroids.

SHORT NOTES

1. Classify the vesiculobullous lesions of oral cavity. (or) Group the oral vesiculobullous lesions based on their etiology.

Vesiculobullous Lesions Caused by Viral Infections

1. Herpes simplex infection (HSV type 1)

2. Herpes zoster infection
3. Coxsackievirus infection
   a. Hand-foot-and-mouth disease
   b. Herpangina.

Vesiculobullous Lesions Caused by Autoimmune Disorder

- Bullous lichen planus
- Pemphigus vulgaris
- Mucous membrane pemphigoid
- Bullous pemphigoid
- Paraneoplastic pemphigus.

Vesiculobullous Lesions Caused by Hereditary Disorder

Epidermolysis bullosa.

Vesiculobullous Lesions Caused by Hypersensitivity Drug Reactions

- Erythema multiforme
- Drug eruption.

Miscellaneous Causes for Vesiculobullous Lesions

Aphthous stomatitis.

2. Discuss about the primary herpetic gingivostomatitis or primary herpes infection.

Primary gingivostomatitis is a HSV type 1 infection usually occurring in preschool children. The incubation period is 7–10 days. Prodromal symptoms like fever, chills, malaise, fatigue, and nausea may be present for 10–14 days.

The viral particles multiply in epithelial cells and cause local inflammation. The gingiva is the usual site of involvement. It appears erythematous with mild discomfort for brushing and chewing. Small ulcers may also present on the palatal mucosa. The formation of vesicles and ulcers is known as cold sores.

Children may become dehydrated because of the pain associated with swallowing.

Many times the primary infection is subclinical and the child may not experience any symptoms or very mild symptoms often left unnoticed.

Viral shedding characterizes the initial episode. The amount of virus shed is unrelated to the severity.

After the primary infection, the virus reaches the sensory ganglion and remains in a dormant state.

Treatment

Adequate rest is advised. Fluid and nutritional supplement is sufficient.

3. List the complications of herpes zoster infection.

The VZV causes varicella (chickenpox) in childhood. Once the primary illness subsides, the virus remains dormant (latent) in the dorsal ganglia. VZV when becomes reactivated in later life, it causes a painful, maculopapular rash called herpes zoster.

Complications

- The most common complication is PHN. It is pain persisting after 3 months of the healing of mucocutaneous lesions. PHN is characterized by a shooting pain that lasts for short period in an episode. Multiple pain episodes may occur on a single day. The risk of having PHN increases with age. PHN is rare in individuals less than 40 years and is common above 60 years of age. Elderly patients may have long-lasting lesions and more severe pain.
- Ocular involvement with acute or chronic herpes zoster ophthalmicus.
- Secondary bacterial contamination of the oral lesions, *Staphylococcus aureus* and, less commonly, group A β-hemolytic Streptococcus.
- Cranial and peripheral nerve paralysis.
- Meningoencephalitis, pneumonitis, hepatitis, and acute retinal necrosis.
- Ramsay Hunt syndrome; facial paralysis, painful unilocular vesicular eruptions of the external auditory meatus, pinna of the ear and oral mucosa.

Immunocompromised individuals are more prone to herpes zoster infection. They develop disseminated, chronic form of zoster with severe rashes.

4. Describe the Ramsay Hunt syndrome.

Herpes zoster involvement of geniculate ganglion may lead to Ramsay Hunt syndrome which includes:

1. Facial paralysis (Bell's palsy)
2. Painful vesicular eruptions of external auditory meatus and pinna of ear
3. Unilateral vesicles on the oral mucosa.

Pain develops before the vesicles and rash in 14–50% of patients. The pain resembles that of acute otitis. The possible associated findings are:

- Otalgia and loss of hearing
- Dizziness and nystagmus
- Altered taste
- Dry eyes
- Hoarseness of voice due to vocal cord palsy
- Weakness of the masseter and temporal muscles
- Asymmetry of the soft palate due to scaring, deviation of the uvula and tongue, dysphagia, and dilated pupil.

Treatment

Antiviral drug combined with corticosteroid is effective.

Acyclovir 15 mg/kg/day for 1 week and prednisone 100 mg trice daily with decreasing dose for 1 week.

Or

Famciclovir 250 mg three times/day for 3 weeks and prednisone 1 mg/kg/day for 2 weeks, decreased by 10 mg/day until lesions subside.

5. Discuss about the Behçet's syndrome or Behçet's disease.

Behçet's disease is a chronic, inflammatory multisystem disorder. It was first reported by a Turkish dermatologist Hulusi Behçet as a triad of recurrent oral, ocular and genital ulcers.

Etiopathogenesis

The cause disease remains unclear. Genetic predisposition, environmental factors and immunological abnormalities associated with HLA-B are the proposed possibilities.

The following pathogenesis is well accepted which are as follows:

- Inflammation of blood vessels (vasculitis) and epithelium due to the deposition of T-lymphocytes and plasma cell
- Increased neutrophil activity.

Oral Manifestation

Oral ulcer is seen in 98% of affected individuals and is a significant finding for diagnosis. Oral ulcers are painful and occur on the tongue, pharynx, mucous membranes. Clinically, ulcers are well-defined, round or ovoid with raised erythematous border, vary in number from single to many, each measuring few millimeters to 1 cm in diameter, but more extensive lesions can also occur. Yellow, pseudomembranous slough covers the surface. When they are numerous and larger, eating and speaking will be painful. No scar evident after healing and there is no lymph node enlargement. The ulcers resemble RAS, but their number, size, recurrence rate suggest to look for the other manifestations of Behçet's disease.

Diagnostic Criteria

Presence of one required criteria and two minor criteria is necessary to confirm the diagnosis.

Required Criteria

Recurrent oral ulcerations: Minor, major or herpetiform aphthous ulceration with a recurrence of minimum three times in a year.

Minor Criteria

- Current genital ulceration
- Eye lesions: Uveitis, and retinal vasculitis
- Skin lesions: Erythema nodosum, pseudofolliculitis, papulopustular lesions and acneiform nodules
- Positive pathergy test.

Treatment

- The treatment varies among patients, depending on the severity and organ involvement.
- For oral ulcerations, topical steroid or sucralfate solution is useful.
- Colchicine is helpful to prevent mucocutaneous relapse.
- For severe mucocutaneous lesions, systemic corticosteroid and azathioprine, combination are preferred.
- Pentoxifylline, dapsone, interferon-alpha, colchicine, and thalidomide drugs also demonstrated good prognosis.

6. Discuss about the pathergy test.

Pathergy phenomenon is a skin hyper-reactivity reaction to trauma and pathergy test is performed to observe the pathergy phenomenon as a diagnosis for Behçet's disease.

Procedure

Skin Pathergy Test

- Skin over the forearm is thoroughly rubbed with povidone-iodine 10% antiseptic solution.
- Three needle pricks should be made on the sterile skin by inserting interdermally. One prick should be with a 25-gauge disposable needle, the second one with a 21-gauge disposable needle, and the third one with 25-gauge disposable needle and the injection of one or two drops of normal saline. This type of multiple needle prick increases the probability for positive pathergy test.
- After 24 hours, the appearance of a papule or a pustule with an erythematous boundary at the needle prick sites suggests positive result.

Oral Pathergy Test

A 20-gauge blunt disposable needle should be used to prick the lower labial mucosa and results should be observed after 48 hours. Evidence of ulcer or pustule will confirm the diagnosis. The ulcer or a pustule of any size is considered as positive hence it is not necessary to measure the size of the lesion.

Positive pathergy phenomenon is seen in:

- Behçet's disease
- Patients treated with interferon alpha for chronic myeloid leukemia
- Sweet's syndrome (sudden onset of fever, an elevated number of white blood cells, and well-demarcated, red, tender papules and plaques).

7. Describe the contact stomatitis or allergic stomatitis.

Contact stomatitis or allergic stomatitis is an inflammatory response of the oral mucosa to various substances. These substance are potential to induce an allergic response when contact the mucosa. These substances include dental materials, preservatives and flavoring agents in foods or oral hygiene products. Cinnamon, cinnamic aldehyde, menthol, peppermint and eugenol are some of the common oral flavoring allergens.

Oral mucosa is less commonly prone to contact allergic reactions when compared to skin, though the latter is exposed to a wide variety of antigenic stimuli. This may be due to:

- Saliva acting as a solvent that dilutes and digest the allergens and thereby limiting the duration and number of molecules that contact oral mucosa.
- Limited keratinization makes hapten binding more difficult.
- The less number of antigen presenting cells in the oral mucosa reduces the possibility of antigen recognition.
- The high vascularity and rapid rate of epithelial renewal in oral cavity removes the allergens immediately in contrast to the keratinized skin.

The allergic response may be acute or chronic. Clinical presentations depend on the nature of the reaction, type of allergen, site and duration of contact. *Burning sensation and redness* of mucosa are the features of acute lesions. Edema, itching or tingling sensation is present in some patients.

- Acute lesions develop soon after antigenic exposure and diagnosis of this is based on cause-and-effect relationship.
- Chronic lesions manifest as areas of erythema, edema, desquamation, and sometimes ulcer. Rarely, irregular erosions with a rough surface and an erythematous halo may also present.

Three common oral manifestations of allergic reagents:

1. Lichenoid lesion
2. Plasma cell gingivitis
3. Cheilitis and glossitis.

Investigation

If the causative agent is not recognized, cutaneous patch testing may be useful.

Differential Diagnosis

Drug reaction, EM, erosive lichen planus, atrophic candidiasis.

Treatment

- The primary mode of treatment is the elimination of the allergen. Lesions resolve once the antigenic stimulus is eliminated.
- Antihistamines and topical corticosteroids may be used in sever conditions.

8. Write about the hand-foot-and-mouth diseases.

Hand-foot-and-mouth disease is a viral disease affecting children less than 5 years of age. The symptoms are mild and include blisters on the hands, feet and in the mouth that are short-lasting. The infection may rarely affect adults also. An enterovirus, coxsackievirus A16, is the causative agent. Coxsackievirus A6 is responsible for the atypical hand-foot-and-mouth disease.

As it is a contagious disease, it may affect several members of the family and friends. The mode of spread is by direct contact with nasal and oral secretions or fecal contamination. The outbreak is frequent during summer and autumn months.

The manifestation of first symptoms after exposure to the causative agent may take 3–5 days. Symptoms include fever, restlessness, pharyngitis, lymphadenitis, hungerless state and dysentery. The dorsal and palmar surfaces of the hands and feet reveal pale red or pink color rashes that soon turn to small blisters. Healing occurs within a week with no scar formation.

Few small, painful oral blisters and ulcers occur. This causes difficulty in chewing and swallowing. Vesicles also develop at the angle of mouth. Atypical hand-foot-and-mouth disease presents the features of widespread rash, larger blisters, peeling of skin and shedding of nails.

Diagnosis

The diagnosis is based on the characteristic sites involved.

Blood tests may show:

- Raised white cell count
- Atypical lymphocytes
- Elevated serum C-reactive protein (CRP)
- Positive serology report for the suspected virus.

To confirm the diagnosis, viral culture is necessary but usually not advised.

9. Describe the oral ulcers due to chemotherapy.

Chemotherapy-induced damage to the mucosa of the mouth, throat and gastrointestinal (GI) tract is called as mucositis. Erythema and ulcers develop within 3–10 days of starting chemotherapy. The patient experiences a burning sensation followed by pain. The soreness compromises the quality of speech. Chewing and swallowing become difficult, thereby interfering with food intake, resulting in weight loss. Mucosa is prone for opportunistic bacterial and fungal infections. The chemotherapy drugs with high potential to cause oral ulcers are:

- Actinomycin
- Busulfan
- Cytarabine

- Daunorubicin
- Doxorubicin.

Treatment

- Proper oral care.
- Regular use of alcohol-free, antiseptic mouth rinses or saline gargle three to four times/day.
- A mix of salt and soda mouthwash will relieve mouth sores.
- *Cryotherapy (ice chips)*: Sucking ice chips will provide symptomatic relief. Cryotherapy works by decreasing the local blood flow thereby minimizing the drug exposure and the risk of developing mouth ulcers.
- An advanced approach toward prevention and treatment is the use of growth factors, which are natural body substances that stimulate cell growth.

10. Describe the acute necrotizing ulcerative gingivitis or trench mouth.

Acute necrotizing ulcerative gingivitis (ANUG) is an acute gingival infection characterized by interdental papillary necrosis, punched out ulcerated papillae, gingival bleeding, and pain.

The distinctive characteristics of the diseases are:

- Rapid onset
- Ulcerated and necrotic papillary and marginal gingiva and cratering (punched out) of papillae
- Intense gingival pain
- Bleeding gingiva with little or no provocation.

Secondary features:

- Fetid breath, yellowish-white "pseudomembrane" covering the ulcerated papilla, lymphadenopathy, fever and malaise.

Etiology

Fusiform bacteria, *Prevotella intermedia*, and spirochetes invade the gingival tissues.

Predisposing Factors

- Psychological stress and anxiety
- Smoking
- Poor oral hygiene
- Nutrition deficiency
- HIV-positive.

Clinical Features

- Gingiva will be tender, painful and bleeds spontaneously.
- Profuse salivation, loss of taste, or metallic taste.
- Teeth will be slightly extruded and tender or have a woody sensation.
- Diminished pleasure from smoking
- Ulcers rarely may spread to lips, buccal mucosa, and tongue.

Treatment

- Wound debridement under local anesthesia
- Removal of pseudomembranous slough using cotton pellet soaked in chlorhexidine rinse
- Antibacterial mouthwash: Chlorhexidine 0.12% twice daily
- Analgesics: Ibuprofen 400 mg three times/day
- Adequate rest and appropriate fluid intake
- After the acute condition subsides, follow-up care should be initiated with comprehensive periodontal evaluation
- For systemic signs and symptoms, antibiotics should be prescribed:
  - Amoxicillin, 500 mg, three times daily for 1 week and
  - Metronidazole, 200 mg three times daily for 1 week.

Treatment outcome should be monitored for first 24 hours, and then every other day until the signs and symptoms are completely resolved.

11. What is salt split skin test?

Direct immunofluorescence techniques are not helpful in differencing diseases like bullous pemphigoid and epidermolysis bullosa acquisita (autoantibodies against collagen VII). The test result for both these condition is a linear band of IgG and complement at the dermal-epidermal junction. In such circumstances, splitting the skin specimen before evaluation allows the accurate location of target antigens.

The procedure includes incubation of the skin specimen with 1 m sodium chloride that splits the skin at the lamina lucida. The dermal side of the split surface will keep the collagen VII immune complexes whereas the epidermal side of the sample will retain the BP180 immune complexes. In this way, it is possible to differentiate the two diseases.

12. What is immunofluorescence test?

Immunofluorescence technique utilizes fluorescent-labeled antibodies to detect the specific target antigens. Its applications include the evaluation of cells, tissue, beads, and microarrays for the detection of specific proteins. Both fresh and fixed samples can be used for IF techniques. Chemical conjugation of the antibodies with fluorescent dyes like fluorescein isothiocyanate (FITC) or tetramethylrhodamine isothiocyanate (TRITC) is used.

- In the direct IF test, fluorescent-tagged antibodies bind directly to the target antigen in the skin or mucosa. The tissue specimen is washed and rapid freezing is performed. The frozen sample is cut into 5–6 μm sections and placed on the glass slides. The slides are incubated with the fluorescent-tagged antibodies directed against the target antigen that can be viewed on fluorescence microscope. Diagnosis is based on the binding pattern (e.g. intercellular, linear at the dermal-epidermal junction) as well as the isotype (e.g. IgG, IgA) of the antibody is detected.
  Advantages include rapidity and simple.
  Disadvantages are higher cost, and difficulties in labeling procedure.
- Indirect IF detects the circulating antibodies in immune-mediated vesiculobullous diseases. Being a two-step serological procedure, it uses an unlabeled antibody (primary antibody) and a second fluorescent-labeled antibody.

  The serum is incubated with thin sections of the disease-free human skin or other animal tissues that bind the particular target antibody. Monkey esophagus is a suitable substrate for detecting anti-desmoglein antibodies. When autoantibodies in the serum bind with the target antigen in the tissue sample, the test is positive. The fluorophore-labeled antibody then binds to the Fc portion of the autoantibody allowing it to be visualized with the fluorescence microscope.

  Advantages include high sensitivity than direct IF. Commercially produced secondary antibodies are relatively inexpensive and available in an array of colors.

  Disadvantage—it has a potential for cross reactivity. The need to find primary antibodies that are not raised in the same species.

13. Mucormycosis.

Mucormycosis is caused by saprophytic fungi, Zygomycetes. It is a rare opportunistic fungal infection, rapidly progressive and fulminant with a fatal outcome. It seldom causes an infection in immunologically competent patients but frequently affects immunosuppressed individuals, especially uncontrolled diabetic patients. The most common form of mucormycosis is rhinocerebral type. Following the entry of the fungi by inhalation, they travel along and breach the nasopalatine arteries. This leads to compromised blood supply, thrombus formation and necrosis (dry and dark eschar) of palate and alveolus.

Cavernous sinus thrombosis is a severe complication of maxillary infections.

Treatment

- The use of amphotericin B in patients with mucormycosis has been a widely accepted.
- Hyperbaric oxygen (HBO) has also been used to treat rhinocerebral mucormycosis.

14. Herpangina.

Herpangina is an epidemic viral infection caused by coxsackievirus A4. It primarily affects children between 3 years and 10 years of age. The infection begins with fever, chills, and anorexia followed by a sore throat and dysphagia.

- Macules, papules, and vesicles will appear on posterior pharynx, tonsils, faucial pillars and soft palate.
- The blisters will rupture in 24–48 hours and leave 1–2 mm ulcers which heal within a week.
- The clinical onset and course are similar to HSV, but herpangina tends to be milder than HSV and occurs in posterior mouth unlike acute generalized gingivitis in HSV.

Treatment

It is a self-limiting disease hence supporting treatment including adequate rest and hydration is sufficient.

15. What is patch test?

The diagnosis of allergic contact stomatitis, a patch test is the "gold standard". Patch test relies on provoking skin inflammation (dermatitis) less than 1 cm^2 area under close monitoring. Patch testing helps in identification and avoidance of causative allergens thus help to control the symptoms.

The commonly used patch test devise is the round aluminum Finn Chambers. Finn Chamber consists of circular-shaped aluminum chambers on a acrylate-based adhesive and to be filled with test substances immediately before the application.

Test substances should be selected based on clinical history, and include suspected allergens. Finn chamber should be placed using a nonallergic adhesive tape on the hairless body region mostly at back. The exposed area reveals an inflammatory reaction in positive patients. The intensity of the response is scored and recorded. The analysis and interpretation of patch results require training and experience.

16. Explain the photodynamic therapy.

Photodynamic therapy (PDT) is a therapeutic technique of light-induced inactivation of the cell, microorganism, or biological molecules. At the appropriate combination of photosensitive drug and light wavelength (630–700 nm), the photosensitizer is transformed from its ground state (low energy level) to triplet state (high energy) with the release of reactive oxygen species (free radicals) that in turn causes tissue necrosis. The light is generated by lasers, arc lamp, and fluorescent source.

Topical 5-aminolevulinic acid (5-ALA) is commonly used for PDT of intraoral lesions like leukoplakia, verrucous leukoplakia, verrucous carcinoma, and lichen planus, dysplastic lesions. 5-ALA is converted as protoporphyrin in the target tissue and leads to cellular death. The photodynamic action is short spanned, and the drug will be metabolized within 48 hours. Intravenous (IV) and oral administration forms of photosensitizers are also available.

Advantages

- Highly selective tissue necrosis (lesion)
- No scar formation
- Daycare procedure.

17. Discuss about the Koch's postulates for autoimmune disease.

Koch's postulates for infectious disease are adapted for describing autoimmune diseases.

- The first hypothesis is the demonstration that the adaptive immune system directed to self-antigens present in the affected tissue.
- The second hypothesis requires that this autoreactivity should be localized within the affected tissue.

For both first and second hypothesis, the immune system comprises antibodies and T cells.

- The third hypothesis states that the transfer of the autoreactive components from a patient to a healthy individual should induce similar disease manifestations in the recipient as observed in the donor.
- The third hypothesis demands the expression of autoimmune disease features in a healthy recipient who received the autoreactive B cells and T cells from a donor suffering with an autoimmune disease.
- The fourth hypothesis states about the inducement of the autoimmune disease in laboratory animals by immunization procedure.
- The last hypothesis is about therapeutic efficacy; the only therapy that directly targets the adaptive immune system should result in betterment or even cure of the disease.

Pemphigus vulgaris, pemphigus foliaceus, and bullous pemphigoid fulfill all of the adapted Koch's postulates and hence considered as classic autoimmune disorders.

MULTIPLE CHOICE QUESTIONS

1. A well circumscribed, flat lesion with different hue from normal counterpart is known as ***macule***
   a. Macule b. Papule
   c. Plaque d. Purpura
2. Solid, raised lesions, smaller than 1 cm is known as ***papule***
   a. Macule b. Papule
   c. Plaque d. Purpura
   (**Note:** Papules are seen in EM, rubella, systemic lupus erythematosus and sarcoidosis).
3. Larger papules measuring more than 1 cm are known as ***plaque***
   a. Macule b. Purpura
   c. Plaque d. Petechiae
4. Solid lesions present beneath the dermis are known as ***nodules***
   a. Tumor b. Nodules
   c. Nodes d. Epidermal mass
5. Blisters measuring more than 1 cm in size is known as ***bulla***
   a. Bulla b. Vesicles
   c. Pustule d. Cysts
   (**Note:** Elevated blisters containing clear fluid measuring less than 1 cm are known as vesicles and more than 1 cm in size are known as bulla).
6. Superficial moist red lesions are known as ***erosions***
   a. Ulcer b. Erosions
   c. Erythema d. Aberrations
7. Blisters containing purulent material are known as ***pustule***
   a. Bulla b. Vesicles
   c. Pustule d. Infected cysts
8. Lesion with exposure of connective tissue due to break in overlying epithelium is known as ***ulcer***
   a. Ulcer b. Erosions
   c. Burns d. Aberrations
9. Flat purplish lesions due to blood spill in subcutaneous tissue is known as ***purpura***
   a. Hematoma b. Angioma
   c. Purpura d. Petechiae
10. Blanching is present in ***purpuric lesions***
    a. Purpuric lesions
    b. Petechial lesions
    c. Fibrotic lesions
    d. Normal mucosa
    (**Note:** Purpura of 1–2 cm in diameter is known as *petechiae* and larger than 2 cm are known as *ecchymoses*).
11. Herpes viruses are ***DNA viruses***
    a. DNA viruses b. RNA viruses
    c. mRNA viruses d. dsRNA viruses
12. Coxsackieviruses are ***RNA viruses***
    a. DNA viruses b. RNA viruses
    c. mRNA viruses d. dsDNA viruses
13. Kaposi's sarcoma is caused by ***HHV-8***
    a. HHV-8 b. HPV-16
    c. HSV-2 d. CMV-5
14. The most common cause for Bell's palsy is ***reactivation of HSV***
    a. Trauma to facial nerve
    b. Reactivation of HSV
    c. Exposure to cold
    d. Corticosteroid intake

15. Herpetic whitlows can be prevented by ***wearing gloves***
    a. Antiprophylactic drugs
    b. Disinfectants
    c. Alcohol hand rub
    d. Wearing gloves
    (**Note:** Herpetic whitlows are *HSV infection of the finger* and health professionals are commonly affected to this).
16. Peak incidents of HSV infection is at the age of ***2–3 years***
    a. 20–30 years b. 40–50 years
    c. 2–3 years d. Birth to 6 months
17. The common clinical sign of primary HSV infection is ***acute marginal gingivitis***
    a. Multiple acute ulcers
    b. Koplik spots
    c. Acute marginal gingivitis
    d. Coated tongue
18. Gold standard diagnosis for viral infection is ***virus isolation and culture***
    a. Sampling
    b. Virus isolation and culture
    c. Tzanck test
    d. Polymerase chain reaction
19. Cancrum oris is a severe type of ***ANUG***
    a. ANUG
    b. Major aphthous
    c. Erythema multiforme
    d. NOMA
20. Herpangina affects the ***posterior part of mouth***
    a. Anterior part of mouth
    b. Posterior part of mouth
    c. Hard palate
    d. Floor of mouth
21. Group A coxsackievirus causes ***herpangina***
    a. Nasopharyngeal carcinoma
    b. Chickenpox
    c. Herpangina
    d. Kaposi's sarcoma
    (**Note:** Group A coxsackievirus causes herpangina, acute lymphonodular pharyngitis and hand-foot-and-mouth disease).
22. Varicella-zoster virus is a human ***neurotropic herpes virus***
    a. Neurotropic herpes virus
    b. Heterotropic herpes virus
    c. Hemotropic herpes virus
    d. Plasmatropic herpes virus
23. One of the following is seen in Von Recklinghausen's disease—***Crowe's sign***
    a. Crowe's sign b. Red streaks
    c. Chvostek sign d. Facial rashes
    (**Note:** Crowe's sign is also known as axillary freckling).
24. Most activated T cells in the inflammatory infiltrate of oral lichen planus are ***CD8+ cells***
    a. CD4+ cells b. CD8+ cells
    c. T-helper cells d. T-regulatory cells

VIVA VOCE

1. List the blistering diseases of the oral mucosa.

Most common blistering conditions of the oral mucosa are viral infections, especially herpes simplex virus, varicella-zoster virus and various forms of coxsackievirus infections.

Erythema multiforme is a mucocutaneous disorder with oral manifestations that heals in 2–3 weeks. Epidermolysis bullosa, typically have onset in infancy. Bullous lichen planus is an uncommon variant of lichen planus, and other blistering conditions include contact or systemic allergic reactions, bullous pemphigoid and linear IgA disease.

2. What is Nikolsky's test?

Applying tangential pressure to apparently unaffected oral mucosa adjacent to lesions leads to the development of new bulla.

Note: Nikolsky's test is positive in bullous pemphigoid, epidermolysis bullosa and linear IgA diseases.

3. List the periodontal diseases associated with AIDS.

- Linear gingival erythema: Involves only marginal gingival. Do not respond to routine oral hygienic procedures but resolves antifungal therapy.
- Necrotizing ulcerative gingivitis.
- Necrotizing ulcerative periodontitis.

These conditions are caused by HIV by altering the neutrophil functions.

4. What is cancrum oris?

It is a fulminating type of ANUG associated with malnutrition, poor oral hygiene, and simultaneous another infectious disease like measles. *Fusobacterium necrophorum* is the causative pathogen. Initially, it starts as extensive gingival necrosis with a rapid involvement of cheek, facial skin and causes severe disfigurement. Treatment includes debridement of necrotic tissues, irrigation, antibiotic and nutritional support.

5. What is Vincent's angina?

Acute necrotizing ulcerative gingivitis is also called as Vincent's angina by the name of a French physician Henri Vincent, who reported first. The word "angina" is Latin, "angere" meaning "to choke or throttle".

6. List the infections caused by herpes simplex virus type 1.

Oral and pharyngeal infections, meningoencephalitis and dermatitis above the waist.

7. What is latency?

Latency (resting phase) is a feature exhibited by herpes group of viruses. After primary infection or initial contact with the host mucosa or skin, the virus traveled along the mucosal and cutaneous nerve endings and transmitted to the ganglia. In the ganglion, *the viral genome remains inactive in a nonreplicating stage* until it gets reactivated by factors like local trauma, tissue injury, fever or immunosuppression.

8. What is primary herpes simplex virus infection?

The first incidence of HSV infection in persons, who are not yet exposed to the virus.

9. Herpes simplex virus infections are uncommon in newborns. Why?

Placental transfer of HSV antibodies will protect the infants during first 6 months of life.

10. What are prodromal symptoms?

Prodromal symptoms are patients' experience before onset of the clinical appearance of a lesion or disease. They may be either local like itching, pruritus or more generalized like fever, malaise.

11. Which test will differentiate primary and recurrent herpes simplex virus infections?

Primary form of herpes simplex infection is differentiated from the recurrent type by testing the antibody titer.

Acute serum specimen collected within 3–4 days of onset of symptoms should be analyzed for HSV antibodies.

Convalescent sera should be obtained on 3rd weeks and subjected to HSV antibody test (antiHSV antibodies will start appearing within a week of infection and reach a peak value in 3 weeks).

If antiHSV antibody titers in convalescent sera are increased four times than that of primary sera, then it confirms primary HSV infection. If antiHSV antibody titers in acute and convalescent sera are similar, then the diagnosis is recurrent HSV infection.

12. What is zoster sine herpete?

Zoster sine herpete (ZSH) or zoster sine eruption refers to a condition in which pain occurs along the affected dermatome in the absence of rash. PCR provided definitive virologic confirmation.

13. What is macule?

Macule is a flat, circumscribed abnormal coloration of skin which is not raised and hence not palpable.

14. What is papule?

A papule is a solid raised lesion on the skin which may be normal or abnormal in color and smaller than 1 cm in size.

15. Name few conditions associated with vesicle formation.

- Herpes simplex and Herpes zoster infection
- Chickenpox
- Drug eruptions
- Eczema

- Dermatitis herpetiformis
- Hand-foot-and-mouth disease.

16. Name few conditions associated with bulla formation.

- Erythema multiforme
- Pemphigus
- Pemphigoid
- Bullous lichen planus
- Epidermolysis bullosa
- Toxic epidermal neurolysis.

17. What is Koebner phenomenon?

Occurrence of new lesion within scratch marks is known as Koebner phenomenon and is present in:

- Lichen planus
- Psoriasis
- Acute eczema
- Discoid lupus erythematosus.

18. Name the conditions associated with café au lait spots.

- Neurofibromatosis
- Albright's syndrome
- Ataxia telangiectasia
- Epidermal nevus syndrome
- Bloom's syndrome.

19. What is ballooning degeneration?

Ballooning degeneration (also known as koilocytosis) is the pathological changes that occurs in viral infections which manifest clinically as vesiculobullous lesions. The viral replication in the infected cell causes intercellular edema and acantholytic changes (loss of cell to cell contact). When the volume increases, cells burst and release their content into surroundings. Following this, the cells are contained in a small surface area and become a vesicle or bulla.

BIBLIOGRAPHY

1. Arduino PG, Porter SR. Oral and perioral herpes simplex virus type 1 (HSV-1) infection: review of its management. Oral Dis. 2006;12(3):254-70.
2. Bascones-Martinez A, Munoz-Corcuera M, Bascones-Ilundain C, et al. Oral manifestations of pemphigus vulgaris: clinical presentation, differential diagnosis and management. J Clin Exp Dermatol Res. 2010;1:112.
3. Belenguer-Guallar I, Jiménez-Soriano Y, Claramunt-Lozano A. Treatment of recurrent aphthous stomatitis. A literature review. J Clin Exp Dent. 2014;6(2):e168-74.
4. Burket LW, Greenberg MS, Glick M, Ship JA. Burket's Oral Medicine, 11th edition. Ontario, Canada: PMPH-USA; 2008.
5. Criteria for diagnosis of Behçet's disease. International Study Group for Behçet's Disease. Lancet. 1990;335(8697):1078-80.
6. Damoiseaux J. Bullous skin diseases: classical types of autoimmune diseases. Scientifica (cario). 2013;2013:457982.
7. De Rossi SS, Greenberg MS. Intraoral contact allergy : a literature review and case reports. J Am Dent Assoc. 1998; 129(10):1435-41.
8. Johnson RW, Rice AS. Clinical practice Postherpetic neuralgia. N Engl J Med. 2014;371(16):1526-33.
9. Konopka K, Goslinski T. Photodynamic therapy in dentistry. J Dent Res. 2007; 86(8):694-707.
10. Léaute-Labréze C, Lamireau T, Chawki D, et al. Diagnosis, classification, and management of erythema multiforme and Stevens-Johnson syndrome. Arch Dis Child. 2000;83(4):347-52.
11. Scully C, Gorsky M, Lozada-Nur F. The diagnosis and management of recurrent aphthous stomatitis: a consensus approach. J Am Dent Assoc. 2003;134(2):200-7.
12. Sequeira FF, Daryani D. The oral and skin pathergy test. Indian J Dermatol Venereol Leprol. 2011;77(4):526-30.
13. Tontodonati M, Ursini T, Polilli E, et al. Post-herpetic neuralgia. Int J Gen Med. 2012;5:861-71.
14. White JM. Patch testing: what allergists should know. Clin Exp Allergy. 2012; 42(2):180-5.

CHAPTER 3

Orofacial Pain

HIGHLIGHTS

Pain is the most common symptom that makes the patients, seek dental treatment. Dental students should be confident in diagnosing the underlying pathophysiology based on patients' symptoms, direct them for appropriate investigations and provide treatment. This chapter summarizes the important aspects of pain originating from orofacial structures and helps the students to understand the course outline easily.

Students are expected to learn about:

- Classification of orofacial pain.
- Characteristics of different types of pain.
- Trigeminal neuralgia
- Atypical facial pain
- Atypical odontalgia
- Burning mouth syndrome.

ESSAY QUESTIONS

1. Enumerate the causes of orofacial pain.

Pain

Pain is a complex phenomenon, described as unpleasant sensory and an emotional experience caused by definite or potential tissue damage.

Classification Proposed by Academy of Orofacial Pain

- *Pain originating from intracranial lesions:*
  - Neoplasm
  - Hemorrhage
  - Hematoma
  - Edema
- *Pain arising from extracranial structures*
  - Teeth
  - Ears
  - Eyes
  - Nose
  - Throat
  - Tongue
  - Sinuses
  - Salivary glands
- *Musculoskeletal disorders*
  - Temporomandibular disorders
  - Masticatory muscle disorders
  - Fibromyalgia
  - Cervical disorders
  - Generalized polyarthritis
- *Neurovascular disorders*
  - Paroxysmal neuralgia
    - Trigeminal neuralgia
    - Glossopharyngeal neuralgia
  - Continuous neuralgia
    - Atypical odontalgia
    - Traumatic neuroma
    - Neuritis
    - Postherpetic neuralgia.

Classification Based on the Pathogenesis

- *Dental pain originating from tooth*
  - Pulpitis
  - Apical periodontitis
  - Pulp stone
  - Periapical abscess, dentoalveolar abscess
  - Faulty restorations
  - Cracked tooth syndrome

- *Pain from supporting structures of teeth*
  - Pericoronitis
  - Periodontal abscess
  - Acute necrotizing ulcerative gingivitis
  - Acute necrotizing ulcerative periodontitis
- *Ulcers*
  - Aphthous ulcers
  - Traumatic ulcers
  - Pemphigus
  - Erythema multiforme
- *Physical, chemical, thermal and radiation injuries*
  - Aspirin burn
  - Thermal burn
  - Radiation stomatitis
- *Neurological pain*
  - Trigeminal neuralgia
  - Glossopharyngeal neuralgia
  - Sphenopalatine neuralgia
  - Postherpetic neuralgia
  - Atypical facial neuralgia
- *Sinusitis*
  - Maxillary sinusitis
  - Frontal sinusitis
  - Ethmoid sinusitis
- *Facial bone fracture*
  - Dentoalveolar fracture
  - Maxillary fracture
  - Mandibular fracture
  - Nasal complex fracture
  - Zygomatic arch fracture
- *Vascular disorders*
  - Migraine headache
  - Cluster headache
  - Tension headache
  - Temporal arteritis
- *Salivary gland origin*
  - Sialadenitis—bacterial parotitis, mumps
  - Sialolithiasis
- *Associated with syndrome*
  - Eagle syndrome
  - Trotter's syndrome
  - Frey's syndrome
- *Referred pain*
  - Angina pectoris
  - Otitis media
  - Coronary thrombosis.

A simple working classification proposed for orofacial pain (OFP) commonly encountered in dental practice, 2013

- *Neurologic*
  - Trigerminal neuralgia
  - Glossopharyngeal neuralgia
  - Sphenopalatine neuralgia
  - Postherpetic neuralgia
  - Lacrimal neuralgia
  - Multiple sclerosis
  - Auriculotemporal syndrome
  - Malignant neoplasm
  - Short-lasting, unilateral, neuralgiform headache attacks with conjunctival injection and tearing (SUNCT) syndrome
  - Anesthetic dolorosa (post-traumatic trigerminal neuropathy)
- *Vascular*
  - Temporal arteritis
  - Migraine headache
  - Cluster headache
  - Paroxysmal hemicranias
  - Neuralgia induced cavitational osteonecrosis
- *Musculoskeletal*

Muscle disorders
  - Myositis
  - Muscle neoplasms

Tempromandibular joint disorders (Congenital and developmental)
  - Disc derangement disorders
  - TMJ dislocation
  - Inflammatory disorders
  - Ankylosis and fractures
  - Eagle syndrome
- *Dental and oral diseases*
  - Pulpal disease
  - Periodontal disease
  - Salivary gland disorder
  - Oral ulcer
  - Lesion of jaws
- *Head and neck diseases*
  - Lesions of pharynx
  - Ocular lesions

- Lesions of nose and sinus
- Lesion of ear

- *Psychosomatic*
  - Myofascial pain dysfunction syndrome
  - Phantom pain
  - Atypical facial pain
  - Atypical odontogenic pain
  - Burning mouth syndrome
  - Glossopyrosis imperial
  - Glossodynia
  - Idiopathic xerostomia
  - Idiopathic dysgeusia
- *Connective tissue disorders*
  - Rheumatoid arthritis
  - Systemic lupus erythematosus
  - Polyarthritis nodosa
- *Referred pain*
  - Neck—cervical vertebral disease
  - Heart—angina pectoris
  - Lungs—lung cancer
  - Esophagus—esophageal lesions
  - Eyes—glaucoma
  - Ears—middle ear disease.

2. What is neurogenic pain? Describe the etiology, clinical signs and symptoms, investigations, and medical management for trigeminal neuralgia.

Neurogenic Pain

- Pain originating from the nervous system that does not require nerve receptor or fiber stimulation.
- They are characterized by:
  - Bright burning pain with stimulating quality.
  - Good localization.
  - Good correlation between site of pain and lesion.
  - Associated with other sensory or motor symptoms.

Facial Neuralgia

Neuralgia is a unique group of pain involving any of the cranial nerves.

Trigeminal Neuralgia

- A unilateral pain characterized by brief electric shock-like symptoms, sudden in onset and cessation, restricted to the distribution of one or more branches of the trigeminal nerve. (Definition by International Headache society).
- Also known as *tic douloureux*, and *Fothergill's disease.*

Etiology and Pathogenesis

- The following causes are considered:
  - In the majority of cases, etiology is idiopathic.
  - Around 10% cases are associated with:
    - Tumor of cerebellopontine angle (or)
    - Multiple sclerosis.
    - Vascular malformation.
    - Vascular abnormalities pressing the nerve.
    - Meningioma of the posterior cranial fossa.
- The most *widely accepted theory* is:
  - Atherosclerotic plaques developing in the superior cerebellar blood vessels, presses and grooves the trigeminal nerve (V cranial nerve). This causes demyelination of nerve fibers which in turn becomes hyperexcitable and react to mild pressure by pain sensation that persists for a short duration.
  - This theory is supported by the MRI finding of close approximation between the blood vessel and VII nerve on the involved side.

Clinical Features

- Acute experience of severe shooting pain for few seconds.
- Pain characteristically has an *electric shock-like* quality and is unilateral. (In 3% of cases, bilateral occurrence is seen).
- Most commonly affected branch is maxillary, followed by mandibular and then ophthalmic. In some cases, more than one branch is affected.

- Pain is precipitated by *trigger zones* present on skin or mucosa along the distribution of involved division. Common trigger point sites:
  - Nasolabial fold
  - Corner of mouth

    Activities like face shaving, chewing, talking and exposure to cold trigger the pain experience.
- *Intraoral trigger zones* may confuse the diagnosis by suggesting dental pain. The stabbing pain may mimic the pain of cracked tooth syndrome.
- The pain is characterized by episodes occurring for few weeks or months followed by periods of complete remission.
- The occurrence of pain varies between one or two incidents in a day to many incidents per minutes.

Diagnosis

- History of shooting pain along the branch of the fifth nerve, which is precipitated by touching the trigger zones.
- Routine cranial nerve examination will be normal in idiopathic trigeminal neuralgia, whereas sensory or motor changes may be evident in patients with a tumor, or other intracranial pathology.
- The local anesthetic block may temporarily eliminate the trigger zone pain.
- MRI—to rule out the presence of a tumor, multiple sclerosis, and vascular malformations.

Medical Management

- Anticonvulsant—carbamazepine.
  - It is the most effective *drug of choice* in 85% cases. It has both anticonvulsion and antineuralgic properties.
  - Carbamazepine is specific in relieving the trigeminal neuralgic pain and no other types of pain. Hence, it can be used for therapeutic diagnosis.

Dosage

Initially started as a small dose of 100 mg twice daily. In case of no side effects, the gradual increase of 100 mg every 48 hours up to maximum of 1,200 mg/day. The antineuralgic effect occurs at the serum concentration of 24–43 μmol/L.

Side Effects

Generalized erythema multiforme is the severe side effect. Others include bone marrow depression, nausea, vomiting, dizziness and double vision.

Baclofen

Skeletal muscle relaxant with CNS depressing property.

Dosage

- Initial dose—5 mg thrice daily for three days, followed by increasing 10–20 mg/day, up to a maximum dose of 80 mg/day.
- Baclofen is usually initiated after carbamazepine and is combined with carbamazepine for synergetic effect and thereby reducing the dose of carbamazepine and its adverse effects.

Others

Phenytoin—antiepileptic and is given 100 mg three times/day.

Gabapentin—300 mg/day as initial dose and increase 300 mg every day up to the maximum daily dose of 2,400 mg/day.

Prognosis

Since trigeminal neuralgia may have temporary recovery or permanent spontaneous remission, drug therapy should be gradually withdrawn if there is a pain free period of 3 months.

3. What is burning mouth syndrome? Describe the possible causative factors, clinical manifestations, and management of burning mouth syndrome.

- *Burning mouth syndrome* describes oral burning without any evidence of clinical abnormalities like mucosal lesions or neurologic disorders. It does not follow any anatomical course and does not show any radiographic or biochemical abnormalities.
- It is otherwise known as glossopyrosis.

Etiology and Pathophysiology

- The exact cause is unknown.
- *Proposed factors include:*
  - Hormonal disturbances
  - Allergic disorders
  - Salivary gland hyposecretion
  - Chronic low-grade trauma
  - Psychiatric abnormalities
  - Parafunctional habits
- Hypersensitive response to certain food, dentifrices, mouth rinses, dental restorative materials are also suspected as a cause.
- A change in taste sensation is associated with burning mouth syndrome. Dysgeusia (abnormal taste) is more frequently reported in these patients mainly for bitter taste. This taste abnormality associated with burning mouth syndrome is due to a defect in the *sensory peripheral neural mechanism*.
- Psychological disorder: Patients with burning mouth syndrome often report with depression. The role of depression as a cause or result of this syndrome is uncertain.
- Chronic low-grade trauma due to parafunctional habits like rubbing the tongue across the teeth also considered as a possibility.
- Hormonal changes like menopause, diabetes, thyroid and parathyroid disorders are also proposed as causative factors.

Clinical Manifestations

- Women are affected more. (F:M is 7:1)
- Postmenopausal women are most frequently affected and occur between 3–12 years of postmenopause period.
- Any part of the oral cavity may be affected, but the tongue, lips, and palate are frequently involved.
- Burning sensation may be persistent but eating, swallowing, drinking and placing a candy, or chewing gum can relieve the symptom.
- Patients experience the *burning sensation typically upon awakening*, that increases in severity with the progression of a day but do not interfere with sleep.
- The patients may express the symptom as *fire on the mouth*.

Differential Diagnosis

- Conditions that cause burning symptoms like:
  - Oral lichen planus
  - Early stage of oral submucous fibrosis
  - Diabetic neuropathy
  - Anemic stomatitis.

Diagnosis

- There is no definitive diagnostic test for burning mouth syndrome. The following investigations are helpful to confirm the proposed contributing factors:
  - Exfoliative cytology for candidiasis.
  - Hormonal assay
  - Test for nutritional and vitamins deficiencies, anemia.
  - Diabetes (FBS, PPBS, HbA1C).

Management

- No single and promising treatment modalities are available. The condition can be managed but not cured.
  - Counseling and reassurance for individuals with mild burning sensation
  - Low doses of tricyclic antidepressants in moderate to severe symptomatic conditions.
    - Amitriptyline 25 mg twice daily for 15 days.
    - Clonazepam 2 mg once daily at bedtime for 15 days.
- These antidepressants can be given in combination with a sialagogue like buffered citrate or nortriptyline (25 mg at night) which is highly beneficial.
  - Topical anesthetics like lignocaine and benzydamine hydrochloride may also be used.
  - Multivitamins can also be instituted as a placebo, supportive measure.

SHORT NOTES

1. Atypical odontalgia (or) phantom tooth pain.

Definition

- Atypical odontalgia is a severe throbbing type of dental pain with no clinical or radiographic evidence for any pathology.
- The term *phantom pain* is used to denote specifically for persistent pain in endodontically treated tooth or edentulous areas where no radiographic or clinical evidence for pathology is present.
- The etiology and pathophysiology are not specified and is considered as a component of the psychosomatic disorder.

Clinical Features

- Patients present with a complaint of toothache.
- More common in middle and older age women.
- The patient will point out specific single tooth or rarely a group of adjacent teeth in the same quadrant.
- More frequent in maxillary premolar, and molar region.
- Involvement of mandibular teeth are infrequent.
- Pain cannot be provoked by probing or palpation and is not altered by posture.

Diagnostic Criteria

- Pain in an edentulous arch.
- Continuous pain persisting for more than 4 months.
- No evidence for referred pain.
- Absence of radiographic and laboratory findings to support the pain.

Treatment

- Tricyclic antidepressants—amitriptyline 25–75 mg/day. In case of no immediate remedy, medication should be continued for 3 months.
- Phenothiazines can be used as a supplement to tricyclic antidepressants.

2. Describe the referred pain in orofacial region (or) describe the systemic diseases that may cause pain in orofacial region.

- Pain or other unpleasant symptoms in the orofacial region sometimes denote underlying severe condition. Systemic conditions can be diagnosed based on their characteristic pain on specific orofacial site.
- Pain originating from distinct organ and experienced in a different region is called as referred pain.
- Various systemic conditions may produce a pain symptom in the orofacial region (Table 1).

Table 1: Referred pain in orofacial region.

Pain or symptoms in orofacial region (referred pain)	Disease
Pain experienced at the *angle of mandible* that worsens with exertion and relieves at rest	*Cardiac ischemia*
Trismus, distinct sensation experienced in the region supplied by mandibular nerve, and earache	*Carcinoma of infratemporal fossa*
Trigeminal neuralgia in individuals above 50 years	*Multiple sclerosis*
Severe throbbing, temporal pain, *tenderness, and swelling in temporal artery region,* transient visual abnormalities	*Temporal arteritis*
Sudden onset of a headache associated with nausea and vomiting, precipitated by changes in posture	*Intracranial tumor*
Pain in facial region associated with *altered sensation*	*Tumor invading the nerve*

3. Glossopharyngeal neuralgia.

Glossopharyngeal Neuralgia

- It is a sudden onset pain like trigeminal neuralgia but less intense. Common *causes for this neuralgia* are intracranial and

extracranial tumors, and vascular abnormalities that can compress IX cranial nerve.
- The pain occurs along the course of glossopharyngeal nerve (IX) and involves *pharynx, posterior tongue, ear, infra-auricular region, retromandibular part.*

Trigger Zones

- These are located along the course and pain is *triggered by* stimulating pharyngeal mucosa during *chewing, swallowing and talking.*
- This neuralgia also associated with *vagal symptoms* like syncope and arrhythmia due to the close proximity of glossopharyngeal and vagus nerve.

Differential Diagnosis

Geniculate neuralgia and temporomandibular disorders (due to pain associated with mandibular movements in glossopharyngeal neuralgia).

Treatment

Carbamazepine 100 mg twice daily and baclofen 5 mg thrice daily.

4. Describe the chemical mediators of pain.

Chemical mediators are biochemical factors associated with pain.
- Bradykinin: Endogenous polypeptides released from inflammatory cells and ischemic tissues. It serves as powerful vasodilator and acts by increasing vascular permeability. It excites all types of receptors and sensitizes some high threshold receptors to respond to otherwise innocuous stimuli.
- Histamine: It is a vasoactive amine which acts as a vasodilator and increases small vessels permeability.
- Prostaglandin: It sensitizes nociceptors to all types of stimuli and thus lowering their pain threshold for all kinds of stimulation.

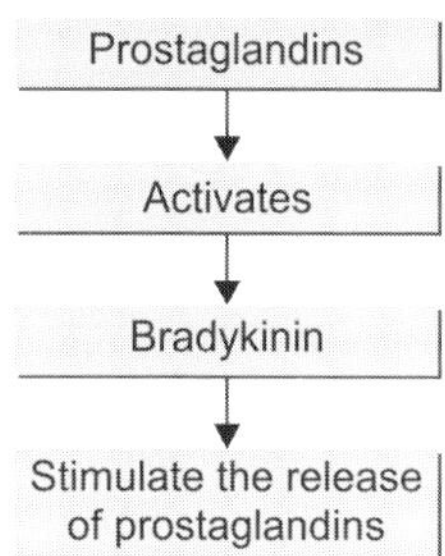

- Serotonin: It is a monoamine algogenic agent and is associated with peripheral vascular pain.
- Substance P
  - It is a polypeptide, acts centrally as an excitatory neurotransmitter for nociceptive impulses.
  - It is released from spinal cord cells by A-delta and C fibers and excites dorsal horn neurons when stimuli trigger them.
  - Substance P modulated pain is non-rapid and of short duration.

5. Describe the clinical findings, diagnosis, and treatment of atypical facial pain.

- Atypical facial pain denotes no muscle or joint pain and has no detectable neurological cause. It produces continuous and variable intensity pain migrating, nagging, deep and diffuse pain which cannot be diagnosed with any other condition.
- So, the terminology atypical facial pain is reserved for painful condition that does not fulfill the criteria for other orofacial pain conditions.

Clinical Features

- Facial pain typically manifests in the middle-aged women.
- The pain is described as kind of vague, burning, aching or cramping, occurring on one side of the face, preferably in the areas supplied by the trigeminal nerve that may spread to the upper neck or backside of the scalp.

- The duration of pain is continuous, and remission is rare.
- The pain will not respond to any medications.
- There will not be any detectable pathology clinically as well as in any investigatory methods.

Diagnosis

- When all the possible causes of facial pain like dental causes, paranasal sinuses related, myofascial and temporomandibular joint related origin, traumatic and inflammatory aspects are ruled out, atypical facial pain should be considered.
- Conventional and advanced imaging modalities should be performed to rule out any possible pathology in the orofacial region.
- Through neurological examination should be carried out to eliminate neurological disorders.

Management

- Medical management includes gabapentin and amitriptyline.
- Alternative therapies like acupressure and acupuncture.
- Transcutaneous electric nerve stimulation (TENS).

6. Nervus intermedius neuralgia (or) Geniculate neuralgia.

- Nervus intermedius neuralgia is a rare type of paroxysmal neuralgia.
- Pain will be experienced along the sensory distribution of nervous intermedius like ear, anterior tongue and soft palate.
- The patient complaints pain in the anterior region of tongue, soft palate, and ear.
- Trigger zones are present within the ipsilateral distribution of the nerve which on provocation causes pain.
- Pain is not sharp as similar to trigeminal neuralgia.
- There may be facial paralysis associated with this neuralgia indicating the simultaneous involvement of motor root of the facial nerve.
- Herpes zoster infection of geniculate ganglion and the nervous intermedius branch of facial nerve (VII N) results in geniculate neuralgia and is known as Ramsay Hunt syndrome. High potent steroid therapy for 2–3 weeks duration is effective. Acyclovir, carbamazepine, and antidepressants are also used for management of this condition.

7. Describe visual analog scale.

- The visual analog scale is used to determine the intensity pain. It is a 10 cm line on which:
  - 0 cm denotes no pain.
  - 10 cm denotes severe pain. (extremely severe pain).
- The patients need to mark a point on the scale that best quantify their pain. The interpretation is made from the score on the numerical scale (1–10) or on descriptive scale (e.g. no pain, mild pain, moderate pain and severe pain) (Fig. 1).
- Visual analog scales are helpful to understand the patient's pain threshold potential and *assess the treatment effects*.

8. Eagle's syndrome (or) elongated styloid process (or) stylohyoid syndrome.

- The stylohyoid ligament connects the styloid process of the temporal bone to hyoid bone. Elongation of the styloid process impinges or compresses the adjacent structures and cause *Eagle's syndrome*.
- It is also called as *diffuse intraosseous skeletal hypertrophy syndrome* (*DISH* syndrome).

Types

- *Classic type*—occurs after tonsillectomy, where surgical exposure of the styloid process heals by *scar formation*. This scar tissue exerts pressure on the adjacent nerve and causes *pain on swallowing*.
- *Carotid artery syndrome—elongated styloid process or calcified stylohyoid ligament* compresses the external or internal carotid artery and cause pain.

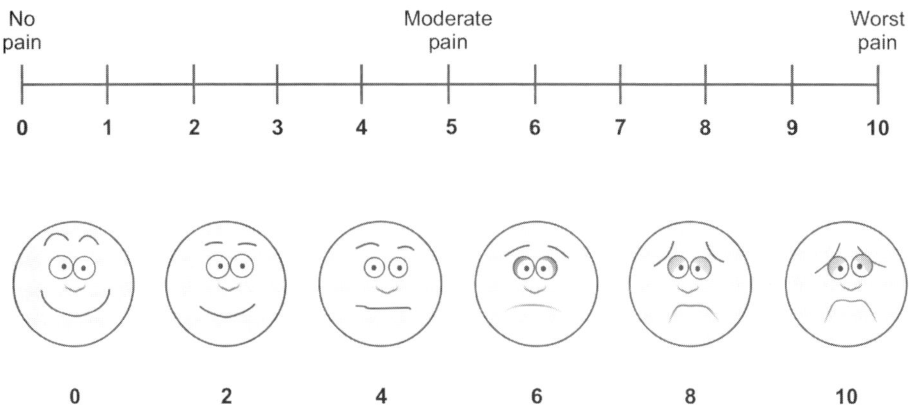

Fig. 1: Visual analog scale.

- *Traumatic Eagle's syndrome*—fracture of calcified stylohyoid ligament causes this type of pain.

Clinical Features

Commonly occurs in middle-age group. Pain is experienced along the lateral pharyngeal wall, side of lower face and neck. There will be difficulty in swallowing, sore throat, painful tongue, and headache. Blurred vision and vertigo also be associated.

Investigation

Orthopantomograph reveals elongated styloid process.

Treatment

- Injection of corticosteroid at the styloid process.
- Surgical segmentation of elongated process.

9. Cracked tooth syndrome (or) greenstick fracture of crown.

Cracked tooth syndrome is a condition associated with the partial fracture of a vital posterior tooth that extends up to the dentine or into the pulp.

Pathogenesis

- Masticatory pressure applied to the cracked crown will separate the tooth components along the line of the crack. If the separation occurs in dentine, movement of dentinal fluid will stimulate odontoblasts in the pulp and subsequently stimulate pulpal nociceptors.
- Movement of saliva through the crack line also increases the sensitivity of dentine.

If the crack extends to the pulp, then direct stimulation of pulp tissues occurs.

Clinical Features

- Age group involved—between 30 years and 50 years of age.
- Gender—men and women are equally affected.
- Commonly affected teeth—mandibular second molar, mandibular first molar, maxillary premolars.
- The centrally located crack may extend to pulp whereas peripherally situated crack cause cuspal fracture alone.
- Pain provoked on biting and disappears after the pressure relief is a typical sign.

Diagnosis

- *Bite tests:* Instruct the patient to bite on various objects like a toothpick, cotton roll, or wooden stick by placing them between the teeth will elicit pain. Pain increases when the occlusal force increases, and relieved once the pressure is withdrawn.

This test is the confirmatory test for cracked tooth diagnosis.

- Vitality testing usually gives a positive response.

Differential Diagnosis

Galvanic pain associated with amalgam restorations—galvanic pain occurs on bringing the teeth together (resting position) but decreases when full contact is made.

Treatment

- Peripherally located crack which is relatively small, can usually be restored.
- Tooth with centrally located crack should be stabilized with an orthodontic stainless steel band with occlusal adjustment will provide immediate pain relief. Provisional, full acrylic crown may also be used for stabilization. The tooth should be examined 2–4 weeks later, and if symptoms of irreversible pulpitis present, endodontic treatment should be performed.
- When vertical cracks occur, the tooth should be extracted.

MULTIPLE CHOICE QUESTIONS

1. *Spontaneous pain* is one that occurs ***without any stimuli***.
   a. In response to stimuli
   b. Without any stimuli
   c. Following provocation
   d. With no organic damage
2. *Induced pain* is one that arises ***in response to stimuli***.
   a. Without provocation
   b. In response to tissue damage
   c. In response to stimuli
   d. Without organic damage
3. *Intractable pain* is one that ***does not respond to treatment***.
   a. Does not respond to treatment
   b. Cannot be diagnosed
   c. Radiate to different sites
   d. Does not require treatment.
4. *Dull pain* is characterized by ***depressing quality***.
   a. Exciting quality
   b. Exhilarating quality
   c. Stimulating quality
   d. Depressing quality
5. *Sharp pain* is characterized by ***stimulating quality***.
   a. Exciting quality
   b. Exhilarating quality
   c. Stimulating quality
   d. Depressing quality
6. Sharp intermittent pain of short duration is known as ***pricking pain***.
   a. Pricking pain
   b. Stimulating pain
   c. Stinging pain
   d. Intractable pain
7. Continuous, high intensity pain characterizes ***stinging pain***.
   a. Pricking pain
   b. Stimulating pain
   c. Stinging pain
   d. Intractable pain
8. Free nerve ending receptors are for ***tactile sensation***.
   a. Cold sensation
   b. Tingling sensation
   c. Tactile sensation
   d. Creeping sensation
   (**Note:** Free nerve ending receptors are for tactile sensation and superficial pain).
9. Krause's corpuscles are ***cold receptors***.
   a. Cold receptors
   b. Pressure receptors
   c. Pain receptors
   d. Touch receptors
10. Ruffini corpuscles are ***warmth receptors***.
    a. Cold receptors
    b. Warmth receptors
    c. Pain receptors
    d. Mechanoreceptor
    (**Note:** Ruffini corpuscles are pressure and warmth receptors).
11. Merkel's corpuscles are ***tactile receptors***.
    a. Cold receptors
    b. Tactile receptors

c. Pain receptors
d. Warmth receptors
(**Note:** Merkel's corpuscles are tactile receptors in oral mucosa and submucosa of the tongue).

12. Golgi tendon organs are ***mechanoreceptors***.
a. Cold receptors
b. Warmth receptors
c. Pain receptors
d. Mechanoreceptors
(**Note:** Golgi tendon organs are mechanoreceptors in muscles and tendons).

13. Pain sensation is predominantly carried through ***small fibers***.
a. Small fibers b. Large fibers
c. Thick fibers d. Thin fibers

14. Nociceptors are ***pain receptors***.
a. Cold receptors
b. Tactile receptors
c. Pain receptors
d. Warmth receptors

15. Pain produced by stimuli that are not painful is known as ***allodynia***.
a. Hyperalgesia
b. Allodynia
c. Costalgia
d. Algedonic

16. Orofacial pain revealing elevated erythrocyte sedimentation rate is ***temporal arteritis***.
a. Temporal arteritis
b. Lupus vasculitis
c. Polyarteritis nodosa
d. Giant cell arteritis

17. Orofacial pain that is associated with abnormal laboratory finding is ***temporal arteritis***.
a. Temporal arteritis
b. Lupus vasculitis
c. Polyarteritis nodosa
d. Giant cell arteritis

18. The significant risk associated with the prolonged use of nonsteroidal anti-inflammatory drugs (NSAIDs) is ***gastrointestinal bleeding***.
a. Hepatic damage
b. Bronchospasm
c. Gastrointestinal bleeding
d. Nephritic syndrome

19. Visual analog scale measures the ***pain intensity***.
a. Depression state
b. Pain intensity
c. Blanching property
d. Patch test result

20. The sensory experience of pain is measured by ***McGill pain questionnaire***.
a. McGill pain questionnaire
b. Numerical rating scale
c. Verbal descriptor scale
d. McMonnies screening questionnaire
(**Note:** McGill pain questionnaire measures the sensory experience of pain with affective and cognitive qualities).

21. *Glossodynia* refers to ***burning pain in the tongue***.
a. Burning pain in the tongue
b. Referred pain in the tongue
c. Swollen and painful tongue
d. Painful bleeding tongue.

22. Glossopyrosis refers to ***burning pain in the oral mucosa***.
a. Burning pain in the tongue
b. Burning pain in the oral mucosa
c. Atrophic and painful tongue
d. Atrophic and painful oral mucosa

23. Sudden attack or outburst of pain is known as ***paroxysmal pain***.
a. Nocturnal pain b. Diurnal pain
c. Paroxysmal pain d. Excruciating pain

VIVA VOCE

1. What is an intermittent pain?

Intermittent pain is characterized by the pain of a short duration that is separated by entirely pain-free periods.

2. What is a continuous pain?

Intermittent pain is characterized as the pain of longer duration even though variable in intensity.

3. What is a recurrent pain?

Two or more painful episodes per day with periodic pain-free intervals.

4. What is a periodic pain?

Pain at regularly recurring episodes.

5. What is throbbing or pulsatile pain?

An intermittent quality of pain coincident with cardiac systoles.

6. What is superficial pain?

The patients accurately describe the pain that is precisely localizable to a superficial lesion or structure with timing and intensity of symptoms.

7. What is a deep pain?

Pain originating from visceral organs with symptoms being diffuse often referred to other regions or as muscle spasm.

8. Pain in orofacial region that mimic dental pain.

Trigeminal neuralgia, maxillary sinusitis, masticatory muscle spasm, atypical odontalgia, atypical facial pain.

9. Systemic conditions that cause headache and orofacial pain.

Paget's disease, hyperthyroidism, hyperparathyroidism, multiple myeloma, metastatic lesions, vincristine therapy for cancer, vitamin B, folic acid and iron deficiencies.

10. Why nonsteroidal anti-inflammatory drugs cause intestinal bleeding (or) why NSAID's should be avoided in patients with gastric ulcer.

- Nonsteroidal anti-inflammatory drugs work by inhibiting the enzyme cyclooxygenase (COX) which is essential for the synthesis of prostaglandins (PG's). PG sensitizes the peripheral sensory nerves to experience pain.
- Prostaglandins maintain the protective layer of gastric mucosa also. In the deficiency or absence of prostaglandins, gastric mucosa becomes more vulnerable to erosion and bleeds.

11. What is the mode of action of capsaicin?

- At the site of application, capsaicin causes neurogenic inflammation and burning sensation followed by hyperalgesia (increased sensitivity to painful stimuli).
- After multiple applications, capsaicin blocks C-fiber conduction and depletes the stores of substance P in C-fibers and decreases their input into the central nervous system.

12. What is barodontalgia (aerodontalgia)?

Pain experienced in the teeth because of alteration in the atmospheric pressure gradient. Individuals may experience a sharp or squeezing pain at an altitude of approximately 3,000 m with 0.75 standard atmosphere pressure and a water depth of 10 m with 1 atm.

13. What is acute pain?

Acute pain is one that subsides within the period required for the process of normal healing. It persists only as long as the stimuli persist.

BIBLIOGRAPHY

1. Chen J, Sindou M. Vago-glossopharyngeal neuralgia: a literature review of neurosurgical experience. Acta neurochir (Wien). 2015;157(2):311-21.
2. Coculescu EC, Radu A, Coculescu BI. Burning mouth syndrome: a review on diagnosis and treatment. Journal of medicine and life. 2014;7(4):512-6.
3. Lynch CD, McConnell RJ. The cracked tooth syndrome. J Can Dent Assoc. 2002; 68(8):470-5.
4. Okeson JP. Bell's orofacial pains: the clinical management of orofacial pain. Chicago, Ill, USA: Quintessence Publishing Company; 2005.
5. Piagkou M, Anagnostopoulou S, Kouladouros K, et al. Eagle's syndrome: a review of the literature. Clin Anat. 2009;22(5):545-58.
6. Toda K. Trigeminal neuralgia—symptoms, diagnosis, classification, and related disorders. Oral Science International. 2007;4(1):1-9.
7. Woda A, Pionchon P. A unified concept of idiopathic orofacial pain: pathophysiologic features. J Orofac Pain. 2000;1;14(3):196-212.

CHAPTER 4

Pigmented Lesions of Oral Mucosa

HIGHLIGHTS

Normal mucosal color depends on melanogenesis and distribution of melanin pigment, keratinization, thickness of epithelium and vascularity, Pigmented lesions are commonly found in the mouth. Such lesions represent a variety of clinical entities, ranging from physiologic changes to manifestations of systemic illnesses and malignant neoplasms. Although biopsy is a helpful and necessary aid in the diagnosis of focally pigmented lesions, with diffuse presentations lesions require a thorough history and laboratory studies to establish a definitive diagnosis.

Learners are expected to learn about:

- ❖ Causes for mucosal pigmentation
- ❖ Differential diagnosis of pigmented lesions
- ❖ Investigation and management.

ESSAY QUESTIONS

1. Define pigment. Classify the pigmented lesions of oral mucosa and briefly describe the pathophysiology of Addison's disease pigmentation.

Pigment is a substance that gives a particular color when it is present in something or is added to it. Pigmentation is the abnormal skin or mucosal coloration due to excess deposition of normal pigments or ectopic pigment deposition.

Oral pigmentation may be exogenous or endogenous in origin. Exogenous pigmentation is commonly acquired from foodstuffs, tobacco products, and foreign-body implantation in the oral mucosa. Endogenous pigments include melanin, hemoglobin, hemosiderin and carotene.

Classification of Pigmented Lesions

I. Oral pigmentation is broadly classified into *diffuse and focal.*

Diffuse pigmentation:

- ❖ Developmental
  - ■ Racial and physiologic pigmentation
  - ■ Peutz-Jeghers syndrome
- ❖ Predominantly adult onset
  - ■ With systemic signs and symptoms:
    - ♦ Addison's disease
    - ♦ Heavy metal pigmentation
    - ♦ Kaposi's sarcoma
  - ■ No systemic signs and symptoms:
    - ♦ Drug-induced pigmentation
    - ♦ Postinflammatory pigmentation
    - ♦ Smoker's melanosis.

Focal pigmentation:

- ❖ Red-blue-purple discoloration
  - ■ Hemangioma
  - ■ Varix
  - ■ Thrombus
  - ■ Hematoma
- ❖ Blue-gray discoloration
  - ■ Amalgam tattoo
  - ■ Blue nevus
- ❖ Brown discoloration
  - ■ Melanotic macule
  - ■ Pigmented nevus

- Melanoacanthoma
- Melanoma.

II. Classification based on exogenous and endogenous pigmentation.

Exogenous pigmentation:

- Silver amalgam
- Graphite
- Lead, mercury and bismuth
- Chromogenic bacteria.

Endogenous pigmentation:

- Hemoglobin
  - Varix
  - Hemangioma
  - Kaposi's sarcoma
  - Angiosarcoma
  - Hereditary hemorrhagic telangiectasia (HHT)
- Hemosiderin
  - Ecchymosis
  - Petechia
  - Thrombosed varix
- Melanin
  - Melanotic macule
  - Nevus
  - Melanoma
- Carotene
  - Carotenemia.

Pigmentation in Addison's Disease (Hypoadrenalism)

Addison's disease or hypoadrenocorticism is an endocrinopathic disease due to progressive bilateral destruction of the adrenal cortex by autoimmune disease, infection, certain medications or malignancy. The destruction results in a decreased level of corticosteroid hormone.

Pathophysiology

When there is a decrease in corticosteroid secretion, the anterior pituitary gland is stimulated to increase the production and secretion of adrenocorticotropic hormone (ACTH) which acts on the adrenal cortex to stimulate corticosteroid production. This feedback mechanism causes the pituitary to slow ACTH secretion. But when the low corticosteroid levels persist, there is a continual ACTH secretion. The alpha-melanocyte-stimulating hormone (α-MSH) gene is also originating from the same host gene that produces ACTH. Hence, when serum ACTH levels rise, there is a concomitant rise in α-MSH secretion which directly stimulates melanocytes, increases the melanin production, and causes diffuse mucocutaneous pigmentation.

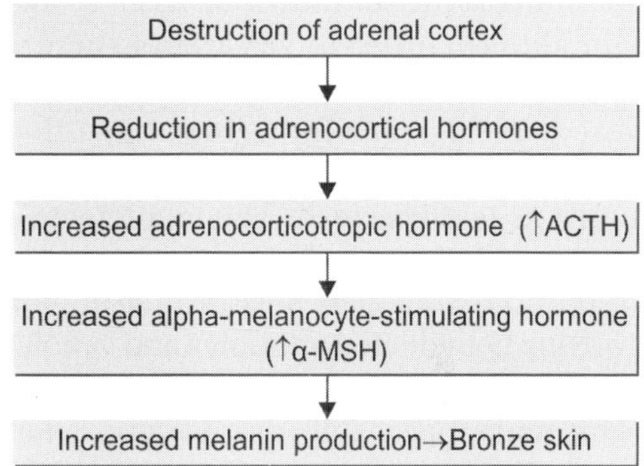

Oral involvement presents as diffuse brown patches on the gingiva, buccal mucosa, palate and tongue which may resemble physiologic pigmentation. Oral mucosal pigmentation is the first sign of Addison's disease and is usually accompanied by systemic manifestations including weakness, nausea and vomiting, abdominal pain, constipation or diarrhea, weight loss and hypotension.

Diagnosis

Laboratory tests to assess the level of ACTH, plasma cortisol and serum electrolytes.

Treatment

Addison's disease can be fatal if left untreated. Management involves treatment of the underlying cause and corticosteroid replacement therapy.

2. Write about the pathogenesis and clinical manifestations of hereditary hemorrhagic telangiectasia.

Hereditary hemorrhagic telangiectasia also known as Rendu-Osler-Weber syndrome is a autosomal dominant disorder. Gene mutations lead to the multisystem vascular dysplasia and development of abnormal vascular structures, which may vary from dilated microvessels to arteriovenous malformations (AVMs) of skin, mucosa and viscera. It affects individuals over a wide geographic distribution with an overall occurrence rate of 1/5,000–10,000 persons.

Pathogenesis

The clinical presentation of HHT results from abnormalities of vascular structure. Fragile walls and turbulent blood flow make these vessels prone for hemorrhage than normal vessels. The individual lesion is known as *telangiectasis*. The telangiectasis appears as 1–2 mm red spot in the skin and disappears upon a slight pressure due to shunt involving both dilated arterioles and venules. As the lesion increases in size, the capillary segments disappear and a direct arteriovenous communication is formed.

Clinical Features

- Telangiectases are most evident on the lips, tongue, buccal mucosa, nasal mucosa, face and fingers. They appear as pink to red, pinpoint lesions, or occasionally as larger purple lesions.
- It blanch with pressure and then immediately refill and are distinguished from petechiae and angiomata by this blanching property.
- It can rupture and bleed at the proximity to the skin surface or to a mucous membrane.
- As the vessel walls are lacking capillaries (contractile elements), bleeding from telangiectases is vigorous and difficult to stop.

Dental Complications

- Vascular lesions in the brain predispose patients to cerebral abscesses. This condition requires special care during invasive dental procedures. Antibiotic prophylaxis is mandatory especially in treating periodontal infections, and dental abscess.
- Patients with severe anemia (hemoglobin level <10 mg/dL) have risk of exacerbation of anemia due to invasive dental treatment and should avoid invasive procedures.

Curacao's Diagnostic: Criteria for Hereditary Hemorrhagic Telangiectasis

Criteria

1. Spontaneous, recurrent epistaxis. Nocturnal nose bleeds increase the risk for HHT.
2. Mucocutaneous telangiectases
3. Internal AVM (pulmonary, cerebral, hepatic, gastrointestinal, spinal).
4. First degree relative with HHT according to these criteria.

Diagnosis

- Definite: Three or more features of Curacao's.
- Possible: Two features of Curacao's.
- Unlikely: Less than two features of Curacao's.

Laboratory Tests

- Significant changes in red blood cell count—hypochromic anemia with anisocytosis.
- High level of liver enzymes.
- No changes in coagulation.

Management

- Systemic therapy: Tranexamic acid and antifibrinolytics
- Local ablation:
  - Laser: Argon, neodymium-doped yttrium aluminum garnet (Nd:YAG)
- Cauterization
  - Embolization.

SHORT NOTES

1. Enumerate the port-wine stains or sturge-Weber syndrome.

Sturge-Weber syndrome (SWS) is a nonfamilial neurocutaneous syndrome characterized by facial port-wine stains and occipital leptomeningeal angiomatosis with resulting neurological abnormalities. Other features associated with this condition include ocular and rarely internal organ involvement.

Etiology

- It is a *congenital malformation* resulting from changes in the ectoderm, mesoderm and neural crest derivatives.
- Persistence of a vascular plexus around the cephalic neural tube portion, characterizes the leptomeningeal angiomatosis and facial port-wine stains.

Classification

- *Type I (Classic) SWS*: This is the most common form with both facial and leptomeningeal angiomas. Seizures usually occur in the first year of life, and ocular involvement (glaucoma) is likely to be present.
- *Type II SWS*: This type manifests with facial angioma and may be glaucoma, but with no evidence of intracranial disease.
- *Type III SWS*: This type only involves leptomeningeal angioma, with no facial nevus and no ocular manifestation.

Clinical Features

The port-wine stain (nevus flammeus) is the most characteristic finding and present since birth. It affects half of the face, and may extend to the neck with a characteristic to darken with age, ranging from reddish to purple over time. Only persons manifesting the nevus flammeus along the ophthalmic branch develop the syndrome in its classical form.

Oral Manifestations

- Oral findings include hemangiomatous lesion in the lip, oral mucosa, gum, tongue, palatal region.
- The oral manifestations are generally unilateral and disappear abruptly in the middle line.
- Ipsilateral gingival hyperplasia and gingival hemorrhage even for the minimal traumatisms may also present.
- The macroglossia and the maxillary bone hypertrophy may present in some patients leading to facial asymmetry.
- Dilantin therapy for convulsive crises may exacerbate the gingival enlargement.

Investigations

- The intraoral radiographic findings reveals horizontal and vertical bone resorptions with loss of lamina dura of the teeth in lesion side obviously confirm diagnosis with the clinical observation of other changes, such as gingival hyperplasia.
- Computer tomographic image reveals the intracranial calcifications and unilateral cerebral atrophy.
- Magnetic resonance image shows cerebral vascular malformations.

Management

Usually, the port-wine nevus in the face may be improved by the use of new techniques of laser therapy.

- Periodic oral examination is necessary for the patients presenting with oral changes.
- Oral infections should be eradicated since it may aggravate the vascular picture.
- Extreme care is essential during oral surgical procedures due to the possibility of intense hemorrhage.

2. What is Peutz-Jeghers syndrome?

Peutz-Jeghers syndrome is a rare genetic disease associated with mutations in the few tumor suppressor genes. It characterized by hamartomatous polyps in the gastrointestinal tract (mostly in the small bowel), and pigmented mucocutaneous lesions with increased risk of carcinomas of the gastrointestinal tract, pancreas, breast, and thyroid.

Black-to-brown spots of less than 1 mm in size are typically localized on the lower lip and in the perioral area. Intraoral, intranasal, and conjunctival pigmented lesions may also be present. The oral lesions are benign and histologically characterized by an increase in melanin in the basal layer without an obviously increased number of melanocytes.

A fading or a disappearance of the spots is usually observed in older age.

Dental practitioners when come across the characteristic oral pigmentation should advise the patients for needful medical examination to reduce the potential later complications.

3. Describe about drug-induced pigmentation.

Certain drugs may cause an intraoral inflammatory reaction and subsequently induce postinflammatory hyperpigmentation which is the basis of pigmentation seen in fixed drug reactions.

- Clotrimazole was the most common drug associated to oral pigmentation followed by tetracycline; however, many others have been implicated including colchicines, ketoconazole, pyrimethamine and barbiturate.
- Arsenic drugs can directly induce pigmentation by combining with sulfydryl groups in the epidermal cells causing increased action of tyrosinase.
- Phenothiazines and minocycline may be deposited in the skin or mucosa and directly react with melanin to form a drug-pigment complex.
- Fixed drug eruptions are more commonly seen in people with dark skin and often present as a slate brown color due to pigmentary incontinence of melanophages in the upper dermis. Pigmented macules of the tongue may also manifest as a result of a fixed drug eruption.
- A dark pigmented macular area on the dorsum of the tongue is noted following inhalation of the heroin and methaqualone.
- Oral brownish pigmentation has also been reported in human immunodeficiency virus (HIV)—positive patients receiving treatment with zidovudine (AZT), ketoconazole and clofazimine.

4. What is exogenous pigmentation or metallic pigmentation?

Many metals have been implicated in the production of pigmentation in the oral region. These include:

Lead, which produces plumbism—characteristic generalized cutaneous "lead hue" (Described as a combination of pallor and lividity), and *"lead lines" (Burtonian line)* on the gingiva as gray areas of discoloration below the gingival margins. The intake of lead is possibly from the cooking vessels, containers, and glass vessels. The ingested lead is secreted in saliva and deposited along the free gingival margin of teeth. Chelating agents are helpful in removing lead from the body.

Mercury can cause *slate-gray* gingival pigmentation. The actual mercury poisoning is called pink disease or acrodynia characterized by excessive salivation and difficulty in mastication.

Amalgam tattoo is caused by the presence of metallic restorative material in the oral tissues that are spilled and implanted during the treatment procedures. Amalgam tattoos are painless, *gray-blue macules* that range in size from a few millimeters to greater than 1 cm. The tattoo can be single or multiple. Most amalgam tattoos are located on the gingiva and edentulous mucosa, but can also be seen on the hard palate, buccal mucosa, and floor of the mouth. Radiographic evaluation may be positive. On histopathological examination, fine black granular or fibrillar material embedded in the connective tissue or in a perivascular location with little or no inflammatory response is seen.

5. Describe the heme-associated lesions of oral mucosa or ecchymosis and petechiae.

Ecchymosis and petechia are extravascular lesions of varying sizes. They occur due to the extravasation of red blood cells into submucosa and appear as a bright red macules. They do not blanch and typically resolve within a month.

Ecchymosis

- Ecchymosis appear as multiple red brown macules measuring 1 cm or larger in size. In case of trauma, ecchymosis will disappear within 2 weeks.
- Patients on anticoagulants may predispose to trauma on chewing and often present with ecchymosis on tongue or cheek.
- Hereditary coagulation disorders and chronic liver failure also causes ecchymosis of skin and mucosa. In such cases, prothrombin time (PT), partial PT (PPT) and clotting time should be evaluated.

Petechiae

- Petechiae are pin size flat hemorrhagic spots usually less than 2 mm in size and initially appearing as red and within few days turn into brown due to lysis of extravasated erythrocytes.
- They occur on soft palate due to excessive or aggressive self-inflicted suction of soft palate against posterior tongue. Usually occur in a cluster of 10–30 spots.
- They also precipitated by viral or allergic pharyngitis which stimulate the action of click on palate with tongue to get relief from pruritus.

Petechiae may also be secondary to:

- Autoimmune or idiopathic thrombocytopenic purpura
- HIV-related thrombotic thrombocytopenic purpura
- Platelet aggregation disorders
- Aspirin toxicity
- Myelosuppressive chemotherapy.

Diagnosis

Platelet count and platelet aggregation test.

Management

If trauma or suction is the cause, then patient should be educated to stop the habit. For hemorrhagic conditions, referral to hematologist is necessary.

6. Describe the café au lait pigmentation.

Café au lait spots are present in neurofibromatosis (type 1), an autosomal dominant disease characterized with nodular and pendulous neurofibromas of skin and oral cavity and concomitant cutaneous pigmentation.

Café au lait spots, or café au lait macules are hyperpigmented lesions that may vary in color from light brown to dark brown; this is reflected by the name of the condition which means "color of coffee with cream". They appear in late childhood as multiple small macules or as broad diffuse lesions overlying the surface of neurofibromatous swelling.

This type of pigmentation also associated with McCune-Albright syndrome, tuberous sclerosis and Fanconi's anemia.

This pigmentation does not require any treatment and only monitoring of underlying associated condition is sufficient.

7. What is black hairy tongue or hairy tongue?

Black hairy tongue is a benign disorder characterized by hypertrophy and discoloration of the middle and posterior third of dorsum of tongue. This condition is characterized by abnormal hypertrophy and elongation of filiform papillae on the surface of the tongue due to defective desquamation of the tongue papillae resulting in excessive growth and thickening of the filiform papilla.

The elongated papillae will subsequently collect debris, bacteria, fungi or other foreign materials contribute to the discoloration.

The proposed precipitating factors include smoking or chewing tobacco, drinking alcohol, poor oral hygiene using peroxide containing mouthwash, radiation therapy, trigeminal neuralgia, using drugs that cause xerostomia like anticholinergics, antihypertensives and antidepressants, and antibiotics, such as tetracyclines and penicillins.

Hairy tongue is usually asymptomatic, but occasionally patients may complain of tickling or burning of the tongue, nausea, halitosis, dysgeusia and unattractive appearance of the tongue.

Diagnosis

Visual identification of discolored tongue with elongated papilla.

Management

Discontinuation of the offending agent alongside practicing good oral hygiene usually resolves the problem. Gentle tongue debridement can be accomplished by cleaning the tongue with a soft toothbrush and a solution of baking soda also help.

8. What is diascopy?

Diascopy (Fig. 1) is a chairside investigation to check the blanching and changes in the color of a lesion. This test is applied to differentiate the vascular lesion from other pigmented, nonvascular lesions. A thin, transparent glass slide is used to apply pressure on the lesion by pressing over the surface.

In hemangioma, there will be complete blanching of the lesion. The blood within the vessels is completely poured out when firm pressure is applied.

9. What is blue nevus?

A blue nevus is a benign, acquired melanocytic lesion that typically presents as an asymptomatic, slate-blue or blue-black smooth-surfaced macule or papule. Size is usually less than 6 mm in diameter. The melanotic cells are located deep in the connective tissue giving the lesion a bluish tint. Oral mucosa is rarely affected by blue nevus.

The intraoral variant of blue nevus is typically identified between third and fifth decades of life, females tend to be more commonly affected than males. Two-third of all intraoral blue nevi are found on the hard palate, and buccal mucosa is the second most common site of presentation.

Blue nevus is characterized by a variety of histologic subtypes, although most are classified as either "common" or "cellular". Common blue nevi are almost always innocuous lesions and rarely recur. Rare cases of malignant melanoma have been reported to arise in cellular blue nevi.

10. Describe the malignant melanoma.

In head and neck region, melanoma occurs on facial skin and oral mucosa. On facial skin, malar region is the common site as it is more exposed to sunlight. Facial melanoma appears as nodular or macular lesion with irregular margins and possesses varying shades from brown to black to blue with some areas of depigmentation.

Mucosal melanoma is rare. It is characterized by proliferation of malignant melanocytes along the junction between the epithelial and connective tissues, as well as within the

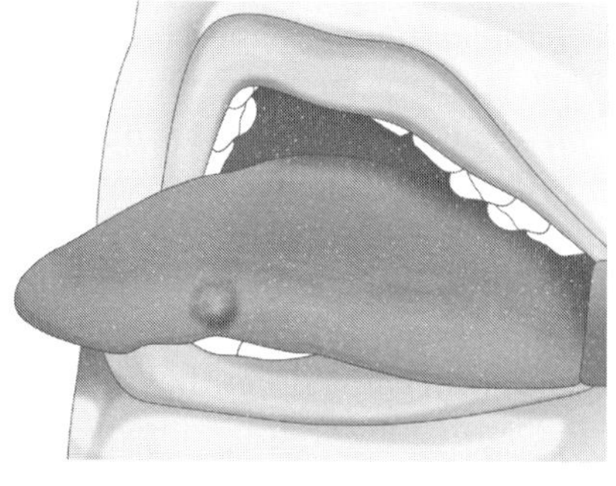

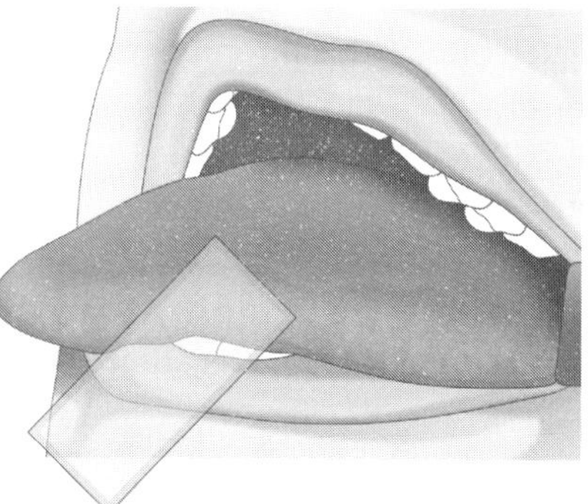

Fig. 1: Diascopy test.

connective tissue. The most common sites are anterior labial gingival and the hard palate.

Oral melanoma occurs between the fourth and seventh decades of life with a greater incidence in men than in women. Clinically, oral melanoma may present as an asymptomatic, slow-growing brown or black patch with asymmetric and irregular borders or as a rapidly enlarging mass associated with ulceration, bleeding, pain and bone destruction.

Malignant melanomas are characterized by:

- A prolonged radial growth phase where it grows superficially and laterally followed by a vertical growth phase where there is deep connective tissue invasion takes place or
- A direct vertical growth phase.

The tumor, nodes, metastasis (TNM) clinical staging system for oral melanoma recognizes three stages:

- Stage I, primary tumor (T, any N0, M0)
- Stage II, metastatic tumor to regional lymph nodes (T, any N1, M0)
- Stage III, metastatic tumor to distant sites (T, any N, any M1).

Treatment involves radical surgical excision with clear margins. Distant metastases often affect lungs, brain, liver, or bones. The prognosis for patients with oral melanoma is much worse than for those with cutaneous lesions.

11. Describe the hemochromatosis.

Hemochromatosis is a condition in which hemosiderin pigments are deposited on multiple organ and tissue.

It is characterized by increased intestinal absorption of iron and subsequent iron deposition in liver, pancreas, heart and pituitary leading to organ damage, iron storage pigmentation, diabetes mellitus, liver and cardiac impairment and arthropathy.

Liver is the first organ to be affected in 95% of cases and hepatocellular carcinoma is common.

Diabetes mellitus and skin pigmentation together known as *"Bronze diabetes"*.

Oral Pigmentation

Diffuse brown to gray macules occur on the palate and gingival due to submucosal iron deposition.

Diagnosis

Blood tests for serum iron. Either total iron binding capacity or transferrin are done as screening tests. Serum ferritin test also indicated which is elevated in patients with hemochromatosis.

Incision biopsy and prussian blue staining of the pigmented tissue will color the iron.

Management

Medical referral is advisable. Parenteral administration of desferrioxamine is used to remove excess iron deposition.

12. What is hemangioma?

Hamartomatous proliferation of vascular channels is known as hemangioma. It is a developmental disorder and usually regresses at puberty.

Oral hemangiomas are present within the connective tissue of mucous membrane and appear reddish blue if the proliferating vessels are closer to epithelium and deep blue if they are at the deeper level. They are raised and nodular or diffuse, flat and macular.

Frequently affected organ is tongue and appear as diffuse, raised, multinodular blue deep racemose. Labial mucosa is the second common site and appears as localized, raised blue lesion.

They are asymptomatic and blanch under pressure. When a microscopic glass slide is placed on the surface of hemangioma and adding pressure will demonstrate blanching and relieving the pressure will cause refilling and original color.

Management

Many cases undergo spontaneous involution after puberty. In persisting cases laser surgery or cryotherapy may be carried out.

For larger lesions, sclerosing agents like 1% sodium tetradecyl sulfate can be administered by intralesional injection.

13. Describe the Kaposi's sarcoma.

Kaposi's sarcoma is a multicentric angioproliferative disorder of endothelial origin with a slowly progressive growth. It predominantly affects mucocutaneous sites, but may also affect visceral organs. This is associated with human herpes virus type 8 (HHV-8).

Kaposi's sarcoma can be primarily categorized into four types:

1. Epidemic of AIDS-related
2. Immunocompromised
3. Classic or sporadic
4. Endemic (African).

Oral lesions occur as blue, red and purple at the hard palate, gingiva, (Fig. 2) oropharynx (upper and lower retromolar area, and soft palate, alveolar mucosa, and the dorsum of the tongue) with decreasing order of frequency. It does not have a tendency for metastasis and is not fatal.

- Kaposi's sarcoma is prevalent in HIV seropositive patients, most cases of HIV-related Kaposi's sarcoma occur when patients have a CD4 cell count below 200 cells/mm^3.

Investigations

- CD4 count and viral load.
- Punch biopsy and histopathological examination.

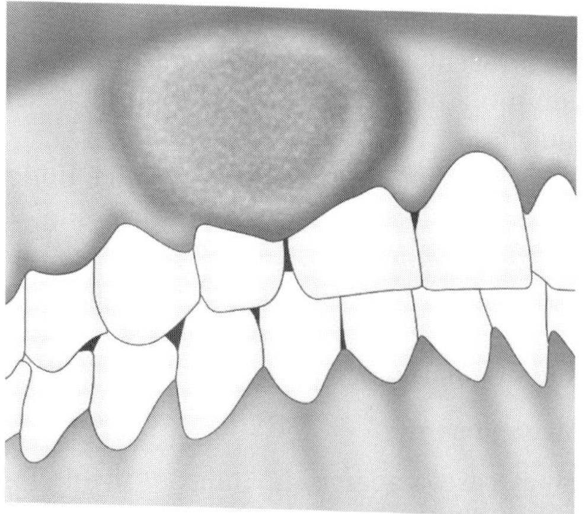

Fig. 2: Kaposi's sarcoma.

Management of HIV-related Kaposi's Sarcoma

Antiretroviral Therapy

Optimal control of HIV infection using highly active antiretroviral therapy (HAART) is an integral part of successful Kaposi's sarcoma therapy.

Local Therapy

Local therapies can be used for palliation of locally advanced symptomatic disease or in individuals who have cosmetically unacceptable lesions:

1. Radiation therapy
2. Cryotherapy
3. Laser therapy
4. Surgical excision
5. Intralesional vinca alkaloid therapy.

- Multiple biweekly injection of vinblastine is administered for eradication of this tumor.
- Intralesional injection of 1% sodium tetradecyl sulfate causes tumor necrosis.
- Topical retinoids.

Immunomodulation

Immunomodulation with interferon-alpha is effective through its antiangiogenic, antiviral, and immunomodulatory properties.

MULTIPLE CHOICE QUESTIONS

1. Moon face is a feature of ***Cushing's syndrome***
   a. Addison's disease
   b. Cushing's syndrome
   c. Acromegaly
   d. Myxedema
2. Endocrine disorders associated with oral pigmentation is ***Addison's disease***
   a. Addison's disease
   b. Cushing's syndrome
   c. Conn's syndrome
   d. Myxedema
   (**Note:** Endocrine disorders manifesting oral pigmentation are Addison's disease and Cushing's syndrome).

3. *Cushing's syndrome* is caused by ***adrenocortical hyperactivity***
   a. Adrenocortical carcinoma
   b. Multiple endocrine neoplasia
   c. Adrenocortical hyperactivity
   d. Adrenocortical insufficiency
   (**Note:** Addison's disease is adrenocortical insufficiency).
4. The appropriate diagnosis for oral pigmentation associated with cutaneous bronzing is evaluation of serum ***steroid and adrenocorticotropic hormone***
   a. Steroid and melanocorticotropic hormone
   b. Steroid and catecholamine
   b. Steroid and adrenocorticotropic hormone
   d. Steroid and aldosterone
5. "Bronze diabetes" is associated with ***hemochromatosis***
   a. Hemosiderosis
   b. Heme peroxidase
   c. Heme oxygenase
   d. Hemochromatosis
   (**Notes:** "Bronze diabetes" is associated with and is characterized by diabetes mellitus and skin pigmentation).
6. Tram-line calcifications are radiographic appearance seen in ***Sturge-Weber syndrome***
   a. Rendu-Osler-Weber syndrome
   b. Maffucci syndrome
   c. Von Hippel-Lindau syndrome
   d. Sturge-Weber syndrome
   (**Note:** Tram-line calcifications are radiographic appearance of *vessel wall calcification* seen in Sturge-Weber syndrome or encephalotrigeminal angiomatosis).
7. Varix is a focal dilation of ***vein or group of venules***
   a. Arteries and capillaries
   b. Arteries or group of arterioles
   c. Arteries and veins
   d. Vein or group of venules
   (**Note:** Varix is a focal dilation of vein or group of venules and once formed they would not enlarge further and *do not regress*).
8. Etiology for varix formation is ***trauma***
   a. Developmental disorder
   b. Congenital malformation
   c. Trauma
   d. Old age
9. Kaposi's sarcoma is caused by ***human herpes virus type 8***
   a. Human herpes virus type 8
   b. Epstein-Barr virus (EBV)
   c. Human papillomavirus type 16
   d. Group B coxsackievirus
10. Nevi are associated with increase in ***melanocyte number***
   a. Melanin synthesis by melanocytes
   b. Melanocyte number
   c. Hypertrophy of melanocytes
   d. Hyperplasia of melanocytes
   (**Note:** Nevi are associated with increased number of melanocytes and increase in melanin production. Melanotic macule and ephelis are associated with increase in melanin synthesis by melanocytes but without any increase in melanocyte numbers).
11. Common sites for intraoral nevi are ***gingiva and palate***
   a. Mucosa and tongue
   b. Lip and vestibule
   c. Tongue and floor of mouth
   d. Gingiva and palate
12. Hutchinson's freckle is otherwise known as ***melanoma in situ***
   a. Melanotic macule
   b. Melanocytic nevus
   c. Café au lait pigmentation
   d. Melanoma in situ
   (**Notes:** Hutchinson's freckle or lentigo maligna melanoma is otherwise known as melanoma in situ or atypical melanocytic hyperplasia of facial skin).
13. Common oral site of graphite tattoo is ***palate***
   a. Lip b. Gingiva
   c. Palate d. Floor of mouth
   (**Note:** Graphite tattoo is due to traumatic implantation of graphite from lead pencil).
14. In hairy tongue, the papilla commonly becomes elongated and is ***filiform papilla***
   a. Fungiform papilla
   b. Filiform papilla
   c. Foliate papilla
   d. Circumvallate papilla
15. Oral pigmentation due to ingestion of heavy metal is common in ***free gingival margin***
   a. Attached gingiva
   b. Free gingival margin
   c. Lower labial mucosa
   d. Hard palate

VIVA VOCE

1. What is pigmented lichen planus?

Erosive form of lichen planus is occasionally associated with overlying diffuse brown macular foci. This pigmentation is due to direct stimulation of melanocytes by inflammatory mediators (T lymphocytes) and also caused by an excess of melanin production and deposition within the basal layer of the epithelium and connective tissue of areas affected by chronic inflammatory nature of lichen planus.

2. What is smoker's melanosis?

Diffuse, irregular, flat brown macule seen on the buccal mucosa, palate, floor of mouth and lateral tongue of cigarette smokers is known as smoker's melanosis. It has no premalignant potential and is due to increased melanogenesis stimulation by tobacco smoke products.

3. What is hemangioma?

Hemangioma is a hamartomatous proliferation of vascular channels. It is a developmental condition and usually regresses after puberty.

4. What are lingual varicosities?

Torturous, serpentine, blue, red, purple elevations seen on the ventral surface of the tongue of elderly individuals are known as lingual varicosities. They are painless and not subjected to rupture and hemorrhage.

5. What are nevi?

Nevi are due to benign proliferation of melanocytes and increase in melanin production.

6. What is drug-induced pigmentation?

- Long-term use of *phenothiazine* may leads to skin deposition of metabolite and cause slate-gray color.
- *Phenytoin* use in females may cause chloasma like pigmentation.
- *Clofazimine may* cause red color discoloration of skin.
- *Large dose of nicotinic acid* causes brown pigmentation.
- *Amiodarone* causes violaceous hyperpigmentation in sun-exposed skin.
- *Oral contraceptives* produce chloasma.

7. What is Laugier-Hunziker pigmentation?

Laugier-Hunziker pigmentation is characterized by multifocal pigmentation of the labial and buccal mucosa with melanotic streaks of the fingernails.

BIBLIOGRAPHY

1. Alawi F. Pigmented lesions of the oral cavity: an update. Dent Clin North Am. 2013; 57(4): 699-710.
2. Cicek Y, Ertas U. The normal and pathological pigmentation of oral mucous membrane: a review. J Contemp Dent Pract. 2003;4(3):76-86.
3. Dummett CO. Oral pigmentation-physiologic and pathologic. NY State Dent. 1959; 25(9):407-12.
4. Ghom AG, Ghom SA. Textbook of Oral Medicine, 3rd edition. Jaypee Brothers Medical Publishers (P) Ltd; 2014 New Delhi, India.
5. Govani FS, Shovlin CL. Hereditary haemorrhagic telangiectasia: a clinical and scientific review. Eur J Hum Genet. 2009; 17(7):860-71.
6. Kaur H, Jain S, Mahajan G, et al. Oral pigmentation. Int Dent Med J Adv Res. 2015; 1:1-7.
7. Kopacova M, Tacheci I, Rejchrt S, et al. Peutz-Jeghers syndrome: diagnostic and therapeutic approach. World J Gastroenterol. 2009;15(43):5397-408.
8. Regezi JA, Sciubba JJ, Jordan RCK. Oral Pathology: Clinical Pathologic Correlations, 7th edition. Elsevier Health Sciences; 2016. St. Louis, MO

CHAPTER 5

Salivary Gland Diseases

HIGHLIGHTS

Salivary glands are *exocrine* (release their secretion through ducts in contrast to ductless endocrine glands) and *mesocrine* (cell walls lose their cytoplasm when secretary products pass through them) in nature and produces serous, mucus and seromucous types of secretion. There are three major salivary glands in pairs and approximately 600–800 minor salivary glands in our oral cavity. The major salivary glands primarily contribute to the total salivary secretion, whereas minor salivary glands are responsible for up to 8% of total secretion. The secretion takes place only in the *acinar* cells of the gland, and their destruction reduces the amount of salivary production and transport. The role of saliva in health and diseases is the prime topic for dental health professionals.

Learners are expected to know about:

- Classification of salivary gland diseases and disorders.
- Diagnostic methods for various salivary gland diseases.
- Quantitative abnormalities in salivary secretion.

ESSAY QUESTIONS

1. Classify salivary gland diseases.

Salivary glands are affected by a range of diseases and disorders and are broadly classified as follows:

- Congenital disorders:
  - Aplasia/agenesis—uni- or bilateral missing of one or more types of major salivary glands.
  - Aberrancy—salivary glands that develop in uncommon sites.
  - Atresia—absence of one or more major salivary gland ducts.
  - Accessory ducts—presence of additional duct.
  - Diverticuli—small pouches from the wall of major salivary gland duct. It causes pooling of saliva and recurrent sialadenitis.
- Developmental disorders:
  - Hyperplasia—increase in size of gland due to endocrinal disorders, metabolic disorders (diabetic mellitus). Alcoholism, hepatic diseases, starvation.
  - Darier's disease—strictures of salivary glands which may leads to obstructive sialadenitis.
- Physical causes:
  - Sialolithiasis
  - Sialodochitis
  - Radiation
- Infection:
  - Bacterial and viral sialadenitis
  - HIV-related salivary gland disorders
- Inflammatory and reactive lesions:
  - Cheilitis glandularis
  - Necrotizing sialometaplasia
  - Chronic sclerosing sialadenitis

- Cysts:
  - Mucocele
  - Ranula
- Tumors:
  - *Benign tumors:*
    - Pleomorphic adenoma
    - Warthin's tumor
    - Basal cell adenoma
  - *Malignant tumors:*
    - Mucoepidermoid carcinoma
    - Adenoid cystic carcinoma
    - Malignant mixed tumor
- Autoimmune disorders:
  - Sjogren's syndrome
  - Mikulicz's disease
- Granulomatous disorders:
  - Tuberculosis
  - Sarcoidosis
  - Orofacial granulomatosis
- Miscellaneous:
  - Drug-induced sialadenosis—e.g. antihypertensive drugs
  - Anorexia/bulimia.

2. Describe the etiology, clinical features, investigations, and management aspect of Sjogren's syndrome.

Sjogren's syndrome (SS) is a chronic autoimmune disorder causing dry mouth and dry eyes by lymphocytic infiltration, and destroying the exocrine glands (salivary and lacrimal glands, lungs, and kidney).

Etiology

- Circulatory autoantibodies against the ribonucleoproteins Ro and La.
- Antinuclear antibodies against DNA histones.
- B lymphocytes hyperactivity
- Circulating immune complexes
- Genetic
  - Primary Sjogren's syndrome: HLA-B_8 and DR_3
  - Secondary Sjogren's syndrome: HLA-B_8 and DR_4

Clinical Features

- Age group—commonly between 40–50 years.
- Females are affected more than males, and the ratio is 9:1. Postmenopausal women are prone to this syndrome.
- Types:
  - Primary Sjogren's syndrome—sicca syndrome; sicca complex: Dry mouth and dry eyes (xerostomia and xerophthalmia).
  - Secondary Sjogren's syndrome—symptoms of primary Sjogren's syndrome together with another autoimmune disorder like rheumatoid arthritis or systemic lupus erythematosus.

Signs and Symptoms

- Xerostomia or dry mouth is the principal disturbing factor causing difficulty in chewing, swallowing and speaking.
- Scanty, thick and ropey saliva.
- Chronic salivary gland enlargement.
- Frequent salivary gland obstruction and gland infections.
- Dry, cracked lips and angular cheilitis.
- Total or partial depapillation of tongue will give a typical red and lobulated appearance.
- Altered taste due to decrease in number of taste buds.
- Oral mucosa will appear dry and glossy.
- Accumulation of food debris leading to increased incidence of dental caries.
- Opportunistic candidal infection.

Investigations

For salivary gland:

- Minor salivary gland biopsy — most accepted criterion.
  - The infiltrated mononuclear cells are counted with a collection of 50 or more cells are considered as a *focus*. Then the focus score is calculated by the sum of foci in 4 mm^2 of the specimen. The focus score may range between 0–12. A focus score 1 confirms the diagnosis of Sjogren's syndrome.

- Histopathological evidence of degenerative changes in the acinar cells and the maintenance of architectural pattern of ducts in minor gland is also a useful diagnostic factor.
- Salivary flow rate (sialometry):
  - The stimulated salivary flow rate will be less than 1 mL/min.
  - (Normal: 1–1.5 mL/min) and unstimulated salivary rate will be less than 0.1 mL/min.
- For lacrimal glands:
  - Rose bengal dye test: Keratotic spots on the cornea will stain pink.
  - Schirmer's test: To measure the reduced tear flow, a filter paper strip should be placed in lower conjunctival sac. The extent of wetting will be less than 5 mm in Sjogren's patients, whereas in normal eyes the wetting will be up to 15 mm length.
  - Lab investigation of antibodies: Presence of antinuclear antibodies SS-A/Ro or SS-B/La.

Radiographic Diagnosis

- Sialography:
  - Obstruction of ducts may appear as, *cherry blossom* or *fruit laden branchless tree.*
  - Sialectasia due to leakage of contrast medium from the weakened ducts produces *snowstorm* appearance.
- Magnetic resonance imaging: Salt and pepper appearance of the salivary glands.
- Salivary scintigraphy: Use of Tc-99m pertechnetate may indicate impaired salivary function by slow and decreased excretion of the dye.

Management

- For dry mouth:
  - In case of *salivary glands with some amount of secretary function,* stimulate the salivary flow using:
    - Sugar-free gum.
    - Cholinergic medications (sialogogues)
    - Cevimeline, pilocarpine hydrochloride and bromhexine.
    - Pilocarpine hydrochloride — 0.5–7.5 mg in 3–4 divided doses/day.
    - Contraindications: Asthma, narrow-angle glaucoma, cardiovascular diseases. In case of complete absence of secretion, artificial saliva can be used with frequent oral rinse.

For other complications, multispecialty medical team approach is necessary.

3. Enumerate the cysts of salivary gland and briefly describe them.

- Cysts of salivary glands are:
  - Mucoceles
  - Ranula

  Mucoceles are broadly classified into (Fig. 1):
    - Mucous retention type
    - Mucous extravasations type.

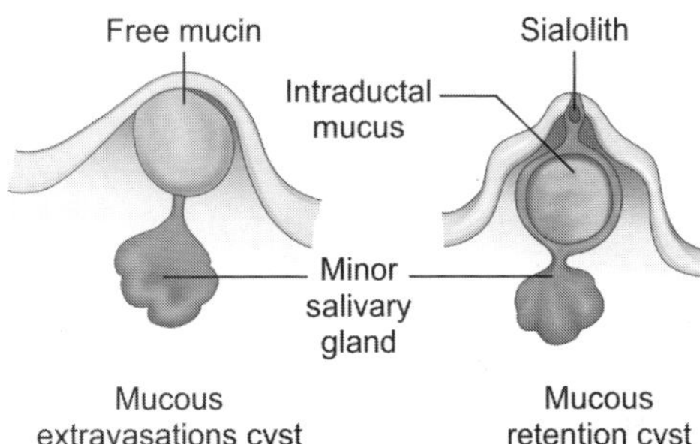

Fig. 1: Types of mucocele.

Retention Mucocele

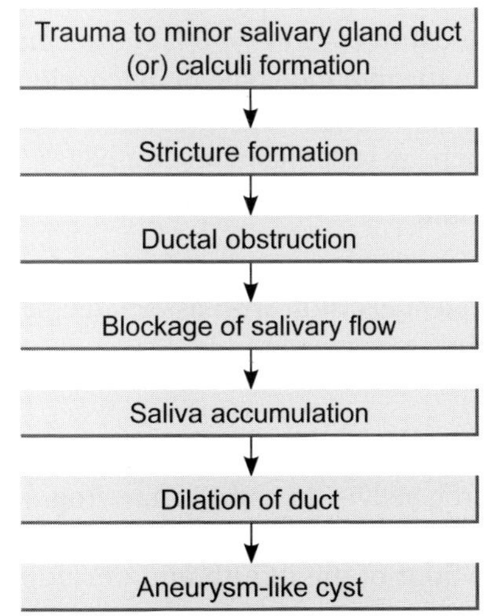

Retention type mucocele is a true cyst because of the dilated duct epithelial lining.

Extravasation Mucocele

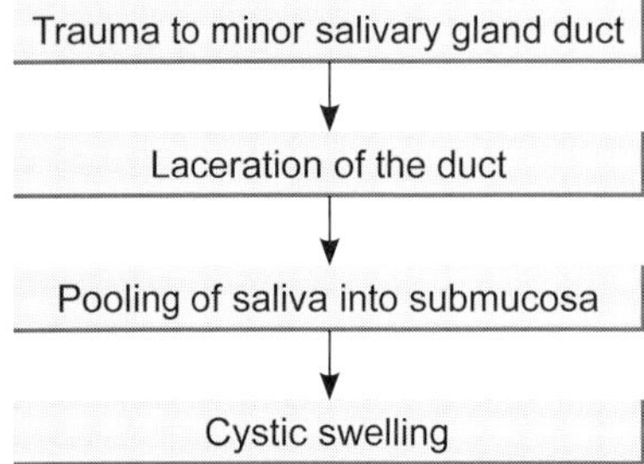

Clinical Features of Mucocele

- Mucoceles are well-circumscribed dome-shaped swellings measuring few millimeters to several centimeters in size. It may occur at any age, but prevalence for the younger age group is common.
- The superficial cysts show a distinct bluish hue due to translucent mucin, and the deeper cysts are covered by normal appearing mucosa. They are fluctuant and non-tender.
- Mucous extravasation type frequently occurs in lower lip (where chance for trauma is higher). The other sites include buccal mucosa, tongue, floor of the mouth and retromolar area. Mucous retention type is common in palate and floor of mouth.
- The extravasation type is more common than the retention type of mucocele.
- *Biopsy findings:* Characteristic *muciphages* which are vacuolated macrophages.

Treatment

- Intralesional injections of corticosteroids.
- Surgical excision with associated salivary gland.

Ranulas

- The name is derived due to its resemblance to frog belly — in Latin, rana = frog.
- Ranulas are larger sized mucoceles on the floor of the mouth and develop from sublingual salivary glands. They may be either extravasation or retention type.

Etiology

- Trauma
- Ductal obstruction
- Ductal aneurysm

Clinical Features

- Common in children and young adults.
- Painless, slowly enlarging, freely movable, soft and fluctuant swelling.
- Usually located on the floor of the mouth, on right or left side of the lingual frenum. However, deep-seated lesions may cross the midline.

Plunging Ranula

Deeper swellings may herniates mylohyoid muscle and appear in the suprahyoid or infrahyoid region.

Diagnosis

- Radiographs are necessary to rule out sialolith.
- Bidigital palpation for plunging ranula—placing one digit over the intraoral surface of the ranula with another finger over the submandibular or cervical counterpart, application of pressure through one finger will cause fluctuation sense on the another finger.

Treatment

- Intralesional injections of corticosteroids.
- Marsupialization of smaller lesion.
- Excision of the gland in recurring cases.

4. List the causes of xerostomia. Add a note on management of xerostomia. (or) What is dry mouth? Discuss the various causes of dry mouth and its management.

- Xerostomia or hyposalivation or dry mouth is a major functional defects of salivary glands and their ductal system. The subjective feeling of dry mouth is called as xerostomia, is a symptom and not a primary cause. Changes in the salivary composition also cause xerostomia.

Causes of xerostomia:

- Developmental:
  - Agenesis:
    - Atresia
    - Darier's diseases (strictures of salivary gland ducts).
- Physical:
  - Sialolith
  - Radiation injury
- Infection:
  - Fever — dehydration
  - Viral (mumps)
  - Bacterial
  - HIV-induced salivary gland disorders
  - CMV infection
- Inflammatory and reactive conditions:
  - Necrotizing sialometaplasia
- Cysts:
  - Mucocele
  - Ranula
- Tumors:
  - Benign: Pleomorphic adenoma
    - Monomorphic adenoma
    - Warthin's tumor
  - Malignant: Mucoepidermoid carcinoma
    - Adenoid cystic carcinoma
    - Carcinoma ex pleomorphic adenoma
- Autoimmune disorders:
  - Sjogren's syndrome
  - Mikulicz's disease
  - Sarcoidosis
- Metabolic disorder:
  - Uncontrolled diabetes
- Chemicals and drugs:
  - Tricyclic antidepressants
  - Antipsychotic medications
  - Antihistamines
  - Anti-HIV drugs
  - Opioids
  - Decongestants
  - Benzodiazepines
  - Proton pump inhibitors and H2 antagonists
- Nutritional deficiencies:
  - Vitamin A and B complex deficiencies
  - Iron deficiency anemia
  - Megaloblastic anemia
- Psychological disorders:
  - Psychosis
  - Manic depression
- Miscellaneous:
  - Anorexia and bulimia
  - Alcoholism.

Management of Xerostomia

- Preventive: Topical application of fluoride
- Symptomatic: Frequent sipping of water throughout the day will hydrate the mucosa and clear the debris.
- Local stimulation:
  - Sugarless chewing gums.
  - Xylitol sweetened gums.
- Systemic medications:
  - Pilocarpine Hcl increases salivary output by stimulating remaining gland tissue.
    - Dose: 0.5–7.5 mg in 3–4 divided doses/day.
    - Contraindications: Patients with uncontrolled asthma, narrow-angle glaucoma, cardiovascular diseases, and pulmonary diseases.
  - Cevimeline Hcl.
  - Bromhexine—mucolytic agent.
- Salivary substitutes (artificial saliva) — contain lubricants like carboxymethyl cellulose or hydroxyethyl cellulose, artificial sweeteners like sorbitol, preservatives, chloride and fluoride salts.

5. What is ptyalism? Enumerate the etiology, clinical findings, and treatment of ptyalism.

An increased salivary flow characterizes ptyalism or sialorrhea.

Causes

- Infection:
  - Herpes simplex infection
  - Ludwig angina
  - Fuso-spirochetal infections

- Inflammation:
  - Aphthous stomatitis
  - Teething
  - Erythema multiforme
- Physical:
  - New dentures
  - Instruments in oral cavity
- Chemicals:
  - Mercury
  - Iodine
  - Plumbism
- Drugs:
  - Clozapine
  - Risperidone
  - Lithium
  - Digoxin
- Hormonal changes: Pregnancy.

Clinical Features

- Saliva may drool spontaneously as well as during speech, chewing, and swallowing functions that disturb the affected individuals to varying extent.
- Infection arising from repeated salivary pooling is also a common problem at the corners of the mouth.

Management

- *Removal of the cause:* In case of infection, inflammation and ill-fitting dentures, possible measures should be taken to treat the underlying problem.
- *Self-awareness and education:* Patients should be educated and trained to improve their motor coordination. Biofeedback may be used for this purpose which will motivate the patients and make them swallow more frequently.
- Antisialagogues:
  - Atropine is an anticholinergic drug that antagonizes the action of acetylcholine in acinar cells and reduces salivary secretions.
    - Dose: Adults—it is 0.4 mg/4 times/day at 4–6 hour intervals.
    - Children—it is 0.01 mg/kg/day but should not exceed the total dose of 0.4 mg/day.
  - Scopolamine—0.4–0.6 mg/day.
  - Propantheline—15–30 mg/day in divided dose.

---

6. Describe the clinical features, investigations, and management of:
a. Bacterial sialadenitis
b. Viral sialadenitis

(or)

Describe in detail about bacterial and viral parotitis.

Sialadenitis is an inflammatory condition, and it is the sequel of bacterial or viral infections.

Bacterial Sialadenitis

It occur in individuals with reduced salivary gland secretion. It results from the retrograde spread of oral microorganism into salivary gland through the salivary duct.

Acute Bacterial Sialadenitis

- Most commonly affected gland is parotid (acute parotitis). The common organism associated with suppurative type is *Staphylococcus aureus.*
- *Streptococcus pyogenes, Streptococcus pneumoniae, E. coli, Prevotella, Porphyromonas, and Fusobacterium species* are also potential causative factors for sialadinitis.

Predisposing Factors

- Poor oral hygiene
- Dehydration
- Malnutrition
- Antihistaminic drugs
- Diuretics
- Ductal obstruction
- Major surgical procedures.

Clinical Features

Sudden, enlargement of salivary glands with erythematous overlying skin will be the early manifestation (Fig. 2). One or both the glands may involve, and the affected glands are indurated and painful. Upon milking the duct

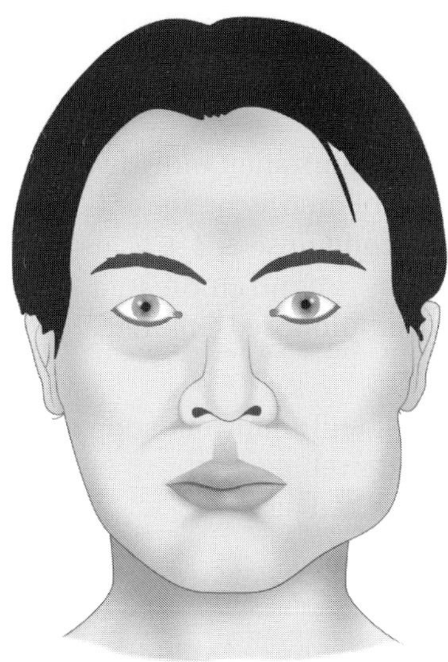

Fig. 2: Acute bacterial sialadenitis.

orifice, a purulent discharge may be released. There may be associated symptoms of fever, and lymphadenopathy.

Diagnosis

- Leukocytosis
- Culture the salivary exudate for aerobes and anaerobes.
- Ultrasonography: Hypoechoic swelling with increased vascularity.
- Computed tomography.

Treatment Plan

- Penicillinase-resistant antistaphylococcal antibiotics should be initiated.
- Frequent intake of water.
- Improved oral hygiene measures.
- Salivary stimulation by sucking a lemon or sour candy.

Postoperative Parotitis (Postsurgical Parotitis)

- Patients undergone for surgeries (especially abdominal surgery) under general anesthesia may develop sialadenitis on 5–7th day of the postoperative period.
- This condition is due to ascending bacterial infection as a result of decreased salivary flow caused by anticholinergic drugs and dehydration from the restricted fluid intake.

Pathogenesis of Acute Bacterial Sialadenitis

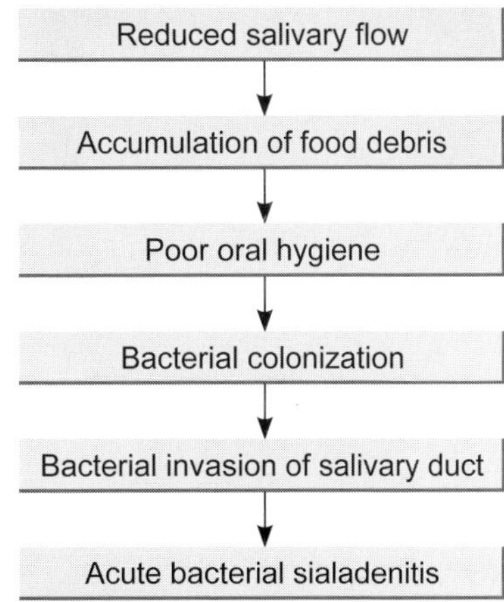

Clinical Features

Sudden onset of a firm and painful swelling at the angle of the jaw with restricted mouth opening.

Management

- Postoperative maintenance of fluid and electrolyte balance.
- Antibacterial mouth rinse (chlorhexidine 0.2%).

Viral Parotitis

Salivary gland infection is caused by paramyxovirus, cytomegalovirus, coxsackievirus and human immunodeficiency virus. Among these viruses, paramyxovirus infection is most common.

Mumps or Epidemic Parotitis

Paramyxovirus is a RNA virus and is transmitted by salivary droplets. The incubation period is 2–3 weeks.

Clinical Features

- Mumps occurs in 4–6 years age group children, but adult age onset can also occur.
- Prodromal symptoms: Salivary gland enlargement is preceded by fever, malaise,

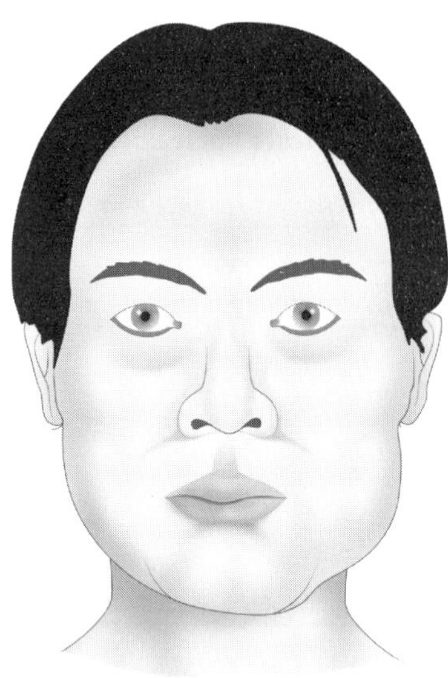

Fig. 3: Epidemic parotitis.

headache, myalgia, and preauricular pain. These symptoms will persist for a week.

- Salivary gland inflammation and enlargement will follow this period and parotid is the commonly affected gland (Fig. 3). Submandibular infection may occur in 10% of cases. Though the swelling occurs in both glands, the gland will become symptomatic on one side 24–48 hours before the other side gland. Swelling will last for 7 days. Inflammation of ductal orifice is common but no purulent discharge on milking the gland.

Complications

- Mumps in adult males cause inflammation of testis (orchitis) and leads to sterility.
- Acute pancreatitis with elevation of serum lipase
- Meningitis and encephalitis
- Myocarditis, thyroiditis
- Deafness, oophoritis, and mastoiditis.

Investigations

Demonstration of:

- Antibodies against mumps antigens V and S.
- Antibodies to hemagglutination antigen.
- Elevated serum amylase level.

Preventive Care

Enhance immunization with a live-attenuated vaccine in children at the age of 12–15 months and the second dose at 4–6 years of age. But vaccination is contraindicated in severely immunocompromised children.

Treatment

- Analgesic and antipyretic support to relieve pain and swelling.
- Adequate bed rest.

SHORT NOTES

1. Discuss features of Mikulicz's disease.

- Mikulicz's disease is a benign lymphoepithelial condition of symmetric, bilateral, painless, enlargement of lacrimal and salivary glands due to lymphoid infiltration. Etiology is nonspecific but autoimmune, viral and genetic causes are considered. It shows both inflammatory and neoplastic features. It affects middle-aged women more frequently with the typical signs of diffuse enlargement of salivary gland with mild local discomfort, pain, and xerostomia.
- Diagnosis is by salivary gland biopsy and treatment is palliative. Malignant transformation is the potential complication.

2. Briefly describe sialolithiasis (or) sialolith.

Lith = stone

Formation of calcified bodies in the duct of the major salivary glands or rarely within the major salivary gland itself is known as sialolith.

Pathogenesis

- Small organic foci deposition due to:
  - Local irritation
  - Inflammation
  - Irregular ductal course
  - Anticholinergic medications
  - Altered salivary flow

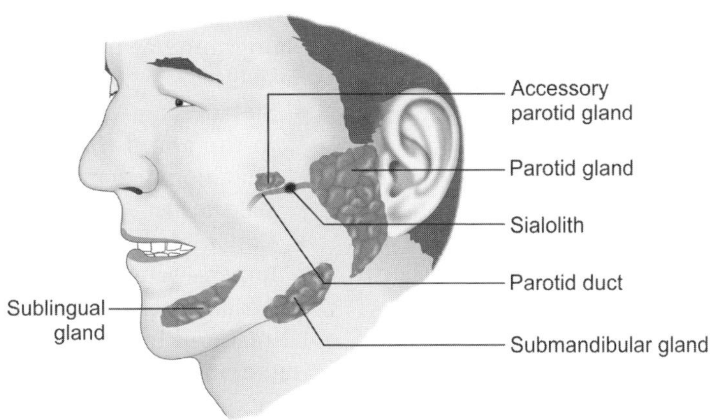

Fig. 4: Sialolith in parotid gland duct.

- Increased serum calcium and phosphorus

❖ It may act as central nidus and calcification may take place in a concentric manner around the nidus.

Composition

Hydroxylapatite crystals composed of calcium phosphate and carbon with less quantity of magnesium, potassium chloride and ammonium. About 50% parotid calculi and 20% submandibular calculi may not be calcified and will not be visible on radiographs.

Clinical Features

Sialoliths primarily form on the submandibular gland duct (80–90%) and then in the parotid (5–15%) and sublingual (2–5%) glands (Fig. 4). Acute, painful, intermediate swelling of affected gland are the characteristic symptom. Eating will initiate the swelling because the stone blocks the increased amount of salivary flow associated with eating and leads to pooling within the duct and gland. Since glands are encapsulated, it allows only little expansion and enlargement causes pain.

Complication

Atrophy and fistula also occur in some cases.

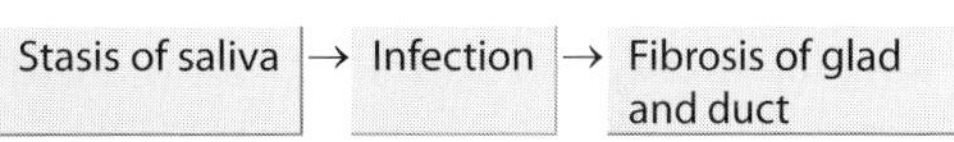

Diagnosis

❖ Clinical: Bidigital palpation.
❖ Radiographs: Occlusal view for submandibular gland and PA view for parotid.
❖ Noncontrast computed tomography for calcified stone and contrast CT for noncalcified sialolith.
❖ Ultrasound imaging.
❖ Rarely sialographs.

Treatment

❖ For acute condition—supportive therapy with analgesics, antibiotics, and increased fluid intake.
❖ If stones are near the duct orifice, removal is by massaging and manipulation of gland or by peripheral ductotomy.
❖ Larger stones and those away from orifice are removed by:
  - Excision of the duct and gland
  - Lithotripsy
  - Sialoendoscopy.

3. Describe necrotizing sialometaplasia.

It is a benign, reactive, inflammatory disease of the minor salivary gland that mimics both clinically and histopathologically as a malignant condition.

Etiology

- Local ischemia precipitated by administration of local anesthesia during oral surgical procedures and restorative treatment.
- Also, occur in patients suffering from bulimia and practice induced vomiting.

Clinical Features

- More prevalent in the posterior hard palate. Other sites of occurrence include retromolar pad, buccal mucosa, lower lip, and tongue.
- The sudden appearance of the firm nodule with intact mucosa causing a feeling of obstruction is the early symptom. Within 2-week period, the nodule will break, and surface ulceration will occur with a dull pain.

Investigation and Treatment

- It is a self-limiting condition and heals by secondary intention within 6 weeks. Debridement with saline rinse may accelerate healing. In symptomatic cases, analgesics can be prescribed.
- To rule out the malignant, histopathological examination of the biopsy specimen can be carried out.

4. Describe Kuttner's disease (tumor).

- Chronic sclerosing sialadinitis is known as kuttner's disease (tumor), and it frequently affects the submandibular gland.
- The suspected etiological factors include autoimmune sialadenitis, sialolithiasis, and idiopathic nature.

Pathogenesis

Chronic inflammation leads to atrophy of serous and mucous acinar cells, and hyperplasia of glandular connective tissues resulting in tumor-like mass.

Clinical Features

It is a firm enlargement of the affected side gland with mild or no pain.

Investigations

- Sialography of the enlarged gland may reveal:
  - Sialectasia—leakage of contrast agent in the gland from the duct produce dilatation of acinar cells and known as sialectasis.
  - Constricted ductal course with dilated lumen—sausage like *appearance.*
  - Absence of terminal branches
- Ultrasound image: Enlarged gland with numerous hypoechoic regions.
- CT and MRI.

Treatment

Surgical removal of the gland.

5. Briefly describe HIV-salivary gland disease (HIV-SGD).

- Dry mouth and enlarged salivary glands in HIV-infected individuals are collectively called as HIV-induced salivary gland disease. The uni- or bilateral enlargement of the gland is caused by both neoplastic and non-neoplastic lesions.
- Xerostomia in this condition is associated with cytomegalovirus (CMV) infection, and neoplastic conditions include kaposis's sarcoma and lymphoma.

Clinical Features

- Parotid gland is affected in 98% of cases and 60% of patients show bilateral enlargement.
- In the later stage of HIV, benign lymphoepithelial lesions (BLEL) or AIDS-related parotid cysts (ARPC) may develop a single or bilateral, soft to firm cystic enlargement of the glands. Xerostomia may present with ocular dryness. This condition is termed as BLEL-HIV.

Investigations

- *Lab diagnosis:*
  - Elevated levels of salivary IgA.
  - Immunohistochemical analysis of minor salivary gland biopsy reveals CD8 positive cells.

- The biopsy specimen from major salivary gland reveals lymphocytic infiltrates, cystic cavities and hyperplastic lymph nodes.
- *Imaging studies:* Ultrasonography, CT, MRI.

Treatment

- Symptomatic management for xerostomia—frequent sipping of water, chewing sugar-free gum or using salivary substitutes.
- For cystic lesions—aspiration of cysts followed by injecting tetracycline solution into cystic spaces to induce sclerosis.
- External radiation therapy for benign enlargements.

6. Describe cheilitis glandularis.

It is a rare, chronic, suppurative, inflammatory condition of the minor salivary glands of lower labial mucosa.

Pathology

The mucous secreting minor salivary glands become swollen with dilated duct orifice.

Suspected causes: Smoking, actinic damage, and bacterial infection.

Clinical Features

- Swelling and eversion of lower lip (Fig. 5).
- Inflamed ductal opening.
- On palpation, mucopurulent discharge through duct orifice.

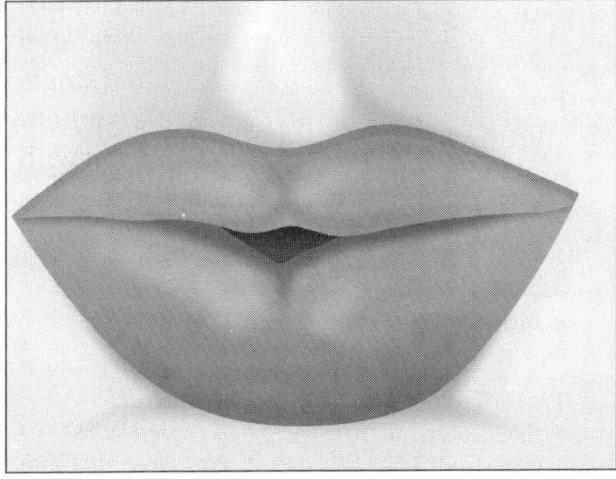

Fig. 5: Cheilitis glandularis.

Three types of cheilitis glandularis are:
Type 1: Simple
Type 2: Superficial suppurative—swelling with superficial ulceration and crusting.
Type 3: Deep suppurative—swelling with deep seated infection and spontaneous pus discharge from duct orifice.

Diagnosis

Biopsy of minor salivary gland.

Treatment

- Topical steroid application (0.1% triamcinolone acetonide).
- Intralesional steroid injection.
- Antibiotics and anti-inflammatory drugs.
- Surgical management for nonresponsive cases.

7. Discuss sialadenosis.

- Sialadenosis is a noninflammatory and non-neoplastic, bilateral enlargement of parotid and submandibular glands. It is associated with a systemic disorder like diabetes, hypothyroidism, obesity, anorexia, and bulimia. Alcoholism is also a common cause. Drugs like bronchodilators, antihypertensive agents, and psychotropic medications are also associated with sialadenosis.
- The enlargement will be gradual and usually asymptomatic.
- *Autonomic neuropathy which diminishes sympathetic innervations* is the proven mechanism in all these associated conditions. The altered innervation reduces the secretary mechanism of acinar cells. The acinar cells become hypertrophic with eventual glandular enlargement to compensate the functional demands.

MULTIPLE CHOICE QUESTIONS

1. The only imaging technique to find the functional capacity of salivary glands is ***scintigraphy***.
   a. Sialography b. Ultrasonography
   c. Scintigraphy d. Fluoroscopy

2. The possible alternate to sialography contra-indication is ***scintigraphy***.
   a. CT sialography b. Scintigraphy
   c. MRI sialography d. Ultrasonography
   (**Note:** Scintigraphy or Tc-99m scan).
3. The best imaging choice to evaluate salivary gland tumor is ***magnetic resonance imaging***.
   a. High-resolution ultrasonography
   b. Computed tomography
   c. Radionuclide scintigraphy
   d. Magnetic resonance imaging
4. In suspected cases of Sjogren's syndrome, the preferred site for biopsy is ***labial minor salivary gland***.
   a. Von Ebner's gland
   b. Parotid gland
   c. Labial minor salivary gland
   d. Glands of Blandin and Nuhn
   (**Note:** Glands of Blandin and Nuhn are minor salivary glands located on the anterior ventral aspect of tongue. Von Ebner's minor salivary glands are located anterior to the sulcus terminalis on the dorsal aspect of tongue, around the circumvallate papilla).
5. The pouch or sac projecting from the walls of major salivary gland ducts is known as ***diverticulum***.
   a. Diverticulum b. Atresia
   c. Salivary fistula d. Lingual thyroid
6. Complication of diverticuli is ***recurrent sialadinitis***.
   a. Recurrent sialadinitis
   b. Obstructive sialadenitis
   c. Sialolithiasis
   d. Sialadenosis
7. *Darier's disease* cause ***obstructive sialadenitis***.
   a. Recurrent sialadinitis
   b. Obstructive sialadenitis
   c. Diverticulosis
   d. Sialadenosis
8. Salivary gland abnormality in Darier's disease is a ductal dilation with ***recurrent stricture of main ducts***.
   a. Aplasia of major glands
   b. Aberrant minor salivary glands
   c. Recurrent stricture of main ducts
   d. Recurrent parotid abscess
   (**Note:** Salivary gland abnormality in Darier's disease is duct dilation with recurrent stricture of main ducts).
9. Contrast CT and sialographs diagnose ***non-calcified sialoliths***.
   a. Gland inflammation
   b. Minor salivary gland tumor
   c. Noncalcified sialoliths
   d. Deep seated mucocele
10. Most efficient method for removal of sialolith is ***sialoendoscopy***.
    a. Lithotripsy b. Sialoendoscopy
    c. key-hole surgery d. Gland removal
11. Salivary gland virus disease is the name for ***cytomegalovirus infection***.
    a. Paramyxovirus infection
    b. Infectious mononucleosis
    c. Epstein-Barr virus infection
    d. Cytomegalovirus infection
12. The PH range of saliva in health is between ***6.7 and 7.4***.
    a. 5.0 and 9.0 b. 6.7 and 7.4
    c. 0 and 7.0 d. 4.5 and 11.3
13. Increased caries rate occurred when salivary pH range goes below, ***5.5***.
    a. 0 b. 7
    c. 5.5 d. 3.2
14. Schirmer's test is done for measuring the ***tear production***.
    a. Serum vitamin B^{12} level
    b. Tear production
    c. Salivary flow rate
    d. Serum folate level
15. Computed tomographic image of parotid gland in intermediate stage of Sjogren's syndrome patients reveal ***multiple cysts***.
    a. Parotid atrophy
    b. Multiple cysts
    c. Parotid hypertrophy
    d. Multiple tumors
16. Intermediate postprandial salivary gland swelling is a diagnostic symptom of ***sialolith***.
    a. Mucocele
    b. Pleomorphic adenoma
    c. Sialolith
    d. Mumps
17. The most prevalent type of salivary gland neoplasm is ***pleomorphic adenoma***.
    a. Pleomorphic adenoma
    b. Warthin's tumor
    c. Mucoepidermoid carcinoma
    d. Adenoid cystic carcinoma

18. Tumor occurring only in parotid gland is ***Warthin's tumor (Papillary cystadenoma lymphomatosum)***.
    a. Pleomorphic adenoma
    b. Warthin's tumor
    c. Mucoepidermoid carcinoma
    d. Adenoid cystic carcinoma
    (**Note:** Warthin's tumor also known as *papillary cystadenoma lymphomatosum*).
19. Developmental salivary gland defect *is* known as ***Stafne's cyst***.
    a. Mucocele
    b. Ranula
    c. Stafne's cyst
    d. Plunging ranula
    (**Note:** Stafne's cyst does not require any treatment).
20. Pseudomembranous candidiasis is common in ***Xerostomia***.
    a. Anemia
    b. Avitaminosis
    c. Xerostomia
    d. Anorexia nervosa

VIVA VOCE

1. Contraindications for sialography.

a. Active salivary gland infection—in this condition sialography procedure further aggravate the inflammatory condition. The contrast media when injected forces the bacteria to spread throughout the ductal course and potentiate the infection.
b. Allergy—iodine (contrast agent) may induce an allergic reaction in suspected people.

2. Indications for contrast CT images of salivary glands.

To diagnose more defined lesions like tumors, abscesses, and inflamed lymph nodes.

3. Indications for nonenhanced (without contrast) CT images of salivary glands.

To diagnose, sialoliths, glandular enlargements and asymmetry, and lymph node involvement.

4. Serological markers (lab tests) for diagnosis of Sjogren's syndrome.

- Antinuclear antibodies (SSA/Ro or SSB/La), rheumatoid factors, elevated levels of IgG, and elevated ESR.

5. Where lithotripsy is used and what are the merits and demerits of using it?

Lithotripsy is used for removal of larger sialoliths and sialolith located away from the duct orifice.

- Advantage: Noninvasive treatment
- Disadvantages:
  - Several appointments are necessary.
  - Transient hearing change.
  - Pain and hematoma.

5. Why sialographs are not usually advised for the diagnosis of sialolith (or) What are the drawbacks of using sialography for the detection of sialoliths?

- Sialography is an invasive procedure and increases the pain especially in acute cases.
- In case of existing ductal infection due to salivary stasis, sialography may induce retrograde spread of infection to the gland.
- The sialographic procedure may displace the stone deeper into the gland.

6. Functions of saliva.

Lubrication of oral mucosa, buffering the oral cavity, antimicrobial and antifungal protection to the oral cavity, remineralization of tissues, excretion of certain drugs and chemicals and flushing the food debris.

7. What is *cracker sign*?

The inability of a patient to eat cracker (biscuit) without drinking fluid is known as cracker sign. It indicates hyposalivation.

8. What is *lipstick sign*?

Lipstick adhering to the incisal edge of the upper anterior teeth is known as lipstick sign. The positive sign indicates hyposalivation.

9. What is *mouth mirror test*?

If the dentist places the mouth mirror in patients buccal mucosa and unable to move the mirrored surface of the mouth mirror along the buccal mucosa effortlessly, it is the indication for hyposalivation and dry mouth.

10. Name few benign tumors of salivary gland.

Pleomorphic adenoma, Warthin's tumor (papillary cystadenoma lymphomatosum), canalicular adenoma, basal cell adenoma.

11. Name few malignant tumors of salivary gland.

Mucoepidermoid carcinoma, adenoid cystic carcinoma, carcinoma e.g. pleomorphic adenoma.

12. What is Stafne cyst?

Stafne cyst is a radiographic finding (orthopantomogram) on the lingual surface of the posterior body of the mandible. It appears as a round or ovoid radiolucency of 1–3 cm size with radiopaque border located ***above*** *the inferior border of the mandible and below the inferior alveolar canal.* The inclusion of salivary gland tissue in the cortical plate is the reason for this defect. It is asymptomatic and *does not require any treatment.*

13. Sialolith is common in which gland and why?

Sialolith is common in the submandibular gland. The reason is:

- Irregular and tortuous course of Wharton's duct.
- Mucous secretion is predominant hence easily form plug.
- Deeper position of the gland and flow direction opposite to gravity.

Salient Points to Remember

- *Sausage appearance* (dilated lumen and narrow course of the duct) is seen in *chronic sclerosing sialadenitis or Kuttner's disease.*
- *Salivary gland aplasia* is associated with *first branchial arch anomalies, hemifacial microsomia,* and *mandibulofacial dysostosis.*
- *Salivary composition* is influenced by *sympathetic stimulation.*

BIBLIOGRAPHY

1. Burket LW, Greenberg MS, Glick M. Burket's oral medicine: diagnosis and treatment. BC Decker; 2003.
2. Glick M. Burket's Oral Medicine, 12th edition. PMPH-USA; 2015.
3. McQuone SJ. Acute viral and bacterial infections of the salivary glands. Otolaryngol Clin North Am. 1999;32(5):793-811.
4. Moutsopoulos HM, Chused TM, Mann DL, et al. Sjögren's syndrome (sicca syndrome): current issues. Ann Intern Med. 1980;92(2 Pt 1):212-26.
5. Mínguez-Martinez I, Bonet-Coloma C, Ata-Ali-Mahmud J, et al. Clinical characteristics, treatment, and evolution of 89 mucoceles in children. Oral Maxillofac Sur. 2010;68(10):2468-71.
6. Ongole R, Praveen BN. Clinical manual for oral medicine and radiology. Jaypee Brothers Medical Publishers (P) Ltd; 2007.
7. Speight PM, Barrett AW. Salivary gland tumors. Oral Dis. 2002;8(5):229-40.
8. Villa A, Connell CL, Abati S. Diagnosis and management of xerostomia and hyposalivation. Therapeutics and clinical risk management. 2015;11:45-51.

CHAPTER 6

Dental Consideration for Patients with Systemic Diseases/Disorders

HIGHLIGHTS

The dental students should gain a sound knowledge about the systemic diseases as they are handling patients with such conditions. They should able to transfer this knowledge during the practice for better patient care. Diagnosis of oral lesions in systemic disease is only one end of the task spectrum, whereas giving dental treatment by carefully assessing their history, medications and advising needful investigations before providing treatment, prescribing appropriate medications and managing emergency conditions at chair side constitute a series of tasks that should be imparted during the course time. This chapter is a complete compilation of topics need to be familiarized by every dental student for delivering a safety care for medically-compromised dental patients.

Learners are expected to study about dental care for patients with:

- Diabetic mellitus
- Hypertension
- Cardiovascular disorders
- Central nervous system disorders
- Respiratory diseases
- Renal disorders
- Hepatic dysfunction
- HIV and hepatitis
- Immunological diseases
- Gastroesophageal reflux disease.

ESSAY QUESTIONS

1. Briefly describe the oral findings in HIV-infected patients and add a note about specific management.

HIV-associated oral lesions are the result of immune suppression. Depleted CD4 count leads to fungal, viral infections, and neoplastic growths in the oral cavity.

Fungal Infections

- *Pseudomembranous candidiasis* (Oral thrush)—when CD4 count falls below 400 cells/mm^3, asymptomatic, creamy-yellow plaques develop on oral mucosa which can be rubbed-off easily and leave erythematous mucosa.
- *Atrophic (or) erythematous candidiasis*—Reddish or atrophic patch on oral mucosa associated with burning sensation. If tongue dorsum is involved, depapillation will occur.
- *Chronic (or) hyperplastic candidiasis*—Occur only in patients with remarkably low CD4 count and xerostomia. Appear as creamy yellow or yellow-white, non-scrapable plaques. Symptoms include burning sensation, dysphagia, altered taste and feeling of large cotton in the mouth.
- *Angular cheilitis:* Appear as red fissures along the labial commissures of mouth.

Management

- *Topical antifungal drugs* are used if the CD4 count is above 150–200 cells/mm^3.

- *Topical preparations include:*
  - Nystatin oral suspension 100,000 units/mL: 10 mL swish and swallow 4 times/day for 2 weeks
  - Nystatin troche—dissolved in mouth 4 times/day.
  - 1% clotrimazole ointment.
  - 2% ketoconazole cream.
- *Systemic antifungal medications:*
  - Ketoconazole 200 mg tablets twice a day with food.
  - Fluconazole tablets—200 mg on the first day of therapy followed by 100 mg/day for 14 days.
  - Itraconazole 100 mg tablets twice daily.

Viral Infections

- *Herpes virus infection*—occurs during initial acute phase HSV-infection among HIV patients are more severe and involve even nonkeratinized mucosa. Reactivation of latent viruses causes this condition as crops of vesicles which ulcerate, bleed and heal in 7–10 days. Intensely painful linear gingival erythema is characteristic.
- *Cytomegalovirus infection*—occurs when the CD4 count is below100 cells/mm^3. Single painful ulcer with no other vesicles on oral mucosa with delayed healing is the frequent finding.
- *Epstein-Barr virus (EBV) infection*—occurs when CD4 count is below 200 cells/mm^3.
- *Hairy leukoplakia*—asymptomatic, vertically running, white lines along the lateral borders of the tongue.
- *Varicella-zoster infection*—occurs when the CD4 count is below 200 cells/mm^3. Vesicles that rupture quickly leaving multiple shallow, erythematous ulcers unilaterally along the division of 5th cranial nerve. Pain, neuropraxia, and tenderness are the typical symptoms.
- *Human herpesvirus 8 (HHV-8) infection and Kaposi's sarcoma*—asymptomatic, blue or purple nodule on the hard and soft palate. Occurs when the CD4 count is below 200 cells/mm^3. Kaposi's sarcoma is an AIDS-defining lesion.
- *Human papillomavirus (HPV) infection:*
  - Squamous papilloma and verruca vulgaris—exophytic, pedunculated papules.
  - Heck's disease (or) focal epithelial hyperplasia—multiple smooth or pebble-like lesions on the alveolus and labial mucosa.
  - Condyloma acuminatum manifests as single or multiple verrucous lesions that is pale in color, measuring few-millimeters in size in the mucosa of tongue and palate.

Management

For HSV infection:

- Tab. acyclovir 200 mg 4 times/day.
- Foscarnet is used for resistant cases.

For cytomegalovirus (CMV) infection: High dose of acyclovir 800 mg 5 times/day for 2 weeks.

For Hairy leukoplakia (EBV) infection: Acyclovir 800 mg orally 5 times a day for 2 weeks.

For varicella-zoster infection:

- Acyclovir 800 mg orally 5 times a day.
- Famciclovir 500 mg orally 3 times a day.
- Foscarnet is used for resistant cases.

For Kaposi's sarcoma:

- Surgical excision
- Radiation therapy: 800–2,000 rad.
- Intralesional injections of vinblastine sulfate 0.1 mg/mm^2.

For human papillomavirus (HPV) infection:

- Surgical excision
- Laser ablation
- Cryotherapy
- Keratolytic topical agents—25% podophyllum resin.
- Intralesional injections of Interferon alpha.

Bacterial Infections

- Periodontal infections:
  - Linear gingival erythema—atypical gingivitis manifesting as 2–3 mm band of fiery-redness on the marginal gingiva. It is not associated with increased plaque deposits, gingival pockets, or attachment loss.
  - Necrotizing ulcerative gingivitis—spontaneous gingival bleeding with mild to moderate gingival pain.
  - Necrotizing ulcerative periodontitis—rapid bone loss in a specific quadrant or in multiple quadrants with gingival denudation leading to the symptoms of bleeding gums, halitosis, and intense pain. 1–2 mm destruction of bone and gingiva occurs per week.

Management

- *For linear gingival erythema*:
  - Scaling and root planning (with homecare use of 0.12% chlorhexidine gluconate mouth rinses twice daily for 3 months).
  - Simultaneous use of topical antifungal medication.
- *For necrotizing ulcerative gingivitis and periodontitis:*
  - Debridement of necrotic tissues.
  - Antibiotic therapy—tetracycline 500 mg 4 times/day for a week followed by scaling and debridement.
  - 0.12% chlorhexidine gluconate mouth rinses as maintenance therapy.
- *Nonspecific ulcerations:*
  - Aphthous ulcers—all three forms of aphthous ulcers (minor, major, herpetiform) occur in HIV patients. The surrounding erythematous halo may not be seen in severely immunocompromised patients due to lack of inflammatory response. Major aphthous ulcers in HIV patients may occur when CD4 cells fall below 100 cells/mm^3 and appear as a group of up to 10 lesions and persist more than 3 weeks and heal with scar formation.
  - *Management of aphthous ulcers:*
    - *Minor aphthous and herpetiform ulcers:*
    - *Topical corticosteroids*—0.1% triamcinolone acetonide in carboxymethyl cellulose paste, applied 4 times/day. 5% amlexanox oral paste is an active inhibitor of the inflammatory mediators from mast cells, neutrophils, and mononuclear cells. Amlexanox suppress both the formation and release of the mediators.
    - *Major aphthous ulcers:*
      - Topical application of high potent steroids like 0.05% clobetasol or 0.05% fluocinonide gel.
      - Dexamethasone elixir mouth rinse — 0.5 mg/5 mL.

Drug-induced Ulcers

Medications used for HIV-infection like zidovudine, ganciclovir, interferon may induce oral ulcers usually in the nonkeratinized mucosa, but in severely immunocompromised patients, keratinized mucosa also be involved.

SHORT NOTES

1. What are oral manifestations of diabetes mellitus?

- Diabetes mellitus is a metabolic and endocrine disorder with defective glucose metabolism resulting in impaired peripheral utilization of sugar and increase blood glucose value.
- Diagnose of diabetes mellitus is based on the following reference values:
  - Glycated hemoglobin (HbA1c) >7%
  - Fasting blood glucose (FBS) >120 mg/dL
  - Postprandial blood glucose (PPBS) >160 mg/dL

Oral Manifestations

The most commonly affected structures are periodontium and tongue.

Mucosa

- Atrophy of oral mucosa which appears dry and shiny.
- Candidiasis.
- Drug-induced lichenoid lesions
- Ulcers caused by self-bites due to diabetic neuropathy.

Tongue

- Atrophic tongue — bald tongue.
- Fissured tongue.

Lips

Angular cheilitis

Gingiva and Periodontium

- Gingivitis
- Gingival recession
- Multiple periodontal abscesses
- Mobility of teeth

Salivary Glands

Sialadenosis (asymptomatic bilateral enlargement of parotid).

Teeth

Increased incidence of dental caries secondary to xerostomia.

2. Dental treatment for diabetic patients.

The following factors should be considered to minimize the risk during dental treatment:

- Medical history:
  - Frequency of hypoglycemic episodes.
  - Medication, dosage, and schedule.
  - Lab report for plasma glucose value.
- Dental treatment with minor surgical procedures, extractions, scaling can be carried out when postprandial blood sugar is within 160–200 mg/dL and fasting glucose is less than 120 mg/dL.
- The dental appointment should be preferably scheduled in the morning. The patient should be advised to take their usual medications and diet within 2 hours before coming for dental treatment.
- Antibiotic prophylaxis should be considered only for extensive surgical procedures, rapidly spreading infections like cellulitis and necrotizing gingivitis or periodontitis.
- During treatment, the expected complication is the signs of hypoglycemia (sweating, tachycardia, incoherence, hypothermia, unconsciousness) and the emergency management should be instituted with:
  - Oral administration of 15 g of glucose.
  - Intravenous administration of 25–30 mL of 50% dextrose over 3 min period.
- In case of hyperglycemic crisis:
  - Immediate hospital transport is necessary for medical management and insulin administration.

3. Dental management for hypertensive patients.

- The reference measure for normal blood pressure is below 120/80; blood pressure between 120/80 and 139/89 is for *pre-hypertension*, whereas 140/90 and above is referred as high blood pressure.
- Patients with optimal (≤120/80 mm Hg) and prehypertensive (120–139/80–89 mm Hg) blood pressures can take up all dental procedures and can receive local anesthetic with vasoconstrictor (epinephrine) 1:100,000.
- Patients with mild to moderate hypertension (140–180/90–108 mm Hg) require an overall assessment depending on the complexity of dental treatment procedure and patients level of anxiety. Antianxiolytic (5–10 mg of diazepam the night before and 1–2 hours before treatment) can be considered, or elective procedures may be delayed until blood pressure is controlled.
- Patients with a blood pressure greater than 180/95 (systolic/diastolic) should be referred for medical management.

Dental treatment should be delayed for these patients until the values are bringing to near normal. In case of emergency dental care to be provided, the patient should be hospitalized and procedure should be carried in the presence of the medical practitioner. Sedation with benzodiazepine or nitrous oxide should be considered.

4. Discuss prophylactic antibiotic coverage for dental patients to prevent infective endocarditis (or) Antibiotic prophylaxis for dental patients.

Antibiotic Prophylaxis Guidelines Proposed by American Heart Association

- *Conditions that require antibiotic prophylaxis are:*
  - Prosthetic valve
  - Previous history of infective endocarditis
  - Congenital heart diseases (CHD)
- *Standard regime:*
  - For adults: Capsule amoxicillin 2.0 g—1 hour before dental treatment.
  - For children: Capsule amoxicillin 50 mg/kg body weight—1 hour prior to dental treatment.

No second dose is needed for adults and children.

- *The standard regimen for patients allergic to penicillin.*
  - Anyone of the following course can be prescribed.

Antibiotic	Adult	Children
Tab clindamycin	600 mg—1 hour before dental procedure	20 mg/kg body weight 1 hour before dental treatment
Tab erythromycin	500 mg—1 hour before dental procedure	15 mg/kg body weight 1 hour previous to the dental treatment

- *For patients not able to take oral preparation*
  - Adults:
    - Ampicillin—2 g by intravenous (IV) (or) intramuscular (IM) route—30 minutes before the dental procedure.
  - Children:
    - Ampicillin—50 mg/kg body weight by intravenous (IV) or intramuscular (IM) route—30 minutes before the dental appointment.
- *For patients not able to take oral medications and history of penicillin allergy*
  - Adults:
    - Clindamycin 600 mg by intravenous route (IV)—½ hour prior to dental treatment.
  - Children:
    - Clindamycin—20 mg/kg body weight by intravenous route (IV)—½ hour before the dental appointment.
- *Antibiotic prophylaxis is essential for the following procedures:*
  - Extraction
  - Subgingival scaling
  - Semi-surgical procedures—like curettage.
  - Periapical surgery, implant surgery.
  - Rubber dam, wedge placement.
- *Antibiotic prophylaxis is not required for:*
  - Routine endodontic procedures (procedures not extending beyond root apex).
  - Investigative and treatment methods that do not cause bleeding.
  - Suture removal.

5. Dental management for patients with ischemic heart disease.

- A detailed medical history regarding the nature of heart disease, severity, the time between the cardiological event and treatment received should be taken to access the clinical complications.
  - Patients should be advised to continue the medications for cardiac care.

- If *nitrates* are prescribed, then the patient should be asked to take the drug as a preventive therapy before local anesthesia or in case chest pain develops.
- For patients *on* anticoagulant drugs, INR should be determined on the day of treatment.
- For patients *on antiplatelet drugs,* local hemostatic measures should be followed:
  - Only emergency dental procedures can be carried out for patients with *history of recent infarction* (before 4–6 weeks).
  - For very anxious patients, *premedication* should be instituted. (5–10 mg of diazepam the night before and 1–2 hours before treatment).
  - Appointments should be maintained below half-an-hour duration. It is better to avoid early morning and late afternoon hours.

- In case of administering *local anesthesia:*
  - Infiltration should be preferred.
  - Maximum of two carpals with vasoconstrictors should be used.
  - If anesthetic reinforcement is needed: Local anesthesia without vasoconstrictor can be considered.
  - Patient should be made in semisupine position.
  - Patient should get up carefully to avoid orthostatic hypotension.
  - Monitoring of blood pressure and pulse are preferable.

6. Enumerate the oral manifestation of renal diseases.

- Chronic renal failure (CRF) produces oral lesions.
- Renal failure leads to uremic toxicity and almost 90% uremic patients manifest changes in oral soft tissues and jaw bones.

Dental Findings

The incidence of caries is reduced in renal patients even in younger age.

Incidence of dental caries in renal patients.

↑Urea content → ↑Buffering capacity of saliva → ↓Dental caries

- Early onset of chronic renal failure lead to defective metabolism of calcium and phosphorous and hence *enamel hypoplasia.*
- Repeated regurgitation and vomiting caused by uremia, medications, and dialysis induced nausea causes *severe erosions* on the lingual aspect of teeth.
- Impairment of calcium and phosphorus metabolism also causes *narrowing of the pulp chamber* and *increased calculus deposition.*
- *Tooth mobility* and *migration* result in *malocclusion.*
- Periapical radiolucencies and root resorption are the radiographic findings of teeth with mobility.

Soft Tissue Changes

- A sudden increase in the blood urea nitrogen (>150 mg/dL) results in *uremic stomatitis.* The mucosa becomes erythematous, covered by grayish surface and then become ulcerative. Frequently affected sites are base of tongue and buccal mucosa.
- The findings will disappear within 2–3 weeks of initiating medical management to decrease the blood urea nitrogen (BUN) level.
- Increased blood urea nitrogen level (BUN >55 mg/dL) results in *uremic frost* (urea crystals after evaporation of saliva), appearing as white patches.
- Oral mucosa will look pale due to anemia, and dry.
- Salivary gland swelling, xerostomia, and retrograde parotitis in some cases.
- Platelet defect results in gingival bleeding, petechiae and ecchymosis in labial and buccal mucosa, soft palate and on the tongue borders.

Bony Changes

Oral manifestations of renal osteodystrophy occur in late stage. Radiographic features are evident in mandible or maxilla due to bone demineralization and loss of trabeculation. The findings include *ground-glass appearance*, complete or partial *loss of lamina dura*, *irregular healing of socket*, *brown tumors* and metastatic calcification.

7. Dental treatment for renal disorder patients.

- *Pretreatment considerations:*
  - When using drugs eliminated by kidney, dose reduction is necessary (penicillin)
  - If the patient is on renal dialysis, dental treatment should be performed on the next day of dialysis (because dialysis will bring back the levels of serum electrolytes, urea, nitrogen, and creatinine to normal).
  - Serological assay for hepatitis B and C viruses (HBV, HCV) and HIV antibody should also be considered.
  - Patients should be evaluated for hypertension or hypotension.
- *During dental treatment:*
  - Eliminating the potential sources of infection and bacteremia.
  - Drugs toxic to the kidney should be avoided (tetracycline, acetaminophen, steroids, ketorolac, nonsteroidal anti-inflammatory drugs).
  - Local hemostatic measures like oxidized cellulose, gelatine matrix, topical thrombin or tranexamic acid should be used during surgical procedures.
  - Short appointments should be scheduled to avoid cramps.
- *Post-treatment considerations:*
  - Postoperative antibiotics should be prescribed for traumatic procedures.
  - Home care oral hygiene procedures should be encouraged.

8. Describe the dental management for asthmatic patients.

Asthma is a reversible, diffuse stenosis or stricture of the peripheral bronchi in respiratory system as an exacerbated response to allergens.

- *Oral findings associated with asthmatic patients*:
  - Reduced salivary flow—dryness of mouth.
  - Increased incidents of dental caries.
  - Increased episodes of gingivitis (due to mouth breathing habit).
  - Candidal infection in patients using nebulizers.
- *Dental management:*
  - Nonsteroidal anti-inflammatory drugs need to be eliminated in prescription especially for nonallergic or intrinsic asthmatic type.
  - Tetracycline and erythromycin should be avoided since it will potentiate the action of theophylline.
  - Self-cured methylacrylic material is highly contraindicated since it may precipitate an asthmatic attack.
  - For patients on long-term systemic steroid, steroid prophylaxis is necessary to avoid steroid crisis.
  - The appointment should be scheduled in the later day to minimize asthmatic attack.
  - If the patient developed an asthmatic attack on the dental chair, the dental procedure should be stopped immediately and all intraoral devices like suction, rubber dam should be cleared. The patient should be positioned in a comfortable position, and proper ventilation should be provided.
  - For patients taking leukotriene modifiers with coumadin have elevated INR and hence invasive surgical procedures should be planned with medical advice.

- Local anesthetic agents with vasoconstrictors have sulfite preservatives and thus precipitate asthmatic attacks. Using LA without sulfite preservatives is safe.
- Patients should be advised to bring their β-2 agonist inhaler medication during their dental appointment to manage any acute asthmatic attack.

If there is no improvement, subcutaneous injection of epinephrine 1:1,000 concentration should be given. In exacerbated conditions, administration of bronchodilators and oxygen are necessary.

9. Management protocol for dental patients with a history of viral hepatitis (or) precautions to be considered for dental patients with hepatitis B.

- It is recommended for dental healthcare workers to receive vaccination against hepatitis.
- The history of hepatitis should be considered as a risk of infection. *No dental treatment* other than emergency care or absolute necessary service should be rendered for patients with *active viral hepatitis* (HBsAg and HBeAg).
- Aerosols should be minimized and *drugs metabolized in the liver avoided* as much as possible (e.g. antibiotics—ampicillin, tetracycline, metronidazole, analgesics like ibuprofen, acetaminophen).
- In patients with liver cirrhosis *prothrombin time increases and platelet count decreases;* hence a preoperative evaluation should be obtained for surgical procedures.
- Utmost care should be provided to *avoid or minimize the soft-tissue trauma* during dental procedures.
- Universal infection control protocol should be strictly adhered—like disinfection of dental units, proper sterilization of instruments, appropriate personal productive measures.

10. Oral manifestations of HIV infection.

Fungal Infection

Pseudomembrane candidiasis and erythematous (atrophic) types are the common oral manifestations. *Candida albicans* and *Candida krusei* are the prime causative organisms.

Viral Infection

- *Herpes simplex infection* occurs due to reactivation of latent virus and manifests as crops of vesicles which tend to rupture and form painful ulcers on oral mucosa including nonkeratinized surfaces.
- *Human herpesvirus 8*—cause AIDS-defining kaposi's sarcoma on hard and soft palates as blue or purple nodules.
- *Human papillomavirus* can cause lesions like verruca vulgaris, Heck's disease, papilloma, and oral wart (condyloma acuminatum).
- *Epstein-Barr virus* produces hairy leukoplakia along the lateral borders of the tongue.

Bacterial Infections

- Linear erythematous gingivitis.
- Necrotizing ulcerative gingivitis and periodontitis (NUG and NUP).

Aphthous Stomatitis

Aphthous minor, aphthous major, and aphthous herpetiform.

Drug-induced Ulcers

Medications used to treat HIV-infection — zidovudine, interferon.

11. Describe systemic lupus erythematosus.

- Systemic lupus erythematosus is an autoimmune disorder. Autoantibodies are produced against self-antigens, and immune-complexes are deposited in vessels and tissues. Females in 20–40 years age group are affected more.

- Types:
  - Discoid lupus erythematosus (DLE)
  - Systemic lupus erythematosus (SLE)
  - Drug-induced lupus erythematosus.

Systemic Lupus Erythematosus

It involves many organs including heart, kidney, hematological organs, mucocutaneous, and central nervous system due to immune complex deposition in small vessels.

Discoid Lupus Erythematosus

- It is limited to skin and mucosa. Malar or butterfly rash is common.
- *Oral manifestations:*
  - Nonspecific ulcerations
  - Angular cheilosis
  - Mucositis
  - Glossitis
  - Salivary gland diseases
- Lip ulcerations show a central region of atrophy and ulceration, surrounded by a white keratotic border of radiating white lines and dots.
- Differential diagnosis: Lichen planus.

Treatment

- High potent topical corticosteroids — 0.05% clobetasol.
- Intralesional steroid injections.

12. Aspirin.

- Aspirin is an effective antiplatelet drug administered as a preventive drug for cardiovascular collapse for patients with coronary artery or peripheral vascular diseases and cerebrovascular accident. It also prevents stroke and myocardial infarction.
- Aspirin exerts an irreversible inhibitory effect on cyclooxygenase (COX-1) which in turn initiate the antithrombotic effect. COX is an enzyme involved in the thromboxane A2. In high dose (≥1 g/day), aspirin also inhibits COX-2 which is a potent vasodilator, an inhibitor of platelet aggregation, and initiates the synthesis of prostacyclin.
- Daily recommended a dose of aspirin is 75–100 mg for most indications whereas 160 mg is suggested for rapid platelet inhibition.
- Side effects: Gastrointestinal disturbance like dyspepsia, erosive gastritis or peptic ulcers.

13. What factors to be considered for drug usage in patients with hepatic dysfunction?

- Hepatic dysfunction is associated with altered effects on the hepatic metabolism of drugs, and this may lead to unusual manifestations of commonly prescribed drugs.
- A dosage reduction should be considered for drugs metabolized in the liver if any of the following conditions present:
  - Serum albumin level of less than 3.5 g/dL.
  - Serum bilirubin level elevated above 2 mg/dL.
  - Elevated ALT and AST (aminotransferase) levels (more than four times normal).
  - Patients with mild to moderate alcoholic liver disease have increased tolerance to local anesthetics and sedative drugs due to enzyme stimulation and require increased dosage for adequate pain control. Hence the increased dose of local anesthetics is needed before dental extraction or other surgical procedures.
  - For patients suffering from advanced liver disease or cirrhosis, the following drugs should be avoided or minimized:
    - Amide group of local anesthetics.
    - Benzodiazepines and other sedatives.
    - Antibiotics—(ampicillin, tetracycline, metronidazole, erythromycin).
    - Analgesics (NSAIDs and aspirin).
    - Barbiturates
    - Imidazole antifungal drugs (Increases drug-induced hepatotoxicity).

14. Discuss dental management for patients with gastroesophageal reflux disease.

- Gastroesophageal reflux disease (GERD) is a lifelong incurable relapsing disorder.
- Erosive GERD—reflux esophagitis is due to the chronic exposure of the lower esophagus to gastric contents.
- Non-erosive GERD or silent GERD—patients with minimal or no mucosal injury but same symptoms of GERD.

Etiopathogenesis

- Motor dysfunction of the lower esophageal sphincter and retrograde flow of the gastric contents through the gastroesophageal junction.
- *Dental consideration:*
  - GERD patients presents with a complaint of hypersensitivity due to dental erosion.
  - Cimetidine and ranitidine are toxic to bone marrow and cause defective marrow function which in turn leads to pale oral mucosa secondary to anemia, mucosal ulcerations due to agranulocytosis, petechiae and gingival bleeding due to thrombocytopenia.
  - Anticholinergic and acid blockers (famotidine) cause xerostomia.
- *Drug interactions to be considered:*
  - Antacids reduce the absorption of tetracycline, erythromycin, and fluoride.
- *Dental management:*
  - Avoid prescribing NSAIDs, aspirin, and steroids which cause intestinal discomfort.
  - Instruct patients to rinse mouth after regurgitation to prevent enamel etching.
  - GERD patients should be advised for periodic dental check-up and topical fluoride application; also to follow good oral hygiene home care practice.
  - Consider premedication of patients with H2 blockers before dental procedures.
  - Advice total and differential blood count for patients with H2 blockers before invasive oral procedures.

15. Define the dental treatment for patients with history of arrhythmia. (or) define dental treatment for patients with a history of congestive heart failure.

- Patients in a state of *controlled angina or congestive heart failure* (angina pectoris) can be treated without any precaution.
- If a patient is reporting with a history of recent episode of angina or angina pectoris (within 6 months), dental treatment should be delayed.
- If patient develops *angina during dental treatment*, the procedure should be discontinued until the cardiac rhythm is stabilized, then treatment should be completed quickly and calmly. (Patient may require hospitalization).
- If *angina pectoris (congestive heart failure) occurs in the midst of dental treatment*, the procedure should be stopped. Oxygen administration should be started, and efforts should be taken to reduce the stress until the pain resolves. Treatment should be continued if necessary, and the patient feels capable of completing it.
- Local anesthetic with vasoconstrictor (epinephrine) 1:100,000 can be used, but 1:50,000 concentration and epinephrine impregnated retraction cords should be strictly avoided.
- *Emergencies to be anticipated:*
  - High blood pressure—patient should be instructed to inform if they develop a sudden headache or feeling jittery.
  - Profuse bleeding beyond what is usual.
  - Sudden arrhythmia—patient may cough or experience catchy feel in the chest.
- *Safety measures to be followed by the dental team:*
  - Be supportive of the patient.
  - Dentist and team members should not be panic, because it will worsen the patient condition by intensifying or prolonging angina.

16. Outline the special considerations for treating dental patients with central nervous system disorders.

Two standard conditions to be considered are stroke and seizures.

1. Stroke

- No special precaution is necessary except for avoiding sudden and rapid movements.
- Psychological support can be provided for better cooperation.
- If oral muscles are flaccid, removable appliances or removable type of dentures should be avoided.
- If swallowing is affected, suction is mandatory.
- If eyelids are affected, eye protection should be given.
- If the patient is on an anticoagulant, lab test should be advised for prothrombin time and INR.
- Patient's guardian should be allowed to stay nearby and asked to inform immediately in case of any signs of stroke is noticed.

2. Seizure

- Patients with a history of poorly-controlled seizures need a medical consultation to carry out the dental treatment.
- Morning appointment is preferred.
- The patient should be asked to take their medication correctly.
- If a patient develops seizures during the treatment, the procedure should be stopped and maximum support should be given to the patient to prevent self-hurts.
- Following the seizure, a decision to continue the treatment depends on patient's status and treatment procedure.

17. Describe the dental management for patients with liver diseases.

Oral Manifestations

- Petechiae, ecchymoses and gingival bleeding due to decreased production of clotting factors.
- Signs of malnutrition like pale oral mucosa, glossitis, and angular cheilitis. (Anemia and vitamin deficiencies).

Dental Management

- The patient should be asked for lab tests; *prothrombin time (PT), partial thromboplastin time (PTT) and INR* to proceed dental treatment like scaling, extraction, and semisurgical procedures.
- Patients with cirrhosis exhibit significant hemostatic defect, hence replacement with fresh frozen plasma and platelets should be considered when planning for surgical procedures.
- Drugs which are metabolized in the liver should be avoided.
- The local anesthetic agent should be used minimally and only if necessary.
- Prescribing mouth rinse containing alcohol should be avoided.
- Easy bleeding for even minor iatrogenic trauma and delayed-wound healing are the potential complications to anticipate.

18. Enumerate the oral changes in post-transplant renal patients.

- Immunosuppressants used to prevent transplant rejection cause gingival enlargement.
- Increased incidents of opportunistic infections.
- Hairy leukoplakia.
- Most common and serious oral complication in these patients is herpes and cytomegalovirus (HSV and CMV) infections.
- Immunosuppression causes mucositis and abnormal bone loss. Petechiae and ecchymosis may also occur.

19. Outline the treatment plan for dental patients with congestive heart diseases.

- Antibiotic prophylaxis should be followed.
- In administering local anesthetics with vasoconstrictors, aspiration should be carried out.
- Gingival retraction cord with epinephrine should be avoided.

- Local hemostatic measures should be followed because of the easy tendency to bleed even for a minor insult (due to platelet dysfunction and increased fibrinolytic activity).

20. Discuss dental treatment for patients with rheumatic heart diseases.

Rheumatic heart disease patients are at the risk of developing infective endocarditis.

Standard regime:

- *For adults:* Capsule amoxicillin 2.0 g—1 hour before dental treatment
- *For children:* Capsule amoxicillin 50 mg/kg body weight—1 hour prior to dental treatment.
- No second dose is needed for adults and children.

The standard regimen for patients allergic to penicillin: Anyone of the following course can be prescribed:

Antibiotic Adult Children

- Tab clindamycin 600 mg—1 hour before dental procedure, 20 mg/kg body weight 1 hour before dental treatment.
- Tab erythromycin 500 mg—1 hour before dental procedure, 15 mg/kg body weight 1 hour previous to the dental treatment.

For patients not able to take oral preparation:

- *Adults:* Ampicillin—2 g by IV (or) IM route—30 minutes before the dental procedure.
- *Children:* Ampicillin—50 mg/kg body weight by IV or IM route—30 minutes before the dental appointment.

For patients not able to take oral medications and history of penicillin allergy:

- *Adults:* Clindamycin 600 mg by IV - ½ hour prior to dental treatment
- *Children:* Clindamycin—20 mg/kg body weight by intravenous route IV—½ hour before the dental appointment.

Antibiotic prophylaxis is essential for the following procedures:

- Extraction
- Subgingival scaling
- Semisurgical procedures like curettage
- Periapical surgery, implant surgery
- Rubber dam, wedge placement.

Antibiotic prophylaxis is not required for:

- Routine endodontic procedures (procedures not extending beyond root apex).
- Investigative and treatment methods that do not cause bleeding.
- Suture removal.

21. Discuss graft-versus-host disease.

- Graft-versus-host disease (GVHD) is a unique side effect of organ transplantation.
- In the oral cavity, it resembles lichen planus and lichenoid reaction, appearing as areas of radiating, fine white lines (hyperkeratosis) on a red base. In severe cases, it seemed eroded and associated with ulceration.
- It is difficult to treat oral lesions and require a change of immunosuppressive agent. However, topical application of cyclosporine or azathioprine may be beneficial. PUVA therapy with ultraviolet irradiation is also useful.
- Other than oral mucosa, GVHD involves gastrointestinal tract, skin, and liver.

22. Discuss angioneurotic edema.

- Angioneurotic edema is an anaphylactic reaction. Blood vessels in the deeper subcutaneous tissues are dilated with increased fluid and leukocyte permeability into tissue space resulting in edema.
- The recurrent type is inherited, but in the majority of cases, it is idiopathic.
- It frequently involves lips, tongue, and surrounding areas of eyes.
- If the posterior part of tongue or larynx is involved, a respiratory arrest may occur.

Management

- Around 50 mg of diphenhydramine hydrochloride—4 times/day till the swelling subsides.
- In severe cases (laryngeal edema), subcutaneous injection of 0.5 mL of 1:1,000 epinephrine (or) 0.2 mL of intravenous administration of epinephrine will be useful.

23. Discuss dental management for patients with chronic obstructive pulmonary disorder (or) dental management for patients with chronic bronchitis (or) dental management for patients with emphysema.

- Chronic obstructive pulmonary disorder (COPD) (chronic bronchitis or emphysema) is a slowly progressive airway obstructive disorder which is not completely curable. Most commonly affected age group is above 40 years and smoking is the potential etiology.
- History should be taken clearly in addition to reviewing of medical records to rule out coexisting cardiac disorders and adrenal insufficiency status (due to corticosteroid therapy).
- For high-risk patients (Patients with dyspnea at rest, chronic respiratory failure, etc.) dental treatment should be given in hospital set-up.
- *Dental consideration:*
  - Precautious steps should be taken to avoid procedures that could compromise respiration (like avoid using rubber dam).
  - Dental procedures should be carried out in an upright or semisupine chair position.
  - The pulse oximeter can be used to check the oxygen saturation rate during dental treatment. (A drop in SaO_2 to 94% indicates impaired oxygen and need for intervention).
  - Nitrous oxide inhalation sedation should be avoided.

24. Discuss dental management for patients with history of congestive heart failure, (or) coronary failure, (or) ventricular failure.

- In congestive heart failure (CHF), the heart is unable to pump the usual amount of blood. The causes include coronary artery diseases, hypertension, cardiomyopathy, valvular heart diseases, and mitral stenosis.
- *Dental management:*
  - Medical consultation with patient's cardiologist is mandatory before dental treatment.
  - For untreated or uncontrolled CHF patients, elective dental procedures should be avoided.
  - For patients with class I or II CHF, under regular medical care, elective procedures can be carried out using a limited quantity of local anesthetics with vasoconstrictors.
  - For patients with class III CHF, local anesthetics without vasoconstrictors should be used.
  - For patients with class IV CHF, emergency and minimally invasive procedures alone can be carried out in a hospital set-up.
  - Change in chair position should be carried out slowly.
  - Dental appointment should be short scheduled.

MULTIPLE CHOICE QUESTIONS

1. Hepatitis B virus infection is known as ***serum hepatitis***.
   a. Yellow fever
   b. Serum hepatitis
   c. Viral hepatitis
   d. Epidemic hepatitis
2. Uremic stomatitis is considered as a ***chemical burn***.
   a. Fixed drug eruption
   b. Renal disorder
   c. Lichenoid reaction
   d. Chemical burn
3. *Socket sclerosis* is associated with ***renal osteodystrophy***.
   a. Renal osteodystrophy
   b. Pulse granuloma
   c. Brown tumor
   d. Osteoradionecrosis

4. Oral changes associated with the use of steroid nebulizers are ***candidiasis***.
   a. Dysgeusia
   b. Numbness
   c. Candidiasis
   d. Herpetiform ulcers
   (**Note:** Oral changes associated with the use of steroid nebulizers are candidiasis and tongue hypertrophy).
5. Anemia in patients with renal disease is the type of ***normocytic and normochromic***.
   a. Normocytic and normochromic
   b. Normocytic and hypochromic
   c. Microcytic and hypochromic
   d. Macrocytic and hyperchromic
6. The necessary precaution in prescribing penicillin for patients with renal diseases is ***dose reduction***.
   a. Avoid penicillin
   b. Dose reduction
   c. Avoid oral route
   d. Drug combination
7. Jaundice occurs when total serum bilirubin level is ≥ ***3 mg/dL***.
   a. <3 mg/dL
   b. ≥3mg/dL
   c. <5 mg/dL
   d. ≥5 mg/dL
8. Oral manifestation of eating disorders (anorexia and bulimia) is ***enamel erosion***.
   a. Coated tongue
   b. Enamel erosion
   c. Dry mouth
   d. Sialectasia
   (**Note:** Oral manifestation of eating disorders (anorexia and bulimia) is enamel erosion on the lingual surface of maxillary teeth).
9. Anorexia is the condition of ***intentional starvation***.
   a. Binge eating
   b. Orthorexia nervosa
   c. Intentional starvation
   d. Rumination syndrome
10. Plummer-Vinson syndrome is also referred as ***hysterical dysphagia***.
    a. Hysterical dysphagia
    b. Nutritional anemia
    c. Spastic motility disorder
    d. Cooley's disease
11. HIV-2 is associated with the ***indolent course***.
    a. Rapid spread
    b. Active phase
    c. *Short incubation period*
    d. *Indolent course*
    (**Note:** *HIV-2 is associated with the more indolent course and less efficient transmission*).
12. The median time for AIDS in HIV-2 infection is ***20 years***.
    a. 10 years
    b. 20 years
    c. 5 years
    d. 6 months
    (**Note:** The median time for AIDS in HIV-1 infection is 10 years, and HIV-2 infection is 20 years).
13. Average CD4 cell count is ***≥500–600 cells/mm³***.
    a. ≥10,000–12,000 cells/mm³
    b. ≥5,000–8,000 cells/mm³
    c. ≥100–300 cells/mm³
    d. ≥500–600 cells/mm³
14. AIDS occur when CD4 count is ***<200 cells/mm³***.
    a. <500 cells/mm³
    b. <400 cells/mm³
    c. <200 cells/mm³
    d. <10 cells/mm³
15. The immune level in HIV-infected individuals is assessed by ***CD4 cell count***.
    a. CD4 cell count
    b. Viral load
    c. Drug response rate
    d. Morbidity rate
16. Acute HIV-infection develops ***2–6 weeks after exposure***.
    a. Immediately after exposure
    b. 3–6 months after exposure
    c. 2–6 weeks after exposure
    d. At the time of exposure
17. In the acute stage of HIV infection, patients establish ***high plasma levels of virus***.
    a. Low plasma levels of virus
    b. High plasma levels of virus
    c. Proactive phase of virus
    d. Dormant phase of virus
18. Antibodies to HIV develop after ***2–3 months of exposure***.
    a. 2–3 weeks of exposure
    b. 2–3 months of exposure

c. 6–12 weeks after exposure
d. After 12 months of exposure

19. Diagnosis of primary HIV-infection is positive ***HIV-RNA test with negative HIV-antibody test***.
a. Positive HIV-RNA test with positive HIV-antibody test
b. Negative HIV-RNA test with positive HIV-antibody test
c. Negative HIV-RNA test with negative HIV-antibody test
d. Positive HIV-RNA test with negative HIV-antibody test

20. Heck's disease is caused by ***human papilloma-virus***.
a. Human herpes virus
b. Human immunodeficiency virus
c. Human zoster virus
d. Human papilloma virus

21. Tuberculous lymph node is known as ***scrofula***.
a. Metastatic node
b. Sentinel node
c. Cold abscess
d. Scrofula

22. Wiskott-Aldrich syndrome is characterized by ***lymphocyte abnormalities***.
a. Elevated platelet count
b. Altered red cells
c. Absence of eosinophils
d. Lymphocyte abnormalities

23. Butterfly rash is common in ***seborrheic dermatitis***.
a. Erythema multiforme
b. Systemic lupus erythematosus
c. Seborrheic dermatitis
d. Rosacea
(**Note:** Butterfly rash is common in *discoid* lupus erythematosus and seborrheic dermatitis).

24. Restricted movement of mandible in scleroderma is due to ***pseudoankylosis***.
a. Condylar atrophy
b. Disk degeneration
c. Muscle spasm
d. Pseudoankylosis

25. The mask-like face is seen in ***scleroderma***.
a. Trigeminal neuralgia
b. Bell's palsy
c. Risus sardonicus
d. Scleroderma
(**Note:** The mask-like face is seen in scleroderma is due to loss of skin folds around the mouth).

26. Heparin is an ***anticoagulant***.
a. Anticoagulant
b. Antithrombotic
c. Vitamin K agonists
d. Promote angiogenesis
(**Note:** Heparin acts by *activating the enzyme antithrombin* (Antithrombin inhibits the clotting enzymes thrombin and factor Xa).

27. Drug contraindicated in patients with the liver disorder is ***acetaminophen***.
a. Acetaminophen
b. Doxycycline
c. Amoxicillin
d. Tramadol
(**Note:** Drugs to be avoided in patients with the liver disorder are erythromycin, tetracycline, ketoconazole, and acetaminophen).

28. The common dental findings in cystic fibrosis is ***anterior open bite***.
a. Premature eruption
b. Delayed exfoliation
c. Anterior open bite
d. Multiple unerupted teeth
(**Note:** Enamel hypoplasia and anterior open bite are common dental findings in cystic fibrosis).

29. Salivary gland involvement in cystic fibrosis leads to ***altered sialochemistry***.
a. Thick and scanty saliva
b. Altered sialochemistry
c. Salivary gland cysts
d. Sialadenosis
(**Note:** *Altered sialochemistry* is the altered level of salivary electrolytes, proteins, and enzymes).

30. Oral mucosal manifestation of Crohn's disease is ***mucosal tags***.
a. Mucosal tags
b. Fibroepithelial polyps
c. Squamous cell carcinoma
d. Pyostomatitis vegetans
(**Note:** Cobblestone appearance and mucosal tags are the oral mucosal manifestation of Crohn's disease).

VIVA VOCE

1. Why NSAIDs should be avoided in patients with renal diseases?

NSAIDs should not be used because they may induce:

- Sodium retention
- Impairment of diuretics functions
- Inhibition of aldosterone production
- Decreased perfusion of renal arteries
- Acidosis.

2. What is bulimia nervosa?

Bulimia is the condition of consuming large amount of food and immediately acts against weight gain by inducing forcible vomiting, using laxatives or diuretics, and aggressive physical workouts.

3. Enumerate the causes for periodontitis in diabetic patients.

- Defective neutrophil chemotaxis
- Increased collagen breakdown
- Microangiopathy causing poor peripheral circulation.

4. What are the complications expected in dental treatment of diabetic patients?

If extraction was carried out, there are increased chances for:

- Delayed wound healing (Due to microangiopathy).
- Dry socket.

5. Name few immunosuppressive drugs.

- *Cyclosporine*—reversibly inhibits immunocompetent lymphocytes and calcineurin.
- *Tacrolimus*—suppress T-cell activation.
- *Azathioprine*—inhibits DNA and RNA synthesis
- *Corticosteroids*—suppresses activated macrophages.

6. What is autoimmune disorder?

It is a condition where the body reacts against self components (Its own cells, and tissues).

7. What is immunnocomplex disease?

It is a type of autoimmune disease in which antigen-antibody complexes combine with complement and cause conditions like vasculitis, systemic lupus erythematosus, glomerulonephritis, Behcet's syndrome and erythema multiforme.

8. What is hypersensitivity reaction?

It is a state where immune system reacts against a risk-free antigen in out of proportion.

9. Enumerate systemic conditions that require antibiotic prophylaxis for dental treatment.

- Previous history of bacterial endocarditis
- Prosthetic cardiac valves
- Acquired valvular dysfunction
- Mitral valve prolapsed with regurgitation
- Congenital cyanotic cardiac diseases
- Cardiomyopathy
- Pulmonary shunts.

BIBLIOGRAPHY

1. Abel SN, Fischman SL, Glick M, Phelan JA. Principles of Oral Health Management for the HIV/AIDS Patient. Dental Alliance for AIDS/HIV Care (DAAC). 2000.
2. Aframian DJ, Lalla RV, Peterson DE. Management of dental patients taking common hemostasis-altering medications. Oral Surg Oral Med Oral Pathol Oral Radiol Endod. 2007; 03:S45.
3. Bramante RM, Rand M. Angioedema. New England Journal of Medicine. 2011; 365(2):e4.
4. Bricker SL, Langlais RP, Miller CS. Oral diagnosis, oral medicine, and treatment planning. Lea and Febiger; 1994.
5. Claramunt Lozano A, Sarrión Pérez MG, Gavaldá Esteve C. Dental considerations in patients with respiratory problems. J Clin Exp Dent.2011;3(3):e222-7.

6. Douglas LR, Douglass JB, Sieck JO, et al. Oral management of the patient with end-stage liver disease and the liver transplant patient. Oral Surg Oral Med Oral Pathol Oral Radiol Endod. 1998;86(1):55-64.
7. Field EA, Longman LP. Tyldesley's oral medicine. 5th edition, 2003, Oxford University Press; Oxford.
8. Scully C, Carrozzo M, Gandolfo S, et al. Update on mucous membrane pemphigoid: a heterogeneous immune-mediated subepithelial blistering entity. Oral Surg Oral Med Oral Pathol Oral Radiol Endod. 1999;88(1):56-68.
9. Scully C. Medical problems in dentistry E-Book. 2010, Elsevier Health Sciences.
10. Tong DC, Rothwell BR. Antibiotic prophylaxis in dentistry: a review and practice recommendations. J Am Dent Assoc. 2000;131(3):366-74.

CHAPTER 7

Bleeding Disorders

HIGHLIGHTS

This chapter deals with the management of dental patients with various bleeding disorders. Hemostatic disorders have characteristic findings in the mouth and the facial structures. Many of these signs are nonspecific, but instruct the dental surgeon about the chances for a coexisting hematological disease. It is essential in dental practice to understand the risk of bleeding when performing semisurgical and surgical procedures with consideration of their medication and provide safe care.

Learners are expected to know:

- The various causes of oral bleeding.
- The presence of a systemic pathologic process.
- The precautions to provide the preventive, conservative and invasive treatment procedures for dental patients with bleeding disorders.
- Laboratory tests of the hemostatic system.
- Various hemostatic agents.

ESSAY QUESTIONS

1. Classify the common bleeding disorders and add a note on oral manifestations in different conditions.

- Classification of bleeding disorders:
  - Coagulation factor deficiencies
  - Platelet disorders
  - Vascular disorders
  - Fibrinolytic defects

Coagulation Factor Deficiencies

Congenital

- Factor VIII and IX deficiencies (hemophilia A and hemophilia B)
- von Willebrand disease (deficiency in factor VIII protein complex)
- Other factor deficiencies (factor XI, XII, X, V, XIII — rare).

Acquired

- Liver disease
- Vitamin K deficiency
- Heparin and coumarin therapy
- Disseminated intravascular coagulation.

Platelet Disorders

Quantitative disorders —thrombocytopenia

- *Congenital*
  - Immune-mediated
  - Collagen vascular disease
  - Sarcoidosis
- *Acquired*
  - Idiopathic thrombocytopenic purpura
  - Disseminated intravascular coagulation
  - Microangiopathic hemolytic anemia
  - Leukemia
  - Myelofibrosis
  - Aplastic anemia
  - Systemic lupus erythematosus
  - Infection — HIV, malaria, mononucleosis
  - Cytotoxic chemotherapy
  - Drug-induced — rifampin, quinine.

Qualitative disorder (nonthrombocytopenic or functional platelet defect)

- *Congenital*
  - Glanzmann's thrombasthenia
  - Platelet-type von Willebrand disease
  - Bernard-Soulier syndrome
- *Acquired*
  - Drug-induced
  - Liver disease
  - Alcoholism

Vascular disorders (vessel wall disorders)

- Scurvy
- Purpura
- Hereditary hemorrhagic telangiectasia
- Cushing's syndrome
- Ehlers-Danlos syndrome

Fibrinolytic defects

- Disseminated intravascular coagulation
- Streptokinase therapy

Oral manifestations of bleeding disorders

- Spontaneous gingival bleeding, petechiae, ecchymosis—multiple, small.
  - Characteristic of vascular and platelet disorders.
  - Unusual in coagulation disorders.
- Bleeding from surface injuries and scratches due to:
  - Continuous and profuse bleeding in vascular and platelet disorders.
  - Minimal in coagulation disorders.
- Delayed bleeding, hematomas:
  - Characteristic of coagulation disorders
  - Rare in vascular and platelet disorders.

2. Briefly describe the anemic conditions associated with orofacial manifestations.

- Anemic conditions with orofacial manifestations are:
  - Iron-deficiency anemia
  - Plummer-Vinson syndrome
  - Megaloblastic anemia
  - Sickle cell anemia
  - Thalassemia
  - Aplastic anemia

Iron-deficiency Anemia

- It is the most prevalent type of hematological disorder and manifests in the orofacial region as:
  - Tongue atrophy (atrophic glossitis)
  - Pale mucosa
  - Angular cheilitis

Atrophic glossitis is characterized by patchy, or diffuse, atrophy of papilla on the dorsal aspect of the tongue (*flattening of the tongue papillae*), giving the appearance of a smooth, red and shiny tongue. In the advanced state, tenderness and burning sensation of the tongue will be present.

Angular stomatitis is a condition characterized by painful fissures at the corners of the lip. The common etiology include iron deficiency and candidal infection. Treatment must focus on iron supplementation and anticandidal therapy. Iron deficiency state may also lead to peeling of superficial peeling of epithelium at the lips and at the angle of mouth associated with dryness known as *Cheilosis*.

Plummer-Vinson Syndrome

It is also known as Paterson-Brown-Kelly syndrome and sideropenic dysphagia. It is caused by iron deficiency. Women are frequently affected.

The features of this syndrome include atrophic glossitis, angular cheilitis, and difficulty in swallowing. The formation of esophageal web (a ring-like membrane of 2–3 mm thick composed of normal esophageal structure (mucosa and submucosa and protrudes into esophagus) causes dysphagia. Other associated findings include koilonychia (or spoon nails), pharyngoesophageal ulcerations and white, keratotic lesions in the oral mucosa. This syndrome may rarely lead to carcinoma of the esophagus and throat due to the increased turnover rate of epithelial cells in the upper digestive tract. Barium swallow study and fluoroscopic evaluation will confirm the diagnosis.

Megaloblastic Anemia

It is caused by vitamin B12 and folic acid deficiency and is slowly progressing condition. The oral manifestations include glossitis, stomatitis, and recurrent aphthous ulcers. These findings are associated with the altered-metabolic status of oral epithelial cells.

Magenta tongue or Beefy red tongue is due to decreased epithelial thickness and is a characteristic of B12 deficiency. Oral changes are the early manifestations and occur before the sign of anemic symptoms or macrocytosis.

Sickle Cell Anemia

It is a hereditary disorder with the presence of the abnormal hemoglobin S. There is a genetic replacement of valine by glutamic acid of the β-polypeptide chain of DNA at the sixth position. This change alters hemoglobin and subsequently the structure of red cells which acquires a sickle shape.

- Hemoglobin value in sickle cell patients is reduced and is in the range between 5–9 g/dL. The white blood cell count ranges is elevated and between 12,000–20,000 cells/mm^3.
- The life expectancy is variable because these patients may undergo sickle cell crisis due to microvascular occlusion and multisystem complications.
- Facial changes include increased thickening of skull and osteoporotic changes, tendency for a protruding maxilla and mandible, osteomyelitis of mandible, and mental nerve paresthesia.
- Oral and dental findings include pale mucosa, late eruption, malocclusion, hypoplastic enamel, midline diastema, and asymptomatic pulpal necrosis. The radiographic changes comprise coarse-trabecular pattern of mandible, step-ladder appearance of alveolar bone.
- Radiographic findings include:
  - The sparse and coarse trabecular pattern gives rise to the generalized radiolucent appearance jaw bones.
  - Inferior border of the mandible appears thin.
  - Generalized osteoporosis commonly caused by salmonella infections.
  - Step-ladder appearance in the interdental bone is due to the horizontal trabeculation.

Thalassemia

Thalassemia is a hereditary hemolytic anemia. There is a defective synthesis of α or β polypeptide chains of hemoglobin (α-thalassemia, β-thalassemia).

Classification:

1. Homozygous thalassemia
2. Homozygous β-thalassemia (Cooley's anemia or Mediterranean anemia, or thalassemia major) is prevalent among the Mediterranean population (Greece, Turkey, Cyprus and Southern Italy).
3. β-thalassemia is characterized by significant orofacial malformations and severe anemia. Hypoxia and cardiac failure in early infancy lead to a short span of life. To overcome the anemic changes, bone marrow produces more red cells and shows hyperplasia and expansion.
4. The marrow changes result in following facial malformations:
   - The affected individuals have a pathgnomonic *chipmunk face* due to larger and prominent maxilla, frontal bossing, and prominent malar processes.
   - The maxilla-mandible discrepancy leads to class II malocclusion with increased overjet and spacing between maxillary teeth.
5. Heterozygous thalassemia (thalassemia minor)
6. Heterozygous thalassemia is a minor form and is asymptomatic. On peripheral smear analysis, it shows hypochromic and microcytic pattern.
7. Compound heterozygous thalassemia

3. Classify hematological malignancies of white blood cells. Describe the etiopathogenesis, oral manifestations, investigations and dental consideration for leukemia.

Hematologic malignancies are leukemia, lymphoma and plasma cell tumors.

Leukemia

- Leukemia is associated with excessive exposure to ionizing radiation, certain chemicals (benzene), and some viral infections (e.g. Epstein-Barr virus, human lymphotropic virus). The result is the abnormal proliferation of white blood cell-forming tissues which leads to increased number of immature and abnormal white blood cells in the circulation.
- *Classification of leukemia:* Based on the type of hematopoietic stem and progenitor cells affected:
  - Acute myelogenous leukemia (AML)
  - Acute lymphocytic leukemia (ALL)
  - Chronic myelogenous leukemia (CML)
  - Chronic lymphocytic leukemia (CLL)
- *Oral manifestations:*
  - *Gingival enlargement:* Leukemic cells infiltrate into the gingival tissue and cause gingival hyperplasia. The inter-dental papillae, marginal, and attached gingiva become progressively enlarged. In severe form, the crowns are covered by gingiva. Gingival hyperplasia is prevalent in acute leukemia than the chronic variety. Leukemic chemotherapy will helps to control the hyperplastic growth to a greater extent.
  - Gingiva appears swollen, pale pink to purple color, and with loss of stippling.
  - Ulceration: Atypical mucosal ulcers are present.
  - Unprovoked bleeding from gingiva and petechiae.
  - Herpetic infections and candidiasis.
- *Lab investigations*
  - The peripheral granulocyte count is strikingly increased in chronic leukemia, whereas in acute leukemia, the count may either increased (with numerous blast forms), decreased, or normal.
  - Atypical hematopoietic cells in the bone marrow.
  - Cytogenetic analysis of chromosomal abnormalities.

Oral complications in leukemic patients:

- Spontaneous, severe bleeding gums.
- Pulpal and periodontal infections may lead to osteonecrosis of the jaw bones.
- Corticosteroid therapy may results in opportunistic candidal infection.

Dental care for leukemic patients:

- A detailed-history, comprehensive oral examination, and full mouth radiographic examination are necessary for treatment planning. Treatment should be carried out after consulting the hematologists.
- Preventive dental care need to be started prior to leukemic treatment (chemotherapy or radiotherapy).
- Patients in long-term remission can go for any dental treatment, but patients in severe or relapse condition should be provided with palliative or emergency dental treatment alone.

4. Dental treatment for patients with bleeding disorders.

- The severity of the bleeding disorder and the invasiveness of the dental procedure will determine the course of dental treatment in these patients.
- If the dental treatment is minimally invasive and the bleeding disorder is a *milder form*, only minor or no changes are needed.
- For patients with *severe bleeding disorders*, revising the hemostatic system to satisfactory level and hemostatic measures using local and adjunctive methods are necessary. The hematologist should be consulted before planning for invasive dental procedures.
- *Oral surgical procedure:* For coagulation disorders, transfusion of right factors with, 50–100% of normal levels is mandatory.

Local hemostatic techniques like pressure, surgical packs, sutures, and surgical stents may also be applied independently or in combination.

- *Periodontal procedures:* Gingival probing and supragingival scaling can be carried out safely. Subgingival scaling and root planning may also be carried out carefully without inducing bleeding. Factor replacement is necessary only for extensive periodontal surgery and to give nerve blocks. Bleeding can be controlled at the surgical site by using local hemostatic materials and conventional mouthguards. Postoperative bleeding can be control with the use of hemostatic mouth rinse containing tranexamic acid or aminocaproic acid.
- *Restorative and endodontic procedures:* Dental restorations do not carry the bleeding risk. Appropriate care should be taken to avoid soft-tissue injury when using instruments and rubber dam. Routine endodontic therapy can be performed without any special attention but, surgical endodontic procedures require factor replacement therapy.
- *Prosthodontic procedures:* Careful post-insertion adjustments will minimize trauma. Oral tissue should be handled carefully during prosthesis fabrication to reduce the risk of ecchymosis.
- *Orthodontic procedures:* Orthodontic treatment can be carried out without any modification. The appliances should not impinge on soft-tissues, and good oral hygiene practice should be encouraged.
- *Medical management:*
  - Nonsteroidal anti-inflammatory drugs should not be prescribed for patients with antiplatelet and anticoagulant medications because of their increased risk of bleeding.
  - Penicillins, erythromycin, metronidazole, tetracyclines, and miconazole potentiate the action of warfarin.
  - Physician's advice is mandatory before prescribing these drugs.
- *Patients on antiplatelet drugs:* In most cases, no need to stop antiplatelet drugs like aspirin (ASA), clopidogrel and dipyridamole. Local hemostatic measures are adequate to control bleeding. Before modifying the drug regimen, the patient's physician should be consulted.
- *Patients on anticoagulant drugs:*
  - For patients taking *warfarin*, the international normalized ratio (INR) should be checked before invasive procedures. The normal range is 2.0–3.0. When INR is below 3.0, dental surgery can be carried out routinely and no need to revise warfarin dose.
  - Heparin is administered for end-stage renal patients undergoing dialysis. Dental procedure should be carried out on the days when the patient is not posted for dialysis.

5. Describe the pathogenesis and orofacial manifestations of lymphomas.

- Lymphoma is a solid malignancy of the reticuloendothelial system which cares the body's immune mechanism. Lymphocytes are the affected cells.
- Lymphomas are of two types: Hodgkin's and non-Hodgkin's. About 90% of cases are non-Hodgkin's type, while about 10% is Hodgkin's type.
- In non-Hodgkin's type, both B and T lymphocytes are affected, whereas, in Hodgkin's lymphoma, only an abnormal type of B lymphocyte named Reed-Sternberg cells are involved.
- *Non-Hodgkin's lymphoma (NHL):*
  - Non-Hodgkin's lymphoma is the second prevalent oropharyngeal tumor next to squamous cell carcinoma. It occurs at an extranodal site in 40% of cases and 2–3% of these cases occur in the mouth and jaw bones. Waldeyer's ring, salivary glands, and maxilla are the

common sites, although any region may be affected. Oral lesions appear as a red and painless enlargement. Surface ulceration occurs when subjected to trauma. However, deep oral ulcerations are rare. The mobility of teeth is common in the affected jaw, and rarely paresthesia will occur. The characteristic *symptoms* include a fever of unknown origin (>38°C), weight loss (>10% over 6 months), drenching night sweats, visceral pain, and malaise.

- Radiographic findings include generalized bone resorption and loss of the lamina dura. The *loss of the lamina dura* in lymphoma patients may be related to the effects of *tumor cell infiltration* and in some cases may be because of the release of *osteoclast-activating factors* from the lymphoid cells.
- *Non-Hodgkin's lymphoma* is classified as indolent, aggressive, and highly aggressive.
  - *Indolent lymphoma* accounts for 40% of all NHL with the most common type being follicular lymphoma. Aggressive lymphoma approximately represents 50% of cases and occurs as diffuse large B-cell lymphoma and T-cell natural killer (NK) cell lymphoma. The highly aggressive form includes Burkitt's lymphoma and lymphoblastic lymphoma.
  - *Burkitt's lymphoma:* It is a fast-growing tumor. Three types are recognized:
    1. Endemic (African): Primarily affects African children in the age group of 4–7 and has a preference for boys with 2:1 ratio.
    2. Sporadic (non-African): It occurs worldwide and accounts for 1–2% of adult lymphoma cases.
    3. Immunodeficiency-associated: This variant of Burkitt's lymphoma occurs in HIV or AIDS patients. It represents 30–40% of non-Hodgkin's lymphoma in HIV-patients and also an AIDS-defining disease.

Symptoms

The symptoms of Burkitt's lymphoma vary among subtypes. The endemic variant starts with tumors involving the jaw or other facial bones.

Investigations

- Computed tomography (CT) and magnetic resonance imaging (MRI): If neurologic signs or symptoms are present.
- Bone scanning and plain radiography: When associated with bone symptoms.

Treatment

Intensive chemotherapy is the main treatment.

- Cyclophosphamide
- Cytarabine
- Doxorubicin
- Etoposide
- Methotrexate
- Vincristine

- *Hodgkin's lymphoma (Hodgkin's disease):*
  - The frequent manifestation is cervical lymphadinopathy and extranodal Hodgkin's lymphoma is extremely rare. The tumor spreads via the lymphatic channels in a characteristic pattern and hence the treatment results in good prognosis.
  - If extranodal Hodgkin's lymphoma occurs, it presents as swelling and ulcers on oral mucosa of the palate, tonsils, floor of mouth, vestibule, and alveolus.

SHORT NOTES

1. International normalized ratio (INR).

The prothrombin time (PT) is highly variable because different thromboplastins are derived from different sources are nonstandardized. Prothrombin time performed on the same sample at different laboratories revealed different results. To standardize the PT, the INR was introduced by World Health Organization (WHO) in 1983.

Method

- The INR is a ratio and has no units.
- The first point in the INR calculation is to *normalize* the PT by comparing it with the mean standard prothrombin time (MNPT—the mean prothrombin time of the healthy adult individuals).
- In the next step, the ratio is raised to a power nominated by international sensitivity index (ISI). The ISI is a function of the thromboplastin reagent. Two data groups are used to obtain the ISI:
  1. Healthy adult people.
  2. Patients stabilized on warfarin.
- The normal INR is typical of 1.0 but varies from 0.9–1.1. During Warfarin administration, the INR increases between 2 and 3.5.
- This test assesses the extrinsic pathway of coagulation and measures factors I, II, V, VII, and X.

Purpose

International normalized ratio is helpful in evaluating the effectiveness of warfarin. Warfarin therapy is indicated to prevent clot formation and at the same time to avoid excess bleeding. The INR is used to adjust a person's warfarin dose and to bring the PT into an acceptable range.

Inference

- No dental surgical procedure is recommended when INR is >3.5–4.
- For full mouth extraction, INR should be <2–3.
- For flap surgery and multiple transalveolar extractions, INR should be <1.5.

2. Outline the medical consideration for dental patients with liver diseases.

- In liver diseases, the production of clotting factors (factor II, VII, IX and X, vitamin K) is reduced due to parenchymal damage and obstruction. These patients exhibit bleeding tendency depending on the extent of their liver disease.
- Viral hepatitis patients are a source of cross-infection, and so necessary precautions should be taken during procedures.
- Management of hemostatic defects in liver disease:
  - Vitamin K and freshly frozen plasma infusion for prolonged prothrombin time and partial thromboplastin time.
  - Cryoprecipitate is the choice for replacement for factor VIII deficiency and disseminated intravascular coagulation.
  - The impaired liver function necessitates dose modification before drug administration in these patients. The patient's physician should be consulted for the same.

3. Dental consideration for patients with platelet disorders. (or) dental management for patients with thrombocytopenic purpura.

Thrombocytopenia is a platelet disorder manifest due to the following abnormalities:

- Decreased bone marrow production of platelets
- Increased platelet destruction
- Platelet sequestration due to enlarged spleen.

There are two types of platelet disorders:

1. Idiopathic thrombocytopenic purpura (ITP).
2. Thrombotic thrombocytopenic purpura.

Idiopathic thrombocytopenic purpura is characterized by mild to a severe decrease in platelet count, with bone marrow in relatively healthy condition, and by mucocutaneous bleeding with the absence of other abnormalities.

Pathogenesis

The reason for platelet reduction is idiopathic (unknown). The autoimmune reaction of platelet destruction seems to participate in this process.

Signs and Symptoms

- An important general symptom is the presence of petechiae and indicates capillary bleeding.
- Oral manifestations—in advanced or severe stage:
  - Gingival bleeding is the first indicator of thrombocytopenia many times. Profuse bleeding occurs either spontaneously, or following a minor trauma induced by tooth brushing and flossing.
  - Hematomas and hemorrhagic bullae.
  - Petechiae and ecchymosis in the soft palate and buccal mucosa.

Investigations

- The complete blood count (CBC) is useful in the diagnosis.
- The reduced number of platelets supports the diagnosis of thrombocytopenia.
  - When platelet levels are between 50,000/mm^3 and 100,000/mm^3, mild clinical manifestations can occur because the platelets still maintain the capacity for hemostatic equilibrium.
  - When the platelet number is below 50,000/mm^3, it suggests purpuric manifestations.
  - Below 30,000/mm^3, the symptoms and signs are more intense; when between 10,000/mm^3 and 5,000/mm^3, the hemorrhagic phenomena can be critical.
- Platelet function is evaluated by bleeding time (BT) and is prolonged in thrombocytopenia (>5 min). Clot retraction may be deficient or absent with only a slight absorption of prothrombin 1 hour after coagulation.

Dental Consideration

- Dental treatment of ITP patients should correlate with the presentation of disease and physicians help should be taken to proceed.
  - Dental treatment is indicated when the platelet counts above 50,000/mm^3.
  - If the platelet count is very low (10,000–20,000/mcL), dental treatment is contraindicated. In emergency situations, the patient should be supported with IV Immunoglobulin (IVIg) combined with IV methylprednisolone to provide the needful assistance.
  - In routine condition, prednisone 1–2 mg/kg/day is the initial treatment option.

4. What is tourniquet test? (or) capillary fragility test (or) Rumpel-Leede phenomenon.

- Tourniquet test is a marker of capillary fragility.
- *Method:*
  - Record of the patient's blood pressure by covering 2/3rd of the arm with a sphygmomanometer.
  - Calculating the mean blood pressure—systole+diastole/2.
  - The cuff should be retained at mean blood pressure for 5 minutes.
  - About 2 minutes following cuff deflation and removal, petechiae should be counted in 4 cm distal surface of antecubital fossa.
  - A positive test is 10 or more petechiae per 1 square inch.
- In normal conditions, for men, the number of petechiae is up to 5, whereas in women and children up to 10 petechiae appear but do not go beyond 10.

5. Enumerate the dental management for hemophilic patients.

- *Hemophilia A*—invasive dental procedures need physician's assistance. Factor VIII replacement may be necessary.
  - Desmopressin (DDAVP) is valuable to achieve a transient rise in factor VIII level. This drug is adequate to meet hemostasis in mild hemophilia. Desmopressin is administered along with

antifibrinolytic agents to enhance its effectiveness. Hemostatic mouth rinse is helpful in postoperative care. Epsilon aminocaproic acid and tranexamic acid are the frequently used antifibrinolytic hemostatic oral rinses.

- *Hemophilia B* is factor IX deficiency disease. Replacement therapy manages it with highly purified, virally inactivated factor IX concentrates.

6. Briefly describe the systemic management of patients with bleeding disorders.

For irreversible coagulopathies, systemic replacement of missing factors may be necessary.
The standard agents used are:

Platelets

- *Platelets:* 1 unit = 50 mL; and raise count by 6,000.
- *Indications:* Platelet count:
  - It is less than 10,000 in nonbleeding individuals.
  - It is less than 50,000 in presurgical level.
  - It is less than 50,000 in actively-bleeding individuals.
- Nondestructive thrombocytopenia.

Fresh Frozen Plasma

Fresh frozen plasma: 1 unit = 150–250 mL, contains factors II, VII, IX, X, XI, XII, XIII and heat-labile V and VII.

- *Indications:*
  - Undiagnosed bleeding disorder with active bleeding.
  - Severe liver disease.
  - When transfusing is greater than 10 units of blood.
  - Immune globulin deficiency.

Cryoprecipitate

- Cryoprecipitate: 1 unit = 10–15 mL.
- *Indications:*
  - Hemophilia A, von Willebrand disease
  - When specific factor concentrates are unavailable.
  - Fibrinogen deficiency.

Factor VIII Concentrate

- *Factor VIII concentrate:* 1 unit raises factor VIII level by 2%
- *Indications:*
  - Hemophilia A with active bleeding state or before surgery.
  - von Willebrand disease.

Factor IX Concentrate

- *Factor IX concentrate:* 1 unit raises factor IX level by 1–1.5%.
- *Indications:* Hemophilia B with active bleeding or before surgery.

Desmopressin

- Synthetic analog of antidiuretic hormone, —intranasal application mode.
- *Indications:*
  - Active bleeding state in von Willebrand disease or before surgery
  - Uremic bleeding in liver disease
  - Bleeding in esophageal varices.

Tranexamic Acid

- It has 4.8% mouth rinses for antifibrinolytic effect following oral surgical procedures.
- Oral dose: 25 mg/kg 8 hourly.
- Indications: To maintain clot formation.

7. Discuss local hemostatic agents.

- Absorbent gelatin sponge material
- Microporous polysaccharide hemispheres
- Oxidized cellulose
- Fibrin sealant (glue)
- Topical thrombin
- Tranexamic acid
- Epsilon-aminocaproic acid
- The use of absorbable hemostatic materials helps in clot formation and maintaining clot stability. But these materials should be avoided in immunosuppressed patients as they carry a risk of infection and delay the healing period.
- Topical thrombin products fasten the hemostasis when applied at the surgical site. They convert soluble fibrinogen to

insoluble fibrin and arrest bleeding. When using thrombin products in conjunction with absorbable collagen or cellulose (gelform) or with fibrinogen (fibrin glues), the hemostasis is very efficient and this minimizes the chances for factor replacement.

8. Multiple myeloma.

- Multiple myeloma (MM) is a *malignant neoplasm of plasma cells* characterized by the synthesis of pathologic M proteins, bony lesions, kidney disease, hyperviscosity of blood, and hypercalcemia.
- *Oral manifestations:*
  - The patient may experience pain, swelling, and numbness of the jaws, gingival epulis, and mobility of the teeth.
  - More than 30% of MM patients develop osteolytic jaw lesions. These lesions are common in the mandible than in the maxilla and occur in the posterior teeth region, ramus and condylar process, because of the increased hematopoiesis in these sites.
- *Radiographic features:*
  - Normal bone pattern
  - Multiple radiolucent lesions
  - Diffuse rarefaction
  - Osteoporotic changes.

Skull lesions frequently occur than jaw lesions. Multiple punched out radiolucent lesions of varying size with ill-defined margins is pathognomonic and suggest the diagnosis.

- *Dental treatment:*
  - Dental procedures are routinely indicated for myeloma patients on recovery phase. For patients in active phase or relapse state, hemato-oncologist guidance is mandatory to proceed with dental treatment.
  - It is advisable to start dental treatment before the chemo-or radiotherapy.
  - If hematopoietic cell transplant is planned for a patient, dental procedures should not be carried out in the immediate pre and postprocedure days (minimum of 72 hours) to avoid transient bacteremia.

9. Basic physiology of hemostasis.

- Hemostasis is a physiological process of arresting the blood flow or blood loss following an injury (hemo = blood; stasis = standing).
- It has four basic steps:
  1. Vascular phase
  2. Platelet phase
  3. Coagulation cascade
  4. Fibrinolytic phase
- When a blood vessel is injured, the first 3 phases play the major role to stop bleeding and prevent blood loss.
  - Vasoconstriction—vasoconstrictors like serotonin are released from platelets.
  - Platelet plug formation—the platelets attach to the collagen in the damaged vessels. These attached platelets release an enzyme, adenosine diphosphate (ADP) which attracts more platelets and form a plug that temporarily stops bleeding.
  - Blood coagulation—fibrin deposition will reinforce the loose plug into a definitive plug.
- *Physiology of coagulation:*
  - The clotting process is known as coagulation and involves the following steps:
    - Formation of fibrin from fibrinogen.
    - Formation of unstable fibrin mesh—fibrin monomers polymerizes to form a loose mesh.
    - Formation of intact fibrin mesh (clot stabilization)—formation of covalent cross-linkages within fibrin mesh will result in a dense and stable mesh.
- *Fibrinolytic system:* Once healing occurs, the clot formed within the vessel is disposed of fibrinolysis which involves the dissolution of the clot. This step needs the presence of a proteolytic enzyme called plasmin.

MULTIPLE CHOICE QUESTIONS

1. Platelet count and bleeding time are used to check the ***primary hemostasis***.
   a. Vascular spasm
   b. Primary hemostasis
   c. Clot formation
   d. Secondary hemostasis
   (**Note:** In primary hemostasis, the platelets adhere to the damaged endothelium and forms platelet plug).
2. Spontaneous clinical hemorrhage occurs when platelet count is ***10,000–20,000/mm³***.
   a. 10,000–20,000/mm^3
   b. Below 50,000/mm^3
   c. 50,000–1,00,000/mm^3
   d. Below 10,000/mm^3
3. Surgical or traumatic hemorrhage occur when platelet count is below ***50,000/mm³***.
   a. 50,000/mm^3
   b. 1,00,000/mm^3
   c. 10,000/mm^3
   d. 20,000/mm^3
4. Normal bleeding time by modified Ivy's test is ***between 1 minute and 6 minutes***.
   a. Between 10 minute and 15 minutes
   b. Between 1 second and 6 seconds
   c. Between 10 seconds and 15 seconds
   d. Between 1 minute and 6 minutes
5. Bleeding time is considered as prolonged if it is greater than ***15 minutes***.
   a. 5 minutes
   b. 15 minutes
   c. 5 seconds
   d. 15 seconds
6. Platelet transfusion is given ***30 minutes before the surgery***.
   a. 1 hour before surgery
   b. 1 day before surgery
   c. 30 minutes before surgery
   d. 4 hours before surgery
7. The most common inherited coagulopathy is ***von Willibrand disease***.
   a. Hemophilia C
   b. Hemophilia A
   c. von Willibrand disease
   d. Stuart disease
8. The rate-limiting step in clotting is ***fibrinolysis***.
   a. Endothelial damage
   b. Platelet aggregation
   c. Thrombin activation
   d. Fibrinolysis
9. Normal range of prothrombin time is ***11–13 seconds***.
   a. 11–13 minutes
   b. 1–7 minutes
   c. 11–13 seconds
   d. 1–7 seconds
10. Vessel wall integrity or platelet disorders is diagnosed by ***tourniquet test***.
    a. Tourniquet test
    b. Coagulation test
    c. Hematocrit
    d. IVY method
11. Rumple-Leede phenomenon is used for measuring ***capillary fragility***.
    a. Bleeding time
    b. Capillary fragility
    c. Factor deficiency
    d. Clot integrity
    (**Note:** Tourniquet test uses Rumple-Leede phenomenon for measuring capillary fragility).
12. Scurvy results when daily intake of vitamin C falls below ***10 mg/day***.
    a. 90 mg/day
    b. 75 mg/day
    c. 500 mg/day
    d. 10 mg/day
13. Hypermobility of temporomandibular joint is a feature of ***Ehlers-Danlos syndrome***.
    a. Temporomandibular dysfunction syndrome
    b. Laskin's syndrome
    c. Ehlers-Danlos syndrome
    d. Myasthenia gravis
14. Stunted teeth with pulp stones is a finding in ***Ehlers-Danlos syndrome***.
    a. Taurodontism
    b. Regional odontodysplasia
    c. Klinefelter syndrome
    d. Ehlers-Danlos syndrome
15. Glanzmann's thrombasthenia is a qualitative defect of ***platelets***.
    a. Platelets
    b. Factor IX
    c. Thrombocytes
    d. Factor II
    (**Note:** Deficiency in platelet membrane phospholipids).

16. Bernard-Soulier syndrome is a qualitative disorder of ***platelets***.
    a. Platelets
    b. Factor IX
    c. Thrombocytes
    d. Factor II
    (**Note:** Defect in platelet membrane glycoprotein).
17. The expected complications of using cryoprecipitate and fresh frozen plasma are the ***transmission of viral infection***.
    a. Hypersensitive reaction
    b. Hypothermia and bradycardia.
    c. Transmission of viral infection
    d. Transfusion hemolysis
18. Ischemic tissue injury is a characteristic of ***sickle cell anemia***.
    a. Thalassemia major
    b. Intravascular coagulation disorders
    c. Herpes zoster infection
    d. Sickle cell anemia

VIVA VOCE

1. What is the range of normal platelet count?

The normal range is 1,50,000–4,50,000/mm^3.

2. What are the guidelines for treating dental patients on warfarin?

For patients taking warfarin, their INR should be checked before any invasive procedure. The therapeutic range is 2.0–3.0. Many of the minor surgical procedures can be carried out without any alteration in warfarin dose when INR is less than 3.0.

3. What are the guidelines for treating dental patients on heparin?

Heparin is given for end-stage renal disease patients on hemodialysis. Heparin has a short half-life of 5 hours, and patients can be treated safely on the days between dialysis.

4. Name the inherited coagulopathies.

von Willibrand disease (deficiency of von Willibrand factor), hemophilia A and hemophilia B.

5. What are the complications of factor replacement therapy?

- Allergic reactions.
- Viral disease (hepatitis B and C, HIV, cytomegalovirus).
- Development of antibodies to factor concentrates.
- Disseminated intravascular coagulation.
- Thromboembolic diseases (especially for factor IX complex concentrate).

6. How aspirin affects hemostasis?

- Aspirin is an antiplatelet drug that causes a functional defect in platelets as follows:
  - Aspirin inactivates the enzyme prostaglandin synthetase resulting in inactivation of cyclooxygenase catalytic pathway. This decreases the biosynthesis of prostaglandin and thromboxanes which are essential for the interactions between platelets and endothelium for hemostasis.

7. What is pagophagia?

Pagophagia is a craving for ice chewing or iced drink. It is an occasional symptom of Plummer-Vinson syndrome (iron-deficiency anemia) due to pharyngoesophageal ulceration.

BIBLIOGRAPHY

1. Adeyemo TA, Adeyemo WL, Adediran A, et al. Orofacial manifestations of hematological disorders: anemia and hemostatic disorders. Indian J Dent Res. 2011;22(3):454-61.
2. Deliverska EG, Krasteva A. Oral signs of leukemia and dental management-literature data and case report. J of IMAB. 2013;19(4):388-91.
3. Gupta A, Epstein JB, Cabay RJ. Bleeding disorders of importance in dental care and related patient management. J Cant Dent Assoc. 2007;73(1):77-83.
4. Israels S, Schwetz N, Boyar R, et al. Bleeding disorders: characterization, dental considerations and management. J Can Dent Assoc. 2006;72(9):827.

CHAPTER 8

Cervicofacial Lymphadenopathy

HIGHLIGHTS

Lymphadenopathy is the term used to denote enlargement of lymph nodes. It may be a primary or secondary manifestation of various disorders and may be a presenting sign or symptom of patient's illness. The involvement of nodes may be localized or generalized.

Lymphadenitis is an acute infectious condition where lymph nodes are swollen, tender, soft, and isolated, while chronic infection gives a firm, nontender and freely mobile nodes. Lymph nodes that are gradually enlarging, hard in consistency and fixed to the underlying or adjacent tissues are malignant.

Soft, flat palpable submandibular nodes which are smaller than 1 cm size are normal in children.

This chapter highlights the reasons for cervicofacial lymphadinopathy and diagnostic clues for various diseases based on lymph node examination.

ESSAY QUESTIONS

1. Outline the various causes of cervicofacial lymphadenopathy.

Infection

- *Bacterial*
  - *Streptococcus* and *Staphylococcus* infection.
  - Cat-scratch disease
  - Tuberculosis
  - Atypical mycobacterial infection
  - Primary and secondary syphilis
  - Diphtheria
  - Leprosy
- *Viral*
  - Herpes simplex infection
  - Herpes zoster infection
  - Rubella
  - Measles
  - Infectious mononucleosis
  - Adenovirus infection
  - Acquired immune deficiency syndrome
- *Fungal*
  - Rhinocerebral mucormycosis
  - Histoplasmosis
- *Parasitic*
  - Toxoplasmosis
  - Leishmaniasis

Immunologic Diseases

- Rheumatoid arthritis
- Systemic lupus erythematosus
- Sjogren's syndrome
- Mikulicz's disease
- Serum sickness
- Drug hypersensitivity
- Graft-versus-host disease

Malignant Diseases

- Leukemia
- Hodgkin's lymphoma
- Non-Hodgkin's lymphoma
- T-cell lymphoma
- Multiple myeloma
- Metastatic tumors of head and neck

Lipid Storage Disease

- Gaucher's disease
- Niemann-Pick disease

Other Disorders

- Castleman's disease (giant lymph node hyperplasia)
- Sarcoidosis
- Lymphomatoid granulomatosis
- Kawasaki's disease (mucocutaneous lymph node syndrome)
- Histiocytosis X
- Severe hypertriglyceridemia

Drugs

- Allopurinol
- Atenolol
- Captopril
- Carbamazepine
- Gold
- Hydralazine
- Phenytoin
- Primidone
- Quinidine.

2. Clinical evaluation of cervical lymphadenopathy.

The following features need to be checked:

- Location: Anatomical site of involvement. (cervical, submandibular, submental, supraclavicular, occipital, preauricular, auricular, axial inguinal).
- Number of nodes—single or multiple.
- Enlargement of nodes—localized or generalized.
- Involvement—unilateral or bilateral, if bilateral nodes are present, the symmetry should be checked.
- Consistency—firm, soft, rubbery, rock hard and bone hard.
- Nature—movable or fixed.
- Size: <1 cm, or >1 cm
- Symptoms: Tenderness and associated systemic symptoms.

Diagnosis

- Complete blood count
- Lymph node biopsy and fine needle aspiration cytology
- Ultrasonography
- Computed tomography
- Magnetic resonance imaging
- Positron emission tomography.

SHORT NOTES

1. Write simplified numerical classification system for cervical lymph nodes.

Cervicofacial lymph nodes are presented in the Figure 1 and Table 1.

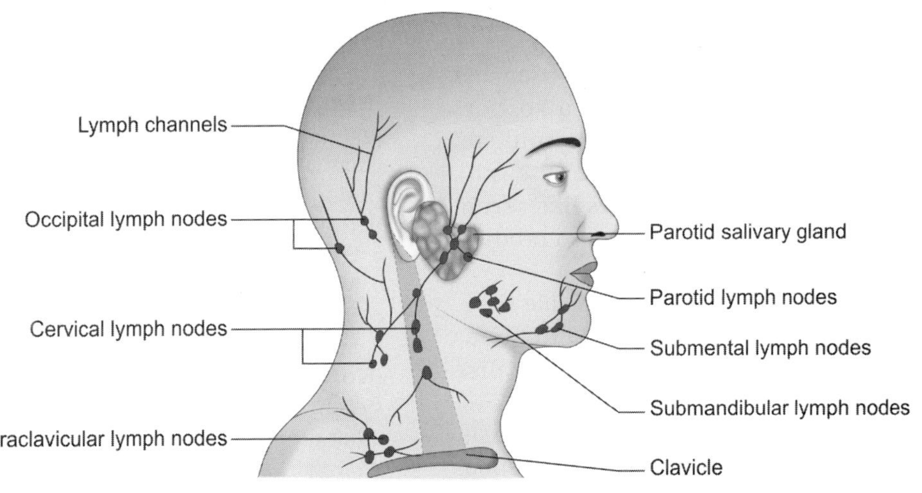

Fig. 1: Cervicofacial lymphnodes.

Table 1: Classification system for cervical lymph nodes.

Level	Location
IA	Submental lymph nodes
IB	Submandibular lymph nodes
II	Internal jugular chain from skull base to inferior hyoid bone.
III	Internal jugular chain from hyoid bone to the inferior border of the cricoid arch
IV	Internal jugular chain between the inferior border of the cricoid arch and the supraclavicular fossa
V	Posterior triangle or spinal accessory nodes
VI	Central nodes from the hyoid bone to the suprasternal notch
VII	Nodes inferior to the suprasternal notch in the upper mediastinum

2. Enumerate the conditions that cause generalized lymphadenopathy.

- Generalized lymphadenopathy occurs in systemic conditions where the symptoms are widespread.
  - AIDS-related complex due to severe immune deficiency by HIV-infection results in unexplained, generalized lymphadenopathy.
  - Disseminated carcinomatosis and lymphomas can cause generalized adenopathy.
  - Inherited metabolic disorders (Gaucher disease) and endocrine disorders (Graves' disease—hyperthyroidism, and Addison's disease hypocortisolism).
  - Immunological disorders like serum sickness and sarcoidosis also produce widespread adenopathy.
  - Connective tissue disorders like rheumatoid arthritis and systemic lupus erythematosus also tend to cause generalized lymphadenopathy.
  - Infectious diseases like tuberculosis, hepatitis, toxoplasmosis, and infectious mononucleosis lead to generalized lymph node enlargement.

MULTIPLE CHOICE QUESTIONS

1. Lymph node of <1 cm^2 size denotes ***nonspecific reactive nodes***.
   a. Anatomical nodes
   b. Inflammatory response nodes
   c. Nonspecific reactive nodes
   d. Granulomatous disease
2. Lymph node of >2 cm^2 size is probably due to ***malignancy***.
   a. Malignancy
   b. Tuberculosis
   c. Parasite infection
   d. Reactive lesions
   (**Note:** Lymph node of >2 cm^2 size is probably due to malignant or granulomatous disorders).
3. Metastatic nodes are ***hard and nontender***.
   a. Soft and tender
   b. Tender and mobile
   c. Mobile and hard
   d. Hard and nontender
4. The approximate total number of lymph nodes in a body is ***600***.
   a. 300
   b. 1200
   c. 600
   d. 80
5. The organ devoid of lymphatic supply is ***brain***.
   a. Brain
   b. Liver
   c. Kidney
   d. Limbs
   (**Note:** *Bone, cartilage, brain, spinal cord and retina* are the organs that do not have lymphatic vessels).
6. During development, lymphatic system is the derivative of ***mesoderm***.
   a. Endoderm
   b. Mesoderm
   c. Bone marrow
   d. Spleen
   (**Note:** During development, lymphatic system is the derivative of *mesoderm* but the adult progenitor cells are derived from *bone marrow*).

7. Stone hard consistency of lymph node suggests ***metastasis***.
   a. Tuberculosis
   b. Lymphoma
   c. Metastasis
   d. Syphilis
8. Firm and rubbery nodes are characteristic for ***lymphoma***.
   a. Tuberculosis
   b. Lymphoma
   c. Metastasis
   d. Syphilis
9. Buckshot nodes are the cervical nodes in children with ***viral infections***.
   a. Primary complex
   b. Malnutrition
   c. Congenital syphilis
   d. Viral infection
10. The cartilage-like consistency of lymph node denotes ***syphilis***.
    a. Tuberculosis
    b. Lymphoma
    c. Metastasis
    d. Syphilis
11. Inflammatory lymph nodes are ***soft and mobile***.
    a. Soft and mobile
    b. Hard and mobile
    c. Soft and fixed
    d. Hard and fixed
12. Group of coalesced nodes that move as a single unit is denoted as ***matted nodes***.
    a. Buckshot nodes
    b. Matted nodes
    c. Caseous nodes
    d. Granulomatous nodes
13. Matted nodes are seen in ***tuberculosis***.
    a. Tuberculosis
    b. Syphilis
    c. Hodgkin's disease
    d. Non-Hodgkin's disease
    (**Note:** Matted nodes are seen in tuberculosis, sarcoidosis, and lymphomas).
14. Positive monospot test confirms ***infectious mononucleosis***.
    a. Hodgkin's lymphoma
    b. kaposi's sarcoma
    c. Sarcoidosis
    d. Infectious mononucleosis
    (**Note:** *Monospot test* is a *positive heterophilic antibody test* that confirms infectious mononucleosis).
15. Localized lymphadenopathy with constitutional symptoms should be advised for biopsy when persist more than ***3–4 weeks***.
    a. 6 days
    b. 3–4 weeks
    c. 6 months
    d. 2–3 weeks
16. In benign lymphadenopathy, the nodes are ***freely mobile***.
    a. Freely mobile
    b. Fixed
    c. Nonpalpable
    d. Nonenlarged
17. Left side supraclavicular nodes are known as ***Virchow's nodes***.
    a. Virchow's nodes
    b. Sentinel nodes
    c. Waldeyer's ring
    d. Castleman's nodes
18. Lymphadenopathy that indicates dangerous sign is ***supraclavicular lymphadenopathy***.
    a. Sacral lympadenopathy
    b. Subclavian lymphadenopathy
    c. Supraclavicular lymphadenopathy
    d. Inguinal lymphadenopathy
    (**Note:** *Supraclavicular lymphadenopathy* is an alarming sign for the clinician).

VIVA VOCE

1. What are Virchow's nodes?

- Left supraclavicular lymph nodes are called as Virchow's nodes, by the name of a German pathologist "Rudolf Virchow and enlargement of these nodes is called as Troisier's sign.
- The enlargement of these nodes denotes malignant metastasis from the distant organs like stomach, esophagus, testis, and breasts; hence they are also called as signal nodes.

2. What is lymph?

Lymph is an interstitial fluid composed of cellular fluids, extravasated leukocytes, extracellular substances, protein, and fat.

3. What are the functions of the lymphatic system?

The lymphatic system delivers the lymphocytes and antigen-presenting cells to regional nodes and encounters the pathogens, maintain the homeostasis of tissue fluid, transport of cell debris and extracellular substances.

BIBLIOGRAPHY

1. Bruch JM, Treister NS. Clinical oral medicine and pathology. 2009, Humana Press; New york.
2. Longo DL, Fauci AS, Kasper DL, Hauser SL, Jameson JL, Loscalzo J. Harrison's principles of internal medicine 18th. New York: McGrow-Hill. 2012.
3. Som PM, Curtin HD, Mancuso AA. An imaging-based classification for the cervical nodes designed as an adjunct to recent clinically based nodal classifications. Arch Otolaryngol Head Neck Surg. 1999; 125(4):388-96.

CHAPTER 9

Oral Cancer—Investigation and Treatment Procedures

HIGHLIGHTS

Oral cancer, in general, denotes squamous cell carcinoma as it comprises more than 90% of all cancers occurring in the oral cavity. In India, among all type of cancers, oral cancer incidence is 12% in men and 8% in women. Early diagnosis and effective treatment of potentially malignant and malignant disorders will significantly reduce the rate of morbidity and mortality. This task exclusively depends on the precise knowledge and investigative skill of dental practitioners.

Learners are expected to study about:

- Etiological factors of Oral squamous cell carcinoma (OSCC).
- Pathogenesis, clinical manifestations, TNM staging of OSCC.
- Chair side investigations, biopsy techniques, and imaging modalities.
- Various treatment, modalities and their risk-benefit assessment.

ESSAY QUESTIONS

1. Describe the principle, mechanism and types of radiation therapy applied for oral cancer.

Radiation Therapy

Principle: Radiation damage the cellular DNA, cell membrane, chromosomes, enzymes and proteins either directly by ionization or indirectly by generating free radicals (H^+, OH^-) from radiolysis of water. Affected cells either die or become incapable of undergoing cell division and maintaining their integrity.

During the treatment course, normal cells get protected because:

- The reparative ability following radiation injury is much higher for normal cells than malignant cells.
- Cancerous cells are in rapidly dividing phase (higher growth potential) which makes them more susceptible to therapeutic effect.
- *Therapeutic effects of radiation depend on:*
  - Total dose
  - Number of fractions/day
  - Dose/fraction
  - Total treatment time (time dose fraction—TDS).
- *Radiotherapy for oral cancer:*
  - Squamous cell carcinoma is radiosensitive and is curable in early stage.
  - Poorly-differentiated tumors respond better than well-differentiated type because of increased cell division rate.
  - Exophytic, well-oxygenated tumors are more responsive than an infiltrative and invasive tumor.
  - Squamous cell carcinoma restricted to mucosa is highly curable than the one with bone involvement.
  - Small cervical nodes are managed with radiotherapy, but the extensive involvement of cervical nodes needs combination therapy.

- *Radiation treatment is determined by:*
  - Site, size and total volume of tissue to be irradiated.
  - Patient's tolerance.
  - Total number of days of treatment.
  - Protecting the normal, uninvolved tissues and organs.

Types of Radiotherapy

Teletherapy (External-beam Radiation Therapy)

- *Indication:* Primary tumors of the posterior-third of tongue, oropharynx, and tonsillar pillar.
- *Treatment planning:*
  - Localization of a tumor and radiation planning: The margins of a tumor are marked with radiopaque lead wire or gold or by a tattoo on facial skin.
  - If multiple fractions are planned, the area of treatment needs to be immobilized by using head holders, bandages or custom acrylic shells. Oral device with or without tongue depressor is combined with these materials to position the mandible into or out of radiation field.
  - Commonly used type is electron beam therapy and is applied in:
    - Parallel opposed field (bilateral)—for more extensive tumors and tumors crossing the midline.
    - Wedged-pair field for unilateral lesions.
  - The usual dose of epithelial neoplasms: It is 1.8–2 Gy/fraction for 5-weeks for total dose of 6,000–6,500 cGy.
  - Hyperfractionation protocol: It is 100–150 cGy twice daily for a total dose of 5,000 cGy in 3-weeks.

Brachytherapy (Implant techniques)

- Implant technique of radioisotopes is used to deliver radiation to a localized lesion.
- *Indications:*
  - A tumor involving anterior 3rd of tongue.
  - Booster dose of radiation to specific site.
  - For recurrent tumors.
- The radioisotopes used are: Cesium, iridium, and gold—192Ir, 137Cs, 125I, 198Au.
- *Treatment method:*
  - Direct implantation technique—to deliver radiation.
  - After loading technique—isotope is implanted using previously inserted guide tubes.
- *Advantages of brachytherapy:* The implanted radio isotopes deliver radiation in a relatively low dose at the immediate locality, and so there is minimal radiation exposure to adjacent structures.

2. Briefly describe the pathogenesis of oral cancer.

Pathogenesis of oral cancer is given in Flowchart 1.

Flowchart 1: Pathogenesis of oral cancer.

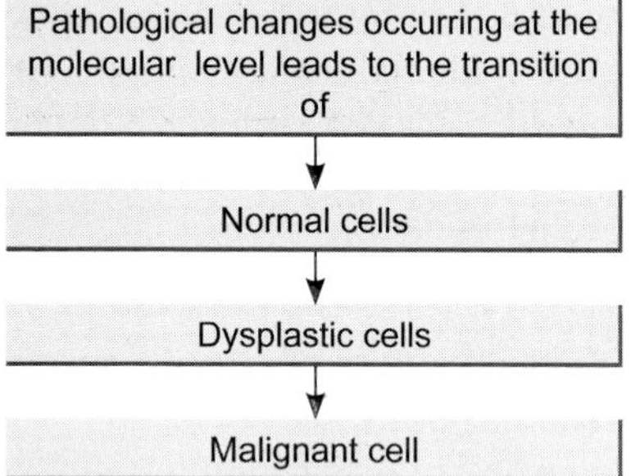

Cellular Level

When the cells are exposed to irritant stimuli, they respond by series of changes like cellular atypia, epithelial dysplasia, carcinoma-in-situ and oral carcinoma (Fig. 1, Flowchart 2).

Molecular Level

- Genetic mutations in proto-oncogenes and tumor suppressor genes results in malignant changes.
- Proto-oncogenes increase cell growth and differentiation thereby provoke carcinomatous changes.
- Proto-oncogenes responsible for oral cancer include ras, *MYC* gene, bcl1, bcl2, CK8, and CK19.

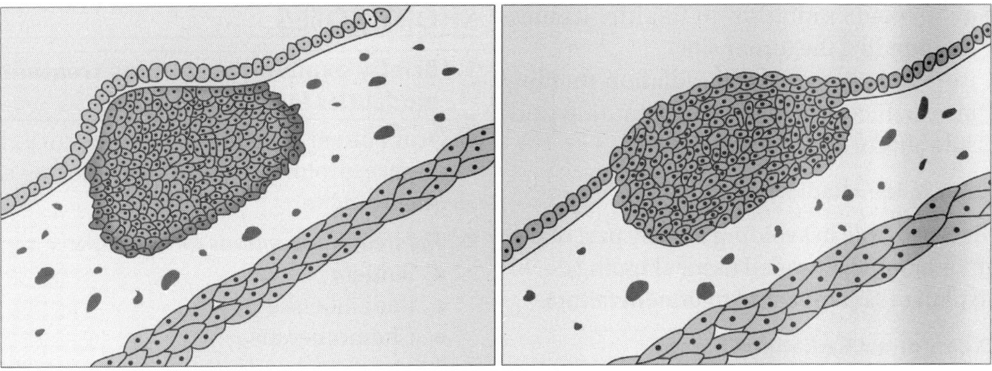

Fig. 1: Cellular changes in oral cancer.

Flowchart 2: Pathological changes in oral cancer.

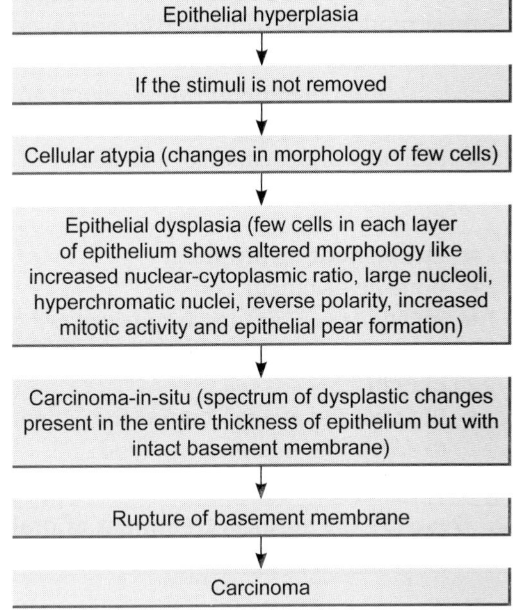

- Tumor suppressor genes (TSG) negatively regulate cell division and differentiation.
- These gene products inhibit the cell cycle when DNA damage occurs following exposure to carcinogen or infection with oncogenic viruses. If DNA damage is severe and irreparable, the TSG proteins may subject these cells to apoptosis (programed cell death).
- Tumor suppressor genes responsible for oral cancer include p53 and p21.
- If p53 is not expressed or mutilated, there will be no break in cell cycle and mitosis progress. Most of the oral cancers have a p53 mutation.

3. Briefly describe the different forms of radiotherapy available for head and neck cancers.

Particle Radiation Therapy

- It is the traditional method of delivering therapeutic radiation and includes both proton and neutron therapy.
- Proton rays are advantageous in their ability to deliver the dose conform to the shape of the tumor.

Stereotactic Radiotherapy

It uses single high dose radiation delivery directly to the tumor mass. The technique is precise and painless, e.g. gamma knife surgery.

Intraoperative Electron Radiation Therapy

- This technique delivers high single dose radiation to the tumor cells during surgery.
- Intraoperative electron radiation therapy (IOERT) is called as precision radiotherapy

as it avoids radiation to healthy tissues surrounding the tumor site.

- Intraoperative electron radiation therapy also reduces the treatment duration and side effects of radiotherapy.

Image-guided Radiotherapy (IGRT)

This is valuable in avoiding the any part of the tumor or tumor-invaded tissue skipping down the path of radiation and treatment failure.

3D Conformal Radiation Therapy

Radiotherapy supported with CT and MRI to deliver the radiation from multiple angles to reach tumor in three dimensional aspects and at same time preserving the healthy tissues.

Intensity-modulated Radiotherapy

- Intensity-modulated radiotherapy (IMRT) is delivered by the use of computer-assisted linear accelerators with static or multileaf collimator or volumetric arc modulated therapy. It provides appropriate radiation dose accurately to the three-dimensional shape of the tumor, by protecting the surrounding healthy tissues. This technique is known as tomotherapy.
- Intensity-modulated radiotherapy is at present used for the treatment of head and neck tumors and tumors of the central nervous system.

Radioimmunotherapy

- It is a form of radiation therapy used with immunotherapy. Monoclonal antibody is combined with a radioactive material (such as iodine-131, yttrium-90) and is injected into the patient's blood. When they reach tumor site, monoclonal antibodies bind to the tumor cells and deliver high-dose radiation. This type of radiation delivery is also known as targeted radiotherapy.
- Currently used in the treating lymphoma cases.

SHORT NOTES

1. Briefly explain the various treatment modalities for oral cancer.

- Oral cancer treatment aims to cure the disease, prolonging life and improving the quality of life.
- *The treatment options for oral cancer are:*
  - Surgery
  - Radiation therapy
  - Chemotherapy
- Surgery and radiotherapy are used as principle curative therapy in oral cancer, whereas chemotherapy is used as an adjunct.
- Either radiation or surgery is used for T1, and T2 stages, whereas combination of these modes is often followed for advanced cases.
- *Selection of specific option depends on factors like:*
  - Site, size, and location of a tumor
  - Cell type and degree of cellular differentiation
  - Lymph node involvement
  - Bone involvement
  - Ability to preserve speech and swallowing
  - Possibility of achieving adequate surgical margin
  - Physical and mental status of the patient to accept the treatment method
  - Potential complications of the therapy.

2. Describe the surgical treatment of oral cancers.

Indications

- A tumor involving bone.
- Radioresistant tumors.
- Recurrent neoplasm following radiotherapy.
- When side effects of surgery is assessed to be less than that of radiation.
- To reduce the bulk of a tumor.
- Existence of clinically positive nodes.

Potential Complications Need to be Considered

- Incomplete excision
- Inadequate margins of resection
- Tumor seeding
- Esthetic compromise due to considerable loss of tissues or part of organ.
- Lymphatic spread, hematogenous spread, neural and perineural invasion may be unrecognized and reduce the rate of treatment success.

3. Describe the use of chemotherapy in oral cancers.

Indications for Chemotherapy

- Advanced stage of a tumor.
- Recurrent tumors.
- Multiple metastasis.
- Palliative therapy for patients who cannot treat by other modalities.
- To decrease the incidents of micrometastasis.
- In combination with radiotherapy and surgery.

Types of Chemotherapy

- Induction chemotherapy—chemotherapy before surgery or radiotherapy to reduce the tumor size.
- Adjuvant chemotherapy—chemotherapy is administered in concomitant with surgery or radiotherapy to limit micrometastasis.
- Concurrent chemotherapy—administration of chemotherapy conjointly with radiotherapy will make tumor cells more susceptible to radiation.

Chemotherapeutic Agents for Oral Cancer

Methotrexate, bleomycin, cisplatin, platinum derivatives, 5-fluorouracil and taxanes (docetaxel).

- Methotrexate is an antimetabolite for folic acid and inhibits the division of cancerous cells and cause cell death.
- Bleomycin is an antibiotic and causes DNA damage.

Adverse Effects of Cancer Chemotherapy

Mucositis, nausea, vomiting and bone marrow depression.

Chemotherapy Cycle

Administration of chemotherapeutic agents followed by a period of rest to help the recovery of normal tissues.

4. Briefly describe fine needle aspiration cytology (FNAC) technique.

It is a diagnostic method in which cellular and fluid content are obtained through a needle attached to the syringe by applying a negative pressure.

Procedure

- The skin on the area to be aspirated is swabbed with an antiseptic solution.
- A thin needle attached to a syringe (21–25 gauge needle and 2–5 mL syringe) is inserted through the skin into the abnormal area.
- Position the needle within the target tissue
- Negative pressure is applied by withdrawing the plunger creating 2–4 mL vacuum.
- The needle should be directed into different tangents.
- The plunger is released to return the vacuum to 0 mL.
- The syringe and needle are withdrawn from the lesion and aspirates are blown on to the microscopic slide.
- The slide should be transported to the pathology lab where fixing is done in 95% alcohol, followed by papanicolaou (PAP) or H and E staining and microscopic examination is carried out.

Indications

- Diagnosis of salivary gland diseases
- Diagnosis of superficial cystic lesions
- To diagnose benign and malignant tumors
- To detect the metastatic cervical nodes.
- To replace extensive biopsy.

5. What is biopsy? List the indications for biopsy.

A biopsy is a process of surgically removing tissue samples from a living individual.

Types of Biopsy

- *Commonly employed types:* Incision biopsy, excision biopsy, punch biopsy, fine needle biopsy (FNB), brush biopsy and trephine biopsy
- *Rarely employed types:* Endoscopic biopsy, core biopsy, pressure biopsy.

Indications

- To evaluate the exact cellular nature of any soft-tissue or intraosseous lesions.
- To diagnose abnormal tissue mass.
- To confirm malignancy.
- To diagnose mucocutaneous lesions like lichen planus, and pemphigus.
- Aid in determining tumor grade.
- To assess therapeutic management.

6. Briefly describe excision biopsy.

Excisional biopsy is the procedure of total cutting out of a lesion for histopathological examination. It is a therapeutic and diagnostic method for smaller sized lesions.

Indications

- Lesions smaller than 1 cm in size which can be removed along with margins of healthy tissue.
- Freely movable tissue located above mucosa just beneath the surface.
- Sessile or pedenculate growth.

Procedure

- A 2% lignocaine anesthetic solution with vasoconstrictor should be injected around the periphery of the lesion.
- BP blade should be kept at an angle of 45° towards the center of lesion and two elliptical incisions should be made on either side of the base of the lesion.
- Tissue forceps should be used at the edge of the lesion to avoid crushing of the tissues.
- The specimen is gently dissected out by using either scalpel or scissors and placed in 10% formalin.
- Suturing should be done over the surgical site.

7. Write about incision biopsy (or) describe diagnostic biopsy.

Incision or diagnostic biopsy is a process of surgical removal of a small wedge-shaped specimen of the lesion tissue along with surrounding healthy zone.

Indications

- To diagnose larger sized lesions with diffused borders where total excision is not advisable before an established diagnosis.
- Any condition where complete removal is inadvisable.
- To determine the nature of the treatment to be carried out—whether conservative or radical.

Procedure

- Selection of biopsy site—it should be away from visible ulceration or area of necrosis or infiltration site.
- Infiltrate 2% lignocaine anesthetic solution around the periphery of the lesion.
- With a scalpel, an elliptical incision with sufficient depth should be made into underlying connective tissue.
- Specimen should be gently removed and placed in 10% formalin or 70% alcohol.
- Suturing should be done over the surgical site.

8. Describe brush biopsy technique.

- By using a specially designed brush, (with a flat end and circular border) which can penetrate to the basement membrane, a complete transepithelial specimen is obtained for histopathological examination (Fig. 2).

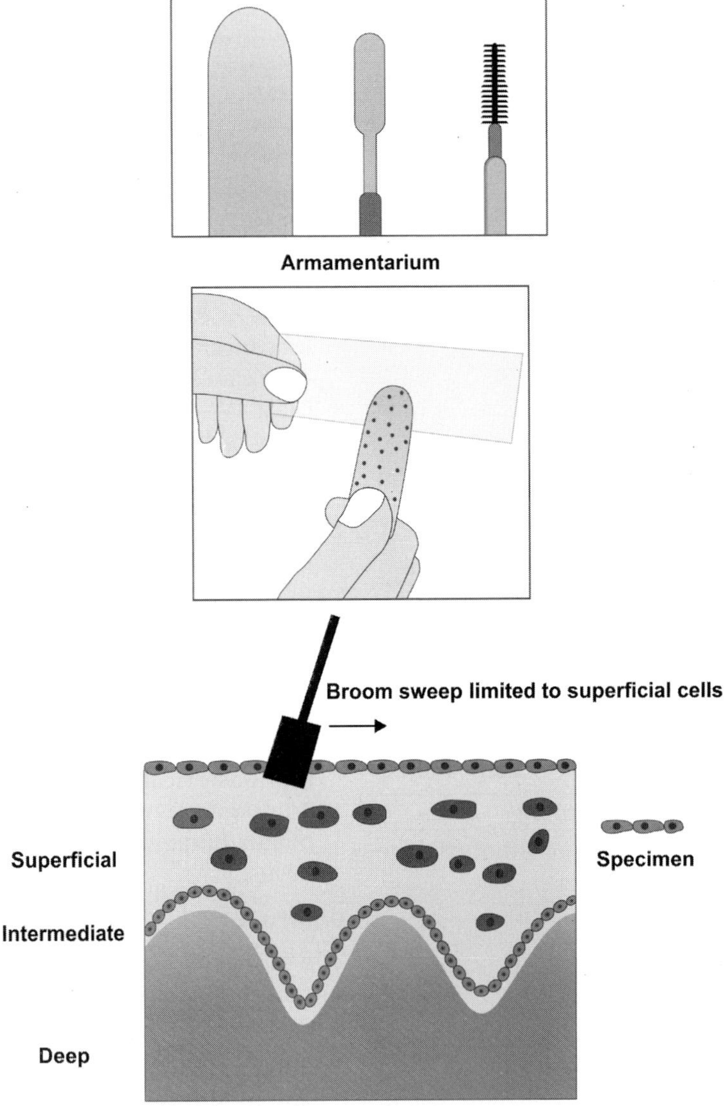

Fig. 2: Brush biopsy procedure.

- The oral CDx test kit with following components are used.
  - Oral brush biopsy instrument
  - Precoded glass slide
  - Alcohol/carbowax fixative pouch
  - Preaddressed container for submitting the contents.

Procedure

The brush rubs the surface of suspected tissues aggressively to the state of minor bleeding.

The cells are subjected to microscopic examination and results are given as:

- Inadequate—incomplete specimen.

- Negative—no abnormality in the epithelial cells.
- Atypical—abnormal changes in the epithelial cells.
- Positive—definite epithelial cell changes or carcinoma.

Advantages

- Specimen represents the superficial, intermediate and basal layer cells of the mucosa.
- Increased acceptance of patients' for the initial diagnostic procedure.

Indications

To diagnose:
- Epithelial lesions like leukoplakia and erythroplakia.
- Chronic ulcerations
- Mucosa that is atrophied, thickened or traumatized or irritated.
- Innocuous looking abnormalities.

Contraindications

- Lesions with intact epithelium.
- Highly suspicious lesion for malignancy.

9. Describe exfoliative cytology.

It is a method of interpreting cells that exfoliate or abrade from body surfaces.

Principle

In pathological conditions, the cells of epithelium lose their cohesiveness and get detached from each other. Hence cells in deeper layer also shed along with superficial cells in contrary to normal epithelium where cells in superficial layer alone shed due to physiological turnover.

Procedure

- Cleaning the surface debris and mucin over the lesion by vigorous gargling followed by gentle wiping with gauze.
- A sample of exfoliated cells is collected using tongue blade or cement spatula by applying firm stroke several times over the surface.
- The collected material is immediately spread over the microscopic slide and fixed with 95% alcohol; air dried and subject to microscopic study.

Cytological Report

- Class I—regular cells.
- Class II—minor form of cellular atypia but no malignant changes.
- Class III—intermediate cells which show wider atypia and may represent precancerous state or carcinoma-in-situ or even cancer. Biopsy is mandatory.
- Class IV—suggestive of cancer. Few cells show malignant features while many cells reveal borderline characteristics. A biopsy is mandatory.
- Class V—positive for cancer. A biopsy is necessary.

Advantages

- Simple, rapid, painless procedure.
- No bleeding or discomfort.
- A valuable method for screening procedures.
- Helpful in the detection of recurrence in previously treated patients.
- To diagnose mucosal lesions like pemphigus, herpes infection, and white sponge nevus.

Drawback

The biopsy is mandatory for all clinically suspicious lesions even if the cytological report is negative.

10. Briefly state about various investigations for oral cancer.

Following clinical examination, the patient with suspected malignant lesion (e.g.—ulcer with the indurated base, rapidly enlarging growth, growth with surface ulceration, deep fissures or ulcer, growth, or fistula with cervical node involvement) should be subjected for the following diagnostic procedures to confirm malignancy.

- Vizilite—chemoluminescent technique used to screen dysplastic cells. On function, the emitted light will be observed by normal tissues and appear dark whereas dysplastic cells glow differently.

- ❖ Vital staining—to screen as well as to select the biopsy site.
  - ■ Toluidine blue test—stains cells with more amount of DNA and RNA
  - ■ (Dysplastic and malignant cells contain more DNA).
- ❖ Incision biopsy—surgical removal of a small wedge-shaped specimen along with surrounding normal zone for pathological examination.
- ❖ Conventional radiographs—to find the bony involvement and alveolar changes. In dentate condition, check for root resorption.
- ❖ Specialized imaging techniques:
  - ■ Ultrasonography—to verify the node involvement.
  - ■ Computed tomography (CT)—to find out bone involvement, soft tissue involvement of maxillary sinus and nasopharynx, to find out smaller masses or lymph node is smaller than 1 cm in size.
  - ■ Nuclear scintigraphy—to find out bony involvement and bone necrosis following radiotherapy.
  - ■ Magnetic resonance image (MRI)—accurately differentiates tumor mass and benign growths. T2 weighted image demonstrates tumor extension in comparison with normal adjacent soft tissues and muscles.

11. Describe toluidine blue staining (or) vital staining procedure.

Toluidine blue test is a vital tissue stain that helps in diagnosis of potentially malignant and malignant disorders.

Principle

- ❖ Metachromatic dye (basic, 4.5 PH) that stains acidic tissue components hence bind rapidly with DNA.
- ❖ The test is comparatively more sensitive 93.5–97.8 with less specificity 73.3–92.9.

Composition

- ❖ Toluidine blue—1 g
- ❖ Acetic acid—1 cc
- ❖ Absolute alcohol
- ❖ Distilled water.

Method

- ❖ Rinse the mouth thoroughly with water twice for 20 seconds then with 1% acetic acid for 20 seconds.
- ❖ Gently dry with gauze.
- ❖ Apply 1% toluidine blue on the lesion using cotton swab and wait for 1 minute.
- ❖ Rinse with acetic acid (150 mL for 1 minute) followed by a thorough rinse with water.

Effect on

- ❖ Normal epithelium: Most of the epithelial surface stains blue, but stain is lost after application of 1% acetic acid.
- ❖ Benign lesions: Well-defined uptake at the margins.
- ❖ Dysplasia or malignancy: Diffuse marginal uptake.

Uses

- ❖ Assist in identifying the biopsy site.
- ❖ Outline the boundaries of the lesion for surgery.

12. What is ViziLite?

ViziLite is a biocompatible, chemoluminescent device used in the chair side diagnosis of oral cancer.

Contents

- ❖ ViziLite rinse—1% acetic acid.
- ❖ VizilLite capsule—chemiluminescent light stick.
- ❖ ViziLite retractor—sheath and handle.

Methods

- ❖ Thoroughly rinse the mouth with rinsing solution.
- ❖ On exposing ViziLite on oral tissues.

- Normal tissues absorb the light and appear dark.
- Dysplastic cells glow differently because their nuclei become larger resulting in reflection of light.

Advantages

1. No need for staining
2. Simple procedure.

13. What are the chair side investigations for oral cancer and precancer?

Light-based, chair side, screening tools have been developed for the diagnosis of precancerous and cancerous lesions. These noninvasive in vivo tools detect the tissue alterations. They are:

- Chemical method: Toluidine blue
- Light-based systems:
  - Chemiluminescence (ViziLite Plus)
  - Tissue fluorescence imaging (VEL scope)
- Spectroscopy: Autofluorescence and chemiluminescence
- Autofluorescence spectroscopy consists of a small optical fiber that produces different excitation wavelengths and a spectrograph which receives and analyzes the reflected fluorescence from the tissue with the help of software. It helps in the identification of an optimal location for biopsy.
- Autofluorescence spectroscopy also monitors the treatment response to oral submucous fibrosis.

14. TNM staging of oral cancer.

Tumor—Node—Metastasis (TNM) staging system:

T—size of primary tumor in centimeters

TX—primary tumor cannot be assessed
T0—no evidence of primary tumor
Tis—carcinoma-in-situ
T1—tumor 2 cm or less in greater diameter
T2—tumor >2 cm but ≤4 cm in greater diameter
T3—tumor >4 cm in greater diameter
T4—tumor >4 cm in greater diameter with invasion of adjacent structures like cortical bone, muscles of tongue, maxillary sinus, and skin.

N—cervical lymph node metastasis

NX—regional lymph nodes cannot be assessed
N0—no regional lymph nodes metastasis
N1—single ipsilateral node <3 cm
N2a—single ipsilateral node <6 cm
N2b—multiple ipsilateral node >3 cm but <6 cm
N2c—bilateral or contralateral node <6 cm
N3a—Lymph node >6 cm

M—distance metastasis

M0—no metastasis
M1—metastasis present

TNM clinical staging:

Stage I - T1-N0-M0
Stage II - T2-N0-M0
Stage III - T3-N0-M0 (or) T1-T2 or T3-N1-M0
Stage IV - T4 any N, M0 (or) any T-N2 or N3-M0 (or) any T or N with M1.

15. What is the prognosis of oral cancer?

- Squamous cell carcinoma (SCC) of the lip, hard palate and maxillary gingiva are slowly progressive. They seldom metastasis and hence the treatment outcome is favorable.
- The SCC occurring on the tongue, the floor of mouth and the gingiva are highly destructive and has unfavorable outcome.
- The well-differentiated, low-grade oral SCCs spread to the adjacent structures like bone and muscle before reaching the lymph nodes. The delayed metastasis results in good prognosis.
- The poorly-differentiated, high-grade oral SCCs are very destructive and tend to metastasize to regional lymph nodes during the early phase of the disease and have unfavorable prognosis.
- The histological grading of oral SCC reflects the aggressive nature of a tumor, but does not influence on the prognosis. The depth of the tumor infiltration determined histopathologically significantly predicts

the progress. Oral SCCs that have penetrated more than 5 mm into the underlying tissues have a poorer prognosis.

16. Enumerate the etiology of oral cancers. (or) list the risk factors associated with oral cancer.

The following are the predisposing factors for oral cancer (squamous cell carcinoma):

- *Tobacco and Alcohol Habits*
  - Both smoking and smokeless forms of tobacco are responsible for inducing oral cancer. The carcinogenic components of smokeless tobacco like polycyclic aromatic hydrocarbons, nitrosoproline, nitrosamines (nicotine) and ingredients of the smoking form of tobacco like carbon monoxide, hydrogen cyanide, thiocyanate and nicotine dramatically increases the risk of developing primary oral cancers. These components cause an impaired T-cell activation, generating reactive oxygen species (O^2, H^2O^2, OH), and cell damage through DNA single-strand break.
  - When tobacco use is combined with frequent alcohol intake, the risk of developing cancer is increased due to their synergetic harmful effects.

Genetic Susceptibility

The genetic hypothesis states hyperactivity of a tumor promoting genes (oncogenes, e.g. c-myc, ras) and reduced function of tumor suppressor genes (e.g. p53, p21) is the probable cause for oral cancer.

- *Viruses:* Herpes simplex virus and human papillomavirus (HPV 16 and 18) are capable of inducing cellular mutations and act either as proto-oncogenes or oncogenes in the pathogenesis of oral cancer.
- *Immune suppressed conditions:* The incidence of increasing oral cancers in elderly individuals is associated with reduced host resistance in advancing age.
- *Chronic trauma and nonhealing ulcers:* Chronic trauma or irritations related to ill-fitting dentures, broken restorations and sharp cusps may potentiate the effects of other carcinogens.
- *Potentially malignant disorders:* Premalignant lesions and conditions like erythroplakia, speckled leukoplakia, submucous fibrosis and lichen planus may also progress to oral cancer.

17. Describe punch biopsy.

- The punch biopsy is a substitute to incisional biopsy. The punch biopsy kit consists of a circular blade with diameters of two to ten millimeters attached to a plastic handle are available.
- On applying a firm stroke, the blade removes a core of tissue from the base which is simply released using curved scissors. It is rarely indicated for oral lesions.

18. Describe frozen section biopsy.

It is carried out to get the immediate histopathological report.

Indications

- To diagnose whether the lesion is malignant or not.
- To evaluate the margins of an excised carcinoma during surgery to find out whether the entire lesion is removed.

Procedure

The tissue is kept in the deep freeze, and frozen tissue is sectioned and stained to get a diagnosis.

Disadvantage

The slide cannot be preserved for future reference.

19. What is VELscope?

VELscope is a fluorescent screening tool used to delineate abnormal cells in the oral cavity. It is an *adjunctive* device and to be used with other diagnostic tools to examine oral cancer and premalignant lesions.

Method

- VELscope emits a blue excitation light (400–460 nm) on epithelial cells. The shorter wavelength blue light is absorbed by the cells and normal cells fluoresce in response to a bright, homogeneous, apple-green glow. The dysplastic cells reveal no fluorescence response or decreased dull response.
- The fluorescence property depends on the cellular content of flavin adenine dinucleotide, collagen, and keratin.
- Cancerous cells:
  - The increased metabolic rate in cancerous cells decreases the concentration of flavin adenine dinucleotide (FAD) and hence decreases the fluorescence.
  - In dysplastic cells, there is an increased rate of collagen break down; accordingly, there is a reduction in fluorescence.
  - In leukoplakia, there is hyperkeratosis and therefore fluoresce brightly.

Advantages

1. No need for tissue staining.
2. Chair side procedure.
3. Simple technique.

20. Discuss Lugol's iodine test (vital staining procedure).

Lugol's iodine is a vital tissue stain used to diagnose the potentially malignant and malignant conditions.

Principle

Lugol's iodine will bind to glycogen present in normal cells. Hence it is retained in normal epithelial cells but not in dysplastic or malignant cells. (Action is opposite to that of toluidine blue).

Composition

- Iodine—2 g
- Potassium iodide (KI)—4 g
- Distilled water.

Method

- Thoroughly rinse the mouth with plain water and gently dry.
- Lugol's iodine solution should be applied to the lesion site using cotton swab.
- Iodine will react with glycogen in normal cells and produce brown-black color.

Staining Effect

- Proliferating cells—cellular glycogen content is in reverse to the amount of keratinization, so proliferating epithelial cells are poorly stained.
- Inflammatory cells—contain more glycogen and take up more stain, giving dark brown coloration.

21. What is optical coherence tomography?

- Optical coherence tomography (OCT) constructs cross-sectional image of tissues and organ by registering the time and intensity of back scattered light reflections from them. OCT uses low-voltage modular device coupled with software. It is a non-invasive procedure.
- The commonly used technique is known as, the frequency-domain optical coherence tomography that creates three dimensional image of the structure in a short time.
- In oral cavity, OCT is helpful in diagnosing the soft-tissue lesions including inflammation, dysplasia, malignancy, periodontitis and regressive changes of teeth like attrition, abfraction, erosion and demineralization of enamel.

22. What are the recent advances in the management of oral cancer? (or) targeted therapy for oral cancer.

The prime agent is cetuximab; a monoclonal antibody used to focus the epidermal growth factor receptor (EGFR) which is overexpressed in epithelial cancers, such as oral squamous cell carcinoma. Cetuximab inhibits EGFR.

Gene Therapy

Gene therapy is useful in reversing the congenital defects by substituting a mutant gene by a normal functioning gene. Most of the gene therapy studies are aimed at cancers linked to genetic defects. In the future, it will provide a specific treatment for oral cancer and precancerous lesions.

Nutraceuticals

- Research has provided that plant-derived dietary compounds, nutraceuticals are a positive-approach in cancer treatment. Their chemical diversity, multi-targeting action and lack of adverse effects are considered in cancer treatment. The anti-tumor effects of curcumin and green tea polyphones are widely supplemented with standard therapy for oral cancer.
- Polyphenol products of grapes (Resveratrol) and mulberries had many favorable medicinal properties and is utilized in treating cancer.

MULTIPLE CHOICE QUESTIONS

1. Following the complete cessation of smoking, the risks of developing cancer will be reduced after ***5–10 years***.
   a. 1.6 years b. 5–10 years
   c. 15–20 years d. 3.2 years
2. Hit and run effect is associated with ***HSV oncogene***.
   a. Chemical oncogenes
   b. Proto-oncogenes
   c. HSV oncogene
   d. Activated oncogene
3. Most commonly proven viral infection in oral carcinogenesis is ***HPV-16***.
   a. HSV-2 b. HHV-8
   c. HPV-16 d. EBV -2
4. Carcinoma of gingiva-buccal complex is known as ***Indian oral cancer***.
   a. Indian oral cancer
   b. Rodent tumor
   c. Aboriginal cancer
   d. Trigone cancer
5. Indian oral cancer is due to (or) etiology for Indian oral cancer is ***placement of tobacco quid***.
   a. Bidi smoking
   b. Placement of tobacco quid
   c. Eating spicy food
   d. Tobacco and alcohol consumption
6. IMRT is chiefly indicated for ***nasopharyngeal carcinoma***.
   a. Non-Hodgkin's lymphoma
   b. kaposi's sarcoma
   c. Multiple myeloma
   d. Nasopharyngeal carcinoma
   (**Note:** IMRT refers to Intensity-modulated radiation therapy).
7. The most adverse effect in using methotrexate is ***bone marrow depression***.
   a. Bone marrow depression
   b. Folic acid deficiency
   c. Osteonecrosis
   d. Altered taste sensation
8. A biopsy is contraindicated for ***vascular lesions***.
   a. Bony lesions
   b. Necrotic lesions
   c. Vascular lesions
   d. Glandular lesions
9. The preferred imaging modality for head and neck tumor is ***computed tomography***.
   a. Computed tomography
   b. Cone-beam computed tomography
   c. Magnetic resonance image
   d. Ultrasonography
10. The principal field arrangements associated with teletherapy is ***parallel opposed field***.
   a. Focal field
   b. Reverse field
   c. Parallel ipsilateral field
   d. Parallel opposed field
   (**Note:** Wedged-pair field, parallel-opposed field, and three-field technique are the principal field arrangements associated with teletherapy).

VIVA VOCE

1. Define carcinoma or tumor.

Carcinoma is defined as a new growth of tissues or an abnormal mass of tissue, the growth of which is uncontrolled uncoordinated, and exceeds that of normal tissues and persist in the same manner even after the cessation of stimuli.

2. Compare (or) differentiate benign and malignant tumors.

Table 1: Difference between benign and malignant tumor.

Benign tumors	Malignant tumors
▪ Slow growing	▪ Rapidly growing
▪ Well-defined	▪ Ill-defined borders
▪ Most commonly manifest as an asymptomatic growth or swelling	▪ May manifest as growth, ulcer, ulceroproliferative growth and fissure. Ulcers have indurated base
▪ Not associated with pain, bleeding or secondary changes or rarely produces such symptoms in later stages of long-standing lesions	▪ Frequently associated with pain and discomfort like hoarseness of voice, dysphagia, restricted movement of tongue and trismus due to the involvement of adjacent vital structures, blood vessels, nerves, and muscles
▪ Do not involve lymph nodes	▪ Lymph node involvement is common and nodes are enlarged, fixed and nontender
▪ Metastasis is not a feature	▪ Metastasis (spreading to a distant part of the body) is common and usually spread via lymphatic channels

3. How alcohol is increasing the chances of cancer occurrence in tobacco users?

- ❖ Alcohol causes dehydration of oral mucosal epithelium and increases the penetration of tobacco by-products into the underlying mucosa.
- ❖ The liver cirrhosis associated with alcohol reduces the detoxification effect of the liver on carcinogenetic substances.
- ❖ Nutritional imbalance and decreased immunity in alcoholics due to reduced appetite and improper diet indirectly increase the risk of cancer.

4. What is palliative care?

Palliative care includes all efforts given for pain relief and psychological support to the patients and their family from diagnosis, throughout diseases. The purpose is to provide a quality care for life regardless the possibility of a cure.

5. What is sentinel node?

It is the first lymph node receiving lymphatic drainage from a malignant tumor.

6. What is IMRT?

- ❖ Intensity-modulated radiation therapy is called as IMRT. It uses a computer-aided radiation source to target the cancerous tissue more preciously.
- ❖ Advantage of IMRT—maximize the radiation dose to tumor site and significantly reduces the radiation dose on normal structures.

7. Explain about combined therapy in cancer management.

- ❖ Combined therapy is indicated in patients with advanced stage of a tumor or an aggressive tumor. In this method, the benefit of combined the advantages of radiotherapy and surgery intended to increase the survival period.
- ❖ Surgery—reduces the tumor size, remove radiation-resistant hypoxic tissues, and remove the bony part of tumor.
- ❖ Radiotherapy—kills the oxygenated peripheral tumor mass, control the regional metastasis.

BIBLIOGRAPHY

1. Field A, Longman L. Tyldesley's oral medicine. Oxford: Oxford University Press; 2003.

2. Khetrapal S, Jetley S, Jairajpuri Z, et al. FNAC of head and neck lesions and its utility in clinical diagnosis: a study of 290 cases. NJMR. 2015;5:33-8.
3. Naikmasur VG, Sattur AP, Mutalik S, et al. Recent advances in diagnostic oral medicine. J Indian Acad Oral Med Radiol. 2009;21:99-104.
4. Prelec J, Laronde DM. Treatment modalities of oral cancer. Can J Dent Hyg. 2014; 48(1):13-9.
5. Shafer WG, Hine MK, Levy BM, et al. A textbook of oral pathology. Saunders Philadelphia: 1983.
6. Zargaran M. A review of biopsy in dentistry: principles, techniques, and considerations. J Dent Mater Tech. 2014; 3(2):47-54.

CHAPTER 10

Focal Sepsis

HIGHLIGHTS

The oral cavity acts as a source of foci of infection (harbors microorganism with or without the manifestation of disease). Oral foci (viridans group streptococci) may spread via blood or lymphatic system and produce focal infection (generalized state of infection or infection at multiple sites or at a distance organ) like pericarditis, endocarditis, meningitis, otitis media, conjunctivitis, arthritis, sinusitis, lung abscess and so on. The causative organisms are not the primary pathogens in these conditions, but acts as an opportunistic microbe if there is a biological change in these tissues and support the growth of VGS. The focal theory concept is applied in *reverse diagnosis* concept; when no explainable cause exists for a disease or infection, the possibility of oral foci is suspected and necessitated to eradicate all possible oral and dental diseases, and observing for improvement in the general condition. This focal theory concept demand interdisciplinary practice and dental graduates must be trained with adequate knowledge and skill to contribute for the well-being of patients.

The learners are expected to:

- Differentiate the concepts of foci of infection and focal infection.
- List the possible systemic diseases that may arise from oral focal sepsis.
- Explain the mechanism of focal infection.

ESSAY QUESTIONS

1. Define focal sepsis. Describe the possible routes and various systemic infections caused by oral foci of infection.

- The concept of focal infection describes the spread of microbes and their toxic by-products from a confined site which may be asymptomatic to a remote organ of the body and begin a new infection and inflammation.
- Focus of infection is the site from which microbial species or toxin spreads and cause distant infections. Foci of sepsis contribute to the development of inflammatory diseases like arthritis and peptic ulcers.
- The central concept of the focal infection theory is that infection occurs at a site distant from the site of microbial colonization (foci), the foci are usually unrecognizable, and the metastatic infection occurs only in locations that are susceptible to the bacterial species or toxins.
- Oral cavity acts as a site of origin and dissemination of microbial pathogens to distant organs.

Possible Mechanism Proposed for the Spread of Oral Infections

- *Metastatic infection:* The release of microbes from dental infections and dental treatment procedures can cause transient bacteremia. The microorganisms entering into the blood are usually removed by the reticuloendothelial system within short duration (transient bacteremia) and do not cause any symptoms. If the disseminated microbes find favorable conditions, they may settle, and, start to multiply.

- *Metastatic injury:* Endotoxins are released from outer cell wall after bacterial cell death. Endotoxins (a lipopolysaccharide), when released into the bloodstream, produces many pathological symptoms.
- *Metastatic inflammation:* Soluble antigens when entering the bloodstream react with circulating antibodies and form an antigen-antibody complex and begin an inflammatory reaction at the site where they get accumulated.

Systemic Diseases-associated with Oral Foci

- *Metastatic infection from oral cavity through transient bacteremia:*
  - Subacute infective endocarditis
  - Acute bacterial myocarditis
  - Brain abscess
  - Cavernous sinus thrombosis
  - Sinusitis
  - Lung abscess
  - Orbital cellulitis
  - Dermatitis
  - Prosthetic joint infection
- *Metastatic injury from circulation of oral microbial toxins:*
  - Cerebral infarction
  - Acute myocardial infarction
  - Persistent pyrexia
  - Toxic shock syndrome
  - Chronic meningitis
- *Metastatic inflammation caused by oral organisms:*
  - Behçet's syndrome
  - Chronic urticaria
  - Uveitis
  - Inflammatory bowel disease
  - Crohn's disease.

Dental infection as foci of infection:

- Periodontal bacteria enter the blood and invade the blood vessel tissue and cause harmful effects.
- The periodontal infection produces inflammatory mediators that travel through the blood and cause adverse effects on the heart and blood vessels.
- Bacterial products like lipopolysaccharides enter the blood and damage the heart and blood vessels.
- Streptococci species isolated from carious teeth are similar to streptococci cultured from an inflamed joint.

Focal infection theory is accepted because:

- Primary foci are associated with diseases like tuberculosis, syphilis, and sarcoidosis which otherwise cannot occur. When the primary focus is eliminated, there will be betterment in response to secondary disease.
- Patients with primary oral foci and resultant systemic illness experience bacteremia. The persistent focus of infection also leads to recurring bacteremia.
- The bacteria are highly-specific and selective for certain tissues.
- There are aggravated incidence of arthritis and myositis on patients in postsurgical period.
- The elimination of primary focus relives the sign and symptoms of secondary systemic illness.
- A patient may be rendered vulnerable to bacteremic episodes by lowering of his resistance mechanisms.

SHORT NOTES

1. Briefly explain how periodontal diseases trigger systemic diseases.

Periodontal disease predispose to cardiovascular diseases:

- Periodontal infections are associated with gram-negative bacteria (*Streptococcus sanguis* and *Porphyromonas gingivalis*) which induce the release proinflammatory cytokines and thrombus formation through platelet aggregation. These factors lead to vascular pathology (intravascular clot formation) and cardiac disease.

- Periodontal infection stimulates liver to produce an inflammatory marker, C-reactive protein that has the tendency to deposit on the damaged vessels. They contribute to atheroma formation by activating phagocytes and coronary heart disease.
- Chronic periodontal inflammation releases inflammatory cytokines into circulation. These cytokines affect the functions of platelet and prostaglandin synthesis leading to cerebrovascular accident and stroke.
- The gingival microbes like *A.comitans, P.gingivalis* and *Fusobacterium* species can be aspirated into lower airways and cause bacterial pneumonia.
- In pregnancy, the hormonal changes induce more plaque formation and Gram-negative bacterial species. They release cytokines (IL-1, IL-6, and TNF) and the elevated level of circulating cytokines reach amniotic fluid. The cytokines induce prostaglandin synthesis and preterm labor and low birth weight infants.
- Periodontal infections also exacerbate the diabetic condition. The release of TNF-alpha and IL-1 leads to a state of insulin resistance and increased amount of advanced glycation end products.

BIBLIOGRAPHY

1. Li X, Kolltveit KM, Tronstad L, et al. Systemic diseases caused by oral infection. Clin Microbiol Rev. 2000;13(4):547-58.
2. Nayak S, Nayak P. Systemic diseases associated with oral infection-a review. Indian Journal of Dental Sciences. 2010;2.
3. Seymour GJ, Ford PJ, Cullinan MP, et al. Relationship between periodontal infections and systemic disease. Clin Microbiol Infect. 2007;13(Suppl 4):3-10.

CHAPTER 11

Acquired Immune Deficiency Syndrome

HIGHLIGHTS

When human immunodeficiency virus enters the body, it start multiplies in the lymph node and destroys T-helper cells. HIV-induced oral diseases to develop when patients CD4+ cells reduced below 200/µL and plasma HIV-RNA levels exceed 3,000 copies/mL. The presence of characteristics oral lesions in HIV-positive individuals but not under antiretroviral treatment may alarm the progression of HIV, and for those undertreatment, it denotes the elevated plasma levels of HIV-1RNA.

Learners are expected to know about:

- Oral diseases associated with HIV patients.
- Specific management for each condition.

ESSAY QUESTIONS

1. Enumerate the oral findings of HIV-infected individuals and management of each condition.

- There is a substantial association between HIV and oral infections, and so far 10 different types of oral lesions were recognized in HIV-infected individuals internationally. They are:
  - Oral candidiasis, oral hairy leukoplakia, Kaposi's sarcoma, linear gingival erythema, necrotizing ulcerative gingivitis, necrotizing ulcerative periodontitis, non-Hodgkin's lymphoma, oral warts HSV-1 infection in HIV and neutropenic ulcerations.

Oral Candidiasis

The clinical manifestation of candidal infection in HIV patients are of 3 types which are here:

1. Angular cheilitis: Redness, cracking, or fissuring at the lip commissures.
2. Erythematous candidiasis: The lesion appears as a smooth-red surface on the dorsum of the tongue and palates.
3. Pseudomembranous candidiasis (or thrush): Thrush appears as creamy-white plaques on the oral mucosal surfaces. The plaques when rubbed off, leaves an erythematous or bleeding surface.

Management

- Topical application (mild to moderate candidiasis):
  - Clotrimazole troches 10 mg: Dissolve 1 troche in mouth, 5 times/day for 2 weeks.
  - Nystatin oral suspension 500,000 units: Swish 5 mL in mouth then swallow, 4 times/day for 2 weeks.
  - Nystatin pastilles 100,000 units: Dissolve in mouth, 4 times/day for 2 weeks.
- Systemic therapy: Fluconazole 100 mg, 2 tablets on the first day, followed by 1 tablet a day for 2 weeks.

Oral Hairy Leukoplakia

- The Epstein-Barr virus causes hairy leukoplakia, as white, corrugated, vertical lines on the lateral surface of tongue in immune-deteriorated conditions including HIV infection.
- The expected median CD4 count HIV-infected patient with oral hairy leukoplakia

is 468/μL. With each 300 unit decrease in the CD4 count, the possibility of occurrence increases two-fold for hairy leukoplakia.

- ❖ It is often asymptomatic, and patients are unaware of its presence. Some patients may experience the symptoms of mild pain, unpleasant sensation, altered taste, and aesthetic problem.
- ❖ Severe immunodeficiency associated with chemotherapy, organ transplant and leukemia may also present hairy leukoplakia as a finding.

Kaposi's Sarcoma

Kaposi's sarcoma is an HIV-associated oral malignancy, caused by human herpes virus 8 (HHV-8). It can be macular, nodular, or raised and ulcerated, with red to purple coloration. Definitive diagnosis requires biopsy (Fig. 1).

Management

- ❖ Vinblastine sulfate injection at the lesion site.
- ❖ Surgical removal.
- ❖ Systemic chemotherapy.

Linear Gingival Erythema

- ❖ Linear gingival erythema is otherwise known as red band gingivitis. It appears as a red band along the marginal gingiva (Fig. 2).

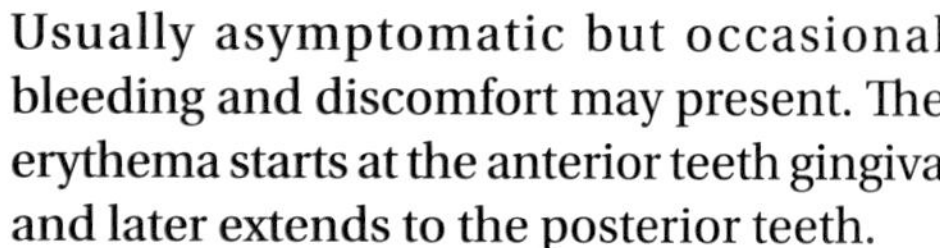

Usually asymptomatic but occasional bleeding and discomfort may present. The erythema starts at the anterior teeth gingiva and later extends to the posterior teeth.

Management

- ❖ Oral prophylaxis.
- ❖ A 0.12% chlorhexidine gluconate rinse twice daily for 2 weeks.

Necrotizing Ulcerative Gingivitis

- ❖ Gingiva appears red and tends to bleed spontaneously. A sudden onset of necrosis in the interdental papilla gives rise to the characteristic punched-out appearance. Pseudomembranous slough covers the necrotic surface. The condition is painful and is resistant to routine periodontal treatment.
- ❖ Lesions were staged as follows:
  - ■ Stage 1: Necrosis at the tip of the interdental papilla.
  - ■ Stage 2: Necrosis of entire papilla.
  - ■ Stage 3: Necrosis of marginal gingiva.
  - ■ Stage 4: Necrosis of attached gingiva.

Management

- ❖ Debridement of the ulcer under local anesthesia.
- ❖ A 0.12% chlorhexidine mouth rinse for home care procedures.

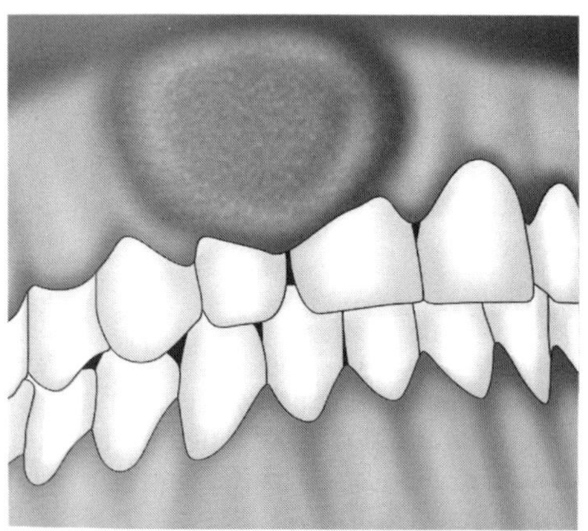

Fig. 1: Kaposi's sarcoma.

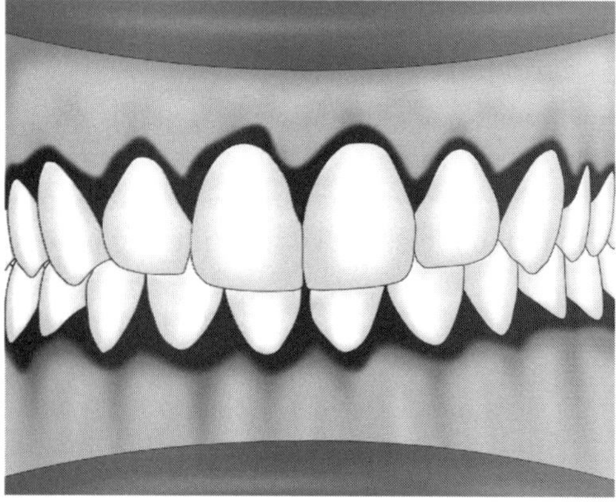

Fig. 2: Linear gingival erythema.

- Analgesics: Ibuprofen 400 mg 3 times/day.
- Antibiotics: Combination of amoxicillin 250 mg and metronidazole 250 mg one tab of each, 3 times/day for 1 week.

Necrotizing Ulcerative Periodontitis

- Pathogens associated with necrotizing ulcerative periodontitis (NUP) in HIV-infection are majorly anaerobic bacteria. The lesion begins as ulceration in the interdental papilla and changes the knife edge contour of the papilla to blunt. The ulceration progress to necrosis and slowly destroys the interdental bone. The condition spreads to involve the entire gingival encircling the teeth and sometimes to adjacent soft-tissues. The patient will experience severe pain (deep jaw pain) and mobility of the teeth.
- Spontaneous bleeding is also characteristic. Alveolar destruction may lead to exfoliation of teeth within 3–6 months of onset, leaving sequestrum.

Treatment

- Chlorhexidine gluconate rinse (0.12%) twice daily after brushing.
- Antibiotic therapy:
  - Metronidazole is the drug of choice, 200 mg 4 times/day for 2 weeks (or)
  - Clindamycin 150 mg 4 times/day can be considered.
- Topical anticandidal therapy
- Scaling, root planning and irrigation with 10% povidone-iodine.

Non-Hodgkin's Lymphoma

- The incidence of non-Hodgkin's lymphoma (NHL) increases when the CD4 cell count falls below 100/mm. NHL frequently occurs in the advanced stage of HIV infection and hence known as AIDS-related lymphoma. Older age group and men are more prone to NHL.
- Patients present with poor prognostic features, such as weight loss is greater than 10% of original body weight, drenching night sweats, and fevers. Clinical features include swollen, painless lymph nodes in the neck, armpits, or groin. Common extranodal involvements include CNS, GIT, liver and bone marrow.
- Lab investigations reveal elevated levels of serum lactate.
- CHOP regimen (cyclophosphamide, doxorubicin, vincristine, and prednisone) is the treatment modality for HIV-associated NHL.

Oral Warts

The warts are caused by human papillomavirus (HPV). It appears as cauliflower-like, spiked, sessile or raised pedunculated growth with a flat surface. The warts are asymptomatic, and the development is related to immune suppression. The histopathological finding of the biopsy specimen reveals epithelial hyperplasia and large vacuoles of cells in the epidermis. Dysplastic changes are rare.

Treatment

- Topical podophyllin
- Alpha interferon injection
- Topical 5-fluorouracil therapy can also be used on external lesions, but hyperpigmentation will be the side effect.
- Laser surgery or cryotherapy.

Herpes Simplex Virus-1 Infection in HIV

- Herpes simplex virus (HSV) causes extensive oral ulceration in HIV-infected patients. Recurrent HSV infection start as tingling and numb sensation followed by the development of multiple small vesicles which immediately break down and ulcerates. These tiny ulcers coalesce and form painful, large ulcers.
- Lesions are usually self-limiting and occur on keratinized mucosa (hard plate and gingiva), but in the severely immunocompromised state, it involves nonkeratinized mucosa as well.

Management

- Topical acyclovir 3% ointment 5 times application/day.
- Antiviral medication acyclovir 800 mg 4 times/day is the treatment to prevent secondary infection and shorten the episode.

Neutropenic Ulcerations

- Neutropenia is a condition where neutrophil count is below 1,500 cells/µL. Neutropenic ulcers develop when absolute granulocyte count is less than 800/µL. Patients under azathioprine (cause neutropenia) are more prone to develop this ulcer.
- Painful ulcerations and appear on both keratinized and nonkeratinized oral mucosa. Ulcers are periodic and occur once in 3 weeks duration. They appear massive, fulminating and indolent.

Management

- Granulocyte colony-stimulating factor substitution.
- Systemic or topical steroid treatment.

SHORT NOTES

1. Briefly describe the dental care protocol for HIV-infected patients.

- For HIV-infected individuals, routine, noninvasive dental treatment like restoration and removable prosthesis can be provided without any precaution. However, care should be taken for sterilization and personal protection.
- For minimally invasive procedures like deep scaling, care should be taken to minimize bleeding and trauma.
- Invasive dental procedures should be performed after obtaining the lab reports for hemostatic function and infection risk. Aseptic technique should be followed.
- Antibiotic prophylaxis before invasive procedures should be started when neutrophil count is less than 500/mm^3.

2. Oral lesions in HIV infection (or) oral manifestations in HIV infection associated with immune suppression.

The new classification of oral diseases of HIV-associated immune suppression (ODHIS) is proposed in 2004.

- Group 1: ODHIS with CD4 <200 cells/mm^3 (severe immune suppression).
  - Kaposi's sarcoma, oral hairy leukoplakia, chronic HSV, CMV ulcers; necrotizing ulcerative gingivitis and periodontitis, neutropenic ulcers, recurrent major aphthous ulcers.
- Group 2: ODHIS with CD4 <500 cells/mm^3 (immune suppression).
  - Recurrent aphthous major, non-Hodgkin's lymphoma, linear gingival erythema, HPV infection, salivary gland diseases.
- Group 3: ODHIS assumed to associate with immune suppression
  - Candidiasis, oral HSV ulcers, minor aphthous ulcers, VZV infection, deep fungal infection
- Group 4: Therapeutically induced oral diseases.
  - Hyperpigmentation, nonspecific ulcers, neutropenic ulcers, hyposalivation, lichenoid drug eruption.
- Group 5: Emerging oral diseases.
  - Erythema migrans, NHL-B cell type, epithelial neoplasm, warts and aggressive proximal caries.

MULTIPLE CHOICE QUESTIONS

1. Red band gingivitis or linear gingival erythema is an oral manifestation of ***HIV infection***.
   a. Necrotizing ulcerative gingivitis
   b. Necrotizing periodontitis
   c. HIV-infection
   d. Desquamative gingivitis
2. Xerostomia in HIV patients occurs as a side effect of ***antiretroviral therapy***.
   a. Salivary gland atrophy
   b. Viral parotitis

c. HIV-associated salivary gland diseases
d. Antiretroviral therapy
(**Note:** Xerostomia in HIV patients occurs as a side effect *of antiretroviral therapy* or as a result of the proliferation of CD8+ cells in major salivary glands).

VIVA VOCE

1. What is AIDS?

- In HIV-infected individuals, CD4 cell count declines gradually and when it becomes less than 200 cells/mm^3 (normal CD4 counts are between 500 cells/mm^3 and 1,600 cells/mm^3), the patients encounter severe immune deficient state and prone for opportunistic infections. This stage of HIV infection is described as AIDS.

2. What are the lab investigations to be performed for HIV infected dental patients?

Before proceeding dental treatment, the investigation should include:

- Complete and differential blood count.
- PT, PTT, INR, hemoglobin%
- CD4 cell count
- Viral load.

BIBLIOGRAPHY

1. Arendorf TM, Bredekamp B, Cloete CA, et al. Oral manifestations of HIV infection in 600 South African patients. J Oral Pathol Med. 1998;27(4):176-9.
2. Aškinytė D, Matulionytė R, Rimkevičius A. Oral manifestations of HIV disease: a review. Stomatologija. 2015;17(1):21-8.
3. Greenberg SM, Glick M. Burket's Oral Medicine: Diagnosis and Treatment. Orofacial Pain, 9th edition. BC Decker Inc, Elsevier India; 2003:pp.230-232.
4. Greenspan JS, Barr CE, Sciubba JJ, et al. Oral manifestations of HIV infection: definitions, diagnostic criteria, and principles of therapy. The USA oral AIDS colloborative group Oral Surg Oral Med Oral pathol. 1992;73(2):142-4.
5. Petersen PE, Bourgeois D, Ogawa H, et al. The global burden of oral diseases and risks to oral health. Bull World Health Organ. 2005;83(9):661-9.

CHAPTER 12

Infectious Disease of Oral Cavity

HIGHLIGHTS

Dental professionals are involved in the diagnosis and treatment of common and rare infections that are either specific to the oral cavity or as a part of generalized or systemic infection or diseases. Dentists are responsible for management of these conditions by developing a promising treatment plan. Selection of appropriate antimicrobials plays a critical role in successful treatment. Though infectious diseases are a large entity, this chapter is a compilation of bacterial, viral and fungal infection that is important from the dentist's perspective with precise diagnostic points and treatment plans.

Learners are expected to study about:

- Hepatitis B infection in dental practice.
- Common bacterial, viral and fungal infections in oral cavity.
- Rare but potential infections like tetanus, actinomycosis, and noma.

ESSAY QUESTIONS

1. Enumerate the risk factors for hepatititis B infection and write the investigation for the same. Add a note on the significance of hepatitis B in dental practice.

- Hepatitis is a hepatic disease affecting the parenchymal cells of the liver leading to necrosis of hepatocytes. It is caused by a DNA virus, hepatitis B.
- Potential risk factors for hepatitis B transmission:
  - Substance abuse (Needle drugs)
  - Hepatitis B infected sexual partner
  - Polyamory practices
  - Traveling to hepatitis endemic areas
  - Exposure to outbreak of hepatitis B
  - Occupational hazards like needle stick injury
  - Hepatitis B infected mother to newborn
  - Transfusion depended illness
  - Nonsterile tattoos/body piercing needles
  - Household contact with hepatitis B infected person.
- In dental practice, hepatitis should be considered on two aspects for patients:
  1. Once the liver gets infected, the functions of liver like synthesis of the enzymes, clotting factors (II, V, VII, IX, X), metabolism of drugs and bilirubin are affected, and these are the points to be noted before dental treatment in a patient with a history of hepatitis.
  2. There are chances for infection spread through infected needles and blood. Hence proper sterilization protocol and protective measures are necessary.

When the patient's medical state hepatitis infection, then it is mandatory to advise the following investigations before dental treatment which are as follows:

Lab Investigation

- Serum bilirubin—raised above 1.2 mg/dL.

- SGOT and SGPT—raised between 400-4,000 IU.
- Prothrombin time—prolonged (Normal PT is 11-16 seconds).
- International normalization ratio (INR)—increased (normal INR is 1.5-2).

Serological Tests

Hepatitis B virus has a surface (s), core (c), and envelope antigens. These three antigens and their antibodies are the diagnostic markers.

1. Hepatitis-B surface antigen and antibody (HBsAg and anti-HBs): Anti-HBs denotes previous infection and immunity to HBV.
2. HBeAg and anti-HBe:
   - HBeAg—denotes viral replication, presence of high titer HBV in serum and serum infectivity.
   - Anti-HBe—denotes carrier state (low serum titer of HBV).
3. Anti-HBc-IgM—denotes recent HBV infection. Detectable in serum up to 4-6 weeks following infection. Anti-HBc—denotes prior infection with HBV.

- Hepatitis B is the most commonly acquired occupational infection among dentists. The exposure occurs as follows:
  - Injuries from contaminated sharp instruments (e.g. bur laceration, needle sticks).
  - Blood or saliva contamination on open wounds of hands and fingers.
  - Splashing of blood or saliva on the open wounds.
- Jaundice is a symptom of raised serum bilirubin level (Normal serum bilirubin level: 0.3-1.2 mg/dL) and is a common response to hepatitis B. It manifests as yellow discoloration of the skin, oral mucous membrane, sclera, and conjunctiva. When the patient's history reveals jaundice, the tests as mentioned above should be asked before proceeding with dental treatment. If the jaundice history is less than month duration, dental procedures should be avoided. In case of 6-12 months duration, emergency procedures alone can be considered after lab investigations with careful precautions.

2. Briefly outline the deep fungal infections of oral cavity.

Mucormycosis

- Mucormycosis (zygomycosis) is a ubiquitous, aerobic, opportunistic fungal hyphae present in nasal mucosa of healthy individuals.
- In rhinocerebral form (that affects facial, oral, orbital, sinuses, and cerebral structures). Rhizopus genera are the pathogen that enters through inhalation. The organisms affect only immunocompromised individuals, and diabetes mellitus (DM) with diabetic ketoacidosis is the associated condition is the majority of reported cases. However, malignancies, cytotoxic drugs, neutropenia, malnutrition, and deferoxamine therapy are also the said conditions.
- The clinical presentation includes facial swelling, extensive intraoral ulcers, and necrosis of palate and alveolar bone. The maxilla is affected more than mandible. The palate is the predominant site but may extend to involve alveolus and cheek mucosa.

Complications

- Untreated condition may lead to orbital cellulitis, proptosis, diplopia, and vision loss.

Investigation

- Incisional biopsy specimen stained with 10% KOH, or eosin and hematoxylin, or periodic acid-Schiff reveals fungal hyphae without septa and necrotic tissues.
- CT and MRI to assess the extension of lesion.

Treatment

- Management of the underlying cause (like DM).

- Intravenous administration of amphotericin B 50 mg for 1 week.
- Surgical debridement and hydrogen peroxide irrigation in the following week.
- Postoperative management of amphotericin B 40 mg/day for 2 weeks.

Aspergillosis

- It is caused by ubiquitous, fungal hyphae, *Aspergillus* species as both noninvasive and invasive diseases. It is the second common fungal infection affecting human next to candida. Inhalation of fungal spores is the mode of entry into sinuses and respiratory system. After their entry, the spores are innocuous but when there is an immune decline, the spores germinate and spread through the blood vessels.
- Rhinosinusitis is the clinical manifestation of fever, headache, facial swelling and nasal congestion. Sinus lesions may perforate and manifest in the oral cavity as a large necrotic ulcers with pseudomembrane slough. In the advanced stage, destruction of gingiva, alveolar bone, osteomyelitis of jaw bones, and facial muscles takes place.

Investigation

Histopathological examination and culture isolation.

Treatment

- Management of underlying immunocompromised state
- Antifungal therapy
- Local tissue debridement.

Histoplasmosis

It is caused by an endemic, saprophytic, dimorphic fungus *Histoplasma capsulatum*. Mode of spread is through the inhalation of spores. The infection occurs in acute, chronic and subacute forms. In the oral cavity, it present as ulcerative lesions resemble the squamous cell carcinomatous ulcers. The ulcers have a central necrosis, indurated base, and rolled margins. The tongue, palate and buccal mucosa are the common sites.

Investigation

Incisional biopsy and histopathological examination.

Management

- The lesion is self-limiting.
- In uncontrolled cases, cap itraconazole 100 mg/day is the drug of choice for 3–12 months.

Blastomycosis

A rare form of infection caused by saprophyte, *Blastomyces dermatitidis* present in the moist soil, decomposed leaves and woods. Oral lesions occur in variable forms including ulcers, verruciform, and granulomatous conditions. The mobility of the teeth and bone loss are the associated findings.

Cryptococcosis

- It is caused by an encapsulated, opportunistic yeasts, *Cryptococcus neoformans* and *Cryptococcus gattii*.
- The infection is commonly seen in AIDS patients. Any severely immunocompromised individuals and organ recipients are also prone to the infection. Oral lesions appear as nodules and granulomas that rupture and form ulcers with sinus orifice. Isolating the organism in culture will confirm the diagnosis.

Treatment

Intravenous amphotericin B or oral fluconazole.

SHORT NOTES

1. Describe Warts.

- Common warts are caused by human papillomavirus (DNA viruses) as keratotic papules on the fingers, hands, knees and rarely on the orofacial region. The virus enters the body through maceration and trauma; infect the basal layer leading to viral replication and DNA synthesis. Protein deposition occurs in different genes.

- There is no viremia, and hence systemic immune plays no role in protection. Langerhans cells evoke local cell-mediated immunity at the basal layer. Warts are difficult to treat, and spontaneous resolution occurs within 2 years.
- The therapeutic options are:
  - Cryotherapy
  - Podophyllin
  - Intralesional bleomycin.

2. Molluscum contagiosum.

- Molluscum infection is common in children, especially children in immunosuppressed and atopic status. The infection is caused by a poxvirus and spread by direct skin contamination. The lesions appear as dome-shaped umbilicated papules commonly on body folds and genitals and rarely on the oral cavity.
- The characteristic histopathological finding is the presence of Henderson-Paterson bodies (intracytoplasmic inclusion bodies).

Treatment Option

- Cryotherapy using liquid nitrogen
- Curettage
- Topical cidofovir.

3. Discuss tetanus (or) lockjaw.

- Tetanus is caused by an anaerobic, gram-positive bacterium, *Clostridium tetani*. The complication of this infection is the muscle spasm and autonomic nervous system disturbance due to the release of a neurotoxin, tetanospasmin by this bacterium.
- In mild cases, local muscle spasm may present. Pharyngeal and laryngeal muscle spasms may cause airway obstruction.
- In severe cases with generalized form, the jaw and face are affected. Trismus, muscle pain, stiffness and difficulty in swallowing are common.
- Prognosis depends on the speed at which infection spreads. Shorter the incubation period, the prognosis will be poor.

Treatment

- Cleaning and wound debridement to prevent further toxin production.
- The preferred antibiotic is — metronidazole 500 mg IV 6 hourly for seven days.
- To deactivate the circulating tetanus toxin, and prevent the neuronal uptake, antitoxin — human tetanus immune globulin (TIG) should be administered as IM dose.

4. Actinomycosis (or) cervicofacial actinomycosis (or) lumpy jaw.

(Actino = ray; mykes = fungus)

- Actinomycosis is an infectious disease caused by the invasion of tissues by fungus-like bacteria called *Actinomyces israelii*. In many individuals, these anaerobic gram-positive *Actinomyces* species are present in polymicrobial flora with other normal commensals, especially in the tonsillar crypts and oropharynx. From these sites, the bacteria may enter an opening in the oral mucosa, probably an extracted wound and cause the characteristic lumpy jaw. Radiotherapy, bisphosphonate therapy, and ulcerative mucosal lesions are the common predisposing factors.
- When the oral mucosal barrier is disturbed, actinomycosis spreads in a slow-progressive mode and cross the facial planes. The cervicofacial form typically affects tissues surrounding maxilla, mandible, cheek, chin, and posterior region of the oral cavity. It starts as a progressive, painless and firm-swelling that develops multiple abscesses and draining sinus tracts on the skin surface or oral mucosa. This is followed by a chronic indolent phase in which single or multiple indurations appear which are in woody consistency. Central necrosis of the induration occurs with sulfur granules. Pain and trismus are the later complications.
- The sulfur granules are the tiny clumps of 0.1–1 mm in diameter in size. Typical microscopic findings include a necrosis and filament gram-positive bacterium that resembles fungi.

Diagnosis

Bacterial culture.

Management

Actinomycosis needs prolonged treatment with high dose of antibacterial drugs. The standard regimen is intravenous penicillin, 18–24 million units/day for 2–6 weeks. The follow-up by treatment is the oral amoxicillin for a total period of 6–12 months.

5. Pyogenic granuloma.

Pyogenic granuloma is a reactive or reparative lesion. It is a connective tissue proliferative response to an irritant stimulus like calculus or injury due to foreign materials like denture clasps. Other factors like hormones, drugs, gingival inflammation due to defective fillings in the proximal tooth surface, food impaction have also been suggested as causative agents.

Clinical Features

Gingiva is involved frequently followed by tongue, labial, buccal mucosa, and hard plate (Fig. 1). It is a sessile or elevated growth, soft in consistency, dark red in early stage and later become reddish-purple. Bleeding is common for even a slight provocation but no pain.

Gravid Tumor (or) Pregnancy Tumor

During the first and third-trimester of pregnancy, the estrogen hormone levels will be highly increased. Gingival tissues have estrogen receptors which respond to the excess level of the hormone when the associated stimulus is present. A pedunculated or sessile, bright-red growth occurs in gingival which is usually asymptomatic.

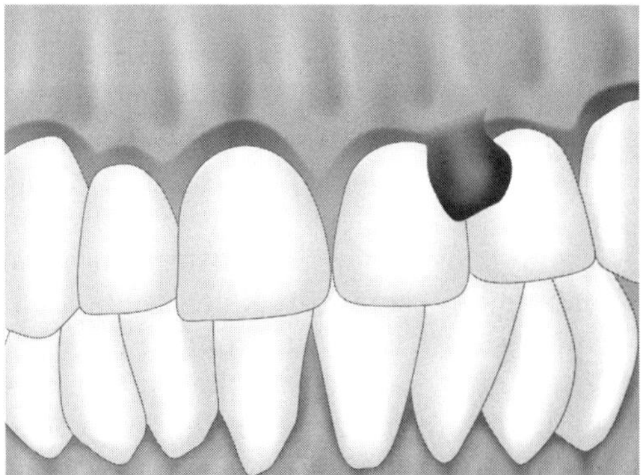

Fig. 1: Pyogenic granuloma on maxillary incisor region.

Radiographic Findings

No specific finding for pyogenic granuloma.

Differential Diagnosis

Fibroma, peripheral giant cell granuloma.

Treatment

- Removal of the irritating factor like calculus, or overhanging restorations or followed by surgical excision of the lesion.
- If it is associated with pregnancy, treatment should be carried out after childbirth. Proper oral hygiene procedure should be recommended.

6. Necrotizing ulcerative gingivitis (or) trench mouth (or) Vincent's stomatitis.

Acute necrotizing ulcerative gingivitis (ANUG) is a relatively rare clinical entity caused by a heterogeneous mixture of fusospirochetal complex consisting of spirochetes, vibrios, *Treponema macrodentium*, fusiform bacilli, and *Borrelia vincentii*.

Predisposing Factors

- Stressful conditions induce changes in the gingival tissue, and the causative organisms exert their pathogenic effects on the altered tissues.
- Immunosuppression (especially HIV infection)
- Smoking
- Poor oral hygiene
- Malnutrition.

Clinical Findings

Gingival ulceration, sharply punched out cratering of the interproximal papillae, necrosis, pseudomembrane formation, pain, bleeding, fetid odor, excess salivation, abnormal sensations of the teeth, lymphadenopathy, and fever are the common clinical presentation.

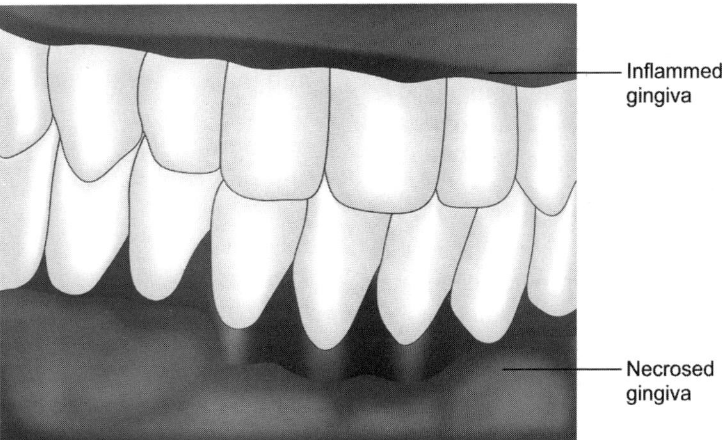

Fig. 2: Acute necrotizing ulcerative gingivitis.

For a clinical diagnosis, three signs and symptoms are essential:

1. Acute necrosis and ulceration of interdental papillae (Fig. 2).
2. Pain
3. Bleeding.

Treatment

- Chlorhexidine (or) hydrogen peroxide mouth rinse for superficial cleaning and debridement.
- Scaling and polishing with the use of topical anesthetics.
- Antibiotics: Amoxicillin (500 mg thrice daily; and metronidazole 400 mg twice daily).

7. Cancrum oris (or) noma.

- Noma is a sudden onset of gangrenous infection of the oral cavity which rapidly involves the adjacent hard and soft tissue structures of the face (lip, nose, and cheek) and then stops spreading further. There is no specific age group, but the affected individuals are usually malnourished and influenced by some infectious disease which weakens the immune system. The children are frequently affected especially those below 5 years of age.
- The condition starts with acute necrotizing ulcerative gingivitis preferably in the premolar-molar region. There will be profuse salivation, fetid odor, and purulent discharge. The ulcerative lesions may expose the underlying alveolar bone and cause spontaneous shedding of teeth. Within 2–3 days, it causes bluish discoloration of lips and cheek. Systemic manifestations include fever, tachycardia, lymphadenopathy, anorexia, edema, and ascites.

Prevotella intermedia and *Peptostreptococcus* are the microbial agents associated with noma.

Complications

Trismus, oronasal fistula, jaw bone sequestration.

Treatment

- Debridement with hydrogen peroxide solution and saline followed by a daily oral rinse of chlorhexidine gluconate (0.12–0.2%).
- Amoxicillin and metronidazole are the choices of antibiotics.
- Supportive therapy with multivitamins and high protein diet.
- Surgical correction for residual damage later.

8. Discuss oral manifestations of tuberculosis.

- Tuberculosis is a granulomatous disease caused by *Mycobacterium tuberculosis*. Involvement of oral cavity is infrequent in tuberculous infection.
- Occasionally, primary TB lesion is present in the oral cavity of young individuals as single, painless ulcer with enlarged regional lymph nodes mimicking oral cancer.
- Secondary oral lesions are rarely present in pulmonary tuberculous patients as single, large, painful ulcer with an indurated base and irregular margins. These types of lesions occur in elderly patients. The tongue is the commonly affected organ (especially lateral border); however, the involvement of buccal mucosa, palate, and floor of the mouth are also possible.
- Tuberculous gingivitis present as erythematous gingiva with ulcerated gingival margins with/without pain. It is common among tuberculous-positive children and adolescents.

Diagnosis

Mantoux skin test, chest X-ray, and biopsy of the oral lesion.

Treatment

Oral tuberculosis lesions are treated as same as systemic tuberculosis. A combination drug therapy (isoniazid, rifampicin, pyrazinamide, and ethambutol also known as, 4D- therapy) is the treatment of choice.

9. Infectious mononucleosis.

- Infectious mononucleosis is caused by Epstein-Barr virus, transmitted through saliva. The infection spread through kissing, or by a cough or sneeze, or by sharing food utensils with individuals infected by infectious mononucleosis. It is also called as kissing disease.
- It is also known as glandular fever and described as a hyperplastic disease of the reticuloendothelial system, lymph nodes, and spleen. Fever, sore throat and malaise are the early symptoms and thrombocytopenia is a later complication.
- Intraoral findings include the erythematous appearance of soft palate with multiple tiny petechiae. White pseudomembrane covers the tonsils.
- Patients may develop generalized faint, nonpruritic, maculopapular rash and disappears rapidly.

Diagnosis

Differential count: Increases number of white blood cells (lymphocytes) and atypical lymphocytes.

Antibody tests

- Monospot test—to check antibodies to the Epstein-Barr virus. This screening test is based on the agglutination of horse RBCs on exposure to heterophile antibodies. The result is given on the day but is not applicable to diagnose during the first week of illness.
- Paul-Bunnell test—infected serum is inactivated by water bath and treated with 0.85% NaCl. Fresh sheep cells are added. The final serum dilution is 1:20 up to 10,240. Sheep RBCs agglutinate in the presence of heterophile antibodies and incubated at 370°C for 4 hours. This is followed by overnight refrigeration. In the next day morning, the test tubes are again incubated for 1 hour at 37°C and then lightly turned upside down to observe the agglutination.

Management

Treatment is nonspecific. Management includes bed rest, proper nutrition and drinking plenty of fluids.

10. Necrotizing ulcerative periodontitis.

- Necrotizing ulcerative periodontitis (NUP) is characterized by extensive soft tissue necrosis and loss of interdental and alveolar bone.

- The microbial component includes Treponema species, Spirochetes, Fusobacterium, Bacteroides melaninogenicus, P. intermedia.

Predisposing Factors

- Immunosuppressed patients especially HIV-positive patients with CD4 count is less than 200 are associated with NUP.
- Severe malnutrition
- Smoking
- Poor oral hygiene
- Necrotizing ulcerative periodontitis starts as blunting or ulceration of the interdental papillae, and progress rapidly to destroy the alveolar bone.
- Severe pain and spontaneous bleeding will be present.
- Extensive destruction of periodontal tissue may lead to the shedding of teeth within 3–6 months of onset with sequestration.
- Metallic taste, bad breath, and deep jaw pain are the associated symptoms.

Treatment

The acute phase is aimed for pain control:

- Gentle debridement of necrotic tissues
- Chlorhexidine gluconate rinse (0.12%), twice daily
- Soft brushing
- Metronidazole, 400 mg BID for 10 days.

In the maintenance phase, treatment is directed to eliminate the causative organisms, prevent tissue damage, and to promote healing.

11. Quincy.

- Quincy denotes the peritonsillar abscess following acute suppurative tonsillitis or abscess in the peritonsillar fossa salivary glands (Weber's glands). The Weber's glands are the minor salivary glands function to clear the debris from tonsils. Any obstruction in the gland may lead to infection and pus formation. The other possible etiology includes infectious mononucleosis. The peritonsillar fossa is composed of loose connective tissue. Any nidus deposited in the region will cause infection and pus formation. The subsequent edema and inflammation may spread to the soft palate, pharyngeal wall, and base of the tongue. The incidence of quincy is frequent in young individuals below 30 years of age.
- The potential complications include pain and difficulty in swallowing, dehydration, fever, foul odor, space infection, trismus, and airway obstruction.

Treatment

- Antibiotic sensitivity test should be performed before selecting the medications. Pus collection is done by fine needle aspiration (FNAC), and the sample should be subjected to sensitivity test.
- A combination of amoxicillin 500 mg TID, and metronidazole 400 mg BID should be started immediately following diagnosis till receiving the sensitivity report.
- Clindamycin 500 mg BID is an alternate drug.

MULTIPLE CHOICE QUESTIONS

1. The causative organism for gastric or duodenal ulcer and low-grade gastric B-cell lymphoma is ***H. pylori***.
   a. *H. pylori*
   b. B. henselae
   c. Epstein-Barr virus
   d. *C. glabrata*
2. The causative organism for cat-scratch disease is ***B. henselae***.
   a. *H. pylori*
   b. B. henselae
   c. Epstein-Barr virus
   d. *C. glabrata*
3. Necrotizing granulomatous lymphadenitis is the manifestation of ***cat-scratch disease***.
   a. Wegener's granulomatosis
   b. Cat-scratch disease
   c. Sarcoidosis
   d. Lymphoproliferative disorder

4. Cat-scratch disease is a ***self-limiting disease.***
   a. Polyangiitis disorder
   b. Self-destructive disorder
   c. Self-limiting disease
   d. Metastatic infection
5. Father of immunology is ***Louis Pasture.***
   a. Antonie van Leeuwenhoek
   b. Robert Koch
   c. Alexander Fleming
   d. Louis Pasture
6. Father of oral microbiology is ***D. Miller.***
   a. Alfred Einhorn
   b. D. Miller
   c. Pierre Fauchard
   d. Charles C. Bass
7. An infection control procedure by destroying pathogens in any fluid by heating it at two different temperatures is known as ***Pasteurization.***
   a. Steam sterilization
   b. Vapor sterilization
   c. Pasteurization
   d. Dry cycle
   (**Note:** Pasteurization is an infection control procedure by destroying pathogens in any fluid by heating it to 63°C (145.4°F) for 30 minutes or to 72°C (161. 6°F) 15 seconds).
8. The recovery phase of an infection is known as ***convalescent stage.***
   a. Incubation stage
   b. Prodromal stage
   c. Convalescent stage
   d. Latent stage
9. Cells infected with virus produce ***interferons.***
   a. Virion
   b. Hepton
   c. Interferons
   d. Inclusion bodies
10. Sulfur granules are present in ***actinomycosis.***
    a. Actinomycosis
    b. Mycosis fungoides
    c. Mucormycosis
    d. Blastomycosis
11. Patients with chronic active hepatitis have the risk of developing ***hepatocellular carcinoma.***
    a. Cirrhosis of liver
    b. Hepatocellular carcinoma
    c. Hepatomegaly
    d. Fulminant hepatitis
12. HBsAg positive, anti-HBc negative results in a single test confirms hepatitis ***carrier state.***
    a. Infectious state
    b. Carrier state
    c. Recovery state
    d. Acute state
13. Positive HBeAg indicates ***highly infectious state***
    a. Inactive state
    b. Carrier state
    c. Highly-infectious state
    d. Passive infection
14. Koplik's spots are pathognomonic for ***rubella.***
    a. Mumps
    b. Rubella
    c. Rubeola
    d. Roseola
    (**Note:** Koplik's spots are seen as blue white specks with erythematous boundaries on the buccal mucosa opposite to the first molar region in measles patients).
15. Lues is the other name for ***syphilis.***
    a. Gumma
    b. Syphilis
    c. Chlamydia
    d. Chancre
16. Gumma is common in ***nasal bone and palate.***
    a. Nasal bone and palate
    b. Tongue and floor of the mouth
    c. Lip and facial skin
    d. Buccal mucosa and masticator muscles
17. Gumma of nasal bones causes ***saddle nose appearance.***
    a. Tabes dorsalis
    b. Saddle nose appearance
    c. Internasal keratitis
    d. Necrosis and disfigurement
18. Hutchinson incisors and mulberry molars or Moon's molars are the findings in ***congenital syphilis.***
    a. Rubella
    b. Congenital syphilis
    c. Turner hypoplasia
    d. Erythroblastosis fetalis
19. Tabes dorsalis is a ***tertiary neurosyphilis.***
    a. Congenital neurosyphilis
    b. Secondary syphilis

c. Tertiary neurosyphillis
d. Primary cardiosyphilis
(**Note:** Tabes dorsalis is a tertiary neurosyphilis or locomotor ataxia in which gait is affected).

20. In cardiovascular syphilis, the pulse is known as ***Corrigan's pulse***.
a. Pulsus paradoxus
b. Pulsus alternans
c. Corrigan's pulse
d. Anacrotic pulse
(**Note:** In cardiovascular syphilis, the high pulse is very high and is known as ***Corrigan's pulse*** or water-hammer pulse).

21. The infection referred as the great imitator is ***coccidioidomycosis***.
a. Geotrichosis
b. Coccidioidomycosis
c. Chlamydia
d. Erythema nodosum

22. Oral lesions of geotrichosis resemble ***candidiasis***.
a. Candidiasis
b. Mucormycosis
c. Actinomycosis
d. Wegener's granulomatosis

VIVA VOCE

1. What is furuncle?

- Furuncle is a deep-seated staphylococcal infection occurring as an inflammatory lesion in the hair-bearing region of the body surface. It occurs as an erythematous swelling, filled with pus and tender. They increase in size until it breaks down and drain out the pus. Diabetes and other immunocompromised states are the associative risk factors in the development of carbuncle and furuncle.
- A carbuncle is a collection of furuncle with sinus orifice.
- Pus culture and antibiotics; incision and drainage are the treatment options.

2. What is sterile pus?

Abscess containing anaerobic organisms which yield no organism on routine culture test but respond to gram staining is known as sterile pus.

3. What is an infection?

It is the multiplication and survival of microorganism in the body. It may or may not cause disease.

4. What is incubation period?

It is the duration of the entry of infectious agent into the body till the first symptom of the disease appears. All infectious disease has an incubation stage, and in this time, the microbes either simply survive in the body or multiply.

5. What is prodromal period?

It is the period in which early symptoms of an infectious disease occur. These symptoms include malaise, fever, headache, and chills. In this time, the causative organism multiplied to the sufficiently large amount.

6. What are the modes of infectious disease transmission (or) spread?

- Direct contact—e.g. herpes infection of fingers (herpetic whitlow).
- Indirect contact—e.g. hepatitis B and C infection (due to contact with contaminated instruments, surface, etc.)
- Droplet infection—e.g. mumps, influenza, rubella and herpes infections.
- Airborne infection—e.g. tuberculosis, measles, chickenpox.

7. How the microorganisms enter the body?

Through ingestion, inhalation or the breach in mucosa and skin.

8. What is cell-mediated immunity?

- The phagocytosis (destruction of microorganisms by neutrophils and macrophages) causes activation of T-lymphocytes and the activated T-lymphocytes will turn into various types of T lymphocytes and involved in:
  - Antibody-mediated response
  - Destruction of virus-infected cells
  - Produce lymphokines to activate phagocytes

- Destroy noninfected but structurally or functionally altered cells (e.g. cancer cells).

9. What is antibody-mediated immunity?

- The phagocytosis causes activation of B-lymphocytes, and the activated B-lymphocytes develop into different types of B-lymphocytes that produce lymphokines, and plasma cells which produce antibodies.
- The antibodies bind to specific antigens (microorganism) and either destroys or inactivates and removes them from the body.

10. Name the diseases in which monospot test will be positive.

Monospot positive test results in infectious mononucleosis, toxoplasmosis, rubella, lymphoma, leukemias and lymphomas.

BIBLIOGRAPHY

1. Auluck, A, Pai KM. Noma: life cycle of a devastating sore- case report and literature review. J Can Dent Assoc. 2005;71(10):757.
2. Greenberg SM, Glick M. Burket's Oral Medicine: Diagnosis and Treatment. Orofacial Pain, 9th edition. BC Decker Inc, Elsevier India; 2003:pp.230-232.
3. Iatta R, Napoli C, Borghi E, et al. Rare mycoses of the oral cavity: a literature epidemiologic review. Oral Surg Oral Med Oral Pathol Oral Radiol Endod. 2009;108(5):647-55.
4. Kamal R, Dahiya P, Puri A. Oral pyogenic granuloma: Various concepts of etiopathogenesis. J Oral Maxillofac Pathol. 2012; 16(1):79-82.
5. Kapoor S, Gandhi S, Gandhi N, et al. Oral manifestations of tuberculosis. Chrismed J Health Res. 2014;1:11-4.
6. Telles DR, Karki N, Marshall MW. Oral fungal infections: diagnosis and management. Dent clin North Am. 2017;61(2):319-49.
7. Valour F, Sénéchal A, Dupieux C, et al. Actinomycosis: etiology, clinical features, diagnosis, treatment, and management. Infection and drug resistance. 2014;7:183-97.

CHAPTER 13

Discoloration of Teeth

HIGHLIGHTS

Teeth become darker with advancing age changes by the secondary dentine deposition, incorporation of extrinsic stains and gradual wear of enamel. The causes of teeth discoloration may be influenced by underlying systemic diseases and many times give a clue to identify the related disease. Environmental factors and drugs also play a role in teeth discoloration. The discoloration may be generalized or may involve a group of teeths.

ESSAY QUESTIONS

1. Enumerate and briefly describe the various causes for discolored dentition.

Generalized Discoloration of Teeth

Two factors may cause generalized discoloration:

1. Intrinsic discoloration—due to structural change in the enamel or dentin by either altered composition or poor mineralization.
2. Extrinsic discoloration—due to the deposition of coloring agents on the teeth surface. It is subdivided into nonmetallic or direct staining and metallic or indirect staining. Combination of intrinsic and extrinsic discoloration.

Generalized Intrinsic Discoloration

- *Genetic diseases:*
  - Amelogenesis imperfecta—yellow-brown discoloration.
  - Dentinogenesis imperfecta and dentinal dysplasia—yellow.
  - Osteogenesis imperfecta—brown opalescent teeth.
- *Drugs:*
  - Tetracycline: Tetracycline staining results from the chelation of calcium ions of the hydroxyapatite crystals as a stable orthophosphate complex. Tetracycline stained teeth have a blue-gray or yellowish brown appearance.
  - Minocycline: A semisynthetic derivative of tetracycline. Its prolonged ingestion causes green-gray or blue-gray discoloration of the teeth.
  - Ciprofloxacin: When given to infants at dosages of 10–40 mg/kg/day give a greenish discoloration to the teeth.
  - Chlorhexidine mouth rinse: Prolonged use of chlorhexidine mouth rinse denatures the acquired pellicle on teeth surface and release sulfur radicals. These free radicals interact with the metal ions and form metal sulfide complex and impart tooth coloration.
- *Environmental:*
  - Fluorosis: A daily fluoride ingestion of more than 0.07 mg/kg body weight/day during early childhood period (at the enamel maturation stage) causes dental fluorosis. It is characterized by symmetrical patterns of discoloration resulting from subsurface hypomineralization.

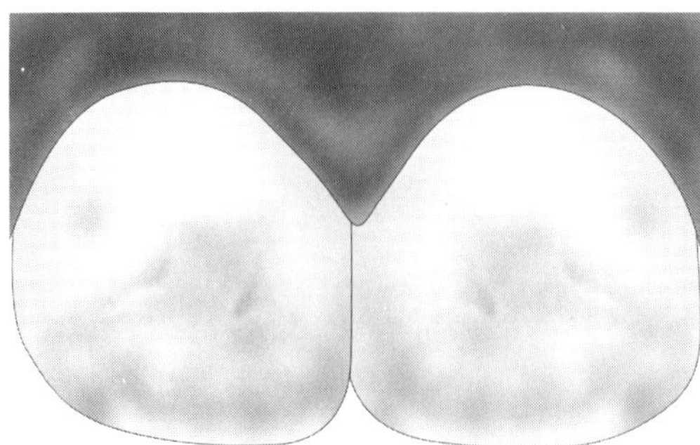

Fig. 1: Chalky white appearance of teeth in dental fluorosis.

- Clinical appearance includes:
  - Generalized chalky white appearance (Fig. 1).
  - Yellow-brown pitting.
  - Horizontal yellow-brown bands.

- *Metabolic disorders:*
  - Hyperbilirubinemia—yellow-green.
  - Porphyria—reddish-brown.
  - Alkaptonuria—brown.
  - Neonatal hyperbilirubinemia may cause bilirubin deposition on the developing tooth buds producing a yellow-green coloration on the teeth known as chlorodontia.
  - Congenital porphyria is an autosomal disorder of porphyrin metabolism, characterized by an increased formation and excretion of porphyrins. The porphyrin pigments have incorporated into the calcium phosphate during tooth development, and these cause a characteristic reddish-brown discoloration of the teeth called erythrodontia. The affected teeth red fluorescence under ultraviolet rays.
  - Alkaptonuria, (also known as phenylketonuria or ochronosis) is an inborn error of tyrosine and phenylalanine metabolism resulting in an increased content of homogentisic acid. This results in a brown discoloration of the permanent dentition.

Molar hypomineralization (or) hypoplastic molars: All first molar may become severely hypomineralized with the appearance of distinct yellow-brown color. The cause is idiopathic but proposed factors include childhood infections, dioxin in mother's milk, or genetic factors.

Hereditary diseases causing tooth discoloration: Defective enamel formation may lead to intrinsic discoloration of teeth in the following conditions:

- Vitamin D dependent rickets
- Epidermolysis bullosa
- Ehlers-Danlos syndrome
- Pseudohypoparathyroidism.

Single Tooth Intrinsic Discoloration

- *Nonvital teeth*
  - Pulp necrosis—rupture of blood vessels in a traumatized tooth leads to leakage of RBC that undergoes hemolysis, and release hemoglobin subsequently. Hemoglobin split into heme and globulin, and the iron in heme imparts blue-black color to the crown.
  - Pulp degeneration—when there is no pulpal bleeding, the necrotic tissue undergo protein degradation and gives a grayish-brown discoloration (Fig. 2).
- *Restorative materials:* Amalgam restoration: The presence of tin in amalgam migrates into dentinal tubules and cause discoloration.

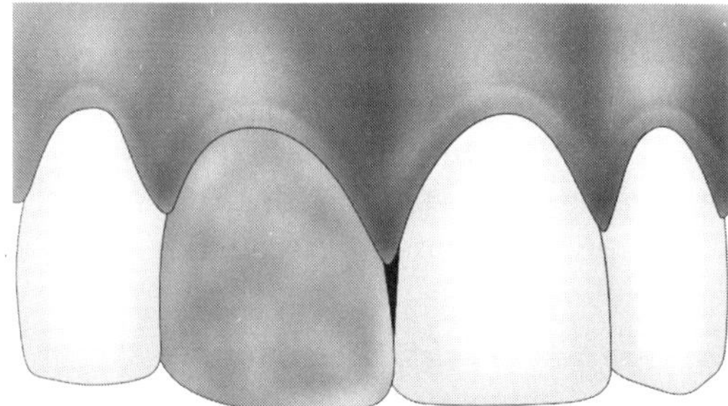

Fig. 2: Black discoloration of tooth due to pulp degeneration.

- *Turner's hypoplasia*
  - Local trauma or infection spread from the corresponding primary tooth may lead to chalky opaque appearance or brown discoloration, or enamel pitting on the permanent successor.
  - The permanent maxillary incisors and maxillary and mandibular premolars are the teeth commonly affected.

Extrinsic Discoloration of Teeth

- *Occupational exposure to:*
  - Iron and silver causes black staining of teeth.
  - Copper and nickel causes a green or blue-green discoloration.
  - Chromic acid fumes cause deep orange staining.
  - Lead dust and mercury imparts a blue-green stain.
- *Poor oral hygiene:* Brown discoloration by a pigmented pellicle deposition occurs on facial surface of upper molars and lingual surface of lower incisors.
- *Tobacco stain:* Deposition of coal-tar by-products of tobacco results in dark brown or black stains on teeth.
- *Black discoloration by chromogenic bacteria:* Black discoloration of teeth at the proximal and gingival margins are produced by *Actinomyces* in individuals with good oral hygiene. The reactions between the hydrogen sulfide released by the bacteria and iron in crevicular fluid causes the black discoloration.
- *Green stain:* A band of green stain is produced by a fluorescent fungus, *Penicillium* that requires sunlight for growth. Hence, it produces discoloration only at the labial surface of the anterior maxillary teeth.

MULTIPLE CHOICE QUESTIONS

1. Parkinson's disease may cause ***blue discoloration of the teeth***.
   a. Blue sclera
   b. Blue discoloration of the teeth
   c. Blue line on gingival margin
   d. Blue tongue
2. *Penicillium* and *Aspergillus* cause ***green staining of teeth***.
   a. Orange-stain of teeth
   b. Slate color of teeth
   c. Green staining of teeth
   d. Brown discoloration of teeth
   (**Note:** *Penicillium* and *Aspergillus* cause green-staining of anterior maxillary teeth).
3. Chlorodontia causes green pigmentation of teeth by ***bilirubin deposition***.
   a. Chloroquine deposition
   b. *P. aeruginosa* colonization
   c. Bilirubin deposition
   d. Porphyromonas colonization
   (**Note:** Chlorodontia is a condition associated with hyperbilirubinemia causing green tint of teeth by bilirubin deposition).
4. Orange discoloration of teeth is caused by ***Flavobacterium and Serratia marcescens***.
   a. Chromobacterium violaceum
   b. *Penicillium marneffei* and *Porphyromonas gingivalis*
   c. Cryptococcus neoformans
   d. *Flavobacterium* and *Serratia marcescens*
   (**Note:** Orange discoloration of teeth is caused by chromogenic bacteria *Flavobacterium* and *Serratia marcescens* in children with poor oral hygiene).
5. Orange-red discoloration of restored teeth is caused by ***Grossman's cement***.
   a. Tricalcium silicate cements
   b. Grossman's cement
   c. Rickert's sealer
   d. Cohen's sealer
   (**Note:** Orange-red discoloration of restored teeth is caused by restorative materials like Grossman's cement and zinc-oxide eugenol cement).
6. The degree of color saturation is ***chroma***.
   a. Hue
   b. Luma
   c. Chroma
   d. Luminance
7. The lightness or darkness on a scale of black and white is denoted by ***value of color***.
   a. Gray scale
   b. Value of color

c. Relative luminance scale
d. Saturation of color

8. Alkaptonuria causes ***brown discoloration of teeth***.
a. Brown discoloration of teeth
b. Yellow discoloration of teeth
c. Brown discoloration of tongue
d. Yellow discoloration of tongue
(**Note:** Alkaptonuria causes brown discoloration of teeth and is a condition of an inborn error in tyrosine and phenylalanine metabolism).

9. Günther's disease causes ***red-brown discoloration of teeth***.
a. Violet-black discoloration of teeth
b. Red-brown discoloration of teeth
c. Yellow-brown discoloration of teeth
d. White-blue discoloration of teeth
(**Note:** Error in porphyrin metabolism known as Günther's disease will cause a red-brown discoloration of teeth due to porphyrin deposition).

10. Usage of a mouth rinse containing potassium permanganate cause ***violet-black discoloration of teeth***.
a. Violet-black discoloration of teeth
b. Red-brown discoloration of teeth
c. Yellow-brown discoloration of teeth
d. Gold-brown discoloration of teeth

11. Stannous fluoride cause ***gold-brown coloration of teeth***.
a. Violet-black discoloration of teeth
b. Red-brown discoloration of teeth
c. Yellow-brown discoloration of teeth
d. Gold-brown discoloration of teeth

BIBLIOGRAPHY

1. Hattab FN, Qudeimat MA, Al-rimawi HS. Dental discoloration: an overview. J Esthet Dent. 1999;11(6):291-310.
2. Mortazavi H, Baharvand M, Khodadoustan A. Colors in tooth discoloration: a new classification and literature review. International Journal of Clinical Dentistry. 2014; 7(1):17-27.
3. Sulieman M. An overview of tooth discoloration: extrinsic, intrinsic and internalized stains. Dent update. 2005;32(8):463-4.
4. Watts A, Addy M. Tooth discoloration and staining: a review of the literature. Br Dent J. 2001;190(6):309-16.

CHAPTER 14

Odontogenic and Nonodontogenic Cysts

HIGHLIGHTS

Odontogenic and nonodontogenic cysts have some characteristic clinical pattern, but their diagnosis largely depends on radiographic interpretation and histopathological examination. This chapter summarizes the relevant clinical aspects of cysts and basic guidelines for accurate diagnosis.

Learners are expected to study about:

- Eruption cysts
- Residual cyst
- Bohn's nodules and Epstein's pearls
- Nasopalatine duct cyst
- Nasolabial cyst
- Traumatic bone cysts of jaw
- Aneurysmal bone cyst
- Stafne's cyst
- Dentigerous cyst and odontogenic keratocyst (Fig. 1):

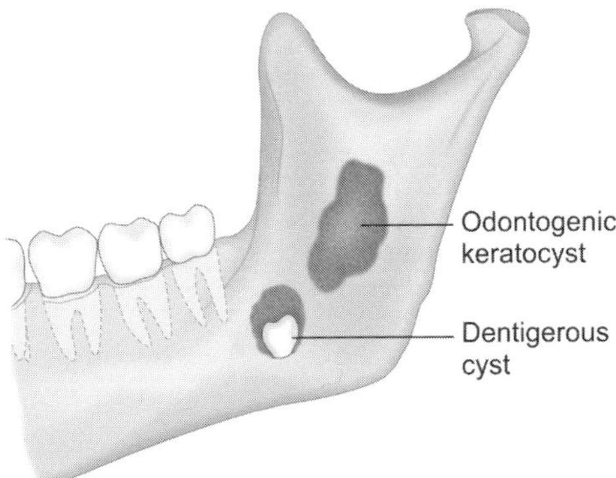

Fig. 1: Dentigerous cyst and odentogenic keratocyst.

SHORT NOTES

1. Classify the cysts of jaw.

Cysts of the jaw are broadly classified into:

- Odontogenic cysts
- Nonodontogenic cysts

World Health Organization Classification (1995)

Further classifies cysts as follows:

- *Developmental odontogenic cysts:*
  - Primordial cyst
  - Gingival cyst
  - Eruption cyst
  - Dentigerous cyst
  - Lateral periodontal cyst
  - Glandular odontogenic cyst
  - Sialo-odontogenic cyst
- *Developmental nonodontogenic cysts (Fig. 2):*
  - Nasopalatine duct cyst

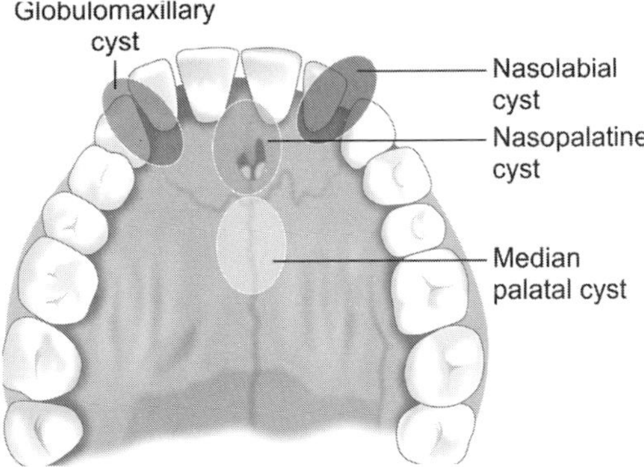

Fig. 2: Developmental nonodontogenic cysts.

- Globulomaxillary cyst
- Median-palatine cyst

❖ *Other cysts of jaw:*
- Aneurysmal bone cyst
- Traumatic bone cyst
- Epithelial jaw cysts

❖ *Other cysts of oral region:*
- Dermoid cyst
- Epidermoid cyst
- Gingival cyst of newborn
- Palatal cyst of newborn
- Nasolabial cyst
- Lymphoepithelial cyst.

2. Describe residual cyst.

- Residual cysts are inflammatory cysts arising as a result of incomplete surgical excision of odontogenic cysts, primarily radicular cysts.
- A residual cyst describes the radicular cysts that are retained after the tooth is extracted or cysts that are left following the incomplete enucleation of an odontogenic cyst (Fig. 3).
- Residual cysts are commonly seen in edentulous areas of mandible or maxilla.
- These cysts are asymptomatic.
- Long-standing cysts may become secondarily infected and turn symptomatic.
- They are diagnosed during routine radiographic examination.
- Size may vary from few mm to several cm.

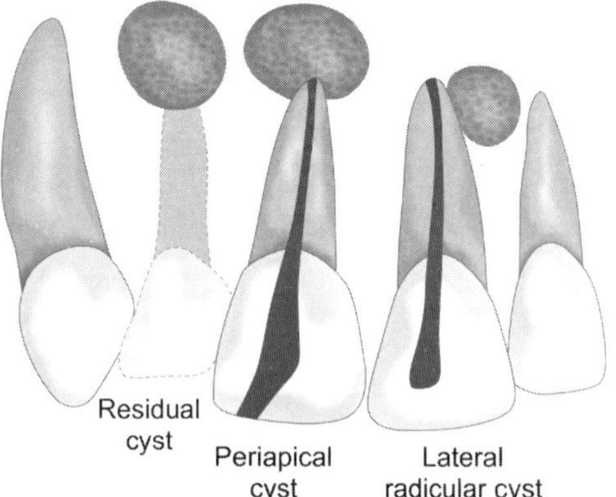

Fig. 3: Periapical, residual and lateral radicular cyst.

- Do not cause any bone expansion.
- Treated by surgical curettage or marsupialization.

3. Discuss periapical cyst (or) radicular cyst.

❖ The periapical cyst is the most frequently occurring type of odontogenic cyst. It is filled with fluid and lined by epithelium, hence true cyst. It is an inflammatory cyst originating from the nonvital tooth with pulpal necrosis.

Clinical Features

❖ Mostly asymptomatic.
❖ Rarely undergo acute exacerbation and become painful.
❖ Commonly involve anterior teeth. Maxillary anterior teeth are frequently affected than the mandibular anterior teeth.
❖ Root resorption and cortical bone expansion are rare.

Pathogenesis of Periapical Cyst (Flowchart 1)

Flowchart 1: Pathogenesis of periapical cyst.

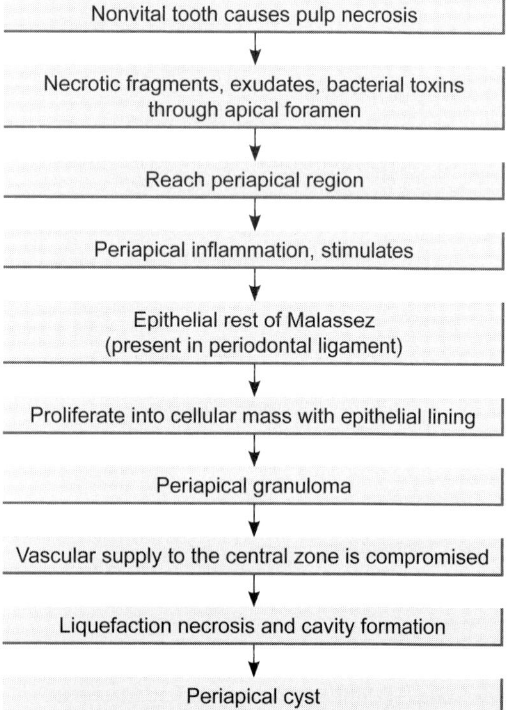

Radiographic Features

At the apical region of the involved tooth, a well-defined radiolucent lesion with a thin-radiopaque line at the periphery is characteristic (Fig. 3). Radiopaque boundary indicates the bone reaction to the slowly expanding lesion.

Treatment

- Endodontic management with or without periapical surgery.
- Extraction of involved tooth.

4. Eruption cyst (or) eruption hematoma.

It is the cyst that develops around the crown of an erupting tooth which is at the level of alveolar crest but not visible clinically.

Pathogenesis

Collection of fluid or blood in the follicular space between the reduced enamel epithelium and crown of erupting teeth leads to cystic swelling. The presence of thick fibrous tissue in the overlying mucosa prevents the eruption.

Clinical Features

- Seen in childhood in the age group of 5–9 years.
- The cyst commonly occurs in association with the eruption of mandibular primary central incisors and permanent mandibular first molars.
- Seen as soft, fluctuant swelling of the alveolus about the emerging tooth and measures about 1–1.5 cm in size, asymptomatic.
- If the cystic cavity contains blood, it appeared purple and called as eruption hematoma.

Radiographic Features

Soft tissue shadow over the crown of erupting tooth. No structural changes evident.

Treatment

In many cases, spontaneous rupture of the cyst is common. Surgically exposing the crown is needful in some cases to accelerate eruption.

5. Nasolabial cyst.

It is a developmental, soft tissue cyst, known as klestadt's cyst or nasoalveolar cyst. It arises as a result of the inclusion of epithelium along the fusion of maxillary process, lateral nasal process, and globular process.

Clinical Features

- Frequently occurs in 4th or 5th decade of life with a female predilection.
- The swelling occurs at the ala of nose over the maxilla with obliteration of nasolabial fold and intraorally manifests at the labial vestibule.
- It is fluctuant and painless unless secondarily infected.
- A large infected cyst may cause referred pain in the anterior maxillary teeth.

Radiographic Features

As it is a soft tissue cyst, after aspirating the cystic fluid and injection of radiopaque dye into cyst followed by taking maxillary occlusal radiograph may reveal the spherically shaped cyst with bracket shaped line indicating the inferior margin of the anterior bony aperture of the nose.

Treatment

Surgical excision.

6. Nasopalatine duct cyst (or) incisive canal cyst.

It is a developmental, nonodontogenic cyst, arises due to the spontaneous degeneration of embryologic remnants of the nasopalatine duct. The cyst develops within the incisive canal in the palatine bone or in the soft tissue covering the incisive foramen.

Clinical Features

- The cyst is characteristically seen at the center of the maxillary central incisor region.
- Usually asymptomatic at the initial stage.

- A salty taste fluid discharge and pain may manifest at later stages.
- Displacement of maxillary central incisors may also occur.

Radiographic Features

- Well-defined, oval or inverted pear-shaped radiolucency located at the inter-radicular region between the apices of maxillary central incisors. The cyst is well-corticated unless secondarily infected.
- Radiographically, if the diameter of the incisive canal exceeds 6 mm, nasopalatine cyst should be considered.

Treatment

Surgical enucleation.

7. Globulomaxillary cyst.

- The globulomaxllary cyst develops due to the entrapment of epithelium between the globular portion of the nasal process and maxillary process.
- Clinically it appears between the lateral incisor and canine teeth. The cyst forms on the bony suture (incisive suture) between the maxilla and premaxilla, hence called premaxilla-maxillary cyst.

Clinical Features

Majority of cases are reported during the routine radiographic interpretation. Very rarely, it shows clinical manifestations. Local discomfort and pain are the symptoms in a secondarily infected cyst.

Radiographic Findings

Inverted peer-shaped radiolucency between the roots of lateral incisor and canine teeth causing divergence of roots.

Differential Diagnosis

- Periapical cyst.
- Teeth associated with a globulomaxllary cyst are vital.

Treatment

Surgical excision.

8. Traumatic bone cysts of jaw.

- This cyst is otherwise known as a hemorrhagic cyst, solitary bone cyst, unicameral bone cyst and simple bone cyst.
- The traumatic bone cyst has no epithelial lining. Hence, it is a pseudocyst.

Etiology

- Trauma-hemorrhage theory: Trauma leads to intraosseous bleeding and hematoma formation. Failure of normal healing process causes liquefaction of clot by enzymatic action and leaves empty cavity within the bone. The trauma may be mild and the time lapse between the traumatic incident and cyst formation may vary from months to years.
- Ischemic necrosis of fatty marrow.
- Result of low-grade infection.

Clinical Features

- Commonly occurs in the second decade of life.
- Posterior mandible is frequently involved than anterior region.
- The associated teeth are vital.
- Swelling will be the complaint. Pain is rare.

Aspiration of Cystic Content

Straw-colored fluid or blood.

Radiographic Features

- A well-defined radiolucent area with/without a sclerotic border.
- Extensive lesions may cause buccal cortical expansion.
- The cyst may extend between roots and produce scalloped margins.

Treatment

Surgical enucleation.

9. Aneurysmal bone cyst.

Aneurysmal bone cyst arises as de novo in bone because definite pre-existing lesion cannot be demonstrated.

Clinical Features

- The cyst occurs in young individuals, predominantly below 30 years of age.
- The cyst has a preference for long bones. Mandible is affected more than maxilla.
- Swelling will be firm and painful.

Pathogenesis

- Initial osteolytic phase.
- Active growth phase: Increased rate of bone destruction and gives a subperiosteal blow out pattern.
- Mature stage: Also known as stabilization stage. Formation of peripheral cortication and internal septa provides soap bubble appearance.
- Healing phase: Gradual calcification and ossification.

Radiographic Findings

Well-defined, multilocular radiolucent cavity. In the mandible, the location of aneurysmal bone cyst is above the inferior alveolar canal.

Treatment

Surgical excision.

10. Stafne's cyst.

It is an unusual form of aberrant salivary gland tissue found within or adjacent to the lingual surface of body of the mandible forming a well-defined depression and therefore known as lingual mandibular salivary gland depression. It is a congenital defect, asymptomatic and detected during routine radiographic examination, hence called as a static bone cavity.

Radiographic Findings

It is a well-defined, ovoid radiolucency, located below the inferior alveolar canal, between the inferior alveolar canal and inferior border of the mandible (Fig. 4).

Complication

Salivary neoplasm may develop rarely.

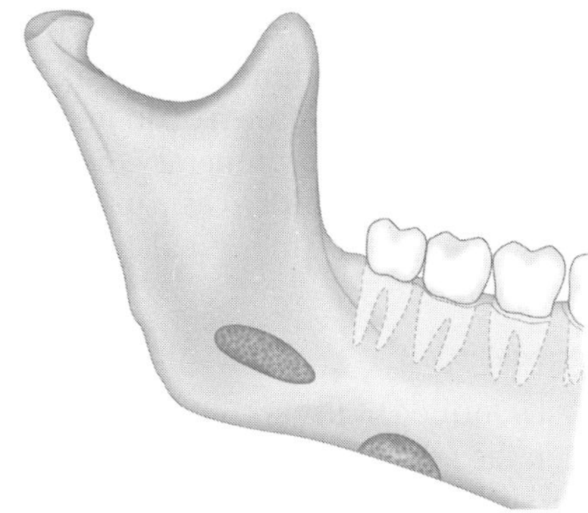

Fig. 4: Stafne's cyst.

Treatment

It is a developmental anomaly hence, do not require any treatment.

11. Dermoid cyst (or) dermoid tumors.

Dermoid cysts are sequestration of skin and subsequent implantation at the line of fusion of embryonic process. It is lined by epithelium and contains all skin appendages like hair follicles, sweat glands and sebaceous glands.

Clinical Features

In head and neck region, dermoid cysts develop as a midline lesion at the scalp, face, neck, and floor of the mouth. Rare site includes lip, tongue, and uvula.

Subclasses

- *Epidermoid cysts:* It is lined by epithelium and devoid of skin structures.
- *Teratoid cysts:* It is lined by epithelium and contains mesodermal components like muscle and bone.

Complications

Development of basal cell carcinoma and squamous cell carcinoma from epidermoid cyst are the remote possibilities.

Treatment

Surgical excision.

12. Dentigerous cyst (or) follicular cyst.

Dentigerous cysts are odontogenic cysts. They are formed around the crown of an impacted tooth or impacted supernumerary tooth. The crown will be characteristically protruding into the cystic lumen. This cyst also develops from odontome.

Pathogenesis

The cyst is formed by the accumulation of fluid between the reduced enamel epithelium and enamel surface.

Clinical Features

- ***Common site:*** Mandibular or maxillary third molar region and maxillary canine region.
- ***Age group:*** 2nd and 3rd decades of life.
- This cyst is aggressive and causes rapid bone expansion, root resorption, displacement of teeth. Mandibular expansion may extend up to coronoid with hollowing out of entire ramus and maxillary expansion usually limited to the anterior region.
- No associated pain until get secondarily infected.
- Bilateral and multiple dentigerous cysts are present in cleidocranial dysplasia and Maroteaux-Lamy syndrome.
- Potential complication—development of mural ameloblastoma.

Radiographic Features

Three types presentation:
1. Central—cyst symmetrically envelops crown.
2. Lateral—cyst develops along the lateral aspect of the crown.
3. Circumferential—the cyst envelops the entire tooth.

Treatment

Surgical removal.

13. Odontogenic keratocyst (or) keratocystic odontogenic tumor.

This cyst develops from the epithelial remnants of dental lamina and resembles an odontogenic tumor. The cyst epithelium produces keratin that fills the cystic lumen. The epithelium is thin and has mitotic property, hence grows like a neoplasm.

Clinical Features

- ***Age:*** 2nd and 3rd decade of life. Uncommon before 10 years of age.
- The mandible is frequently affected than the maxilla. In mandible:
  - Ramus—third molar area is involved more frequently than the first and second molar region followed by mandibular anterior region.
  - In maxilla, the involvement of third molar region and canine region are common in descending order of frequency.
- Soft tissue swelling, pain, expansion of bone, paresthesia of lip are the associated symptoms.
- If associated with nevoid basal cell carcinoma syndrome, this cyst will behave aggressively.
- It is locally destructive and has high recurrence rate.

Radiographic Features

- Well-defined unilocular or multilocular radiolucency.
- Borders are scalloping due to the variation in growth pattern.
- Displacement of adjacent teeth is common
- Rarely produces root resorption

Treatment

Surgical enucleation or marsupialization.

14. Gorlin's cyst (or) calcifying epithelial odontogenic cyst.

A heterogeneous group of cysts showing a variable clinicopathological pattern and includes both non-neoplastic cyst and true neoplasm.

Cystic component
- Type I—typical Gorlin's cyst. Unicystic type with/without calcified material.
- Type II—unicystic odontome type.

- Type III—unicystic ameloblastomatous proliferating type.

Neoplastic component: Odontogenic tumor with ghost cells.

Clinical Features

- Slow-growing, painless, nontender swelling.
- Prevalent in the second decade of life.
- Anterior region of jaws are commonly affected, and maxillary canine region involvement is very common.
- Most commonly associated with the unerupted tooth.

Radiographic Features

The central part of the lesion is radiolucent that may contain foci of calcified material. Margins appear smooth and well-defined or irregular and poorly-defined. The unilocular pattern is typical. It is associated with root resorption and lingual plate expansion.

Treatment

Surgical enucleation and curettage.

15. Describe basal cell nevus syndrome.

- It is an autosomal-dominant condition, comprising cleft lip or palate, frontal bossing, coarse facial features, and hypertelorism. It is also known as Gorlin-Goltz syndrome.
- The classic triad of this syndrome is multiple basal cell carcinomas, odontogenic keratocyst (OKC), and bifid ribs.
  - Odontogenic keratocysts may be the first indicative sign of this syndrome and start manifesting in the 1st and 2nd decade of life and continue to develop in a 3rd decade also. The cysts are asymptomatic initially and later cause jaw expansion, pain, and facial asymmetry.

Clinical Significance

Ameloblastoma or squamous cell carcinoma may arise from these cysts. Other associated neoplasms include Hodgkin's lymphoma, non-Hodgkin's lymphoma, schwannoma, pleomorphic adenoma, tumor of adrenal glands, and salivary adenoid cystic carcinoma.

Management

A multidisciplinary approach including genetic counseling, chemoprevention (vitamin A supplementation) surgical care and life-support measures like a routine examination in every 4 months to identify recurrent lesions is necessary.

16. Describe lateral periodontal cyst.

- The lateral periodontal cyst is a developmental, non-inflammatory, and non-keratinized epithelial cyst presenting lateral to the root of a vital tooth.
- It is seen as a small swelling in the interdental papilla or slightly below the papilla on labial aspect, and is asymptomatic. Pulp vitality tests of adjacent teeth reveal normal response.

Radiographic Features

- Unilocular radiolucent lesion appears between the roots of mandibular canine and first premolar or between premolars. Size is usually less than 1 cm but rarely larger size and polycystic appearance also present.
- The divergence of the roots may also be evident.

Treatment

Cyst enucleation. Recurrence is unusual.

MULTIPLE CHOICE QUESTIONS

1. *Gorlin-Goltz syndrome* is associated with ***multiple odontogenic keratocyst***.
   a. Multiple impacted teeth
   b. Multiple odontogenic keratocyst
   c. Failure of eruption
   d. Delayed ossification
2. Epstein pearls are present in the ***mid-palatine raphe***.
   a. Gingiva
   b. Edentulous alveolar ridge
   c. Mid-palatine raphe
   d. Buccal mucosa
   (**Note:** Epstein pearls are keratin-filled nodules present along the mid-palatine raphe and originate from the epithelial remnants of fusion).

3. *Bohn's nodules* are derived from ***minor salivary glands***.
   a. Epithelial remnants
   b. Palatine vessels
   c. Nutrient canals
   d. Minor salivary glands
   (**Note:** Bohn's nodules are keratin-filled cysts, present at the junction of hard and soft palate, and derived from minor salivary glands).
4. Dental lamina cysts of the newborn are seen on ***edentulous alveolar ridge***.
   a. Gingiva
   b. Edentulous alveolar ridge
   c. Mid-palatine raphe
   d. Buccal mucosa
   (**Note:** Dental lamina cysts of the newborn are solitary, or multiple superficially raised nodules on edentulous alveolar ridge).
5. *Dental lamina cysts of the newborn* are ***asymptomatic***.
   a. Interfere with feeding
   b. Asymptomatic
   c. Interrupting eruption
   d. Severely tender
6. Dental lamina cysts of the newborn require ***no treatment***.
   a. Excision
   b. Incision and drainage
   c. No treatment
   d. Alveoloplasty
   (**Note:** Dental lamina cysts of the newborn require no treatment and disappear during the eruption of teeth).
7. The lateral periodontal cyst is common in ***mandibular premolar region***.
   a. Mandibular molar-ramus region
   b. Mandibular premolar region
   c. Maxillary canine region
   d. Maxillary incisor region
   (**Note:** The lateral periodontal cyst is a developmental cyst).
8. The multilocular pattern of lateral periodontal cyst is known as ***botryoid odontogenic cyst***.
   a. Botryoid odontogenic cyst
   b. Bay cyst
   c. Aneurysmal cyst
   d. Pilar cyst
9. Periapical granuloma with islands of squamous epithelium is known as ***bay cyst***.
   a. Botryoid odontogenic cyst
   b. Bay cyst
   c. Aneurysmal cyst
   d. Pilar cyst
10. Daughter cysts are characteristic for ***odontogenic keratocysts***.
   a. Odontogenic keratocyst
   b. Ameloblastoma
   c. Dentigerous cyst
   d. Follicular cyst
11. Bohn's nodules regress spontaneously within ***3–4 months of age***.
   a. 12–24 months of age
   b. 12 years of age
   c. 3–4 months of age
   d. 4 years of age
12. Single, homogeneous, highly radiopaque dome-shaped lesion with thin radiolucent air space outline in the maxillary sinus denotes ***mucocele***.
   a. Mucoepidermoid tumor
   b. Ciliated cyst of antrum
   c. Pneumatized sinus
   d. Mucocele
   (**Note:** Mucocele or mucous retention cyst of the maxillary sinus).

BIBLIOGRAPHY

1. Lam C, Ou JC, Billingsley EM. "PTCH"-ing it together: a basal cell nevus syndrome review. Dermatol Surg. 2013;39(11):1557-72.
2. Neville BW, Damm DD, Chi AC, Allen CM. Oral and maxillofacial pathology, 4th edition. Elsevier Health Sciences; 2015.
3. Scholl RJ, Kellett HM, Neumann DP, Lurie AG. Cysts and cystic lesions of the mandible: clinical and radiologic-histopathologic review. Radiographics. 1999;19(5):1107-24.
4. Shear M, Speight P. Cysts of the oral and maxillofacial regions. John Wiley & Sons; 2008.
5. Slootweg PJ. Bone diseases of the jaws. International journal of dentistry. 2010;2010.

CHAPTER 15

Odontogenic and Nonodontogenic Tumors

HIGHLIGHTS

A tumor is a nonspecific term and only refers to mass. A tumor may be benign, or a malignant growth originating either from the hard or soft tissue of oral cavity.

Odontogenic tumors develop from the cells or tissues that initiate the tooth development. Their clinical and pathohistological characters are different. The tumors may exhibit hamartomatous proliferation, nonaggressive benign course, or an aggressive and malignant behavior. Nonodontogenic tumors of the jaw are of soft tissue origin like epithelium, connective tissue components, mucosa, and muscles. They arc either benign or malignant.

Learners are expected to learn about:

- Different types of tumors occurring in oral cavity.
- Differentiating benign and malignant tumors.
- Characteristic features of hard and soft tissue tumors.
- Radiographic findings of odontogenic tumors.

ESSAY QUESTIONS

1. Classification of nonodontogenic tumors of the jaws. (or) classification of soft tissue tumors of jaw.

Benign Tumors

- Epithelial tumors:
  - Squamous papilloma
  - Verruca vulgaris
  - Keratoacanthoma
- Fibro-osseous tumors:
  - Ossifying fibroma
  - Juvenile ossifying fibroma
  - Langerhans disease
- Lesions containing multinucleated giant cells:
  - Central giant cell granuloma
  - Giant cell tumor hyperparathyroidism
  - Cherubism
- Neurogenic tumors:
  - Schwannoma
  - Neurofibroma
- Bone tumors:
  - Osteoma
  - Osteoid osteoma
  - Osteoblastoma
  - Ossifying fibroma
  - Desmoplastic fibroma
- Cartilage tumors:
  - Chondroma
  - Chondroblastoma
  - Chondromyxoid fibroma
- Muscles:
  - Leiomyoma
  - Rhabdomyoma
  - Granular cell myoblastoma
- Viral induced tumors:
  - Squamous papilloma
  - Warts

Malignant Tumors

- Malignant epithelial tumors:
  - Basal cell carcinoma

- Squamous cell carcinoma
- Verrucous carcinoma
- Spindle cell carcinoma
- Adenoid squamous cell carcinoma
- Basaloid squamous cell carcinoma
- Malignant melanoma

❖ Lymphoid tissue:
- Hodgkin's lymphoma
- Non-Hodgkin's lymphoma
- Burkitt's lymphoma

❖ Connective tissue:
- Fibrosarcoma
- Liposarcoma

❖ Muscles:
- Leiomyosarcoma
- Rhabdomyosarcoma

❖ Nerve tissue:
- Neurosarcoma
- Neurofibrosarcoma

❖ Vascular:
- Angiosarcoma
- Kaposi's sarcoma

❖ Bone:
- Osteosarcoma
- Chondrosarcoma
- Ewing's sarcoma.

2. Classify odontogenic tumors of the jaw and describe the clinicopathological and radiographic features of ameloblastoma.

World Health Organization Classification (1992)

Benign Odontogenic Tumors

❖ *Odontogenic epithelium without odontogenic ectomesenchyme:*
- Ameloblastoma
- Squamous odontogenic tumor
- Calcifying epithelial odontogenic tumor (Pindborg tumor)
- Clear cell odontogenic tumor

❖ *Odontogenic epithelium with odontogenic ectomesenchyme, with/without dental hard tissue formation:*
- Ameloblastic fibroma
- Ameloblastic fibrodentinoma (dentinoma)
- Ameloblastic fibro-odontoma
- Odontoameloblastoma
- Adenomatoid odontogenic tumor
- Calcifying odontogenic cyst
- Complex odontoma
- Compound odontoma

❖ *Odontogenic ectomesenchyme with/without odontogenic epithelium:*
- Odontogenic fibroma
- Myxoma (odontogenic myxoma, myxofibroma)
- Cementoblastoma, and true cementoma.

Malignant

❖ *Odontogenic carcinomas:*
- Malignant ameloblastoma
- Primary intraosseous carcinoma
- Malignant variants of other odontogenic epithelial tumors
- Malignant changes in odontogenic cysts

❖ *Odontogenic sarcomas:*
- Ameloblastic fibrosarcoma (ameloblastic sarcoma)
- Ameloblastic fibro-dentinosarcoma
- Ameloblastic fibro-odontosarcoma

Ameloblastoma

❖ Robinson defines ameloblastoma as a unicentric, nonfunctional, true neoplasm of enamel organ tissues with intermittent growth; behave as benign lesion but locally aggressive.

❖ Ameloblastoma is the second common type of tumor originating from odontogenic tissues.

Pathogenesis

It may be derived from:

❖ Cell rests of enamel organ.

❖ Odontogenic cystic epithelium.

❖ The basal cells of the surface epithelium.

Clinical Features

❖ It affects individuals in the 4th and 5th decades of life.

❖ The mandible is frequently involved, molar-ramus region being the common site (80%).

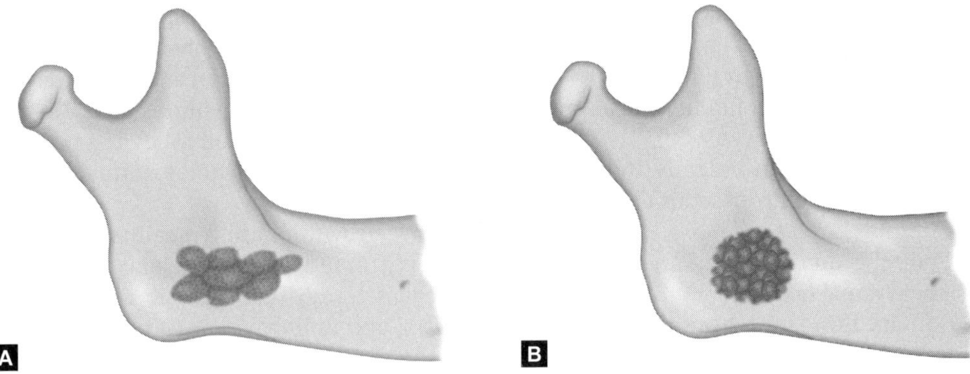

Figs. 1A and B: (A) Soap bubble appearance of ameloblastoma. (B) Honeycomb appearance of ameloblastoma.

- In early stage, it is slow-growing and asymptomatic.
- As a tumor enlarges, it causes expansion of jaw bone and facial deformity.
- The swelling will be hard, and nontender or mildly tender.
- Eggshell crackling may be elicited due to thinning of overlying bone.
- It is not capsulated. Though locally infiltrate into the bone marrow, they do not metastasize. Occur both in maxilla and mandible with a preference to the middle and posterior parts of the mandible.
- Peripheral ameloblastoma is a rare type and occurs on the gingiva. It is a noninvasive type, occurring in younger individuals. Mandibular premolar region is the reported site of preference. It grows up to 2–3 cm in size.

Radiographic Findings

- Multilocular radiolucent lesion with soap bubble or honeycomb pattern (Figs. 1A and B).
- The unilocular type is as a well-defined radiolucent lesion with minimal sclerotic border and resembling dentigerous cyst (Fig. 2).
- Root resorption of adjacent teeth is common.

Treatment

- For unilocular type—curettage or enucleation.

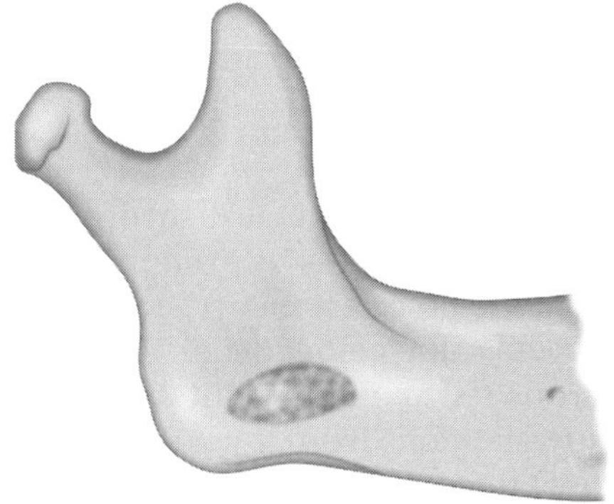

Fig. 2: Ameloblastoma.

- For multilocular type and solid pattern—tumor excision or partial resection of the jaw bone.

3. Classify fibro-osseous lesions of the jaw. Describe the pathogenesis, clinical features and radiographic appearance of fibrous dysplasia.

Fibro-osseous lesions of the jaw: In fibro-osseous lesions, the normal bone is replaced by fibroblasts and collagen fibers with varying amounts of a calcified substance.

World Health Organization Classification (1992)

- Osteogenic neoplasms:
  - Cemento-ossifying fibroma (cementifying fibroma, ossifying fibroma).

- Non-neoplastic bone lesions:
  - Fibrous dysplasia of jaws
  - Cemento-osseous dysplasia:
    - Periapical cemental dysplasia (periapical fibrous dysplasia)
    - Florid cemento-osseous dysplasia
    - Other cemento-osseous dysplasia
  - Cherubism
  - Central giant cell granuloma
  - Aneurysmal bone cyst
  - Solitary bone cyst (traumatic, simple, hemorrhagic bone cyst).

Fibrous Dysplasia

Fibrous dysplasia (FD) is a benign intramedullary genetic disorder of bone that may affect single (monostotic: MFD) or multiple bones (polyostotic: PFD).

Pathogenesis

- Fibrous dysplasia is a disorder in the remodeling process of primordial bone to mature bone. Immature, coarse, bony trabeculae are embedded in a dysplastic fibrous tissue matrix with insufficient mineralization. There is gene mutation in 20q chromosome, and all cell derivatives of the mutant gene manifests dysplastic features.
- McCune-Albright syndrome (MAS) may have a component of fibrous dysplasia. MAS is an intermittent type of syndrome described as a triad of polyostotic, hyperpigmentation (café-au-lait spots), and multiple endocrinopathies like sexual precocity in females.
- Maxillary involvement is common than mandibular involvement. Craniofacial FD describes FD affecting maxilla, maxillary sinus, zygoma, sphenoid, temporal, orbital, nasal, frontal, and occipital bones. FD is unilateral and rarely occurs bilaterally.

Clinical Features

- Fibrous dysplasia arises within the first or second decades of life. It is slow-growing and causes asymptomatic expansion of the affected bone.
- The degree of deformity depends on the site and extent of bone involvement, (mono or polyostotic type). Facial asymmetry is also present. Rapid expansion is rare. There is an acceleration period following the slow growth leading to facial deformity and nerve compression.
- Active growth phase typically slows down during puberty or after skeletal maturation.
- Head is the most common site in monostotic form, and in polyostotic form femur, tibia, and pelvis are involved.
- Prognosis is good, and recurrence following treatment is rare.

Radiographic Diagnosis

The various imaging techniques include:

- Conventional panoramic technique
- Computed tomography
- Magnetic resonance imaging (MRI)
- Scintigraphy

The developmental stage and the quantity of bone deposition in the affected site determine the radiographic pattern of the FD. In conventional tomographic view, well-defined radiolucency represents the early stage of lesion whereas radiodense sclerotic pattern denotes the mature stage of FD. The pathognomonic ground-glass or orange peel image pattern reveals the merged boundaries between the fibrous dysplastic bone and the unaffected bone.

Distinctive Radiographic Features

- Loss of lamina dura of the teeth in the affected region of maxilla and mandible.
- Displacement of inferior alveolar canal in upward direction.
- Arrangement of abnormal trabeculae in a swirling pattern resembling thumbprint.

Differential Diagnosis

- Nonossifying fibroma, low-grade osteosarcoma, simple bone cyst.

Management

- For polyostotic form, referral to an endocrinologist is mandatory for the diagnosis and management of endocrine abnormalities.

Bisphosphonates (pamidronate) is used extensively for treating patients with the polyostotic disease.
- Surgical resection.

SHORT NOTES

1. Describe odontome.

Odontoma is a tumor of odontogenic origin, in which an atypical formation of enamel and dentin occurs. It is considered as a hamartomatous malformation rather than true neoplasm because it has both epithelial and mesenchymal components.

Etiology

Definite etiology is unknown. Local trauma or infection is the most recognized cause.

Types

- Compound composite odontoma: The enamel and dentine are laid down orderly so that they superficially resemble a tooth structure.
- Complex composite odontoma: The calcified tissues are arranged as an irregular pattern without any resemblance to the tooth morphology. This form is rare.

Clinical Features

- There is a male predilection for the occurrence.
- Maxilla is more common (67%) than mandible (33%).
- Compound odontoma occurs in anterior maxilla, whereas complex odontomas have a preference for posterior jaws.
- Odontoma usually remains smaller than a tooth, but rarely it becomes larger and produces bony expansion and facial asymmetry.
- Mostly these are asymptomatic.

Complication

Occasional development of dentigerous cyst.

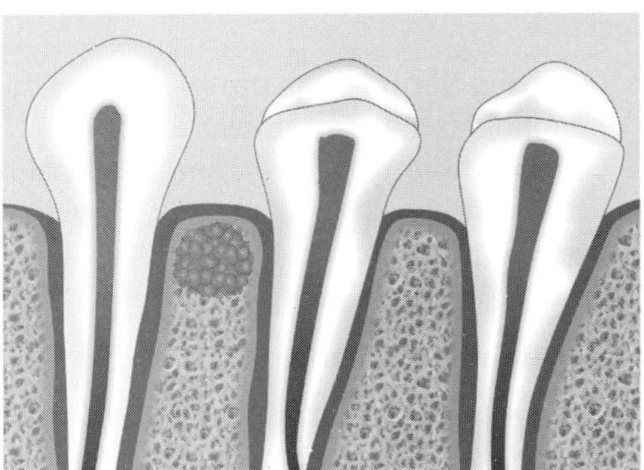

Fig. 3: Intermediate stage odontome on a radiograph.

Radiographic Features

Present as a dense radiopaque mass surrounded by a thin radiolucent boundary.
- Stage I (or) initial stage: Radiolucent due to the absence of calcified structures.
- Stage II (or) intermediate stage: Partial calcification gives rise to mixed pattern of raidiopacity and radiolucency (Fig. 3).
- Stage III (or) mature stage: Radiopaque stage with surrounding radiolucent halo.

Treatment

Surgical excision.

2. Ossifying fibroma.

Ossifying fibroma (OF) is a benign lesion of jaw bones in which the affected site is composed of fibrous tissue and calcified structures like cementum and bone instead of normal bone architecture.

Synonyms

- Cementifying fibroma
- Cemento-ossifying fibroma
- Juvenile ossifying fibroma.

Histological Types

- Juvenile trabecular ossifying fibroma (JTOF)
- Juvenile psammomatoid ossifying fibroma (JPOF).

Location

- Ossifying fibroma has prevalence for the mandibular molar-premolar region.
- Ossifying fibroma presents as a small, painless lesions that are occasionally diagnosed on routine radiographs. They are slow-growing and expansive.

Radiographic Appearance

- They are unilocular lesions with a well-defined, smooth, radiopaque border.
- In the initial stage of development, the lesion resembles a cyst with radiolucent appearance.
- In the later course of the lesion, it appears radiopaque with well-defined radiolucent boundary.

Management

Surgical resection.

3. Describe adenomatoid odontogenic tumor.

- Adenomatoid odontogenic tumor is a tumor originating from the odontogenic epithelium.
- The tumor presents with both intraoral and extraoral swellings in the maxilla (involves both bone and soft tissue). It is referred to as "two-third tumor" because in 2/3rd of reported cases, it occurred in maxilla, in 2/3rd cases, the gender reported is females of young age group and 2/3rd of the diagnosed patients had an unerupted tooth in the affected site and canine is involved in nearly 2/3 cases.
- It is a well-capsulated tumor and hence benign.
- The tumor has a high predilection for females.
- Root resorption, displacement of roots and bone perforation are the rarely associated findings.
- Histological findings reveal calcification in the form of irregular masses or as a pattern of Liesegang rings.

Radiographic Appearance

- Adenomatoid odontogenic tumor occurs as both intraosseous and extraosseous types.
- Intraosseous type takes either follicular (pericoronal) or extrafollicular (extra-coronal) form (Figs. 4A and B).

Intraosseous Type

- Follicular form: Appear as a distinct radiolucent lesion around the crown of an unerupted tooth and hence frequently misdiagnosed as dentigerous cyst (Fig. 4B).
- Extrafollicular form: Appear as a definite radiolucent lesion overlaying the root of an unerupted tooth. Sometimes tiny

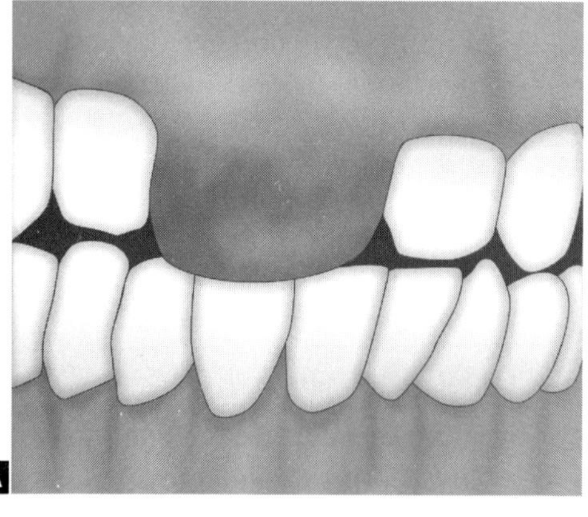

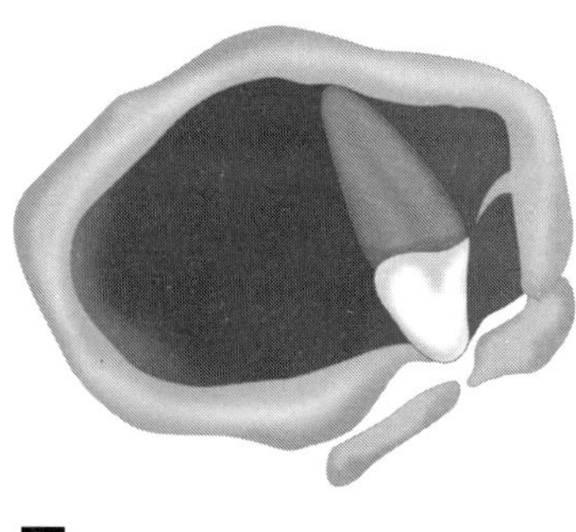

Figs. 4A and B: (A) Extrafollicular form of adenomatoid odontogenic tumor. (B) Follicular form of adenomatoid odontogenic tumor.

radiopaque structures are present within the radiolucency.

Extraosseous (Peripheral or Gingival) Type

- The peripheral type is seldom observed on radiographs. Many times mild erosion of the alveolar bone is the only positive radiographic feature.

Treatment

Curettage is the preferred treatment. Recurrence is uncommon.

4. Calcifying epithelial odontogenic tumor (or) Pindborg tumor.

- This tumor is rare and is known by the name of Dr J J Pindborg, who described first. It is locally invasive and present as a unilocular or multilocular swelling in molar—ramus region and thus resembling ameloblastoma.
- This tumor forms an amorphous amyloid or amyloid-like material. It calcifies in a concentrically lamellar form resembling tree-ring pattern and known as *Liesegang calcifications*. Calcifying epithelial odontogenic tumor (CEOT) is nonencapsulated but does not infiltrate into the deep tissues.
- *Radiographically,* this tumor appears radiolucent but if calcifications present, it appears radiopaque. The central location of the tumor in the jaw with an expansion of cortex and areas of spotty calcification are radiographic characteristics for Pindborg tumor.
- *Enucleation or local block excision* is the treatment of choice.

5. Write about verruca vulgaris (or) oral warts.

It is a focal papillary hyperplasia induced by human papilloma viral infection (HPV-2, HPV-4, and HPV-40). The lesion is contagious and spreading from autoinoculation to other parts of the skin, and mucous membrane in the affected individual is common.

Clinical Features

- Pointed, exophytic surface projection with a narrow stalk, and presents as multiple or clustered lesion.
- It enlarges rapidly and reaches a higher diameter of 5 mm.
- Present on lips and intraoral presentation is rare and seen in palate, gingiva.
- It appears white due to surface keratinization

Diagnosis

- Clinical presentation.
- Histopathological features of thin, long and finger-like projections, hyperkeratosis, koilocytosis (HPV-altered epithelial cells).
- Demonstration of HPV-antigen by immunohistochemistry.

Treatment

- Excision of the lesion with the base in which the stalk is attached.
- Liquid nitrogen cryotherapy.
- Topical keratolytic agents.

6. Discuss condyloma acuminatum.

It is a type of oral wart caused by human papillomavirus-6 (HPV-6). It is a sexually transmitted infection that occurs either single or as multiples.

Clinical Features

- Commonly present on lips, commissure of mouth, and gingiva.
- Coral pink in color with a warty surface.
- The lesions may proliferate and coalesce to form clusters. Size is variable between 2 cm and 3 cm.

Diagnosis

Histopathological features of intranuclear inclusion bodies in epithelial cells.

Treatment

- Surgical excision.
- Topical application of keratolytic agents.

7. Pyogenic granuloma.

It is a localized reactive lesion to mild irritation and manifests as a tissue overgrowth. Pyogenic granuloma is a misused terminology because it is neither associated with pus formation nor with a histological resemblance to granuloma.

Etiology

Low-grade, chronic irritation caused by trauma, calculus, and overhanging restorations.

Clinical Features

- Commonly occur on the gingiva especially in the interdental region of the anterior maxillary teeth. May also occur in lip, tongue and buccal mucosa.
- It appears as an elevated, sessile or pedunculated mass with erythematous overlying mucosa. The surface is smooth or lobulated.
- Spontaneous bleeding is common, and even a slight provocation causes profuse bleeding.
- It is painless and soft in consistency.
- It develops rapidly and reaches full size, few millimeters to several centimeters, then remains static.
- Long-standing pyogenic granulomas may show fibrous changes and undergo dystrophic calcification.

Diagnosis

- Clinical features
- Intraoral periapical radiograph to rule out bone resorption.
- Histopathological features.

Treatment

Surgical excision.

8. Discuss fibroma.

Fibroma is the most prevalent form of benign, soft tissue tumor of the oral cavity. It is a connective tissue, reactive tumor that arises in response to trauma or local irritation.

Clinical Features

- May occur at any site of the oral cavity, but buccal mucosa along the plane of occlusion is the common site.
- It appears as an elevated, sessile, nodular growth with a smooth surface.
- The overlying mucosa is normal in color. It is firm in consistency and nontender.
- Common in 3rd, 4th and 5th decades of life and females are affected more in a ratio of 1:2, male: female.

Differential Diagnosis

Peripheral giant cell granuloma, neurofibroma and mucocele.

Treatment

Surgical excision.

9. Lipoma.

- Lipoma is a slow-growing, benign adipose tissue tumor comprising of mature fat cells. It is relatively rare in oral cavity.
- Intramuscular lipoma arises in the skeletal muscles and occurs in mid and late adulthood.

Clinical Features

- Well-circumscribed, sessile or pedunculated growth with smooth or lobulated surface and slippery margins.
- Soft in consistency, freely movable, and nontender.
- Deeper lesions are more diffuse and only slightly elevated.
- Buccal mucosa, tongue, and floor of the mouth are the common sites.
- Multiple fibromas are associated with:
  - Gardner's syndrome
  - Proteus syndrome
  - Multiple familial lipomatosis syndrome
  - Encephalocraniocutaneous lipomatosis
- Histological types:
  - Fibrolipoma
  - Angiolipoma
  - Myxolipoma
  - Adenolipoma

Treatment

Surgical excision.

10. Hemangioma.

- Hemangiomas are vascular malformation that develops within the first month of life, proliferate rapidly, and then involute within childhood period.
- Types:
  - Capillary hemangioma
  - Cavernous hemangioma
  - Angioblastic hemangioma
  - Racemose hemangioma
  - Port-wine stain
  - Hereditary hemorrhagic telangiectasia.

Oral Manifestations

- Flat or raised, well-circumscribed lesions of the mucosa. Deep red or bluish red.
- Soft and compressible.
- Lip, tongue, buccal mucosa and palate are commonly affected (Fig. 5).

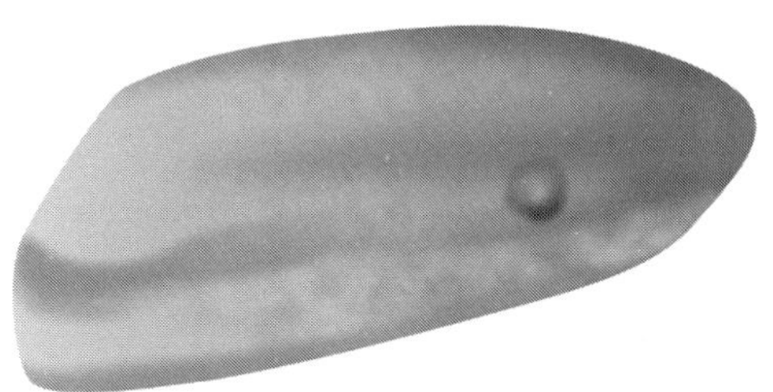

Fig. 5: Hemangioma on the tongue.

- Central hemangioma of the maxilla and mandible may occur but the involvement of mandible is more common.

Syndromes-associated with Hemangiomas

- Osler-Weber-Rendu syndrome
- Sturge-Weber syndrome (Port-wine stain)
- Maffucci syndrome—(Hemangioma of mucous membrane and dyschondroplasia).
- Von Hippel-Lindau syndrome.

Diascopy — chair side investigation

In hemangioma, there will be complete blanching of the lesion when pressure is applied on the surface (Fig. 6).

Radiographic Features

- Central hemangioma show honeycomb appearance on the radiographs with radiating spicules extending at the periphery forming sunray appearance.
- Ultrasonography is useful in determining the angiomatous nature.
- Contrast-enhanced MRI is used to differentiate hemangioma from lymphangioma.

Treatment

Usually undergoes spontaneous remission. In case of failure to undergo remission, treatment option depends on the type of lesion and amount of residual deformity.

- Surgery
- Radiotherapy

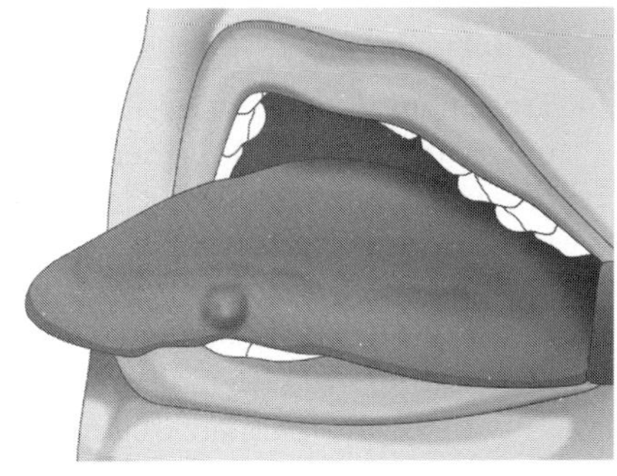

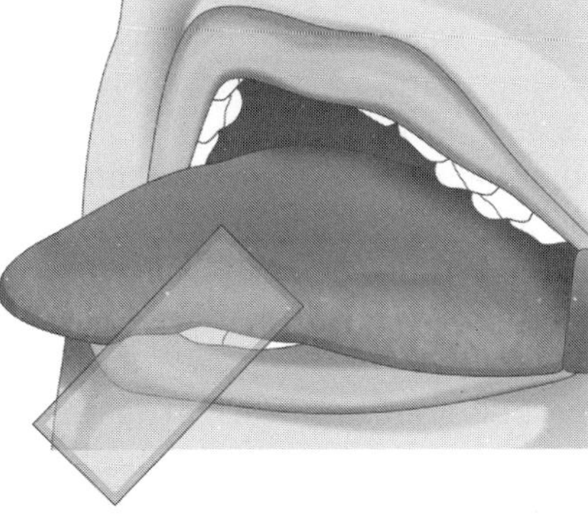

Fig. 6: Diascopy procedure.

- Intralesional injection of sclerosing agents
- Cryotherapy.

11. Paget's disease (or) osteitis deformans.

- Paget's disease is a chronic, noninflammatory, bone remodeling disease that affects adult population (> than 40 years). Males are affected more than females. Its prevalence is worldwide and is the common bone disorder next to osteoporosis.
- It is characterized by excessive bone resorption together with rapid, disorganized bone remodeling. The etiology is unknown but genetic predisposition is noted. The possibility of *slow-virus* infection also considered as a causative factor (paramyxovirus nucleocapsid particles and canine distemper virus have been observed in osteoclasts).
- It preferably involves the axial skeleton (spine, pelvis, femur, sacrum, and skull in descending order of frequency), but may affect any bone. Leontiasis ossea or lion-like face is the term used to characterize the overgrowth of the facial and cranial bones in Paget's disease.
- Involvement of maxilla is two times more than that of the mandible. Progressive enlargement of the maxilla, alveolar bone expansion, and flattened appearance of the palate are the common manifestations. Migration of teeth causes spacing and mobility. Edentulous patient's complaint difficulty in wearing denture because of increasing tightness after the alveolar expansion.
- The common *symptoms* include tinnitus, vertigo, deafness, malocclusion, enlarged maxilla, and cranial nerve disorders.
- Three phases are stated in Paget's disease progression:
  1. Paget's disease starts with the *lytic phase.* Osteoclasts resorb normal bone. Bone turnover rates increase up to 20 times normal.
  2. The second stage is the mixed phase. Numerous osteoblasts are involved in rapid bone formation. The new bone contains haphazardly arranged collagen fibers and appears morphologically abnormal. As the osteoclastic and osteoblastic activities recur, a high-degree bone turnover occurs.
     In the *sclerotic phase,* bone formation is more but in a disorganized pattern (woven bone). The woven bone is weaker than normal adult bone and allows the infiltration of fibrous tissue and blood vessels to the bone marrow leading to a hypervascular state.
  3. After an undefined period, osteoclastic activity decreases, but abnormal bone formation continues. Over a period, osteoblastic activity also reduces, and the bone becomes quiescent known as a *burned-out* phase.
- Sarcomatous changes of pagetic bone are rare but a tedious complication.

Oral Complications

Increased incidents of oral infections and pathological fracture of jaw bone are the associated complications.

Investigation

Serum alkaline phosphatase and bone-specific alkaline phosphatase levels are valuable markers in the diagnosis of Paget's disease.

Management

- Treatment does not cure Paget's disease, but it can control it. Drug therapy for Paget's disease should include:
  - *Bisphosphonate treatment* with serial monitoring of bone markers.
  - Around 1,000–1,500 mg of *calcium* and vitamin D 400 IU, daily in conjunction with bisphosphonate treatments.
  - Chemotherapy and radiotherapy are used to treat neoplasms arising from the pagetic bone.

- Morbidity from Paget's disease can be extensive. A more central lesion carries an unfavorable prognosis.

12. Lymphangioma.

- Lymphangiomatous lesions are congenital malformations of the lymphatic system. It has a predilection for cervicofacial area. The proliferating vessels contain lymph — a clear protein-rich fluid with few cells. They occur either as isolated lesion or in association with hemangiomas. It commonly occurs on tongue like a soft mass without clear boundaries.
- Lymphangioma are classified as *microcystic* (capillary lymphangiomas), *macrocystic* (cavernous lymphangiomas) and *cystic hygromas* based on the size of the lymphatic cavities. When a lymphangioma is confined to solid organs like tongue, it manifests as cavernous lymphangioma, but when it develops in a loose fascia of the neck, a cystic lesion occurs.

Management

- Surgical resection is the preferred treatment.
- Sclerotherapy using dextrose, tetracycline, doxycycline, bleomycin, and OK-432 can reduce the complications of surgery.

13. Schwannoma (or) neurilemmoma.

Schwannoma is a benign tumor of Schwann cells or neurilemma cells.

Clinical Features

- A slow-growing, circumscribed, tumor.
- Occur on tongue, palate, floor of the mouth, buccal mucosa, gingival, and lip.
- Central lesions may occur within mandible and arise from mandibular nerve.
- Central lesions produce significant bone destruction and expansion of cortical palate.
- Usually painless. Pain occurs when they exert pressure on adjacent nerves.

Treatment

Surgical excision.

14. Neurofibroma. (or) Von Recklinghausen's disease (or) neurofibromatosis.

Neurofibroma is a derivative of the nerve sheath cells. It is a benign tumor that occurs either as an independent lesion or as a part of *neurofibromatosis* syndrome.

Clinical Features

- Tumor occurs as discrete nodules with normal mucosal color.
- Involvement trigeminal nerve causes pain.
- In case of multiple endocrine neoplasia syndrome (MEN type II), mucosal neuromas are the early manifestation.
- Central lesions may occur within mandible and associated with mandibular nerve.
- Sarcomatous transformation of neurofibromatosis is also described as fibrosarcoma, neurogenic sarcoma, and spindle cell carcinoma.

Radiographic Findings

Central lesion with mandibular nerve involvement reveals blunderbuss expansion of inferior alveolar foramen with uniformly expanded alveolar canal.

Treatment

- Surgical excision for single neurofibroma.
- Removal of multiple lesions is not possible and should be considered only when malignant transformation is suspected.

15. Hereditary hemorrhagic telangiectasia. (or) *Osler-Weber-Rendu syndrome*.

- It is a triad of telangiectasia, recurrent epistaxsis, and a positive family history of this disorder.
- The major complication associated with this condition is multiorgan arteriovenous malformation. The main organs are GI tract, pulmonary vasculature, brain and nasal mucosa.

- Skin lesions are common on face, neck, and chest. Intraoral lesions involve lip, gingiva, buccal mucosa, tongue and floor of mouth.
- A defect in the perivascular supporting tissue results in weakening of small vessels of skin and mucosa. Both bleeding and clotting time are normal in affected individuals.
- Pressure packs control spontaneous hemorrhage. Telangiectatic areas can be treated with radiotherapy, cauterization or surgery.

16. Sturge-Weber syndrome (or) Encephelo-trigeminal angiomatosis.

- It is a congenital hamartomatous malformation that affects the eye, skin and central nervous system at different time.
- This syndrome is characterized by venous angiomas of leptomeninges over cerebral cortex with ipsilateral angiomatous lesions of face, skull, jaws, and oral soft tissues.
- The facial cutaneous capillary venous angiomas (Port-wine nevi) is the first component of the syndrome to be observed at birth. It is confined to *skin supplied by trigeminal nerve.*
- *Intracranial calcifications* are the second common finding that are noted on radiographs.
- Neurological manifestations are common and include convulsions, spastic hemiplegia with/without mental retardation

Management

Neurological care for seizures.

17. Odontogenic myxoma.

- Odontogenic myxomas are benign tumors derived from embryonic mesenchymal elements of dental papilla, follicle or periodontal ligament. It is an unencapsulated, locally infiltrating tumor.
- They are slow-growing, painless and site-aggressive tumors. Since asymptomatic, the lesions enlarge significantly before the patient reports. Extensive lesions may cause migration of teeth and bone expansion.
- On radiologic examination, the lesions appear either as unilocular or multilocular pattern with well-defined or diffused margins. Fine, bony septa within the radiolucency are known as wispy trabeculations and are characteristic of this tumor. They give a *honeycombed, soap bubble,* or *tennis racket* appearance to the lesion. The tumor is scalloped between the roots, but root resorption is infrequent.
- The preferred treatment is surgical excision by enucleation, curettage, or block resection.

18. Ameloblastic fibroma.

This is a tumor of childhood, seldom is it seen beyond age 20.

- Site: The preferred location for this tumor is the posterior mandible followed by the posterior maxilla.
- Symptoms: Patients present with a painless swelling in the jaw. The lesion may disturb the eruption of teeth in the area. An impacted tooth may often be associated with the tumor in approximately in ¼ of the reported cases. Some lesions are asymptomatic, and detected upon routine dental radiographs.
- Radiographically, ameloblastic fibromas are unilocular lesions, or multilocular if when large. They have smooth well-demarcated borders. Cortical expansion may or may not be seen on radiographs. As lesions are frequently associated with unerupted teeth, often they are misdiagnosed as dentigerous cysts.
- Both odontogenic epithelium and odontogenic ectomesenchyme constitute this tumor.
- Surgical excision with removal of the affected teeth is the treatment of choice. Recurrence is rare.

19. Cementoblastoma (or) true cementoma.

- The cementoblastoma is a benign tumor of odontogenic origin derived from ectomesenchyme. The most common site for occurrence is mandibular molar region with 50% of the cases involving the mandibular first molar. It may be completely asymptomatic or rarely causes pain and swelling.

- This tumor typically occurs around the roots of the lower posterior teeth. When they cause bony expansion, pain is experienced.
- Radiographically, it appears as a well-defined, ball-like radiopacity with a thin halo of radiolucency attached to the root apex. Cementoblastoma continues to grow until it is removed, and hence it is a true tumor—a true cementoma, in contrast to cementoma which is present around the root apices of lower incisor with self-limiting growth.

Treatment

Surgical: Removal of the tumor along with the affected tooth, and peripheral ostectomy.

20. Giant cell granuloma.

- Giant cell granuloma is a benign tumor. The cause of occurrence is unknown and the lesion is uncommon. They may be either centrally located within the jaw, or peripherally located on the gingiva.
- The central lesion of the jaw may be aggressive or nonaggressive. Aggressive lesions are equal to or greater than 5 cm in size and tend to overgrow, and cause tooth displacement, root resorption, cortical bone perforation or thinning out. Recurrence is common following the curettage.
- Non-aggressive lesions are slow growing, asymptomatic, and and do not recur following the surgical treatment.
- Treatment:
  - Curettage
  - Intralesional corticosteroids, calcitonin injections, and interferon-alpha therapy. They are alternatives as well as adjuncts to the surgical procedure.
- Peripheral giant cell granuloma is the frequently occurring extraosseous giant cell lesion. It looks as a bluish-purplish-red nodule and soft in consistency and resembling the pyogenic granuloma in appearance. *Cupping* or superficial resorption of the underlying alveolar crest is present. Treatment comprises surgical resection.

21. Granular cell tumor.

- Granular cell tumor is a nodular hamartomatous lesion occurring on tongue and gingiva (granular cell epulis). The nodular growth has overlying pseudoepitheliomatous hyperplasia and hence leads to a misdiagnosis of squamous cell carcinoma.
- The granular cells are the derivatives of neural crest cells (primitive Schwann cell).
- The lesion may occur as single or multiple. Surface ulceration and pain are common.

Investigation

On immunochemical study, neuron-specific enolase and S-100 protein markers are seen on the tumor cells.

Treatment

Surgical excision. Recurrence is unusual.

22. Nevoid basal cell carcinoma syndrome. (or) Basal cell nevus syndrome. (or) Gorlin syndrome.

It is a hereditary condition characterized by the following major and minor features.

Major Features

- Orofacial structures:
  - Odontogenic keratocysts has predilection for mandibular angle and maxillary 3rd molar region. The affected bone is extensively involved in the cystic cavity before the patient realizing the symptoms like pain and migration of teeth.
  - Ameloblastoma and fibrosarcoma of jaw bones, but the incidence is minimal.
- Bifid ribs and underdeveloped ribs.

- Skin: Epidermoid cysts, multiple basal cell carcinoma, palmar and plantar pits.
- Calcification of falx cerebri.

Minor Features

- Macrocephaly
- Cleft lip and palate, frontal bossing, sunken eyes, broad nasal bridge and mandibular prognathism.
- Syndactyly and pectus deformity.
- Medulloblastoma and cerebellar tumor of childhood.

The presence of any two major or one major and two minor features will establish the diagnosis.

23. Non-Hodgkin's lymphoma.

It is a lymphoproliferative malignancy involving lymph nodes and lymphoid organs as well as extranodal organs and tissues.

Different types of Non-Hodgkin's lymphoma are identified, among which large B-cell lymphoma and follicular lymphoma are common.

- Human T-cell leukemia virus is identified as the cause, and older adults are affected commonly. The other causative factors include immunosupression, *Heliobactor pylori*, and advancing age.
- Lymphadenopathy is a persistent finding.
- Other associated symptoms include fever, night sweats, fatigue, weight loss, chest pain and cough.
- Non-Hodgkin's tumor generally occurs in lymphatic vessels, tonsils, adenoids, bone marrow, spleen, and thymys.
- Oral findings include diffuse swelling in buccal vestibule, hard palate or gingiva that are erythematous, purplish and ulcerated.
- Treatment is radiation and chemotherapy.

24. Langerhans cell histiocytosis.

Langerhans cell histiocytosis (LCH) is an idiopathic histiocytosis disorder characterized by the presence of granulomas. They are composed of proliferating bone marrow-derived Langerhans cells including T-cells, macrophages, eosinophils, and inflammatory cells. It comprises three types of lesions:

1. *Eosinophilic granuloma*: Single or multiple bone lesions are present in affected children and young adults. The extraskeletal sites involvement is not seen.
2. *Hand–Schuller–Christian syndrome*: Extensive lesions involving both skeletal and extraskeletal regions. It affects children and progresses gradually.
3. *Letterer–Siwe disease*: Disseminated acute or subacute condition. It is a fatal disease due to their extensive involvement. Children younger than 3 years of age are affected.

   Jaw lesions are common in Langerhans cell granulomatosis. Mandibular body-angle region is the most common site of involvement. In the oral cavity, localized swelling, pain, ulcers, gingival necrosis, alveolar bone destruction, tooth mobility, and exfoliation are the notable findings. Systemic complications are rare. Hence majority of patients are diagnosed during routine radiological investigation.

Radiographic Findings

Localized, punched-out radiolucent lesion without peripheral sclerosis. Severe alveolar bone resorption produces the appearance of teeth floating in space.

Management

Surgical curettage, radiotherapy, or chemotherapy or combination of these modalities.

25. Nodular fasciitis.

- It is a fibrous proliferative tumor in subcutaneous tissue having a fast-growing tendency.
- It is otherwise known as subcutaneous fibromatosis or pseudosarcomatous fasciitis.
- Head and neck regions, trunk, and hands are frequently involved. Facial skin, parotid, tongue, oral mucosa, and buccinator muscle are the affected sites in orofacial region.

- It is a self-limiting lesion, and the size reaches up to 2 cm, sometimes may exceed but always less than 5 cm. The etiology is unknown, but trauma is considered as a precipitating factor. Histologically it is composed of fibroblasts and myofibroblasts.
- The lesion is well-circumscribed, freely movable, and tender.
- Treatment is surgical excision. The tumor does not recur.

MULTIPLE CHOICE QUESTIONS

1. Self-healing carcinoma is ***keratoacanthoma***.
   a. Basal cell carcinoma
   b. Keratoacanthoma
   c. Nevus melanoma
   d. Sebaceous tumor
2. Yellow epulis are ***intraoral lipoma***.
   a. Bohn's nodules
   b. Adipose adenoma
   c. Intraoral lipoma
   d. Gingival polyp
3. Benign neoplasm of brown fat is known as ***hibernoma***.
   a. Bohn's nodules
   b. Adipose adenoma
   c. Intraoral lipoma
   d. Hibernoma
4. Fibroma molluscum denotes ***neurofibroma***.
   a. Fibrous acanthoma
   b. Neurofibroma
   c. Neurilemmoma
   d. Hibernoma
5. Strawberry hemangioma is the other name for ***capillary hemangioma***.
   a. Cavernous hemangioma
   b. Hemangioendothelioma
   c. Capillary hemangioma
   d. Hemangiopericytoma
6. Cavernous hemangiomas are ***Juvenile hemangiomas***.
   a. Hemangioendothelioma
   b. Juvenile hemangioma
   c. Capillary hemangioma
   d. Hemangiopericytoma
7. Port-wine stain is ***capillary malformation***.
   a. Cavernous malformation
   b. Capillary malformation
   c. Arterial malformation
   d. Venous malformation
8. Cystic hygroma is a ***lymphatic malformation***.
   a. Arterial malformation
   b. Venous malformation
   c. Lymphatic malformation
   d. Capillary formation
9. Sturge-Weber syndrome is also known as ***mother-spot disease*** (phakomatoses).
   a. Mother-spot disease
   b. Nevus flammeus
   c. Dermal nevi
   d. Lentigines syndrome
10. Chinese script writing is the histological appearance of ***fibrous dysplasia***.
    a. Osteosarcoma
    b. Fibrous dysplasia
    c. Fibrosarcoma
    d. Odontogenic myxoma
    (**Note:** Chinese script writing is the histological appearance of delicate and curvilinear appearance of trabeculae in fibrous dysplasia).
11. Osteosarcoma is the most common malignancy associated with ***fibrous dysplasia***.
    a. Angiovenous malformation
    b. Fibrous dysplasia
    c. Fibrosarcoma
    d. Myxoma
    (**Note:** The malignancy tumors-associated with fibrous dysplasia are osteosarcoma, fibrosarcoma, and chondrosarcoma).
12. Pseudosarcomatous fasciitis and giant cell granuloma of bone are example for ***inflammatory hyperplasia***.
    a. Inflammatory hyperplasia
    b. Reactive lesion
    c. Vascular lesion
    d. Epithelial hyperplasia
13. Pile textured carpet mucosal surface is characteristic for ***epithelial hyperplasia***.
    a. Inflammatory hyperplasia
    b. Nevus
    c. Vascular lesion
    d. Epithelial hyperplasia

14. Sessile or pedunculated nodules on the pharyngeal surface of tongue represent ***lymphoid nodule***.
    a. Lymphoid nodule
    b. Varicose vein
    c. Keratin nodules
    d. Adenoid tissue
15. Glomus tumor or glomangioma arise from ***pericytic cells***.
    a. Lymphatic tissue
    b. Neuronal cells
    c. Pericytic cells
    d. Myelinated axons
    (**Note:** Glomus tumor or glomangioma arise from *pericytic cells* (modified smooth muscle cells, occur at the peripheral arteriovenous anastomosis, also known as Abrikossoff's tumor).
16. Dermoid cysts are teratoid cysts and seen on ***floor of the mouth***.
    a. Floor of the mouth
    b. Scalp
    c. Parotid gland
    d. Preauricular region
17. Compound odontomas are common in ***Gardner's syndrome***.
    a. Gorlin syndrome
    b. Gardener's syndrome
    c. Apert syndrome
    d. Carpal tunnel syndrome
18. The oral and perioral papillomatosis with areas of black pigmentation is seen in ***acanthosis nigricans***.
    a. Acanthosis nigricans
    b. Seborrheic dermatitis
    c. Rosacea
    d. Psoriasis
19. Endosteal scalloping is a radiographic feature of ***fibrous dysplasia***.
    a. Ameloblastoma
    b. Odontogenic keratocyst
    c. Central hemangioma
    d. Fibrous dysplasia
20. Polyostotic fibrous dysplasia and intramuscular myxomas is the feature of ***Mazabraud syndrome***.
    a. Cowden's syndrome
    b. *Osler-Weber-Rendu syndrome*
    c. Mazabraud syndrome
    d. Maffucci syndrome
21. *Coast-of-California* is a characteristic feature ***Von Recklinghausen's disease***.
    a. Von Recklinghausen's disease
    b. Paget's disease
    c. Cherubism
    d. Osler–Weber–Rendu syndrome
    (**Note:** Smooth-bordered café-au-lait pigmentations are known as Coast-of-California is a characteristic feature of diffuse neurofibromatosis or Von Recklinghausen's disease).
22. Cafe-au-lait pigmentations with speckled border are known as ***coast of Maine***.
    a. Coast of California
    b. Coast of Maine
    c. Cost of Caribbean
    d. Cost of Mainland
23. The clinical significance of Mazabraud syndrome is the higher risk of ***malignant transformation***.
    a. Malignant transformation
    b. Malignant hyperthermia
    c. Bleeding disorder
    d. Pathological fracture

VIVA VOCE

1. What is fibroma?

Fibromas are sessile, firm-growths occurring on oral mucosal surface. Histologically they are composed of inflamed fibrous and granulation tissues. The primary etiological factor is chronic trauma or irritants.

2. What is epulis?

Epulis refers to small sessile or pedunculated growths occurring on gingiva as a response to inflammatory reaction for chronic trauma or irritants.

3. What is epulis fissuratum?

Epulis fissuratum is the overgrowth of alveolar mucosa associated with periphery of ill-fitting dentures.

4. What is pulp polyp?

Pulp polyp is the proliferation of pulpal connective tissue through a substantial pulpal exposure and fills the cavity with decayed teeth. It is a bright red mushroom-shaped growth with a connecting stalk to the pulp cavity. They bleed on palpation but are asymptomatic due to the presence of fewer nerve endings.

5. What is denture papilloma?

- It is hyperplastic lesion develops on hard palate due to chronic denture irritation. It is also known as denture papillomatosis and palatal papillary hyperplasia. It is very common for denture wearers using maxillary dentures with suction chambers or cut on palatal surface of denture for retention. They are usually excised or removed by electrocautery, cryosurgery or laser surgery.
- Very rarely occurs in individual without wearing dentures.

6. What is pregnancy epulis (or) pregnancy tumor?

It is a pedunculated hemorrhagic nodule seen in gingiva of pregnant women in response to chronic irritation caused by overhanging restorations, calculi, or sharp margins of intraoral appliances. It is the exaggerated response of gingiva to local irritants due to increased level of circulating hormone estrogens. It has increased prevalence toward the end of pregnancy and shrinks after delivery.

7. What is hamartoma?

Greek word hamartia = *fault (or) defect*, and *oma=tumor* gives rise to hamartoma. It is a benign (noncancerous) *tumor-like* malformation; consist of tissues that are specific to that site, but growing as a disorganized mass. It is considered as a developmental error.

8. What is teratoma?

Teratomas are germ cell tumors comprising cells derived from all three germ layers. It may be a benign, well-differentiated cystic lesions or solid and malignant. The findings of various structures like teeth, tissue, hair, and skin in these tumors are characteristic.

9. What is tuberous sclerosis?

It is an inherited disorder characterized by seizure and mental retardation due to neuronal deformity in central nervous system. Fine wart-like lesions known as adenoma sebaceum occurs in a butterfly distribution over cheek and forehead. Pitted enamel hypoplasia is also a common finding.

10. What is Cowden syndrome (multiple hamartomatous neoplasia syndrome)?

There is a hamartomatous involvement of many organs with a potential for neoplastic transformation. Presence of numerous papules and papillomatosis gives a cobblestone appearance to oral mucosa. It is an autosomal dominant.

11. What are xanthomas?

Xanthomas are localized deposition of lipoprotein in skin, subcutaneous tissue, and tendons. They are associated with vascular diseases and internal malignancies.

BIBLIOGRAPHY

1. DiCaprio MR, Enneking WF. Fibrous dysplasia: pathophysiology, evaluation, and treatment. J Bone Joint Surg Am. 2005;87(8):1848-64.
2. Fletcher CD. Pathology and genetics of tumors of soft tissue and bone. World Health Organization Classification of Tumors. 2002;4:35-46.
3. Haddad AJ, Avon SL, Clokie CM, et al. Nodular fasciitis in the oral cavity. J Can Dent Assoc. 2001;67(11):664-7.
4. Praetorius F, Piattelli A. Odontogenic tumors. Surgical pathology of the head and neck. 2009;3:1241-7.
5. Rajendran R. Shafer's textbook of oral pathology. Elsevier India; 2009.
6. Regezi JA, Sciubba JJ, Jordan RC. Oral pathology: clinical pathologic correlations. Elsevier Health Sciences; 2016.

CHAPTER 16

Temporomandibular Joint Disorders

HIGHLIGHTS

Temporomandibular joint (TMJ) is a both hinging and sliding type of joint and hence known as ginglymoarthrodial joint. It is a bilateral joint fused in the midline and hence, influencing the movements of each other. Also, the teeth and muscles of mastication also affect the function of the joint. It has two structural components—the temporal above and mandibular below. A fibrous capsule surrounds TMJ. It has selective sliding movements between the bony joints in addition to hinge movement.

Learners are expected to know about:

- Ankylosis
- Disk derangement, disk displacement, and disk perforation.
- Arthritis changes
- Myofascial pain
- TMJ dislocation
- Trismus.

ESSAY QUESTIONS

1. Define myofascial pain dysfunction syndrome. Describe the clinical features, diagnostic, criteria, and management in detail.

- Myofascial pain dysfunction syndrome is a noninflammatory, musculoskeletal disorder that involves the muscles of mastication. The symptoms include pain, restriction of jaw movements, joint sounds, deviation of the mouth on closing and opening movements, and pain on palpating the affected masticator muscles or their tendons.
- The pain is associated with characteristic myofascial trigger points. The motor and sensory disturbances may be local to the trigger points or may be distant with a referred pain pattern. It often involves the neck and back.
- Myofascial pain dysfunction syndrome is classified as a craniomandibular disorder by American Academy of Craniomandibular Disorders.

Etiopathogenesis

Chronic muscle stress leads trigger points. People undergoing stress and anxiety are more prone for developing myofascial pain dysfunction syndrome (MPDS). This is based on the concept of teeth clenching, in consequence, to stress causes repeated strain on muscles which leads to the development of trigger points.

Predisposing Factors

Psychological disorders, metabolic disorders, sleep disorders, and personality status that prone to parafunctional habits like clenching of teeth predispose to MPDS.

Triggering (or) Precipitating Factors

Trauma to masticator muscles, occlusal disturbance, infection, and iatrogenic causes may trigger MPDS.

Perpetuating Factors or Maintaining Factors

Predisposing and precipitating factors either alone or in combination lead to a myospasm-pain-myospasm cycle.

Pathophysiology

The masticator muscles spasm is the pathogenesis for the clinical features of this syndrome. Muscle spasm is caused by:
- Overextension of the muscle
- Overcontraction of the muscle
- Muscle fatigue.

The myofascial pain dysfunction syndrome (MPDS) so produced causes pain, limitation of movement, changes in jaw position, and occlusal disharmony. Irregularities in occlusion appear to be the precipitating factor in the pathogenesis of myofascial pain dysfunction syndrome. Occlusal interferences, posterior bite collapse, deep overbite, overjet and many other factors tend to restrict movement and predispose the patients to increased parafunctional activity resulting in overuse, and thus fatigue of muscles and pain. The pain may cause muscle spasm and contraction leading to parafunctional habits and forms a cycle of events (Flowchart 1).

Clinical Features

- Myofascial pain is characterized by a deep, diffused, dull quality in contrast to the well-defined dental pain. Trigger points, a rigid and tender muscle, and referred pain are the pathognomonic features associated with MPDS.
- *Four cardinal signs* of this syndrome:
  1. Tenderness with referred pain to the joints and other muscles.
  2. Movements are restricted and limited to relax or fully lengthen the muscle.
  3. Persistent muscle pain, weakness, and stiffness.
  4. Clicking or crepitus sounds during jaw movements.
- It also causes degenerative changes in the joint and muscle contraction as a feature of long-standing spasm.
- Females are affected more. This is due to their less tolerance for pain and tendency for undergoing stressful situation.

Flowchart 1: Cyclic events of myofacial pain.

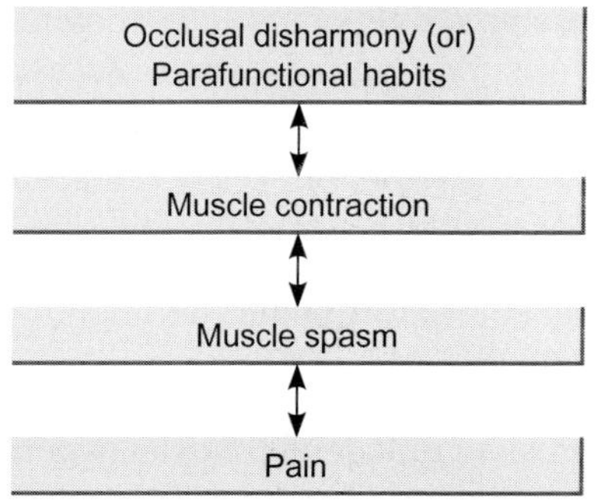

Diagnostic Criteria

- A diagnosis of myofascial pain syndrome (MPS) depends on the clinical examination and palpation. There is no standardized diagnostic tool like lab investigations or radiographic views to make an evidence-based determination.
- Laskin's criteria: Four cardinal signs:
  1. Unilateral pain
  2. Muscle tenderness
  3. Audible clicking
  4. Restricted jaw movements
- Negative characteristics:
  - No radiographic evidence.
  - No tenderness in TMJ area on palpation.

Management

- *Trigger point injection*: Injection of the local anesthetic solution, procaine to the trigger point.
- *Spray and stretch*: It is beneficial to cool the skin over the trigger points and referred sites using ice stick or refrigerant spray. The application should be rapid and for a short duration so that the cooling will not affect the underlying muscle which otherwise will reduce the stretch instead of stimulating it.

The cooling act should be followed by a hot pack application to warm-up the skin.

- *Posture retraining*: Training for maintaining the correct posture and biomechanics will relieve the muscle stress and tension.
- *Electrical stimulation*: Transcutaneous electrical nerve stimulation (TENS) therapy is useful in the management of trigger points and pain control, as they exhibit low resistance to electrical energy.
- *Medical management*:
  - Muscle relaxants and analgesics can be used.
  - Benzodiazepines 2–5 mg — 3times/day with acetaminophen 650 mg —3times/ day.
  - For patients suffering from chronic myofascial pain with proven depression, tricyclic antidepressants (25–75 mg at bedtime) can be administered.

2. Enumerate the various causes of trismus with pathophysiology and treatment.

Trismus is described by a reduced mouth opening due to long-lasting spasm of the muscles. The restriction may range from the simple and nonprogressive to highly morbid.

Classification for Trismus

The mean maximal mouth opening for males is 51.3 mm and for females is 44.3 mm.

- Interincisal distance of greater than 30 mm and less than 35 mm is referred as mild trismus.
- Interincisal distance of 15–30 mm is noted as moderate trismus.
- Interincisal distance of less than 15 mm is noted as severe trismus.

Etiopathogenesis of Trismus

- Infection
- Trauma
- Iatrogenic (Dental treatment like high point restorations)
- TM joint disorders
- Tumors
- Oral submucous fibrosis
- Drug-related
- Radiotherapy and chemotherapy
- Congenital or developmental growth disorders
- Miscellaneous condition like hysteria.

Infection

- The typical finding in space infections is trismus. Both odontogenic and non-odontogenic infections can lead to spreading space infection and trismus. Periapical, periodontal, and pericoronal abscesses, dentoalveolar abscesses and cellulitis are the odontogenic cause of trismus. Among these, pericoronal infections associated with 3rd molar eruption is the most frequent cause of trismus.
- Nonodontogenic infection includes tonsillitis, tetanus, meningitis, and parotid abscess.

Trauma

The fracture of mandible, zygoma, or zygomatic arch can limit the coronoid movement and cause trismus.

Dental Procedures

- Surgical extraction of mandibular 3rd molars.
- Inaccurate needle positioning during mandibular block administration results in trismus, 2–5 days later the process. The needle may penetrate and injure the medial pterygoid muscle or damage the blood vessel. The resulting bleeding and hematoma in the muscle are organized to fibrosis. This type of trismus causes severe symptoms. Application of thermal packs and stretching exercises using wooden spatulas are the needful management. The patient should be reassured about the reversible nature of the condition.

Temporomandibular Joint Disorders

- Fibrosis or unilateral condylar hyperplasia.
- Temporomandibular joint trauma or dislocation.

- Displacement of meniscus anteromedial to the condyle.

Tumors

- Tumors in the pharynx, parotid, mandible or TMJ may lead to trismus. Nasopharyngeal tumors and tumors involving infratemporal fossa may also cause trismus.
- The radiotherapy for oral cancer involving masticator muscles in the field of radiation leads to trismus as a later complication.

Oral Submucous Fibrosis

Oral submucous fibrosis is characterized by chronic inflammation and fibrosis of the submucosal tissues leading to muscle stiffness and difficulty in mouth opening.

Drug-induced

Drugs that cause trismus as a side effect include: Succinylcholine, phenothiazines, tricyclic antidepressants, metoclopramide, and phenothiazines.

Congenital Disorders

Hypertrophy of the coronoid process interferes with the anteromedial border of the zygomatic arch and causes trismus.

Management of Trismus

Treatment depends on the etiological factor:

- For mild pain and dysfunction, heat therapy is indicated by placing moist hot towels on the affected area for 15–20 minutes every hour. Administration of NSAIDs is usually adequate. After the acute inflammation subsides, physiotherapy should be started with opening and closing exercises and lateral excursions of the mandible for 5 minutes every 3–4 hours.
- In case of any dental infection, appropriate endodontic management or extraction should be carried out with antibiotics and analgesic support.
- For oral submucous fibrosis, intralesional corticosteroid injections are the choice of management, but in a severe case of trismus, reconstruction of the buccal pad of fat followed by vigorous physiotherapy is indicated.
- In severe cases, diazepam 2.5–5 mg—3 times/day can be administered as muscle relaxants.
- Treatment should be continued until the patient becomes asymptomatic.

SHORT NOTES

1. Internal derangement of temporomandibular joint. (or) articular disk displacement.

- The articular disk is situated between the condyle and glenoid fossa. It has muscle attachment in the front and connective tissue band at the posterior aspect. These attachments make the disk to move forward and backward in the glenoid fossa when condyle moves (opening and closing movements).
- Disk displacement (*internal derangement*) is described as *a disturbance in the normal anatomic relationship between the disk and condyle that interferes with smooth movement of the joint and causes momentary catching, clicking, popping, or locking.*

Disk Displacement with Reduction

- The articular disk is positioned anterior to the condylar head. The disk remains in anterior position as long as the mouth is closed. When the mouth is opened, the disk is repositioned on the condylar head. The movement of the disk against the condylar head may result in a clicking, snapping, or popping sound but jaw movements are not affected.
- When the disk is displaced anteriorly, there is an excess stretch over the *retrodiscal tissues* by the recurrent forces exerted by condyle. This tissue has an adaptive capacity to these forces and transforms to a *pseudo-disk* state. In this situation, if the disk is recaptured, it

results in complete translational condylar movement and an audible clicking known as disk displacement with reduction. When the condyle is back to the *retrodiscal tissue*, a closing or reciprocal click will result.

Disk Displacement without Reduction (Closed Lock)

- In this, forward translation of condyle is limited by the anterior position of the disk, allowing only rotational and not translational movement. Patients report a sudden onset of pain and inability to open the mouth (mouth opening is restricted to 20–30 mm). The patient may also report that the immediate cessation of joint noise with the onset of the symptoms. Clinically, the mandible deviates to the affected side during mouth opening, due to the translational movement of the unaffected joint.

Treatment

- Stretching exercises
- Occlusal splints
- Arthrocentesis.

2. Describe capsulitis and synovitis.

- Inflammation of the capsular ligament is known as capsulitis and presents as constant pain and swelling over the joint. Trauma or abnormal function leading to inflammation is the causative factor.
- Pain is caused by movements that stretch the capsular ligament. Inflammation may increase joint fluid volume, and when this occurs, the condyle is displaced inferiorly resulting in ipsilateral posterior open bite. The synovial membrane clears the debris through its rich vascular supply. Pain mediators also released at this stage of capsulitis. When this healing response is reduced, synovial membrane gets inflamed and is known as acute synovitis. Inflammation of the synovial membrane is an early sign of degenerative joint disorder.

Treatment

Arthrocentesis and arthroscopy for joint lavage and lysis of adhesions will provide a good therapeutic effect. These procedures eliminate the particulate debris and reduce the inflammation. Steroid injections are also used to reduce synovial inflammation and pain.

3. Describe bruxism.

- Bruxism is defined by American Academy of Orofacial Pain as *diurnal or nocturnal parafunctional activity including clenching, bracing, gnashing, and grinding of the teeth.*
- American sleep disorders association defines bruxism as *tooth grinding or clenching during sleep plus one of the following: Tooth wear, sounds or jaw muscle discomfort in the absence of medical disorder.*

Etiopathogenesis

- Daytime bruxism is associated with anxiousness, depression, and stress-related parafunctions.
- Abrupt sleep disturbance (arousal response) is associated with repulsive changes like involuntary body movements and bruxism.
- Occlusal interference may cause local exaggerated muscle response and bruxism.

Symptoms

- Facial pain, earache, and headache.
- *The International diagnostic grading system for sleep and awake bruxism:*
  - *Possible:* Based on self-report, a questionnaire survey, and clinical history.
  - *Probable:* Based on self-report and the clinical examination.
  - *Definite:* Based on the self-report, clinical examination and polysomnographic record.

Treatment

- No specific treatment is available to stop sleep bruxism. Behavior modification therapy, such as habit reversal therapy, relaxation techniques, and biofeedback, may reduce the daytime bruxism.

- The occlusal splints and night guards minimizes the adverse effects of bruxism.

4. Temporomandibular joint ankylosis.

Ankylosis is defined as stiffness of a joint due to fusion of TMJ condyle with base of skull due to abnormal adhesion, and rigidity of the joint space by bone or fibrous tissue.

Etiology of Temporomandibular Joint Ankylosis

- It may either be congenital or acquired.
- Congenital ankylosis is very rare and obstetric trauma is the cause. Congenital abnormalities like Pierre Robin syndrome and Treacher Collin's syndrome are also associated with TMJ ankylosis.
- Acquired type of TMJ ankylosis arises from trauma, infection, systemic inflammatory disorders, irradiation, previous surgery, and neoplasm. The post-traumatic TMJ ankylosis follows delayed treatment, inadequate surgery, prolonged immobilization or insufficient physiotherapy.
- Temporomandibular joint (TMJ) ankylosis is either fibrous (pseudoankylosis) or bony (true ankylosis).
  - True bony ankylosis occurs in children under 10 years of age due to the fusion of condylar head and the temporal bone. This condition has a preference for children because of the higher osteogenic tendency and incomplete state of disk development. Restricted mandibular movements, deviation of the jaw towards the affected side on opening, and facial asymmetry are the clinical findings.
  - Fibrous ankylosis is characterized by intracapsular fibrous adhesions and fibrous changes in capsular ligaments. The results include severely limited mouth opening, no pain, no joint sounds, deviation to the affected side, and decreased movement to the contralateral side.

Treatment

Surgical correction is the treatment choice. Reankylosis is common complication irrespective of surgical technique used to treat the TMJ ankylosis.

5. Dislocation of mandible (or) condylar dislocation.

- The condyle is positioned in front of the articular eminence and cannot be return to the normal position without manipulation.
- Mandibular dislocation occurs due to the muscular incoordination during wide-opening like yawning. Trauma rarely causes this condition.
- The condition may be either unilateral or bilateral.
- Inability to close the jaws following opening and pain related to muscle spasm are the major symptoms.

Management

- The condyle is repositioned manually by standing in front of the seated patient and placing the thumb lateral to the mandibular molars on buccal shelf of bone. The remaining fingers of each hand are placed under the chin. Simultaneous pressing the posterior mandible in downward and backward movement and raising the chin will reposition the condyle.
- If muscle spasm is severe, diazepam can be advised.
- Recurrent and chronic dislocations are treated with surgery.

6. Osteoarthritis of temporomandibular joint (or) degenerative disorder of temporomandibular joint.

- The temporomandibular joint osteoarthritis (OA) is a unilateral, degenerative disorder.
- It is characterized by a break in the articular cartilage, changes in bone morphology, and disintegration of the synovial tissues causing pain and restricted movements of the jaw.

- The characteristic structural changes are disorganization and loss of articular surfaces and proliferation of tissues in and adjacent to these surfaces.
- The temporomandibular joint is the first joint to get the affected with osteoarthritis. The patients present with symptoms including pain on opening, limited movement, grinding noise on function, history of recently stopped clicking sound, and deviation to the affected side during mouth opening.

Radiographic Diagnosis

Narrow joint space, flat articular surface, bony projection from the degenerated cartilage (osteophytes), anterior lipping of the condyle, and Ely's cysts (irregular radiolucencies near the articular surface).

Management

- Interdisciplinary team approach manages osteoarthritis.
- The physical therapy will relieve inflammation, pain, and functional improvement through various methods like TENS, ultrasound, iontophoresis, ice and stretch exercise, neuromuscular therapy, postural and ergodynamic training.
- Arthroscopic surgery is used to flush out joint tissue fragments and inflammatory mediators.

MULTIPLE CHOICE QUESTIONS

1. Deviation of the jaw towards the affected side occurs in ***unilateral condylar hypoplasia***.
   a. Unilateral fracture of the mandible
   b. Unilateral condylar hyperplasia
   c. Unilateral dislocation of the mandible
   d. Unilateral condylar hypoplasia
   (**Note:** Deviation of the jaw towards the affected side occurs in unilateral condylar agenesis, unilateral condylar hypoplasia, unilateral condylar fracture, and ankylosis).
2. Bilateral condylar fracture results in ***anterior open bite***.
   a. Inability to open the mouth
   b. Inability to close the mouth
   c. Anterior open bite
   d. Posterior open bite
3. In dislocation of mandible, the usual complaint will be ***inability to close the mouth***.
   a. Inability to open the mouth
   b. Inability to close the mouth
   c. Anterior open bite
   d. Posterior open bite
4. Ely's cysts are radiographic findings in ***TMJ osteoarthritis***.
   a. TMJ gouty arthritis
   b. TMJ osteoarthritis
   c. Costen's syndrome
   d. TMJ osteosarcoma

VIVA VOCE

1. What is subluxation?

The condyle moves ahead of articular eminence during wide opening but returns to the original position without any manipulation.

2. What is gouty arthritis?

The accumulation of urate crystals in a joint that leads to inflammation and pain is known as gouty arthritis. This is due to long-term elevation of serum urate levels.

3. What is internal derangement of TMJ?

Internal derangement of the joint comprises conditions like disk displacement, disk dislocation or condylar injury.

4. What is Costen's syndrome (or) mandibular joint neuralgia?

It is complex features of impaired hearing, a stuffy sensation in the ears, tinnitus; mild dizziness, burning sensation in the nose, throat and sides of tongue. The pathology is either malocclusion from any cause or adverse changes of one or both mandibular joints.

BIBLIOGRAPHY

1. Farrar WB. Myofascial Pain-Dysfunction Syndrome. The Journal of the American Dental Association. 1981;102(1):10.
2. Garg AK, Jain S, Gupta S, et al. Myofascial pain dysfunction syndrome: an Overview. Heal Talk. 2013;5(6):12-14.
3. Khare N, Patil SB, Kale SM, et al. Normal mouth opening in an adult Indian population. Journal of maxillofacial and oral surgery. 2012;11(3):309-13.
4. Lynch MA, Brightman VJ, Greenberg MS, (Eds). Burket's oral medicine: diagnosis and treatment. Lippincott Williams & Wilkins; 1994.
5. Reddy SV, Kumar MP, Sravanthi D, et al. Bruxism: a literature review. J Int Oral Health. 2014;6(6):105-9.
6. Scrivani SJ, Keith DA, Kaban LB. Temporomandibular disorders. N Engl J Med. 2008;359(25):2693-705.
7. Thiagarajan B. Trismus an overview. ENT Scholar. 2014.

CHAPTER 17

Oral Manifestations of Endocrine Disorders

HIGHLIGHTS

Endocrine glands secrete hormones that are highly-specific in function by exhibiting a signaling pathway. Hormones (in Greek meaning, *to set in motion*) coordinate the activities of other organs and systems, whereas the hypothalamus regulates the activities of endocrine glands. The synthesis of hormones is affected by glandular diseases (like autoimmune disorders, tumors, etc.) or defect in the hypothalamus-pituitary pathway, characterized by either increase or decrease in the secretion. This chapter highlights the manifestations of hormonal disorders in the oral cavity.

Learners are expected to read about:

- Oral manifestations of hormonal changes associated with puberty, pregnancy, menopausal stages and dental management.
- Early diagnosis of endocrine disorders and advising for proper treatment.
- Oral care for patients with disorders of the thyroid, parathyroid, and adrenal glands.

SHORT NOTES

1. Dental treatment for a pregnant women. (or) dental treatment for a gravid mother.

The physiological changes during pregnancy require special care during dental treatment.

During the first trimester (conception to 14 weeks):

- Elective dental procedures should be avoided.
- In case of emergency, procedures should be carried out with minimum medications or should be avoided if possible.
- Homecare oral hygiene instructions should be given.
- Routine radiographs should be avoided.

During second trimester (14–28 weeks):

- Ideal period to carry out dental treatment.
- Use of medications should be minimized.

During third trimester (29 weeks to childbirth):

- Only emergency dental procedures should be provided.
- During treatment, the patient should be asked to turn on her left side to avoid supine position hypotension.
- Appointment should be of short duration.
- Precautions to be considered:
  - During 2nd and 3rd trimester, cardiac output decreases in the supine position because of the compressive effect of gravid uterus on inferior vena cava, which results in a reduced venous return to the heart. The supine hypotension syndrome (which includes bradycardia, hypotension, and syncope) can be prevented by a left lateral position in the dental chair.
  - Lab reports reveals an elevated counts of RBC and WBC, increased ESR, increased clotting factors VII, VIII, IX, and X leads to increased risk of hypercoagulation state and thromboembolism.
  - Many antibiotics and analgesics cross the placenta and cause adverse effects on the fetus. Macrolides antibiotics

(erythromycin, azithromycin) and COX-2 inhibitors (celecoxib and rofecoxib) do not cross the placenta and harm the fetus. Use of metronidazole also accepted because of its negligible side effects.

2. Oral manifestations of hypothyroidism.

- *Cretinism: Congenital hypothyroidism* is called as cretinism.
  - Delayed eruption of teeth and retained deciduous teeth.
  - Enlarged tongue (macroglossia) and thickening of lips due to deposition of glycosaminoglycans in subcutaneous tissues.
  - Shortened base of skull, broad face with retraction and flaring of nasal bridges.
  - Underdeveloped mandible and overdeveloped maxilla.
  - Protruding tongue leads to malocclusion.
  - Impaction of 2nd molar due to altered ramus growth characterized by less than average resorption of internal aspect ramus and thus failure to create space for eruption.

Radiographic Finding

Thinned out lamina dura.

Clinical Significance

- Delayed wound healing.
- Severe periodontitis.
- *Myxedema: Hypothyroidism in children and adults* is known as myxedema. Orofacial findings are limited to soft tissues:
  - Lips, nose, eyelids and suborbital tissues are swollen and edematous.
  - The tongue is large and edematous leading to speech interference.

Dental Consideration

Patients with hypothyroidism will manifest:

- Increased mucopolysaccharides in the subcutaneous tissues will reduce the contractile properties of blood vessels and cause prolonged mucosal bleeding.
- Delayed wound healing and associated risk for infection.

3. Dental treatment for hypothyroidism patients.

A detailed thyroid function test and endocrinologists opinion should be obtained before starting the dental procedures.

- For patients in a controlled state: Routine dental treatment can be provided. A regular dental check-up is necessary to prevent foci of infection.
- For patients in the uncontrolled state:
  - Surgical procedures in these patients may cause the sudden onset of myxedematous coma characterized by the symptoms of hypotension, hypothermia, slow heart rate, and seizures. If this happens in the dental chair, medical supervision should be immediately provided.
  - There is a probability for these patients to take prophylactic anticoagulation drugs as they are prone to cardiac disorders. Therefore, bleeding time and clotting time should be assessed before procedures that may induce bleeding.
  - Antibiotic prophylaxis is necessary for patients with atrial fibrillation.
  - Local anesthetics with vasoconstrictors should be avoided.

4. Oral manifestations of hyperthyroidism.

Hyperthyroidism

- *In children,* shedding of deciduous teeth occurs earlier than normal with the earlier eruption of permanent teeth.
- *In adults:*
  - Rapidly progressing periodontitis and dental caries.
  - Burning mouth syndrome
  - Dryness of mouth
  - Alveolar atrophy in the advanced state due to osteoporosis.
- *Consideration of dental procedures:* Hyperthyroidism patients may have:
  - Hypertension and tachycardia that require a longer duration of local

pressure application following surgical procedures to stop bleeding.
- Drug-induced leukocytosis require the patients to subject for differential blood count before any invasive procedures.
- Patients taking antithyroid drug propylthiouracil may have increased tendency for bleeding because this drug has vitamin K antagonistic effect.
- Thyrotoxic crisis is also a potential complication in patients undergoing dental surgical procedures due to stress and anxiety.

5. Dental treatment for hyperthyroidism patients.

Before starting the dental treatment, a detailed lab investigation should be carried out (T3, T4, and TSH).

- Patients in controlled situations: Dental treatment can be carried out routinely without any particular alterations. Care should be taken to avoid stressful situation for the patient. High priority is mandatory to circumvent the anchoretic spread of oral infections.
- Patients in uncontrolled situations:
    - A complete blood test should be advised to rule out agranulocytosis and prothrombin time to avoid bleeding problems especially for patients taking polythiouracil drugs.
    - Local anesthetics without vasoconstrictors (epinephrine) should be used. Because in these patients, the myocardium is highly sensitive to vasoconstrictor effect and leads to cardiac arrhythmias, tremors, and chest pain.
    - Surgical procedures should be avoided due to the possibility for stress induced thyroid crisis (sweating, tachycardia, hypertension, nausea, and vomiting). In emergency dental care, if thyroid crisis symptoms develop, treatment should be discontinued, and medical care should be provided by hospitalizing the patient.
    - Adequate pain control is essential to prevent stress-induced complications; hence NSAIDs should be included in the preparatory phase.
    - Oral foci of infection should be eliminated.

6. Describe the oral manifestation of hyperparathyroidism.

Hyperparathyroidism is an endocrine disorder characterized by a generalized disturbance in calcium, phosphate and bone metabolism due to the increased amount of circulating parathyroid hormone (PTH).

Mechanism of Hyperparathyroidism (Flowchart 1)

Flowchart 1: Mechanism of hyperparathyroidism.

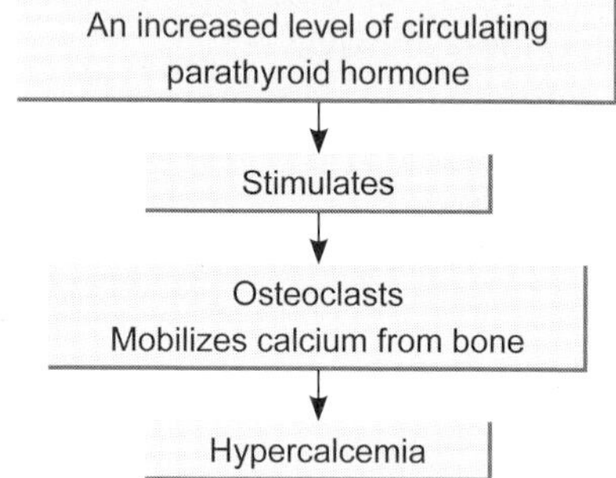

Oral Manifestations

- *Brown tumor (osteitis fibrosa cystic):*
    - Brown tumors are non-neoplastic focal lesion of bone due to abnormal bone metabolism in hyperparathyroid condition. There are localized areas of severe osteoclastic activity and bone resorption. The resorbed bone is filled with fibrous tissues and intermingled with osteoclast-like multinucleated giant cells, hemorrhagic spots, and hemosiderin deposition. The name *brown tumor* derives from the color caused by areas of hemorrhage and hemosiderin.
    - The occurrence of brown tumor has preference for women (3:1, female-male ratio) and elder age group, usually

above 50 years, but may involve hyperthyroidism patients of any age. In the oral cavity, brown tumors appear as asymptomatic or mildly painful, exophytic growth that is hard in consistency.

- *Radiologically*, brown tumors in the jaw bones appear as well-defined unilocular pattern or as multilocular cyst-like lesions known as osteitis fibrosa cystica. Cortical bone expansion and thinning are common in mandible. Thin cortices and loss of trabeculae give the characteristic cystic appearance. Bony trabeculae are replaced by vascular connective tissue with attempted formation of coarse woven bone. Resorbed roots and loss of lamina dura are the associated dental findings.
- *Treatment* of brown tumor depends on the control of hyperparathyroidism. The tumor tends to disappear following the treatment of hyperparathyroid condition. Surgical removal is indicated in resistant cases following the endocrine management.

Alveolar Bone

- Reduction in bone density is due to the replacement of mineralized bony contents by fibrous connective tissues.
- There is loss of cortical bone and a compensatory expansion of trabecular bone. The expansion of trabecular bone may lead to increased occurrence of tori in hyperthyroid patients.

Teeth

- Gradual loosening and drifting of teeth.
- Radiographically:
  - In developing and erupting teeth—loss of crypt wall pointed and tapered roots at apical third are the associated findings.
  - In erupted teeth—large pulp chambers with pulpal calcification and loss of lamina dura around one or more teeth are common. The cortical bone loss in the region adjacent to tooth leads to the discontinuity of lamina dura and widening of periodontal space.
- *Precaution during dental treatment:* Bone fracture is a potential complication, and preventive measures should be taken before extensive dental procedures.

7. Discuss dental consideration for patients on prolonged glucocorticoid therapy. (or) factors to be considered for dental patients on chronic steroid therapy. (or) dental consideration for Cushing's syndrome patients.

Patients on long-term glucocorticoid therapy have:

Defective Hemostasis

- Decreased subcutaneous collagen and fibroblasts derived extracellular proteins. This deficient amount of collagen fibrils and proteins leads to easy bruising and bleeding.
- Defective constriction of small blood vessels during bleeding result in prolonged bleeding.
- Poor wound healing and scar formation.

Risk of Infection

- Increased susceptibility to infection and are considered as immunocompromised.
- More likely to develop candidiasis and other fungal infections.
- Antibiotic prophylaxis should be considered based on immune status, dosage, and duration of steroid and related dental procedure.

Ability to Withstand Dental Treatment

- Patients receiving low dose glucocorticoids (< 30 mg hydrocortisone/day) can withstand dental treatment without additional dose because adrenal suppression will not occur at this dosage.
- Patients on higher dose of corticosteroids (>40 mg hydrocortisone per day) exhibit symptoms of Cushing's syndrome and have minor difficulties with hemostasis, wound healing and infections.

- Patients on prolonged glucocorticoid therapy are prone to adrenal insufficiency due to stressful events like invasive dental procedures or exacerbation of dental infections. In such conditions, the adrenal fails to produce adequate cortisol and experience hypotension, nausea, anorexia, dysphoria, wasting, stress-induced shock and cardiovascular collapse (adrenal crisis). Hence patients with adrenal insufficiency require 100 mg of hydrocortisone acetate intramuscular injection 30 minutes before invasive dental procedures.
- For patients who stopped corticosteroid treatment within 2 weeks period: Maintenance of steroid dose is necessary on the day of treatment for anxious patients and for extensive dental procedures.
- For patients who stopped corticosteroid treatment more than 2 weeks period: No steroid supplement is necessary.
- For patients who are receiving alternate day corticosteroid treatment: No supplement is necessary if dental procedure is carried out on the non-corticosteroid day.
- For patients taking 30–40 mg of daily corticosteroid:
  - The dose should be doubled on the day of extensive dental treatment and if postoperative pain is suspected.
  - General precautions:
    - Dental appointment should be given in morning time to control anxiety.
    - Long-acting anesthetics should be used.
    - Adequate pain control measures should be followed.
    - Patient's anxiety and stress should be relieved or minimized before the procedure.
    - Antacids may reduce the half-life of prednisone should be used with care.
    - Risk of bone fracture should be assessed before doing dental surgery for patients on prolonged corticosteroid therapy.

8. Discuss endocrine pigmentation.

- *Addison's disease* (primary adrenal cortical insufficiency) and Cushing's syndrome (pituitary based cortisol excess) are associated with cutaneous and oral, perioral pigmentations.
- *Addison's disease*: Bronze skin and oral melanotic patches are the characteristic signs.
- Overproduction of adrenocorticotrophic hormone (ACTH has melanocyte exciting action) causes excess melanin deposits on skin and mucosa (Flowchart 2).

Flowchart 2: Pigmentation in Addison's disease.

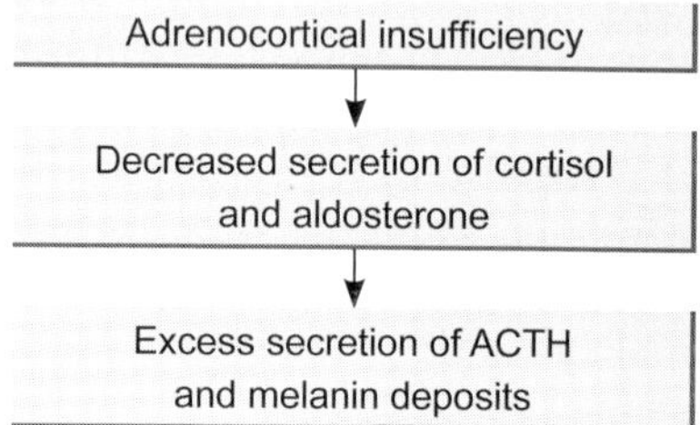

- The pigmentation often starts earlier than other manifestations by months to years. Usually generalized and more prominent in sun-exposed regions. In oral cavity, pigmentation is noted in buccal mucosa, lip, and gingival margins.
- *Cushing's syndrome*: The skin appears tanned, and gingiva, palate, buccal mucosa are blotchy and pigmented (Flowchart 3).

Flowchart 3: Pigmentation in Cushing's syndrome.

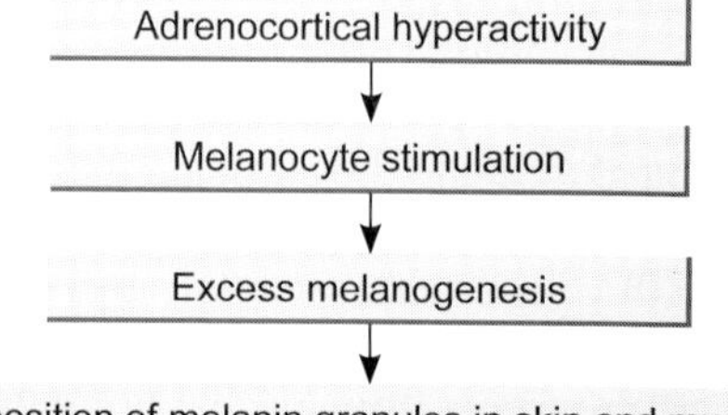

9. Adrenal crisis.

Acute adrenal insufficiency is known as Addison's crisis or adrenal crisis. Acute stress is the cause of adrenal crisis and is due to:

- Acute physiological stress—which increases the metabolic demand for corticoids. Cortex cannot produce this increased amount and the corticosteroid dose (exogenous) should be increased.
- Infection—alters the host's inflammatory response and hence leads to critical condition.
- Acute withdrawal of long-term steroid therapy.
- Adrenal crisis is manifested as nausea, vomiting, dehydration, hypotension and circulatory collapse.
- In patients taking 30 mg or above cortisol equivalent for more than 2 weeks duration, the hypothalamic—pituitary—adrenal axis may become suppressed. A functional ability to respond to stress may return within 2 weeks to 1 month, but for complete recovery, it may take up to 12 months.

Dental Consideration

- When treating dental patients under steroid therapy, the procedures that involve soft tissue manipulation and the chances of developing postoperative wound infection should be minimized by following atraumatic and aseptic protocols.
- Presurgical antibiotic prophylaxis should be considered.
  - Penicillin V potassium 2 g 1 hour before procedure and then 500 mg every 8 hour for 7 days.

Medical Management

- Blood pressure monitoring before, during and after dental procedure.
- Fluid replacement for hypotension.
- Dexamethasone 4 mg IV or IM.

10. Tetany.

- Tetany represents low level blood calcium (hypocalcemia) and is characterized by mild symptoms like perioral numbness, muscular spasm, or paresthesias of extremities and severe symptoms like laryngospasm, generalized muscle cramps, seizures, or even myocardial dysfunction. It can also occur in case of severe alkalosis (When the blood is highly alkaline). Magnesium deficiency is also is a contributory factor and hypokalemia in the absence of alkalosis may also cause tetany.
- Trousseau's sign and Chvostek sign are clinical tests to diagnose latent tetany.

Trousseau's Sign

A blood pressure cuff is placed on the arm and inflated to a pressure higher than the systolic pressure and held in place for 3 minutes. This will occlude the brachial artery and stops blood flow. In hypocalcemic patients, the subsequent neuromuscular irritability will induce spasm of the hand and forearm muscles. This sign is also known as "main d'accoucheur" — (French for *hand of the obstetrician*).

Chvostek Sign

- It is an abnormal reaction to a stimulus on the 7th cranial nerve.
- The simple tapping at the angle of mandible, causes facial nerve to become hyperexcitable and twitching of the same side facial muscles especially of the nose and lips. The underlying mechanism for this is the hypocalcemia due to either hypoparathyroidism, pseudohypoparathyroidism, or hypovitaminosis D.

Management

One or two 10 mL ampoules of 10% calcium gluconate diluted in 50–100 mL of 5% dextrose and infused slowly over 10 minutes as a initial treatment followed by repeated administrations to prevent the recurrence of hypocalcemia.

11. Discuss multiple endocrine neoplasia syndrome.

- Multiple endocrine neoplasia (MEN) syndrome is a group of familial syndromes and is characterized by the occurrence of neoplastic changes in many endocrine glands of the affected person. It has four types:

1. MEN type I—neoplasia of pancreatic islets, adrenal cortex, parathyroid and pituitary glands. In addition, it comprises Zollinger-Ellison syndrome (multiple primary gastrin-secreting adenomas or adenosarcomas in pancreas, duodenum, and extra-abdominal sites).
2. MEN type II A: It is characterized by the occurrence of medullary carcinoma of thyroid, pheochromocytoma, adenoma or hyperplasia of parathyroid gland.
3. MEN type II B or MEN type III: Multiple neuromas of commissural lip mucosa, tongue, buccal, nasal, conjunctival and pharyngeal mucosa in association with endocrine neoplasia hence known as multiple mucosal neuroma syndrome. Thickening of lip giving rise to characteristic bumpy or blubbery lip appearance, cafe-au-lait spots and marfanoid habitus is other characteristic findings.
4. MEN type IV: Rare condition and is characterized by tumors occurring in two or more endocrine glands and sometimes cause tumor occurrence in the non endocrine organs like renal and reproductive organs.

- Oral inference: The presence of oral mucosal neuromas and familial history of carcinoma of thyroid or pheochromocytoma gives a diagnostic clue for MEN III and guidance for early management.

MULTIPLE CHOICE QUESTIONS

1. Ground glass appearance is a radiographic feature of ***hyperparathyroidism***.
   a. Hyperparathyroidism
   b. Hyperthyroidism
   c. Hypoparathyroidism
   d. Hypothyroidism
2. Moth-eaten appearance or mottled appearance in a radiograph suggests ***hyperparathyroidism***.
   a. Hyperparathyroidism
   b. Hyperthyroidism
   c. Hypoparathyroidism
   d. Hypothyroidism
3. Stippled-bone pattern resembling pepper-pot skull in hyperparathyroidism is due to ***osteopenia of skull vault***.
   a. Osteoporosis of the skull vault
   b. Osteopetrosis of skull vault
   c. Osteopenia of skull vault
   d. Osteoid osteoma of skull vault
4. Pitting type of enamel hypoplasia is a feature of ***hypoparathyroidism***.
   a. Hyperparathyroidism
   b. Amelogenesis imperfecta
   c. Hypoparathyroidism
   d. Turner's hypoplasia
5. Persistent oral candidiasis in a young individual is a sign of ***hypoparathyroidism***.
   a. Hyperparathyroidism
   b. Hyperthyroidism
   c. Hypoparathyroidism
   d. Hypothyroidism
   (**Note:** Persistent oral candidiasis in a young individual is a sign of *hypoparathyroidism* and known as endocrine — candidiasis syndrome).
6. Metastatic calcification develops when calcium phosphate solubility product (Ca x P) is ***above 70***.
   a. Above 100 b. Above 70
   c. Equal to 1 b. Zero
7. Normal ion product or calcium phosphate solubility product is ***an average of 35***.
   a. Equal to 100
   b. An average of 35
   c. Equal to 10
   d. An average of 135
8. Patients on corticosteroid therapy are at the risk of developing complications related to ***Cushing's syndrome***.
   a. Noonan syndrome
   b. Borjeson-Forssman-Lehmann syndrome
   c. Comorbid syndrome
   d. Cushing's syndrome
9. Hypothyroid patients are not ***immunocompromised***.
   a. Myxedematous
   b. Immunocompromised
   c. Treated with synthetic thyroxine
   d. Treated with iodine

10. The total amount of body calcium is ***100–170 g***.
    a. 9–11g
    b. 9–11 m
    c. 100–170 mg
    d. 100–170 g
11. Normal serum calcium level is ***9–11 mg/dL***.
    a. 9–11 mg/dL
    b. 9–11 g/dL
    c. 100–170 mg/dL
    d. 100–170 mmol/dL
12. Parathyroid glands control blood ***calcium level***.
    a. Calcium level
    b. Phosphorus level
    c. Calcium-phosphate level
    d. Thyrocalcin level
13. Low serum calcium levels stimulate ***parathyroid glands***.
    a. Parathyroid glands
    b. Thyroid glands
    c. Pituitary gland
    d. Adrenal axis
14. An elevated level of glucocorticoid is associated with ***euphoria***.
    a. Manic depression
    b. Affective disorder
    c. Euphoria
    d. Morphea
15. Glucocorticoid excess causes ***obesity and moon face.***
    a. Hypotension and collapse
    b. Obesity and moon face
    c. Orthostatic hypotension
    d. Disorientation
16. *Adrenal insufficiency causes* ***dysphoria***.
    a. Dysphoria
    b. Euphoria
    c. Cushing's syndrome
    d. Galactorrhea
17. Glucocorticoid withdrawal results in ***mental disturbance***.
    a. Mental retardation
    b. Mental disturbance
    c. Hyperkinesias
    d. Dystonia
    (**Note:** Glucocorticoid withdrawal results in mental disturbances like dysphoria and depression, memory and learning deficits).
18. Alternate day dosage regimen is not applicable for multiple daily dosing with ***glucocorticoids***.
    a. Morphine
    b. Clopidogrel
    c. Insulin
    d. Glucocorticoids
19. The maximum production of pituitary ACTH production is during ***night time***.
    a. Daytime
    b. Night time
    c. Infancy
    d. Pregnancy
20. Congenital hypothyroidism is associated with ***mental retardation***.
    a. Excessive eating
    b. Mental retardation
    c. Warm skin
    d. Microglossia
21. The hormone which depends on dietary intake of micronutrient for its production is ***thyroxine***.
    a. Thyroxine
    b. Cortisol
    c. Estrogen
    d. Insulin
22. Production of thyroxine depends on dietary intake of ***iodine***.
    a. Vitamins
    b. Alanine
    c. Arginine
    d. Iodine
23. Iodine deficiency results in ***goiter***.
    a. Hypoglycemia
    b. Wilms tumor
    c. Goiter
    d. Fibrolamellar adenoma
    (**Note:** Iodine deficiency results in goiter and hypothyroidism).
24. Examination of thyroid gland should be carried out ***superior to the sternal notch***.
    a. Superior to the cricoid cartilage
    b. Inferior to the cricoid cartilage
    c. Superior to the sternal notch
    d. Inferior to the sternal notch
25. An autoimmune diseases of the thyroid is ***Graves' disease***.
    a. Goiter
    b. Graves' disease
    c. Thyroid storm
    d. Riedel's thyroiditis
    (**Note:** Autoimmune diseases of the thyroid are Hashimoto's thyroiditis and Graves' disease).

26. In Graves' disease autoantibodies are produced against ***thyroid-stimulating hormone***.
    a. Thyroxine
    b. Triiodothyronine
    c. Thyrotropin-releasing hormone
    d. Thyroid-stimulating hormone
27. Salivary gland disorder that tends to coexist with Hashimoto's thyroiditis is ***Sjogren's syndrome***.
    a. Sjogren's syndrome
    b. Sialadenitis
    c. Sialadenosis
    d. Carcinoma ex pleomorphic adenoma
28. The primary thyroid screening test for adults is ***TSH testing***.
    a. Thyroid antibody screening
    b. TSH testing
    c. Thyroglobulin test
    d. T3 and T4 tests
29. Diabetes insipidus is caused by decreased secretion or function of ***vasopressin***.
    a. Insulin
    b. Oxytocin
    c. Vasopressin
    d. Glucagon
    (**Note:** Vasopressin is an antidiuretic hormone).
30. The symptom of diabetes insipidus is the production of *large* ***volume of dilute urine***.
    a. Abnormally increased thirst
    b. Large volume of dilute urine
    c. Hunger and dry mouth
    d. Fatigue and blurred vision
31. Multiple neuromas of oral commissural mucosa are characteristics of ***multiple endocrine neoplasia syndrome***.
    a. Lloyd's syndrome
    b. Multiple adenoma syndrome
    c. Multiple endocrine neoplasia syndrome
    d. Goltz syndrome
    (**Note:** Multiple neuromas of oral commissural mucosa are characteristics of MEN IIB (or) MEN III).
32. A salivary steroid hormone that can be correlated to free serum level is and has diagnostic significance is ***cortisol and aldosterone***.
    a. Estradiol and cortisol
    b. Cortisol and aldosterone
    c. Aldosterone and corticosterone
    d. Cortisol and corticosterone
33. Salivary levels of hormones that can be assessed and can be substituted for diagnostic purpose is ***epinephrine***.
    a. Prolactin
    b. Vasopressin
    c. Epinephrine
    d. Growth hormone
    [**Note:** Salivary levels *of lipid hormones* (like estradiol, testosterone, aldosterone, cortisol, tyrosine, tryptophan, epinephrine, and norepinephrine) can be assessed accurately and can be substituted for diagnostic purpose *but not protein hormones* (antidiuretic hormone, growth hormone, follicle stimulating hormone, gonadotrophin, and prolactin)].
34. Fluoride application and fluoridated toothpaste should be avoided in the patients with ***thyroid disorder***.
    a. Thyroid disorder
    b. Turner hypoplasia
    c. Salivary gland disorder
    d. Renal diseases
    (**Note:** Fluoride mimics thyrotropin).
35. Hypoparathyroidism patients are highly susceptible to ***dental caries***.
    a. Sialolithiasis
    b. Dental caries
    c. Periodontitis
    d. Brown's tumor
36. Calcitonin inhibits ***osteoclastic bone resorption***.
    a. Bone calcium content
    b. Blood sodium level
    c. Osteoclastic bone resorption
    d. Osteotropic hormone level
    (**Note:** Calcitonin decreases serum levels of calcium and inhibits osteoclastic bone resorption).
37. Increase in serum calcium increases the secretion of ***calcitonin***.
    a. Parathormone b. Thyroxine
    c. Vitamin D d. Calcitonin
38. Increased urinary phosphoethanolamine level is a diagnostic marker for ***hypophosphatasia***.
    a. Hypophosphatasia
    b. Hyperphosphatemia
    c. Pseudohypoparathyroidism
    d. Primary hyperparathyroidism

39. Osteopetrosis is a ***quantitative bone disorder***.
    a. Qualitative bone disorder
    b. Quantitative bone disorder
    c. Regenerative bone disorder
    d. Degenerative bone disorder

VIVA VOCE

1. What are the precaution for patients with thyroid disorders during dental extraction?

- Chronic *hypothyroidism:* Patients may manifest prolonged bleeding from small vessels and require prolonged local pressure application. This is due to defect in the contracting ability of the small vessels because of excess subcutaneous mucopolysaccharides.
- Patients with long-standing *hyperthyroidism* may have elevated blood pressure. This necessitates the preference for limited use of vasoconstrictors and longer application of local pressure to stop bleeding.

2. State the types of hyperparathyroidism.

High amount of circulatory parathyroid hormone leads to hyperparathyroidism. It is of 4 types:

1. *Primary hyperparathyroidism:* Benign or malignant tumor of the gland is the cause.
2. *Secondary hyperparathyroidism:* The low serum calcium due to either physiological cause or pathological conditions stimulates the parathyroid glands for increased parathyroid hormone production and leads to gland hyperplasia.
3. *Tertiary hyperparathyroidism:* The chronic state of secondary hyperplasia changes to primary type once the underlying cause for low serum calcium is corrected.
4. *Forth type is ectopic hyperparathyroidism,* where parathyroid hormone levels are increased in patients with malignant diseases.

3. Enumerate the various conditions that cause loss of lamina dura.

- Hyperparathyroidism
- Paget's disease
- Osteomalacia
- Fibrous dysplasia
- Cushing's disease
- Addison's disease.

4. What is socket sclerosis?

Abnormal bone repair following dental extraction which radiographically manifests as lack of resorption of lamina dura and the deposition of sclerotic bone at the lamina dura is known as socket sclerosis. This condition occurs in renal disease patients.

5. What are the features of Cushing's syndrome?

- Cushing's syndrome is caused due to the increased amount of ACTH from ectopic secretion (e.g. malignant pulmonary tumor), from adrenal tumors or from iatrogenic glucocorticoids.
- The symptoms include obesity, osteoporosis, hypertension, diabetes mellitus, immunosuppression, psychiatric symptoms, muscle wasting and easy bruising.
- Similar symptoms also characterize Cushing's disease but caused by ACTH secreting pituitary tumors.

6. What is pathological calcification?

Abnormal calcium deposition in tissues is known as pathological calcification. It is associated with deposition of trace amounts of iron, magnesium and other mineral salts. This may occur as dystrophic calcification, metastatic calcification, and calcinosis.

7. What are the actions of corticosteroids when administered in chronic inflammatory diseases?

When glucocorticoid therapy is instituted for chronic inflammatory autoimmune diseases, such as pemphigus, lichen planus, pemphigoid, rheumatoid arthritis, the drug *decreases the production of T-lymphocytes* which leads to the prognosis of these diseases. It also *decreases the production of cytokines* like interleukin-1 (IL-1), interleukin-2 (IL-2), interleukin-6 (IL-6), and TNF-α which precipitate the diseases process.

8. What is an alternate day dosage regimen for glucocorticoids?

Alternate day steroid regimen is given for stable chronic inflammatory diseases like pulmonary fibrosis, rheumatoid arthritis, and asthma. This regimen allows the reactivation of adrenal and pituitary functions on the days when glucocorticoids are not given by *limiting adrenal insufficiency*. For the best beneficiary effect, a *high morning dose* of prednisone or any other short-acting glucocorticoids should be used. Also, this regimen is used to *maintain the total steroid dose constant* by gradually raising *on day* dose and tapering the *off day* dose.

9. Mention the signs and symptoms of hyperthyroidism.

Anxiousness, excess sweating, warm-moist skin, heat intolerance, fine tremors of hands, muscle wasting, weight loss, tachycardia, atrial fibrillation, goiter.

10. Mention the signs and symptoms of hypothyroidism.

Lethargy, dry skin, cold intolerance, decreased hearing, low-hoarse voice, weight gain, increased blood cholesterol level, increased subcutaneous tissue, slow pulse rate, goiter.

11. What is subclinical adrenal insufficiency?

- Subclinical adrenal insufficiency was defined as an elevated ACTH: Cortisol ratio. When patients are on short course (5 days) of high potency glucocorticoid therapy (>60 mg prednisone), may be in the state of adrenal insufficiency but they would not manifest any symptoms, but in acute stressful condition, it produce serious complications.

12. What are the diagnostic tests indicated to assess bone density?

- Dual energy X-ray absorptiometry (DEXA)
- Quantitative computed tomography (Q-CT)

BIBLIOGRAPHY

1. Chandna S, Bathla M. Oral manifestations of thyroid disorders and its management. Indian J Endocrinol Metab. 2011;15(Suppl 2):S113-6.
2. Cooper MS, Gittoes NJ. Diagnosis and management of hypocalcaemia. BMJ. 2008; 336(7656):1298-302.
3. Frederiksen A, Rossing M, Hermann P, et al. Clinical features of multiple endocrine neoplasia type 4: novel pathogenic variant and review of published cases. The Journal of Clinical Endocrinology and Metabolism. 2019. 104(9):3637-3646.
4. McCarthy PL, Shklar G. Diseases of the oral mucosa, 2nd edition. Lea & Febiger; Philadelphia; 1980.
5. Scully C, Kalantzis A. Oxford handbook of dental patient care. Oxford University Press, USA; 2005.
6. Shafer WG, Hine MK, Levy BM, Rajendran R, Sivapathasundharam B. A textbook of oral pathology. Saunders; Philadelphia: 1983.
7. Silverman S Jr, Ware WH, Gillooly C Jr. Dental aspects of hyperparathyroidism. Oral Surg Oral Med Oral Pathol. 1968;26(2): 184-9.
8. Suresh R, Radfar L. Pregnancy and lactation. Oral Surg Oral Med Oral Pathol Oral Radiol Endod. 2004;97(6):672-82.
9. Wiener C, Fauci AS, Braunwald E, Kasper DL, et al. Harrison's principles of internal medicine, self-assessment and board review. McGraw Hill Professional. 2008. 2:1612-5.

CHAPTER 18

Immunological Diseases

HIGHLIGHTS

The immune response consists of an innate system (first-line defense) and acquired or adaptive system (specific response to each infectious agent). The innate (natural) immune response lacks memory hence recognition of previous exposure of the pathogens (no antigen-specific recognition) whereas the acquired immune system is dependent on prior contact of the pathogen to respond. This memory is advantageous for preventing same pathogenic agent causing later infections.

Learners are expected to study the:

- Oral findings in various immunodeficiency diseases.
- Oral complications of autoimmune disorders.

SHORT NOTES

1. Describe oral findings in lupus erythematosus.

- Lupus erythematosus (LE) is an autoimmune disease (in Latin, lupus = wolf, erythematosus = red). It has two types of involvement: Systemic and discoid. The pathognomonic finding is the *facial butterfly rash*, most frequently seen in systemic lupus erythematosus. The typical oral lesion in both systemic and discoid lupus comprises a central atrophic, red mucosa surrounded by a slightly raised, border. This border is composed of white *paint-brush*-like lines that run in the vertical direction. The various sites affected in the oral cavity are palate, buccal, and vestibular mucosa.
- In chronic cases of LE, the oral lesion appears as round, well-circumscribed, scaly, atrophic plaques. The long-standing oral lupus gives a characteristic honeycomb pattern to buccal mucosa due to mucosal scaring with keratotic lesions.
- Lip lesions are a well-circumscribed discoid pattern with diffuse cheilitis. The lesions spread out from vermilion border to the adjacent skin.
- In systemic lupus erythematosus, xerostomia secondary to Sjogren's syndrome is also common.
- In the acute form, palatal erythema, bullous eruption with subsequent ulcerations is common.

Treatment

- Interdisciplinary management is necessary for the prognosis.
- For oral lesions, intralesional injection of 3 mg/mL triamcinolone acetonide is effective.
- Systemic steroids are reserved for more severe cases.
- Methotrexate or azathioprine can be used as a steroid-sparing drug.

2. Oral manifestations of scleroderma.

- Rigid lips with a narrow oral aperture (microstomia) giving the appearance of *fish mouth*.

- Skin folds around the mouth disappear and gives *mask-like* facial appearance.
- *Telangiectasia* on lips and hard palate.
- *Pseudoankylosis* of temporomandibular joints due to involvement of surrounding soft tissues.
- The *rigidity of the tongue* makes speech and swallowing as difficult.
- Pseudoankylosis of TMJ
- Xerostomia
- Radiographic findings include *uniform thickening of periodontal membrane* especially around posterior teeth, involvement of facial muscles cause *pressure-induced resorption on mandible* at angle, coronoid process, and condyle.

3. Behcet's syndrome.

- Behcet's disease or Behcet's syndrome is a triple symptom complex characterized by recurrent oral, ocular and genital ulcers and inflamed blood vessels.
- The underlying pathogenesis is immune-mediated systemic vasculitis and occurs in 3rd or 4th decades of life.
- The lesions are self-limiting with sequelae of remission and recurrence.
- Oral ulcers—most common finding. Both major and minor aphthous ulcers occur in single and crops. Healing of major ulcers takes place with mild scarring. Symptomatic management using topical analgesics and supportive medications may accelerate the prognosis.
- Genital ulcers—both males and females develop genital ulcers. Usually, occur as superficial forms, but sometimes deep ulcers develop leading to fistulous tract formation with unfavorable prognosis.
- Ocular lesions—retina and uvea are affected. Blurred vision, photophobia, and blindness are the complications.
- Apart from these classical traits, involvements of other systems like gastrointestinal, neurological, cutaneous and cardiovascular are also common.

Diagnosis

- Positive pathergy test is associated with the active phase of Behcet's syndrome. The test is performed by pricking a needle on the skin surface or intracutaneous injection of saline. Formation of a sterile pustule or small erythematous papule within 24–48 hours described the hypersensitivity reaction and taken as definite diagnostic criteria for Behcet's syndrome. The positivity did not correlate with the disease severity and related to geographic location (Mediterranean population).
- International study group criteria for diagnosis: Aphthous ulcerations which recur at least three times in a year in addition to any two of the following lesions will confirm the diagnosis.
  Genital ulceration, tender nodules on the skin, eye lesions or positive pathergy test.
- *Treatment* is aimed at reducing the inflammation, relieving the symptoms and minimizing the recurrence.
  Combination therapy of corticosteroids and immunosuppressive drugs are used to reduce the morbidity.
  For oral lesions:
  - Triamcinolone acetonide 0.1% cream 4 times/day is effective.
  - For larger and widespread lesions, 0.5 mg/5 mL dexamethasone elixir 4 times rinse/day is useful.
  - For major ulcers, intralesional 5–10 mg/mL triamcinolone is indicated.
  - Chlorhexidine or tetracycline mouth rinse (250 mg capsule dissolved in 5 mL of water) will reduce the pain and healing period.
  - For severe or resistant oral lesions, systemic prednisone 40–60 mg/day for 2 weeks and then tapering over the next 4 weeks is considered.

4. Sarcoidosis.

- Sarcoidosis is an acquired granulomatous disease affecting multiple tissues and organs. The etiology is unknown. Pulmonary and cutaneous involvements are more common, whereas head and neck involvement occurs in 10–15% of affected individuals.

- Bilateral enlargement of parotid glands and xerostomia are the common findings.
- Oral lesions occur in chronic conditions and appear as nontender, well-defined, brownish red papules or as submucosal nodules. If superficial ulceration occurs, then these nodules or papules become symptomatic. Severe alveolar bone loss and mobility of teeth are also present. Gingiva appears erythematous and swollen in the interdental regions.
- Presence of typical noncaseating epithelioid granulomas on histopathological evaluation will support the diagnosis.
- Glucocorticosteroids with cytotoxic drugs (like methotrexate or cyclosporine) are the primary mode of treatment.

5. Name the different types of immune reactions with examples.

- *Type I immediate hypersensitivity reactions*—anaphylactic shock, angioedema, urticaria, conjunctivitis, rhinorrhea, and rhinitis. It takes 15–20 minutes from exposure time to respond but sometimes may take 10–12 hours. It is mediated by IgE.
- *Type II cytotoxic hypersensitivity reaction*—are mediated by IgG and IgM and takes minutes to hours for manifestation. Examples are drug-induced hemolytic anemia, granulocytopenia, and thrombocytopenia.
- *Type III Immune complex hypersensitivity reaction*—maybe widespread (Serum sickness) or involve single organ like skin (Systemic lupus erythematosus, arthus reaction), kidneys (Lupus nephritis), blood vessels (Polyarteritis), joints (Rheumatoid arthritis). IgM mediates it but IgG also plays a role. The reaction takes 3–10 hours for manifestation.
- *Type IV cell-mediated or delayed type hypersensitivity reaction* — tuberculin (Mantoux) reaction is the example. Injecting the antigen PPD or old tuberculin results in the appearance of erythema and induration after 48 hours in hypersensitive individuals.

MULTIPLE CHOICE QUESTIONS

1. Mask-like appearance of face is seen in ***scleroderma***.
   a. Facial paralysis
   b. Trigeminal neuralgia
   c. Scleroderma
   d. Myofacial pain syndrome
2. Pseudoankylosis of TMJ is common in ***scleroderma***.
   a. Osteoarthritis
   b. Rheumatoid arthritis
   c. Scleroderma
   d. Sarcoidosis
3. Fish-mouth appearance is the finding in ***scleroderma***.
   a. Scleroderma
   b. Submucous fibrosis
   c. Plummer-Vinson syndrome
   d. Angular cheilitis

VIVA VOCE

1. Name the primary immunodeficiency diseases.

Defects in cellular immunity lead to DiGeorge syndrome, severe combined immunodeficiency disease, and Wiskott-Aldrich syndrome.

2. Name the secondary immunodeficiency diseases.

Secondary immunodeficiencies are caused by HIV-infection, immunosuppressive drug therapy, malignancy or granulomatous disorders of lymphoid system and protein depending disorders. It includes: Leukemia, Hodgkin's disease, non-Hodgkin's lymphoma, multiple myelomas, sarcoidosis and acquired immunodeficiency syndrome (AIDS).

3. Give examples of connective tissue diseases.

Also known as, collagen disease, collagen vascular disease, hyperimmune diseases and autoimmune disease. It includes systemic lupus erythematosus, rheumatoid arthritis, scleroderma, dermatomyositis, and polyarthritis nodosa.

4. What is hypersensitivity reaction?

Occurrence of intense and disagreeable (Discomfort and sometimes fatal) responses in a presensitized (Immune) host is known as hypersensitivity reaction.

5. Discuss Wiskott-Aldrich syndrome.

- It is a X-linked recessive disorder characterized by eczema, thrombocytopenia, pyogenic and opportunistic infections and bloody diarrhea. It is due to altered cell surface glycoprotein in lymphocytes and platelets.
- T-cell abnormalities include herpes simplex infection and B-cell abnormalities include recurrent bacterial infection in oral cavity. Neutropenia and neutrophil dysfunction syndrome cause oral ulcers. Maxillary sinusitis, severe asthma, recurrent otitis media, and pneumonia are also common.

6. What is Raynaud's phenomenon?

Paroxysmal vasospasm (reduced blood flow) of the fingers results in color change of the fingertips in response to cold and emotion.

7. What is DiGeorge syndrome (or) what is velocardiofacial syndrome?

- Results from chromosomal deletion 22q11 resulting in defective embryonic growth in thymus, parathyroid glands and greater vessels of the heart. Features include variable immunodeficiency, neonatal hypocalcemia, and congenital cardiac defects.
- Abnormal ear, cleft palate, short palpebral fissures, smallmouth, prominent forehead, and micrognathia give a characteristic facial appearance.

8. What is autoimmune disease?

Autoimmunity is the state where immune system misinterprets the own cells of the body as foreign invaders and sends signal to the immune cells to attack them. Diseases that results from such unusual immune response are called as autoimmune diseases, e.g. lichen planus, lupus erythematosus, and psoriasis

BIBLIOGRAPHY

1. Cawson RA, Odell EW. Cawson's essentials of oral pathology and oral medicine e-book. 8th edition Elsevier Health Sciences; 2017.
2. Kolokotronis AE, Belazi MA, Haidemenos G, et al. Sarcoidosis: oral and perioral manifestations. Hippokratia. 2009;13(2): 119-21.
3. Marmary Y, Glaiss R, Pisanty S. Scleroderma: oral manifestations. Oral surg Oral Med Oral Pathol. 1981;52(1):32-7.
4. Nico MM, Vilela MA, Rivitti EA, et al. Oral lesions in lupus erythematosus: correlation with cutaneous lesions. Eur J Dermatol. 2008;18(4):376-81.
5. Zeidan MJ, Saadoun D, Garrido M, et al. Behçet's disease physiopathology: a contemporary review. Auto Immun Highlights. 2016;7(1):4.

CHAPTER 19

Bone Disorders

HIGHLIGHTS

Bone is a mineralized connective tissue composed primarily (up to 60%) calcium carbonate and calcium phosphate. The organic components (comprise 40%) are protein (collagen) and water. The bone forms skeleton to support the visceral organs. It also provides an attachment site for muscles and aids in their movement. Apporoximately, 90% of the body calcium and 80% of phosphorus are stored in bones. The bone strength is determined by a bone mineral density that measures the weight of the mineral per unit volume of bone. This chapter highlights the bony disorders with characteristic oral lesions.

Learners are expected to study:

- The pathogenesis of different bone disorders.
- Oral manifestations
- Specific investigation and dental management for affected patients.

ESSAY QUESTIONS

1. List the bony disorders with oral manifestations and add brief notes about Paget's disease.

Classification of Bone Disorders

- Developmental diseases:
  - Cherubism
  - Osteopetrosis
  - Osteogenesis imperfecta
  - Cleidocranial dysplasia
- Endocrinal diseases:
  - Hyperparathyroidism
  - Hyperpituitarism
- Idiopathic diseases:
  - Idiopathic osteosclerosis
  - Langerhans cell disease (Histiocytosis-X)
  - Paget's disease
- Reactive diseases:
  - Aneurysmal bone cyst
  - Simple or traumatic bone cyst
- Fibro-osseous lesions:
  - Fibrous dysplasia
  - Cemento-osseous dysplasia
  - Ossifying fibroma
- Inflammatory diseases:
  - Tuberculosis
  - Actinomycosis
  - Osteomyelitis
- Neoplastic diseases
  - Benign: Osteoma, osteoid osteoma, osteoblastoma, chondroma.
  - Malignant: Osteosarcoma—Ewing's sarcoma—chondrosarcoma.
- Metabolic disorders:
  - Osteoporosis
  - Osteopetrosis
  - Osteomalacia and rickets.

Paget's disease is a chronic bone disease characterized by abnormal bone resorption and bone deposition, affecting either single (monostotic) or multiple bones (polyostotic). The etiology is associated with viral infection and inclusion bodies resembling nucleocapsid particles of paramyxovirus, and canine distemper virus are demonstrated in the bone cells of patients. In the initial course, patient will be asymptomatic, and in later stages, pain, facial disfigurement, and fracture of the affected bone may occur. Nerve compression causes neurological symptoms like hearing loss.

Pathogenesis

Phase 1: Severe osteolytic process:
- Aggressive bone resorption.
- Bone turnover takes place at the rate of 20-times of the average rate.

Phase 2: Mixed osteolytic and osteoblastic phase:
- Immature bone formation.
- Poor mineralization.

Phase 3: Active osteoblastic activity:
- More amount of sclerotic bone formation in a disorganized pattern.
- The bone has reduced strength on comparing with the normal bone.

Radiographic Findings

Phase I: Radiolucent resorptive stage
Phase II: Granular or ground glass
Phase III: More opaque late stage.

Management

Calcitonin, bisphosphonate, and mithramycin.

2. Define fibrous dysplasia. Describe the pathogenesis, clinical and radiographic findings with a note on management.

Fibrous dysplasia is a developmental disorder characterized by atypical fibrous tissue which contains small, abnormally arranged bone trabeculae which replaces the normal bone cells. Craniofacial bone is involved in both monostotic and polyostotic form and typically affects the maxilla, mandible, and rarely the calvarium.

Etiology

The etiology of fibrous dysplasia is unknown. The proposed causative factors are linked to a gene mutation where arginine is replaced either by serine or histidine. World Health Organization grouped this as a developmental disorder.

Classifications

- Monostotic fibrous dysplasia
- Polyostotic fibrous dysplasia:
  - Jaffe's type
  - McCune-Albright syndrome
- Craniofacial form.

Clinical Features

- *Monostotic fibrous dysplasia:*
  - This form is characterized by single bone involvement and comprises about 70–80% of the reported cases. The involvement of maxilla or facial bones gave rise to lion-like face to the affected persons and referred as leontiasis ossea.
  - Etiopathogenesis is related to the abnormal activity in the bone forming mesenchymal tissue. Congenital form is an autosomal recessive pattern.
  - The incidence of maxillary lesion is more than the mandibular involvement. Jaw lesions frequently present as painless, hard swelling with intact overlying mucosa that cause bone expansion. Malocclusion and displacement of teeth takes place when the lesion enlarges.
- *Polyostotic fibrous dysplasia: Polyostotic* form affects more than one bone. Genetic mutation is stated as etiology.

Clinical Features

- *Jaffe's type*—affects a variable number of bones. Skin pigmentation, known as cafe-au-lait spots which are light-brown is a notable feature of this form. It is mild and nonprogressive.
- *Albright's syndrome*—McCune-Albright syndrome is an association of polyostotic fibrous dysplasia, precocious puberty, cafè-au-lait spots, and other endocrinopathies.

Oral Findings

- Jaw expansion and delayed eruption are the common findings. The associated endocrine disorder is responsible for late eruption.

Radiographic Findings

Conventional radiographic findings:

- *Pseudotype: Orange or ground-glass appearance*: Grainy appearance of density and radiolucency on radiographs resemble the outer peel of an orange.
- *Whorled plaque*: The core lesion presents radiographically as a radiodense structure intermediate between the bone and soft tissue densities. The amorphous lesion resembles onion peel appearance or whorled pattern.
- *Diffuse sclerotic type*: The lesion is uniformly radiodense and boundaries of the lesion are merged with the normal bone.
- *Cyst-like*: In the early stage, the lesion is poorly mineralized and present as osteolytic cyst-like pattern with peripheral lamellar sclerosis giving a ground-glass appearance.
- *Pagetoid type*: The bony lesion is expansile in nature with alternate radiopaque and radiolucent pattern similar to the picture of Paget's disease. The expanded lower border of mandible demonstrates the characteristic *thumbprint* appearance.
- *Chalky type*: The core lesion is an irregular radiodense mass with well-defined margins. This type occurs rarely.

Computed Tomography Findings

Computed tomography (CT) accurately establishes the diagnosis and extent of bone involvement. CT characteristics of fibrous dysplasia include bone expansion with three variable pattern of densities associated with scattered islands of bone formation.

- *Egg-shell pattern:* Cyst-like core lesion with peripheral radiodense *onion-peel pattern* referred as egg shell lesion.
- *Ground-glass pattern:* In the intermediate stage, mineralization of woven bone takes place and appears as expanded lesion with ground-glass pattern.
- *Pagetoid pattern:* In the later stage, the amount of osseous tissue increases and leads to multiple attenuation of X-ray beam, giving rise to heterogeneous pagetoid pattern.

Laboratory Findings

- Serum calcium, parathyroid hormone, 25-hydroxyvitamin D, and 1,25-dihydroxyvitamin D levels are normal.
- Serum alkaline phosphatase (ALP) is occasionally elevated.

Management

Treatment of fibrous dysplasia is based on their clinical presentation:

- Monostotic fibrous dysplasia tends to stabilize when skeletal growth stops. Hence surgical intervention should be delayed until growth spurts are completed.
- For symptomatic fibrous dysplasia, bisphosphonate therapy is attempted.

3. Describe the classic features of Langerhans cell histiocytosis in jaw bones.

- Abnormal proliferation of Langerhans cell or their precursor cells cause Langerhans cell histiocytosis and 10% of all affected individuals manifest oral lesions.
- Three forms exist, and all demonstrate proliferation of reticuloendothelial cells.

Eosinophilic Granuloma

- It appears in the skeleton either as unifocal or as a multifocal lesion.
- Unifocal type is the common form and has a preference for males. The associated symptoms are recurrent bone pain, swelling, and occasional pathologic fractures. Oral findings include swelling, ulcers, gingival necrosis, alveolar bone destruction, mobility and loss of teeth.

Radiographic Findings

Well-defined lesions with a punched out periphery.

Treatment

- Surgical curettage is the treatment for oral lesions.
- Radiotherapy and chemotherapy should be considered for lesions that are not surgically manageable.

Letterer-Siwe Disease

It is highly morbid and mortal. Involvement of oral cavity is infrequent. Necrosis and ulceration of gingiva covered by grayish-white purulent exudates is the common finding. Both maxilla and mandible are affected with radiographic presentation of multiple radiolucent lesions. Corticosteroids and chemotherapy are the possible treatment options. Prognosis is poor.

Hand-Schűller-Christian Disease

- The classical triad of this disease is exophthalmos, diabetes insipidus, and lytic lesions in the calvarium. Skull is the common site of involvement. It primarily affects infants, children and adults are rarely affected. Facial bone involvement manifests facial asymmetry due to soft tissue swelling, pain, and otitis media. Oral manifestations include sore mouth, halitosis, gingivitis, unpleasant taste, loose teeth. Oral findings are the earliest signs of this disease. Complication includes failure of healing in the extracted sockets.
- Radiographic examination reveals sharply outlined individual lesions. The large serpiginous, punched-out skull lesions give the name *geographic skull*. There is scooped-out pattern of bone loss in the posterior mandibular alveolus starting at the mid-root region. Extensive alveolar involvement causes the teeth to appear as *floating in air*.

Treatment

Surgical curettage or excision correct the localized oral lesions. Intralesional injection of corticosteroids or a low-dose regimen of systemic oral corticosteroids can also be used. Radiotherapy is an alternative treatment for localized bone lesions.

SHORT NOTES

1. Ossifying fibroma.

- The ossifying fibroma (OF) is a benign neoplasm that occurs in adult population (3rd and 4th decades of life). It has a preference for females. Both maxilla and mandible are affected, but mandibular involvement is common. The occurrence of this tumor in children is called as juvenile ossifying fibroma and has aggressive progression.
- It appears as a single, painless and slow-growing tumor in the posterior mandible, specifically in the premolar-molar region.
- Histological features:
  - The excessive proliferation of periodontal ligaments gives rise to this lesion.
  - Both cementum-like calcification and bone materials are present in single lesion.
- Radiographic findings: Ossifying fibroma presents in two patterns:
  1. Cystic lesions, either unilocular or multilocular.
  2. Mixed-density lesions.
  - The radiographic boundaries are well-circumscribed and corticated. Cortical plate expansion is present. The lesion is initially radiolucent and appears as mixed radiolucent and radiopaque areas during maturation. The older lesions are radiopaque surrounded by a radiolucent halo.
  - Loss of lamina dura, root resorption and divergence of associated teeth may also present.

Management

Enucleation treats the small lesions. Larger lesions require radical resection.

2. Cemento-osseous dysplasia (or) florid cemento-osseous dysplasia.

Cemento-osseous dysplasia is the common form of fibro-osseous lesions. By their clinical and radiographic features, it is divided into three groups: Periapical, focal and florid cemento-osseous dysplasia.

Periapical Cemento-Osseous Dysplasia (PCOD)

The term cementoma is often used for this condition. It is an asymptomatic benign lesion occurring in the anterior mandible of patients aged above 30 years. It is common in women, and there is noticeable prevalence for black women. Lesions may be single or multiple. Involved teeth are vital.

Radiographic Findings

It shows three different characteristics:

1. Osteolytic period, circular and elliptical resorption areas.
2. Cementoblastic period or intermediate period, a mixed radiolucent and radiopaque appearance.
3. Late period-Lesions display massive calcifications.

Focal Cemento-osseous Dysplasia (FCOD)

- It is a benign lesion. May occur in any area of the jaws, but posterior mandible is the predominant site. They are asymptomatic.
- Radiographically, the lesion appears as completely radiolucent or completely radiopaque or a mixed pattern. Usually solitary and no treatment are required.

Florid Cemento-osseous Dysplasia (FLCOD)

- It is a reactive type of fibro-osseous lesion. The lesion contains multiple radiopaque cementum-like masses and present at various sites of jaws in all quadrants. The pathogenesis is unclear. It is otherwise known as gigantiform cementoma, chronic sclerosing osteomyelitis, and sclerosing osteitis. It occurs in black adult women, aged above 40 years. It may be asymptomatic and observed on radiographs taken for other purposes.
- *Radiographic findings*: Multiple radiopaque mass surrounded by a radiolucent boundary.

Treatment

This asymptomatic condition does not require any treatment.

Clinical Significance

Extraction of the associated teeth will cause delayed wound healing and sequestrum formation.

3. Differentiate fibrous dysplasia and ossifying fibroma.

Fibrous dysplasia and ossifying fibroma.

Features	Fibrous dysplasia	Ossifying fibroma
Age	1–2nd decades	3–4th decades
Site	Maxilla	Mandible
Symptom	Painless, diffuse swelling	Painless, well-demarcated jaw expansion
Variants	Monostotic and Polyostotic	None
Radiographic findings	Diffuse fine ground glass pattern. Ill-defined borders	Variable — radiolucent, mixed and radiopaque. Well-defined borders.

4. Describe the clinical and radiographic features of cherubism.

- Cherubism is an autosomal dominant disease characterized by fibrous tissue replacement of the bone tissues in affected bones. The prevalence is more among boys than girls with a ratio of 2:1.
- It frequently involves children aged between 2–7 years. There will be an exacerbation immediately after early manifestation followed by a stable period or complete resolution after puberty. The lesion starts as simultaneous enlargement of maxilla and mandible on both sides with characteristic round face, chubby cheeks, and upward-looking eyes (eyes looking

towards heaven). These features give the appearance of *cherubs*. Presence of cervical and submandibular lymphadenopathy is the specific early finding.

Classification

- Grade I—bilateral involvement of the ascending ramus.
- Grade II—bilateral involvement of the ascending ramus and maxillary tuberosity.
- Grade III—complete involvement of the maxilla and mandible.

Dental Alterations

- Early exfoliation of deciduous teeth, impaction, and displacement of permanent teeth.
- Ectopic tooth eruption, agenesis of the second and third molars due to involution of their germs.
- Root resorption of existing teeth.
- Malocclusion

Radiographic Findings

- *Orthopantomographic findings:*
  - Multilocular radiolucent lesions involving the posterior regions of maxilla and mandible, bilaterally.
  - Bone changes start as bilateral radiolucent lesions of body and ascending ramus. Condylar involvement is rare, but lesions extend up to coronoid process. Displacement of mandibular canal is common.
  - Teeth appear as floating in radiolucent areas known as *floating tooth appearance.*
- Computed tomography is useful for treatment planning to locate the extensions of bony involvement.
- MRI is helpful to see the orbital involvement.

Management

- Natural remission by biological stabilization is the preferred choice.
- After regression of disease activity, cosmetic osteoplasty of the affected jaws, and curettage of the lesions may be considered.
- Medical management is provided with calcitonin.

5. Briefly describe rickets and osteomalacia.

- Incomplete mineralization of osteoid tissues due to lack of calcium salts manifests as rickets in children (6–24 months of age) and as osteomalacia in adults.
- Rickets is a metabolic disorder characterized by deficiency or impaired metabolism of vitamin D, phosphorus or calcium.
- In rickets, delayed eruptions, and enamel hypoplasia are the common oral findings. Other notable features include bowed leg, widened epiphyses of long bones, and greenstick fractures in the weight-bearing bones.
- Osteomalacia is caused by poor intestinal absorption of vitamin D. Bone pain, muscle weakness, greenstick fracture, tetany and a waddling gait are the associated symptoms. Cortical thinning and large radiolucency (pseudofractures) are common in long bones, and no radiographic manifestation is seen in the jaws.

6. Describe osteopetrosis (or) marble bone disease.

- Osteopetrosis or Albers-Schonberg disease is a condition in which marrow space is filled with compact bone, resulting in extremely dense, hard and brittle bones. It occurs both in congenital and acquired forms.
- In congenital osteopetrosis, the osteoclasts are defective in either number or function. Multiple bone fractures are common. Neurological symptom like deafness is due to nerve compression at the foramina due to surrounding dense bone. Severe form is fatal, but in mild cases, the child can be expected for average lifespan.

❖ The acquired form is associated with increased fluoride deposition in the bone due to excess consumption.

Dental Complication

Bone fracture is a complication during extraction.

Management

❖ Bone marrow transplantation
❖ Medical management includes gamma interferon and calcitriol.

MULTIPLE CHOICE QUESTIONS

1. Enamel hypoplasia and loss of skull sutures are the findings in ***rickets***.
   a. Paget's disease
   b. Osteopetrosis
   c. Rickets
   d. Cherubism
2. In the jaw bones, osteoporosis is more common in ***alveolar process***.
   a. Anterior maxilla
   b. Anterior mandible
   c. Alveolar process
   d. interdental crest
3. The biochemical values in rickets is characterized by ***lower plasma values of calcium and phosphorus***.
   a. High plasma calcium and low phosphorus
   b. High plasma phosphorus and low calcium
   c. Lower plasma values of calcium and phosphorus
   d. Higher plasma values of calcium and phosphorus
4. Normal level of plasma alkaline phosphatase is seen in ***osteporosis***.
   a. Primary hyperparathyroidism
   b. Osteomalasia
   c. Osteoporosis
   d. Paget's disease
5. Periapical resorption and hypercementosis are the radiographic features of ***Paget's disease***.
   a. Paget's disease
   b. Hyperparathyroidism
   c. Rickets
   d. Osteopetrosis
6. In cherubism, jaw changes occur in the age of ***2–7 years***.
   a. 5–10 months
   b. 1–3 years
   c. 2–7 years
   d. 13–19 years
7. Upward tilting of the eyes is a feature of ***cherubism***.
   a. Fibrous dysplasia
   b. Cherubism
   c. Ossifying fibroma
   d. Hand-Schuller-Christian disease
8. The first radiographic sign of cherubism is seen in the ***angle of mandible***.
   a. Symphysis region
   b. Premaxilla
   c. Alveolar bone
   d. Angle of mandible
9. The common site for ossifying fibroma is ***mandibular premolar-molar region***.
   a. Maxillary canine region
   b. Maxillary premolar-molar region
   c. Mandibular premolar-molar region
   d. Ramus of mandible
10. Destruction of alveolar bone with localized periodontitis and sterile pus discharge is characteristic for ***eosinophilic granuloma***.
    a. Fibrous dysplasia
    b. Florid cemento-osseous dysplasia
    c. Eosinophilic granuloma
    d. Metastatic jaw tumour

VIVA VOCE

1. What are the oral manifestations of hypothyroidism?

In children, delayed eruption and slow exfoliation of primary teeth are common. In adult no dental abnormalities are present.

2. Discuss oral findings associated with hypophosphatemia.

❖ Teeth may have large pulp cavity.
❖ Periapical abscess is common.

3. What are the features of osteopetrosis?

❖ Due to defective osteoclast activity, the normal bone resorption does not happen, leading to increased bone density. Delayed eruption and multiple unerupted teeth are common.

- Radiologic features:
  - High dense appearance of jaw bones
  - In jaw bones, the increased density makes difficult to differentiate teeth and bone.
  - High-bone density hinders the normal eruption.
  - Reduced vascular supply may lead to osteomyelitis and pathological fractures.

4. How to measure the bone marrow density?

- *Dual-energy X-ray absorptiometry (DEXA)*—measures the bone mineral content in grams per square centimeter.
- *Quantitative computed tomography*—assess the right volumetric density by a separate estimation of trabecular and cortical density.
- *Quantitative ultrasound.*

BIBLIOGRAPHY

1. DiCaprio MR, Enneking WF. Fibrous dysplasia. Pathophysiology, evaluation, and treatment. J Bone Joint Surg.Am. 2005; 87(8):1848-64.
2. Lichtenstein L. Histiocytosis X (eosinophilic granuloma of bone, Letterer-Siwe disease, and Schüller-Christian disease). Further observations of pathological and clinical importance. J Bone Joint Surg Am. 1964; 46(1):76-90.
3. Liu Y, Wang H, You M, et al. Ossifying fibromas of the jaw bone: 20 cases. Dentomaxillofac Radiol. 2010;39(1):57-63.
4. Mangala M, Ramesh DN, Surekha PS, et al. Florid cemento-osseous dysplasia: Review and report of two cases. Indian J Dent Res. 2006;17(3):131-4.
5. Özkan Y, Varol A, Turker N, et al. Clinical and radiological evaluation of cherubism: a sporadic case report and review of the literature. Int J Pediatr Otorhinolaryngol. 2003;67(9):1005-12.
6. Ralston SH, Langston AL, Reid IR. Pathogenesis and management of Paget's disease of bone. Lancet. 2008;372(9633):155-63.
7. Triantafillidou K, Zouloumis L, Karakinaris G, et al. Brown tumors of the jaws associated with primary or secondary hyperparathyroidism. A clinical study and review of the literature. Am J Otolaryngol. 2006;27(4):281-6.

CHAPTER 20

Oral Manifestations of Nutritional Disorders

HIGHLIGHTS

The nutritional status of an individual is reflected in their oral mucosa. The oral cavity of the malnourished individuals may reveal the findings of ulcers, microbial infections, dry mouth, and disturbed taste sensation. The deficiency of proteins, vitamins and trace elements produce remarkable changes on the face, lips, tongue, and gingiva. This chapter highlights the oral and dental modifications associated with malnutrition, the pathogenesis associated with a deficient state of different nutrients, and information about the dietary sources of nutrients.

Learners are expected to study:

- Role of nutrients in the development of oral and dental structures.
- Oral changes associated with various nutritional deficiencies.
- Therapeutic implication of antioxidants.
- Kwashiorkor disease and marasmus.

ESSAY QUESTIONS

1. What are water-soluble vitamins? Describe their function, food sources, and oral manifestations of deficiency.

Vitamins are essential nutrients and perform specific vital functions hence crucial for health. *Vitamin B complex and vitamin C* are water soluble. They dissolve in water and eliminated in urine. The body cannot store the vitamins and therefore need to be supplied everyday. Cooking and food processing destroys the vitamins.

- *Vitamin B complex:* B complex group comprises a total of eight vitamins. They are thiamine (B_1), riboflavin (B_2), niacin (B_3), pyridoxine (B_6), vitamin B_{12}, folic acid, pantothenic acid, and biotin.
- *Vitamin B1—thiamine:*
  - Functions: Acts as a coenzyme in the metabolism of carbohydrates, and release energy from food. They are essential for maintaining the proper functioning of muscles and nervous system.
  - Food sources: Most commonly found in whole grains, cereals, legume, liver, and enriched bread.
  - Manifestations of vitamin B1 deficiency:
    - Hyperesthesia (unusual sensitivity) of the oral mucosa.
    - Atypical neuralgias
    - Burning sensation in the oral mucosa and face.
    - Dentinal hypersensitivity.
    - Trigeminal neuralgia and delayed healing after extraction.
    - Gingiva resembles *old rose* in color.
    - Vitamin B_1 deficiencies in infants begin with erythematous papillae over the anterior dorsum and tip of the tongue followed by glossitis.
- *Vitamin B_2—riboflavin:*
  - Riboflavin acts as a coenzyme in oxidation-reduction cycle, metabolism of carbohydrates, proteins, and fat.
  - Food sources: Green vegetables, legumes, milk, whole grain products, egg, and liver.

- The riboflavin deficiency causes angular cheilitis and glossitis. The effects occur within 8 week of deficient status.
    - *Angular cheilitis:* The corners of the mouth become erythematous, and at the advanced stage, it leads to *painful fissures and bleeding*. Lips become red with multiple cracks and known as cracked lip.
    - *Glossitis:* Swollen *fungiform papillae* give a pebbly texture to the tongue and vascular distension gives *magenta color*. Later there is atrophy of the papillae and tongue becomes glazy, shiny, fissured, and painful.
- In young adults, B_2 deficiency causes *interdental bone resorption and mobility of the incisors.*
- Jaws deformities and retardation of condylar growth are the rare complications.

❖ *Vitamin B_3—niacin, nicotinic acid, nicotinamide:*

- It is necessary for energy production, enzyme activities, and function of the nervous system.
- Food sources: Liver, fish, poultry, meat, peanuts, whole and enriched grain products.
- In nicotinic acid or niacin deficiency, the tongue appears *beefy red*, and swollen with papillary hypertrophy. As the deficiency continuous, the fungiform and filiform papillae become atrophic with superficial epithelial desquamation leading to smooth, glossy, and red appearance on the dorsal surface. Diffuse patchy inflammation of the oral mucosa associated with burning sensation, soreness and tenderness also occur. The interdental papillae undergo necrotic changes and spread to involve the other parts of gingiva. Gingival ulceration is also evident.

❖ *Vitamin B_6—pyridoxine:*

- It is essential for protein metabolism, hemoglobin and red blood cell synthesis. B_6 also plays a role in the mechanism of insulin secretion.
- Food sources: Pork, meat, whole grains, cereals, legumes and dark leafy vegetables.
- The pyridoxine deficiency has not yet determined.

❖ *Vitamin B_{12}—cobalamin:*

- It aids in building genetic material, RBC synthesis, and support the functions of nervous system.
- Food sources: It found *only in foods of animal origin,* such as meat, liver, kidney, fish, eggs, and dairy products.
- Addisonian anemia is the severe form of vitamin B_{12} deficiency. The lips, buccal mucosa, and palate become pale yellow. The appearance of brown pigmentation and angular cheilitis with fissuring and yellow crustation are the typical findings.
- Hunter's glossitis—it is the pathognomonic finding of B_{12} deficiency. Atrophic changes of the filiform papillae lead to red, shiny, and smooth dorsal surface of the tongue. The patient reports soreness, burning sensation, and loss of taste sensation.

❖ *Folic acid:*

- It aids in protein metabolism, promoting red blood cell formation and preventing neural tube defects.
- Food sources: Dark leafy vegetables, whole grains, cereals, legumes and citrus fruits, liver, and kidney.
    - Folic acid deficiency causes glossitis, ulcerative stomatitis, and angular cheilitis.
    - Glossitis: The dorsum becomes red, swollen, and tender.
    - Ulcers: Occur either as superficial erosions or minor aphthous. The tongue is very painful and called *beefy tongue*.
    - The filiform and then the fungiform papillae become atrophied. In early stages, the atrophic changes are patchy and involve the lateral borders

of the tongue. Multiple erosions and ulcers develop in the atrophic surface.
    - Gingiva may exhibit exaggerated inflammatory response. There is a remote chance for necrotizing gingivitis. Periodontitis is also a feature of folic acid deficiency.
- *Biotin:*
  - It helps in the metabolism of carbohydrates, fat, and proteins.
  - Food sources: Liver, kidney, egg yolk, fresh vegetables, cereals, and yeast bread.
  - No noticeable oral changes occur in deficient state.
- *Pantothenic acid:*
  - It is involved in the metabolism of fat, proteins and carbohydrates, energy production and hormone synthesis.
  - Food sources: Liver, kidney, meat, egg yolk, whole grains. Intestinal bacteria also synthesize this vitamin.
  - Deficiency may lead to glossitis and cheilosis.
- *Vitamin C—ascorbic acid:*
  - Vitamin C is essential for collagen synthesis, wound healing, bone, and tooth formation, strengthening of endothelial vessel walls. Vitamin C functions as an antioxidant which enhances the body immunity, iron absorption, and utilization.
  - Food sources: Citrus fruits like lemon, kiwi, orange, etc.
    - *Scurvy* is the manifestation of severe vitamin C deficiency. The gingiva becomes swollen, purplish, spongy, and bleed spontaneously. Vitamin C deficiency primarily aggravates the gingival reaction to plaque and manifests the signs of gingivitis.
    - Vitamin C deficiency during the development period causes atrophy of ameloblasts and odontoblasts. This results in the hypoplastic appearance of teeth.
    - In *avitaminosis C,* the osteoblasts exhibit functional deficiency. The bone formation and resorption are affected resulting in the less dense alveolus. Defective collagen synthesis reduces the periodontal integrity. The periodontal fibers tend to break down easily and cause the tooth mobility.

SHORT NOTES

1. Describe orofacial manifestations of kwashiorkor disease.

- *Kwashiorkor is a condition of low quantity protein in children's diet.*
- The child is affected by generalized edema, muscle wasting and shows characteristic *moon face* and *potbelly* appearance (Flowchart 1). They also exhibit apathy, lethargy, and anorexia. The skin appeared thick and cracked with areas of denudation.
- *Dental findings:* If it occurs at the *developmental stage,* the following changes take place:
  - Delayed eruption
  - Retardation of mandible
  - Smaller size molars
  - Enamel hypoplasia
  - Salivary glands:
    - Gland hypoplasia
    - Reduced salivary flow

Flowchart 1: Pathogenesis of edema in kwashiorkor disease.

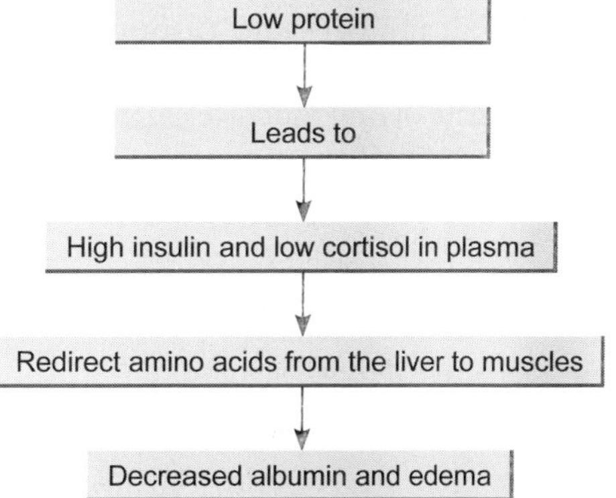

- Decreased salivary immune protection due to less amylase and amino peptides.

2. Describe orofacial manifestations of marasmus.

- Energy deficiency in children due to reduced food intake is known as marasmus.

The affected child manifests low body weight and wasted muscles (Flowchart 2).

Flowchart 2: Muscle wasting in marasmus.

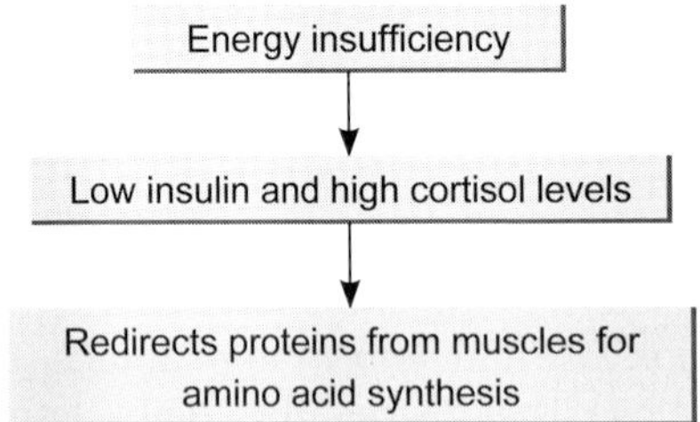

Clinical Findings

- Delayed eruption
- Decreased salivary flow
- Increased incidence of dental caries
- Defective formation of epithelium, bone, and connective tissues
- Reduced level of salivary IgA
- Necrotizing ulcerative gingivitis and noma due to low resistance to infections.

3. Mention the role of vitamin A in oral health.

- *Importance:*
  - Vitamin A is essential for the formation of ameloblasts, odontoblasts, and bone.
  - Also, it is necessary throughout the life for maintenance of the epithelial integrity of oral mucosa.
  - Have antioxidant property.
- Oral manifestations of deficiency in the pre-eruptive stage:
  - Enamel hypoplasia and incomplete enamel calcification.
  - Defective dentin formation.

Therapeutic Consideration

- The scavenging *activity of vitamin A* on free radicals made to use this as a *chemopreventive agent for oral precancer and cancer. Retinoids* are used as a supplement because of their cancer growth inhibiting character (apoptosis) and regulating the immune system. Topical retinoids are used in the treatment of leukoplakia and as adjunctive in the management of reticular and plaque type leukoplakia.

Side Effects

Routine consumption of larger quantity may lead to:

- Dryness of oral mucosa
- Red gingiva
- Cracking and bleeding lips due to epithelial atrophy.

4. State the oral manifestations of vitamin D deficiency.

Vitamin D deficit causes rickets in children and osteomalacia in adults.

Manifestation in Rickets

- The deciduous teeth are not affected. The *permanent central incisors and first molars* and sometimes the lateral incisors and canines show the developmental defects in their crown structures.
- The poor calcification results in moderate to severe *hypoplastic defects* like pits, fissures, and grooves on the crown surface. Improper calcification of the dentine matrix leads to interglobular spaces. The dentine reveals a line of disturbed mineralization. The secondary dentine deposition is retarded.
- The jaw bones are markedly hypocalcified and weak. Open bite and malocclusion are the frequent manifestations.

Oral Manifestation of Vitamin D Deficiency in Adults

Diffuse pain in jaw bones and the tendency for fracture even for mild trauma.

5. Briefly state the importance of antioxidants in oral health.

- Free radicals are reactive oxygen species and are capable of damaging all types of biomolecules. Antioxidants neutralize free radicals throughout the body and are essential for optimum health.

- An antioxidant may be vitamin (beta-carotene, vitamin C, and E), mineral (selenium, zinc, copper), or fatty acids (omega 3 and omega 6) present in food. Other naturally occurring antioxidants include flavonoids, tannins, and phenols. Dietary antioxidants protect the cell membrane molecules from oxidative damage by destroying the oxidative radicals before they injure the tissues.
- They slow down oxidation process and aids in repairing cellular damage. Some antioxidants have anti-inflammatory activity, and some other has antineoplastic properties.
- Antioxidants are provided through several supplements. In dentistry, toothpaste, mouth rinses or oral sprays incorporate antioxidants.

Role of Antioxidants in Oral Diseases

- Antioxidants change the progress of periodontitis, and gingivitis by decreasing the production of collagenase.
- Antioxidants are used as both preventive as well as therapeutic agents in individuals diagnosed with precancer lesions. Tocopherols and carotenoids are the effective antioxidants used for this purpose.
- Vitamin E, carotene, and glutathione inhibit tumor angiogenesis.
- Flavonoids act as histamine blockers and control allergic reactions in the oral cavity.
- Lycopene work to reverse hyperkeratotic changes in oral mucosa and hence used in the treatment of leukoplakia.
- Retinoids had anti-inflammatory property and used to treat lichen planus.

6. Discuss oral manifestations of amyloidosis.

- Amyloidosis develops due to the deposition of insoluble extracellular protein, amyloid in the body tissues. The primary form of amyloidosis affects the oral cavity and is associated with the deposition of AL (amyloid light chain) in the oral tissues.
- *Oral findings:*
  - The tongue is the commonly affected organ. Macroglossia occurs due to amyloid deposition. Enlarged tongue causes difficulty in chewing and talking. Lateral borders of the tongue get pressed against lingual cusps of posterior teeth and show indentations.
  - Other involved sites are buccal mucosa, gingiva and the floor of mouth, minor salivary glands, palate and lower lip.

Investigation

- Incisional biopsy of the affected site. Congo-red staining of the specimen will demonstrate an apple-green birefringence on polarized light microscopy.
- Immunofixation electrophoresis of serum will detect light chain immunoglobulins.

Treatment

Systemic steroids—dexamethasone.

7. Enumerate the oral manifestations of lipoid proteinosis (Urbach-Wiethe disease)

- Lipoid proteinosis is caused by deposition of a hyaline-like substance in various tissues due to mutation in the extracellular glycoprotein.
- Common oral findings:
  - Commonly affected sites are labial, buccal and palatal mucosa, posterior tongue, uvula, tonsils and lingual frenum.
  - Affected mucosa appears thickened and nodular.
  - Yellow white papules are seen in the oral mucosa.
  - The tongue is enlarged (macroglossia) and wood hard in consistency.
  - Lips are enlarged with nodules and fissures.
  - Difficulty in tongue protrusion if lingual frenum is involved.
  - Gingival hyperplasia.

MULTIPLE CHOICE QUESTIONS

1. RDA stands for ***recommended dietary allowance***.
   a. Research and Development Association
   b. Recommended dietary allowance
   c. Radiation diagnostic appliances
   d. Rare Disease Association
2. In India, the body weight of *reference man* is ***60 kg***.
   a. 60 kg
   b. 70 kg
   c. 75 kg
   d. 85 kg
3. In India, the body weight of *reference women* is ***50 kg***.
   a. 60 kg
   b. 70 kg
   c. 50 kg
   d. 65 kg
4. The average weight of Indian men is ***52 kg***.
   a. 60 kg
   b. 70 kg
   c. 52 kg
   d. 45 kg
5. The average weight of Indian women is ***44 kg***.
   a. 55 kg
   b. 37 kg
   c. 44 kg
   d. 65 kg
6. A major source of human energy is ***carbohydrates***.
   a. Unsaturated fatty acids
   b. Carbohydrates
   c. Trace minerals
   d. Proteins
7. Noncariogenic sugar substitute is ***xylitol***.
   a. Aspartame
   b. Saccharin
   c. Xylitol
   d. Corn-syrup
8. Protein malnutrition in children causes ***kwashiorkor***.
   a. Kwashiorkor
   b. Marasmus
   c. Keshan disease
   d. Ketosis
9. Energy deficiency due to reduced food intake is known as ***marasmus***.
   a. Kwashiorkor b. Marasmus
   c. Keshan disease d. Ketosis
10. Keratin accumulation in the skin and oral mucosa occurs due to ***vitamin A deficiency***.
   a. Albumin deficiency
   b. Amino acid deficiency
   c. Vitamin A deficiency
   d. Zinc deficiency
11. Vitamin essential for normal functioning of nerve and muscle is ***vitamin D deficiency***.
   a. Vitamin A deficiency
   b. Vitamin D deficiency
   c. Vitamin K deficiency
   d. Vitamin C deficiency
12. Small noncalcified areas on skull bones are known as ***craniotabes***.
   a. Osteotabes
   b. Craniotabes
   c. Callus
   d. Osteophytes
13. Craniotabes is a feature of ***vitamin D deficiency***.
   a. Vitamin A deficiency
   b. Vitamin D deficiency
   c. Vitamin K deficiency
   d. Vitamin C deficiency
14. Enamel hypoplasia with pitted surface occurs in ***vitamin D deficiency***.
   a. Vitamin A deficiency
   b. Vitamin D deficiency
   c. Vitamin K deficiency
   d. Vitamin C deficiency
15. Gingival bleeding is the first and frequent finding of ***vitamin K deficiency***.
   a. Vitamin A deficiency
   b. Vitamin D deficiency
   c. Vitamin K deficiency
   d. Vitamin C deficiency
16. Type of amyloidosis that is associated with chronic inflammatory destructive diseases is ***secondary form***.
   a. Primary form b. Secondary form
   c. Tertiary phase d. Terminal phase
17. Amyloidosis associated with tuberculosis is characterized by the deposition of ***A amyloid***.
   a. A amyloid b. C amyloid
   c. Alpha amyloid d. Beta amyloid
   (**Note:** Amyloidosis associated with tuberculosis is *secondary form* and is characterized by the deposition of A amyloid).

18. Common biopsy site preferred for the diagnosis of generalized form of amyloidosis is ***gingiva***.
    a. Lip
    b. Gingiva
    c. Skin
    d. Salivary gland
19. Discoloration of teeth in cutaneous porphyria affects the ***cervical region of deciduous teeth***.
    a. Cervical region of deciduous teeth
    b. Cervical region of permanent teeth
    c. Occlusal aspect of deciduous teeth
    d. Occlusal aspect of permanent teeth
20. In cutaneous porphyria, deciduous dentition appears as ***deep red-brown colored***.
    a. Dark red colored
    b. Deep red-brown colored
    c. Deep brown-black colored
    d. Light red colored
21. Porphyria induced dental discoloration is differentiated from other types of discoloration by using ***Wood's lamp***.
    a. Bunsen lamp
    b. Slit lamp
    c. Halogen lamp
    d. Wood's lamp
22. Dental restorative material to be avoided in porphyria patients is ***amalgam***.
    a. Glass-ionomer cement
    b. Amalgam
    c. Gold
    d. Metal-ceramic
23. The wavelength of light that is a hazard to porphyria patients is in the range between ***400–550 nm***.
    a. 100–220 nm
    b. 200–450 nm
    c. 400–550 nm
    d. 500–650 nm
24. Local anesthetic agents contraindicated for porphyria patients is ***lidocaine***.
    a. Lidocaine
    b. Bupivacaine
    c. Procaine
    d. Prilocaine
    (**Note:** Bupivacaine is the choice of local anesthetic drug in porphyria patients).
25. Diclofenac is contraindicated for patients suffering from ***porphyria***.
    a. Sarcoidosis
    b. Tuberculosis
    c. Porphyria
    d. Lupus erythematosus
26. A metabolic disorder associated with intraoral bullae is ***porphyria***.
    a. Amyloidosis
    b. Tay-Sachs disease
    c. Wilson's disease
    d. Porphyria
27. Gargoylism is due to deposition of mucopolysaccharides in ***fibroblasts***.
    a. Epithelium b. Blood vessels
    c. Fibroblasts d. Neurons
    (**Note:** Gargoylism is the presence of clear or gargoylic cells).
28. Hurler syndrome is ***mucopolysaccharidosis type I***.
    a. Mucopolysaccharidosis type I
    b. Mucopolysaccharidosis type II
    c. Mucopolysaccharidosis type III
    d. Mucopolysaccharidosis type IV
    (**Note:** Hurler syndrome is mucopolysaccharidosis type I—gargoylism).
29. Hunter syndrome is ***mucopolysaccharidosis type II***.
    a. Mucopolysaccharidosis type I
    b. Mucopolysaccharidosis type II
    c. Mucopolysaccharidosis type III
    d. Mucopolysaccharidosis type IV
30. Cutaneous ivory-white papules are seen in ***Hunter syndrome***.
    a. Hunter syndrome
    b. Hurler syndrome
    c. Scheie syndrome
    d. Murphy's syndrome
31. Radiographic appearance of dentigerous cyst like radiolucent follicles is seen in ***Maroteaux-Lamy syndrome***.
    a. Hurler syndrome
    b. Hunter syndrome
    c. Maroteaux-Lamy syndrome
    d. Carpal tunnel syndrome
    (**Note:** Maroteaux-Lamy syndrome is mucopolysaccharidosis type VI).

32. Blepharosis moniliformis or eyelid beadings are seen in ***lipoid proteinosis***.
    a. Amyloidosis
    b. Lipoid proteinosis
    c. Krabbe disease
    d. Sphingolipidoses
33. The radiographic appearance of eosinophilic granuloma mimics ***malignancy***.
    a. Hamartoma
    b. Teratoma
    c. Malignancy
    d. Marble bone disease
    (**Note:** The radiographic appearance of eosinophilic granuloma mimics *odontogenic cysts or malignancy)*.
34. Gaucher disease is due to poor function of the enzyme ***β-glucocerebrosidase***.
    a. Phenylalanine
    b. β-glucocerebrosidase
    c. Sphingomyelinase
    d. β-galactosidase
    (**Note:** Metabolic disorder with a short-course and fatal termination are Letterer-Siwe disease, type II Gaucher disease and Niemann-Pick disease. The deposition of glucocerebroside characterizes Gaucher disease).
35. Universal antioxidant is ***α-lipoic acid***.
    a. α-lipoic acid
    b. Carotenoids
    c. Lycopene
    d. Vitamins

VIVA VOCE

1. Are lipids cariostatic or cariogenic? Why?

Lipids are *cariostatic* because:

- Long-chain fatty acids decrease the acid dissolution of hydroxyapatite crystals.
- Fats lubricate the enamel surface and prevent acid penetration through it.
- Dietary fat increases fluoride absorption and increases tissue fluoride concentration.
- Lipid diet also prevents food retention in the mouth.

2. Mention the role of vitamin A in the pathogenesis of potentially malignant oral diseases.

Vitamin A deficiency induces hyperkeratosis and metaplasia of epithelial cells of the oral mucosa and hence related to the pathogenesis of leukoplakia and oral carcinoma.

3. Name few metabolic disorders.

- Disorders of protein metabolism: Amyloidosis, porphyria.
- Disorder of carbohydrate metabolism: Mucopolysaccharidosis.
- Disorders of lipid metabolism: Histiocytosis X
- (Hand-Schuller-Christian disease, and Letterer-Siwe disease).

4. What are free radicals?

Free radicals are chemical substance containing one or more unpaired electrons in the excitable state.

BIBLIOGRAPHY

1. Brown RS, Glascoe A, Feimster T, et al. Vitamins and the treatment of oral and dental diseases. Dent today. 2010;29(12):51-2.
2. Ghom AG, Ghom SA. Textbook of oral medicine. 3rd edition, Japee Medical Publishers, New Delhi; 2014.
3. Odell EW. Cawson's essentials of oral pathology and oral medicine e-book. Elsevier Health Sciences; 2017.
4. Palmer CA. Diet and nutrition in oral health. Upper Saddle River, NJ, USA; Prentice Hall; 2003.
5. Rugg-Gunn AJ. Nutrition and dental health. Oxford: Oxford University Press, USA; 1993.
6. Shafer WG, Hine MK, Levy BM, Rajendran R, Sivapathasundharam B. A textbook of oral pathology. 4th edition. WB saunders; Philadelphia; 1983. p 318.

CHAPTER 21

Dental Caries

HIGHLIGHTS

Dental caries is the noncontagious bacterial disease. The initiation of a carious process is multifactorial including dietary habits, oral hygiene, etc. Caries plays a key role in tooth loss, and the prevention of this deleterious disease is challenging. Both restorative and nonrestorative methods are applied in caries management. This chapter focuses on the role of bacteria in caries process, the ways to diagnose early carious lesions, and prophylactic agents used in caries preventive measures.

Learners are expected to describe the:

- ❖ Action of cariogenic bacteria.
- ❖ Chair side investigation of dental caries.
- ❖ Chemoprevention for dental caries.

ESSAY QUESTIONS

1. Describe the mechanism of different caries preventive agents. (or) Briefly describe the chemoprophylactic agents for caries prevention.

- ❖ Dental caries is a complex process with multifactorial etiological agents. All tooth surfaces are covered with a thin biofilm to which bacteria adhere and mature. These bacteria utilize dietary carbohydrates to produce acid which results in pH drop in the saliva and dissolution of the hydroxyapatite crystals.
- ❖ Preventive measures of dental caries include various mechanical and chemical measures.

Fluoride

- ❖ The use of fluoridated toothpaste, topical fluoride applicants, pit and fissure sealants will prevent dental caries.
- ❖ Fluoride exerts an anticariogenic action by:
  - ■ Preventing tooth demineralization.
  - ■ Promoting remineralization of early carious lesions.
  - ■ Antibacterial effect on cariogenic bacteria.
- ❖ Fluoride is highly effective against smooth-surface caries but very minimal on pit and fissure caries.

Arginine

- ❖ Arginine is an amino acid that occurs in food products and in saliva. It is metabolized by arginolytic bacteria and produces ammonia that increases the pH in the oral biofilm. This neutralizes the acidic environment and controls the growth of aciduric, cariogenic bacteria.
- ❖ It is added in the fluoridated toothpaste for its additive effect for caries prevention.

Sugar Substitutes

- ❖ *Xylitol:*
  - ■ Xylitol is a sugar alcohol, an artificial sweetener which cannot be fermented by cariogenic bacteria. Xylitol functions

by effectively controlling the plaque formation, bacterial colonization, and acid production thereby inhibiting enamel demineralization. It has a direct inhibitory effect on *S. Mutans* (*Streptococcus mutans*).
  - Xylitol chewing gums and xylitol containing lozenges can be used for effective caries prevention. In children, xylitol tablets, and xylitol containing syrup can be used.
- *Sorbitol:* Sorbitol is another artificial-sweetener which can be fermented by oral microorganisms, but the rate of acid production is much slower than that of other dietary sugars and can be considered for caries prevention.

Probiotics

- Probiotic was defined by Stillwell in 1965 as *a substance secreted by one microorganism that promotes the growth of another microorganism.*
- They are primarily bacteria. The live microorganism is safe for consumption and has several beneficial effects. Probiotics develop a biofilm and protect the oral tissues. This biofilm, in turn, prevents the contact of pathogenic bacteria on oral tissues and teeth surfaces. In this way, probiotics compete with the cariogenic bacteria.
- Yoghurts with lactobacilli, probiotic cheese, and probiotic lozenges are used to reduce *S. mutans* colonization on regular consumption.

Novamin—containing Dentifrices

- Novamin is a bioactive glass-ceramic material. They contain calcium sodium phosphosilicate as an active ingredient and releases calcium and phosphate ions when exposed to aqueous media.
- Dentifrice containing 5% novamin and fluoride are effective in remineralization of subsurface carious lesions. NovaMin also has the antibacterial effect.

Antibiotic Toothpaste

The presence of penicillin, triclosan or topical antibiotics like tyrothricin is effective ingredients in destroying acidogenic bacteria and control caries progression.

Chlorhexidine Mouth Rinse

A 0.12% chlorhexidine is active against the cariogenic streptococci strains and thereby provide a bacteriostatic effect. Chlorhexidine also has a retention property in the plaque coated enamel surface and can be released into the mouth after use.

Antimicrobial Peptides

Antimicrobial peptides exhibit a wide range bactericidal effect. They act by binding to the bacterial membrane lipopolysaccharides. After binding, the peptides disrupt cell membrane and kill the microbes by intracellular mechanisms.

Recent Advancements in Caries Prevention

- Casein phosphopeptide (CPP): Casein is a milk phosphoprotein and has cariostatic property. Casein phosphopeptide is casein-derived amorphous calcium phosphate and is used in caries prevention for their remineralization property. CPPs stabilize calcium phosphate ions in solution and form an amorphous calcium phosphate (ACP) complex known as CPP-ACP. The CPP-ACP is taken up by dental biofilms and concentrates it on the enamel surface. Calcium, phosphate, and fluoride released from CPP-ACP, help to maintain the supersaturated state of these ions and assist remineralization.
- Caries vaccines: Vaccine (monoclonal antibody) can control *S. mutans* colonization and prevent caries progression. Allergic reactions should be anticipated when considering nonhuman monoclonal antibodies. However, the concept is at the research level and need a more clinical trial for effective implementation.

- DNA recombination technology (replacement therapy): Replacement therapy uses a harmless effector strain for permanent colonization in the host. This strain, in turn, will prevent the colonization of a specific pathogen.

  S. mutans strain BCS3-L1 is a genetically modified effector strain designed for replacement therapy to prevent dental caries.

SHORT NOTES

1. Write in brief about the caries conductive bacteria. (or) write in brief about the cariogenic bacteria.

- Cariogenic bacteria are those that are directly involved in the dental caries disease (initiation and progression). Members of the Streptococci like *S. mutans* and *S. sobrinus* are the important caries conductive bacteria.
- For the initiation of the carious process, these cariogenic bacteria should exhibit three properties:
  1. Ability to colonize on the tooth surface.
  2. Acidogenic—producing acid from dietary carbohydrates.
  3. Aciduric—ability to live in low salivary pH.
- *S. mutans* are more prone to initiate smooth surface caries by its plaque forming tendency. The plaque on the smooth surface of teeth resists cleansing action and accumulates rapidly on the plaque covered surface in the presence of dietary sucrose.
- *S. mutans* have an enzyme called glucosyltransferases that split sucrose into units of glucose and fructose.
- Fructose is taken up by the bacteria and processes it for fermentation to produce lactic acid.
- The glucose units act as a bridge for new bacterial cells and consistently maintain the plaque formation.
- After the caries initiation and initial destruction of tooth take place by *S. mutans*, *lactobacillus* species like *L. acidophilus* continue the further destructive process of hard tissues. Lactobacillus is both acidogenic and acidophilic but lacks the attachment mechanism on plaque covered tooth surface.
- The lactobacilli species present only in a highly acidic carious environment and in the presence of lactobacilli, *S. mutans* produce more acid from the sucrose and accelerate the caries progression.

2. Discuss advanced chair side diagnostic methods of dental caries.

- *Quantitative light fluorescence (QLF),* also known as laser-induced-fluorescence is used for enhanced visual inspection of dental caries. Laser light provides transillumination to recognize the demineralized zones in the carious lesion. LED laser device apply a specific light wavelength to identify the demineralization spots. Once the demineralization zones are recognized, the LED displays a red color and produces an audible beep tone.
- *Digital imaging fiber-optic transillumination (DIFOTI)* is manufactured with a 655 nm diode and has high sensitivity and specificity for caries detection. This is a chair side tool used by the dentist and has the benefit of identifying changes in density of tooth at proximal surfaces. The device is calibrated to match the reflective index of teeth of a particular patient by moving the camera throughout the patient's mouth, and results are displayed by a two-digit numerical inference and audible report. This tool also helps to identify the early changes of occlusal pits and fissures.
- *The spectra instrument* is a caries illumination apparatus. The device uses a 405 nm blue-violet diode laser and an image capturing mechanism, and analytic software. The device displays the zone of demineralization as a photograph of the tooth with varying color zones in the shades of green, blue, red, orange, and

yellow. The images can be stored. Repeated examinations can demonstrate changes in the tooth, after initiating the preventive or therapeutic measures. The series of images help to predict the caries progression or the effectiveness of remineralization therapy in arresting the caries process.

- *The canary system* uses laser luminescence and photothermal radiometry to identify carious lesion at a depth of 5 mm inside the tooth and to a size as small as 50 µm.

3. Describe caries risk assessment test.

- The caries risk assessment test is carried out to identify the high-risk potential for caries development and for planning the preventive measures. The restorative treatment for the carious tooth only repairs the cavitations due to caries but never arrest the carious activity. Hence appropriate assessment based activities are essential for risk factors elimination or modification to prevent caries progress apart from restorative management.
- For caries-risk assessment, multiple, interlinked factors should be considered for every individual patient like quantity, pH, buffering capacity, and sugar metabolism potential of the patient's saliva.
- The chair side investigatory methods include the quantitative assay of salivary lactic acid produced (LAP) by cariogenic bacteria in the oral cavity. The salivary sample is taken from the dorsum of the tongue.

MULTIPLE CHOICE QUESTIONS

1. The important caries conductive substance in our diet is ***sucrose***.
   a. Glucose
   b. Sucrose
   c. Lactose
   d. Fructose
2. The expected incubation time for clinically detectable caries is ***6 months***.
   a. 6 months
   b. 10 months
   c. 2 years
   d. 6 years
3. The reason for the loss of tooth structure due to dental caries is ***loss of mineral content***.
   a. Microbial colonization
   b. Alkaline pH
   c. Loss of mineral content
   d. Loss of blood supply
   (**Note:** The reason for the loss of tooth structure due to dental caries is prolonged exposure to an acidic environment (low pH) and loss of mineral content).

BIBLIOGRAPHY

1. Agarwal R, Singh C, Yeluri R, et al. Prevention of dental caries-measures beyond fluoride. Journal of Oral Hygiene and Health. 2014 2:2-122.
2. Hallett KB, O'Rourke PK. Oral biofilm activity, culture testing and caries experience in school children. Int J Pediatr Dent. 2009;(19 Suppl 1):4.
3. Kutsch VK. Lasers in dentistry: comparing wavelengths. J Am Dent Assoc. 1993;124(2): 49-54.
4. Schneiderman A, Elbaum M, Shultz T, et al. Assessment of dental caries with Digital Imaging Fiber-Optic Transillumination (DIFOTI): in vitro study. Caries Res. 1997; 31(2):103-10.
5. Young DA, Kutsch VK, Whitehouse J. A clinician's guide to CAMBRA: a simple approach. Compend contin educ denti. 2009;30(2):92-8.

CHAPTER 22

Drugs Used in Dentistry

HIGHLIGHTS

Prescribing drug is a routine act in dental practice. Dental students should acquire adequate knowledge about the commonly prescribed drugs, mode of actions, drug interactions, and safety measures. Before prescribing, it is necessary to review the medical condition, concurrent medications taken by the patient for other illness, and drug allergy. Also, underdosing and overdosing should be avoided as they develop drug resistance and drug toxicity, respectively. This chapter focus on the relevant drugs prescribed in dental practice with drug regimens and dosage.

Learners are expected to study:

- Management of oral disease using medications.
- Dose and duration of the suggested drugs.

SHORT NOTES

1. Antihistamines (or) cetirizine.

Cetirizine is an antihistamine drug used in dentistry to manage acute allergic conditions like allergic stomatitis.

The drug metabolite competes with histamine for H1 receptors and reduces the histamine response.

Dosage:

For adults: 5–10 mg once a day

For children (2–5 years): 5 mg once a day

Adverse effects: Headache, fatigue, abdominal pain, drowsiness, pharyngitis

The drug should be avoided in patients taking anticholinergics and CNS depressants.

2. Saliva substitutes.

Artificial saliva provides symptomatic relief for patients with dry mouth due to minimal salivary gland function. Artificial saliva is composed of buffering agents, cellulose derivatives, and flavoring agents. Cellulose increases the stickiness and aids in moistening capacity.

- **Merits:** It enhances the patient comfort by enhancing the speech, mastication and swallowing actions.
- **Demerits:** The composition of real saliva contains enzymes, immunoglobulins (salivary IgA), antimicrobial proteins and minerals. These substances are not present in artificial saliva. So, the synthetic saliva cannot overcome the effects of reduced salivary flow like increased caries risk and oral infections.

3. Pilocarpine.

Pilocarpine hydrochloride is a systemic sialogogue used in the treatment of xerostomia. It is a parasympathetic drug and stimulates exocrine glands. In salivary gland, it acts by stimulating acinar cells with some residual functioning effects.

Dose: 5–10 mg, three times a day. The action starts in 30 minutes, maximum effect achieved by 1 hour and effects persist for 2–3 hours approximately.

Side effects: Gastrointestinal irritation, sweating, tachycardia, bradycardia, and blurred vision.

Contraindications: Patients with heart diseases, asthma, glaucoma, renal diseases, gallbladder disease, and chronic obstructive pulmonary disease.

4. Orabase.

Orabase is a protective agent for oral mucosa. It stays in close contact with oral mucosa for sufficient time and therefore protects the lesion site from irritations associated with routine activities like speech and mastication. Also acts to prevent secondary infection by forming a protective barrier over the lesion.

It is composed of gelatin, pectin and sodium carboxymethylcellulose in plastibase (plasticised hydrocarbon gel). It is non-irritating and biocompatible.

Indication: Aphthous ulcer, traumatic ulcer, chemical burn.

5. Topical immunomodulators for oral lesions.

Tacrolimus

Tacrolimus is a fungus derived immunosuppressant and is used as a topical ointment for the autoimmune disorder of the oral cavity, such as pemphigus, pemphigoid, lichen planus, psoriasis, desquamative gingivitis and Crohn's disease.

Tacrolimus is a calcineurin inhibitor which inhibits T-helper lymphocyte activation. Calcineurin is responsible for immune response. Tacrolimus inhibition of calcineurin leads to inhibition of IL-2 and other proinflammatory cytokines, such as IL-4 and -IL-5. The result is a failure in the differentiation of inflammatory cells, such as T-lymphocytes, eosinophils neutrophils, and suppression of their action.

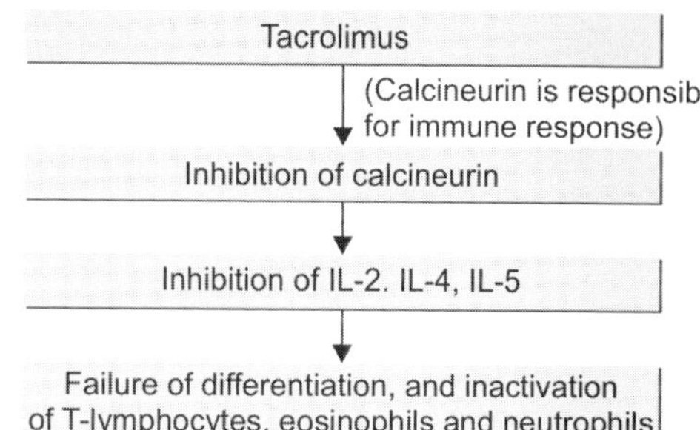

Cyclosporine

Topical cyclosporine A (CsA) is used in the treatment of oral lichen planus, major aphthous ulcer, pemphigus, pemphigoid and lichenoid reaction.

CsA is a polypeptide derived from fungal extracts and selectively inhibits cytokines and the functions of T-cell lymphocytes.

CsA binds with cyclophilins (cellular cytoplasmic proteins), forming a complex that binds to and inhibits calcineurin. The result is the inhibition of T-helper cell activation and suppression of the proinflammatory cytokines release (IL-2, IL-3, IL-4, CD40L, GM-CSF, TNF-α, and IFN-γ), inhibition of T-suppressor and T-cytotoxic cells.

6. Topical corticosteroids.

Topical corticosteroids are primarily used to treat oral mucosal lesions of autoimmune disorders (like lichen planus, pemphigus, and pemphigoid), oral submucous fibrosis, a hypersensitive reaction like erythema multiforme and inflammatory conditions like major and herpetiform aphthous ulcers.

In these conditions, topical steroids are used alone or in combination with systemic steroids.

Topical steroids are available in three different potentials. Based on the severity of lesion the potency of the drug is selected.

Mild Potent Drugs

- Triamcinolone acetonide 0.1% cream

- Fluocinolone acetonide 0.025% cream, ointment
- Betamethasone 0.05% cream

Moderate Potential Drugs

- Fluocinonide 0.5% cream
- Desoximetasone 0.25% cream

High Potency Drugs

- Clobetasol propionate 0.5% ointment
- Betamethasone valerate 0.05% cream.

7. Analgesics (or) NSAIDs in dental practice.

- Nonsteroidal anti-inflammatory drugs indicated for pain control.
- They inhibit COX-2 and COX-1 enzymes or selectively inhibit COX-2 alone. (Pain is mediated by prostaglandins which depend on COX-1 and COX-2 actions).
- Many NSAIDs are not the only analgesic but also possess anti-inflammatory and antipyretic properties.
- Ibuprofen is the frequently prescribed analgesic in dentistry which is administered at 200 or 400 mg, every 4–6 hourly, for the maximum dose of 1200 mg/day. But the major adverse effect associated is gastric ulcer and bleeding in chronic use.
- Selective COX-2 inhibitors are advantageous in reducing the chances of gastric ulcer and bleeding but less effective than Ibuprofen.
- When prescribing analgesics, NSAIDs should be avoided for patients with a history of asthma, renal disorders, and gastric ulcer. It is strictly contraindicated for pregnant women in the 3rd trimester.
- In such contraindicated conditions, acetaminophen should be the drug of choice. Acetaminophen is free of NSAIDs side effects and possess analgesic and antipyretic properties but not anti-inflammatory, at the dose of 500–1,000 mg, 4–6 hourly to a maximum dose of 4 g/day.
- Drug interactions:
  - NSAIDs reduce the effect of ACE inhibitors, diuretics, β-blockers in antihypertensive patients.
  - NSAIDs cause hypoglycemia in diabetic patients taking oral hypoglycemics.
  - NSAIDs reduce the effect of warfarin.

8. Opioids.

- In case of managing moderate to severe pain, like pain due to oral cancer, severe trauma and multiple fractures of facial bones (due to road traffic accidents), and in postsurgical care, opioids are considered in dental practice.
- They are centrally acting drug with peripheral anti-inflammatory properties.
- The potential side effects include drug dependence, sedation, respiratory depression, nausea, vomiting, and constipation.
- The recommended oral dosage:
  - Morphine 100 mg/day, codeine 60 mg/day
- To reduce the side effects, they can be combined with NSAIDs.

9. Carbamazepine.

Carbamazepine is an anticonvulsant drug. Carbamazepine (200–1,200 mg/day) and oxcarbazepine (600–1,800 mg/day) are the most prescribed drugs for treating trigeminal neuralgia.

Their analgesic action is by the sodium channel blockage. This occurs either by stabilization of hyperexcited neuronal membranes, controlling the recurrent firing or by decreasing the synaptic impulses. Initial therapy for pain control should be started with 100 mg two to three times a day, and then gradually increased by 100 mg every other day until adequate pain relief is established. Maintenance doses range from 300–800 mg/day divided into two to three daily doses.

Initial side effects include drowsiness, nausea, dizziness, diplopia, ataxia, hyponatremia. Potentially serious side effects are allergic rash, myelosuppression, hepatotoxicity, lymphadenopathy, Stevens-Johnson syndrome and aplastic anemia.

10. Capsaicin.

Capsaicin is the component of hot chili pepper. This compound is used in a topical form for the management of postherpetic neuralgia. When applied topically, it results in excitation of nociceptive afferent fibers. The frequent application of capsaicin results in desensitization of unmyelinated nerve fibers and pain control.

Low-concentration (0.025 or 0.075%) capsaicin topical creams are efficient in the pain management of postherpetic neuralgia. High-concentration (8%) synthetic capsaicin dermal patches are also available to provide fast and persistent pain relief following a single application. Adverse effects at the application site include erythema and burning sensation.

11. Topical antiviral drugs.

Topical antiviral treatments are used for managing the symptoms rather than treating oral herpes lesions (recurrent herpes labialis). They are effective in reducing the symptoms (itching, tingling burning sensation and pain), the duration of viral shedding and the healing period for ulcers. They also reduce the number of recurrent episodes.

The topical forms available for oral use include: Acyclovir cream 5% and penciclovir cream 1%. Rapid healing and pain relief are possible when applying penciclovir cream at the prodromal period (erythema stages) than start applying at the papule and vesicle stages of the lesion.

The cream should be applied every 2 hours in the daytime for 4 days.

12. Topical antifungal drugs.

The purpose of using topical forms of anticandidal medication is to enhance the drug effectiveness through the direct contact of the drug with the lesion. Topical antifungal treatment is mandatory for minimum 2 weeks to eradicate the infection. But the symptom resolution occurs 3–4 days after application.

- Nystatin is a polyene antifungal antibiotic. Sterols are the component of the plasma membrane of the fungus cells. The antifungal effect of nystatin is due to its physicochemical interaction with sterols resulting in the production of aqueous pores on the cell membrane leading to increased permeability, leakage of cytoplasmic contents, and death of the organism. It is the frequently used topical medication for oral candidiasis. Nystatin preparation includes oral rinse, pastille, and suspension forms.
  - Nystatin oral suspension (100,000 U/mL)—patient needs to rinse 4–6 mL/per dose for 2 minutes and expectorate, four times/day for 2 weeks.
- Ergosterol is a constituent of the fungal cytoplasmic membrane. Clotrimazole interferes with the biosynthesis of ergosterol and provides fungicidal effects.
  - Clotrimazole (10 mg oral troches): Dissolve one troche in oral cavity five times a day.

13. Tricyclic antidepressants.

Antidepressants are used in the management of many chronic pain conditions, even though depression is not caused or precipitating reason. The typical conditions include myofascial pain dysfunction syndrome, atypical facial pain, postherpetic neuralgia, diabetic neuropathy and TMJ disorders especially associated with parafunctional habits.

When the patient is suffering from chronic facial pain, there may be associated state of depression and altered sleep pattern. These conditions further worsen the pain experience. In the presence of parafunctional habits (bruxism), tricyclic antidepressants (TCAs) may bring about muscle relaxation effect.

The analgesic action of tricyclic antidepressants is by blocking the re-uptake of serotonin and norepinephrine. This blockade enhances the inhibition of spinal cord neurons involved in pain perception. Pain relief is not an immediate effect and takes several weeks for sufficient control.

The commonly used antidepressants include amitriptyline (10–30 mg/day), imipramine, clomipramine, nortriptyline, and desipramine.

14. Interferons.

- Interferons are proteins belong to the cytokine group and possess immunomodulatory, antiviral and antiproliferative activities.
- There are three types: Alpha, beta and gamma. Alpha interferons have 24 subtypes, whereas beta and gamma interferons have one subtype each.
- In dentistry, interferons are used in the management of oral premalignant and malignant lesions.
- They bind to specific receptors on the cell surface and exert their effects.
- Antiviral activity: IFNs acts in the viral target cells by either blocking or impairing the viral replication by synthesizing of enzymes that interfere with the cellular and viral processes.
- Anticancer effect: They exert an antiproliferative effect on cancer cells and cause stasis of the tumor growth by inducing certain enzymes.

15. Magic mouthwash.

"Magic mouthwash" is a unique preparation prescribed for oral mucositis induced by chemotherapy or radiotherapy, major aphthous stomatitis, and other mucosal ulcerations. Magic mouthwash is prepared by a mixture of medications to treat oral mucositis and ulcers.

The following medications can be used in combination and preferably any three components can be used as per requirement. Antibiotic (to inhibit the microbial colonization):

1. Antihistamine (to control local allergic reactions)
2. Antifungal (to prevent secondary fungal growth)
3. Steroid (to suppress inflammation)
4. A local anesthetic agent (pain relief), and
5. An antacid (to enhance the coating of the ingredients).

Other preparation includes topical anesthetics, such as lidocaine, viscous diphenhydramine and Maalox (aluminum/magnesium hydroxide) to enhance the adhesion of the ingredients in the mouth.

16. Adverse effects of corticosteroid therapy.

Long-term steroid (glucocorticoids) therapy is associated with:

- Hypertension caused by renal sodium retention and increased response to angiotensin II and catecholamines.
- Inhibition of osteoblast formation leading to osteoporosis by and bone fracture.
- Delayed wound healing due to synthesis of matrix metalloproteinases and collagen.
- It promotes gluconeogenesis and inhibits protein degradation and lipolysis leading to hyperglycemia.
- Gastrointestinal bleeding and peptic ulcer.
- Immunosuppression and reactivation of viral infection.
- In children, the extended use may lead to growth retardation.
- Prolonged topical application of oral mucosa may lead to tissue atrophy and burning sensation.
- Steroid inhalation and topical application may lead to opportunistic candidal infection.

VIVA VOCE

1. Amifostine.

- It has cytoprotective and radioprotective effects on the salivary gland.
- It is used for patients undergoing head and neck radiation therapy.
- IV route administration of the drug before radiotherapy.

2. What are immunomodulators?

Immunomodulators are the drugs that modify the immune reaction by either enhancing (immunostimulators) or reducing (immunosuppressors) the production of antibodies.

- ***Immunosuppressive drugs*** are used to treat autoimmune diseases, such as graft-versus-host, pemphigus, pemphigoid, or lichen planus.
- ***Immunostimulants*** are used to increases, the immune response to immunodeficient conditions (like AIDS) and malignancies.

3. Name few bacteriostatic antibiotics used in dentistry.

Tetracycline, erythromycin, and clindamycin.

4. What is pseudomembranous colitis?

The use of broad-spectrum antibiotics (like penicillin—especially ampicillin, erythromycin, and cephalosporin) alter the gut ecology and leads to the overgrowth of *Clostridium difficile.*

C. difficile and its toxins cause pseudomembranous colitis characterized by diarrhea and abdominal pain, hence otherwise known as antibiotic-associated diarrhea.

The broad-spectrum antibiotic should be immediately discontinued and metronidazole 400 mg, three times/day for 7–14 days should be started to treat this condition.

5. What are requirements for antibiotic prophylaxis?

Dental patients reporting with a history of infective endocarditis, prosthetic heart valves, valvular heart disease, cardiac transplantation, congenital cardiac disorders and total joint replacement should be considered for antibiotic prophylaxis to provide specific dental treatments.

Prophylaxis is not required for patients with pacemakers and implanted defibrillators, and previous history for coronary bypass surgery.

6. What are the dental procedures that require antibiotic prophylaxis in susceptible patients?

Dental extraction, periodontal surgeries, endodontic procedures involving beyond the apices, placement of orthodontic bands, reimplantation of avulsed teeth, subgingival placement of cords or fibers, intraligamentous injections, teeth polishing and implant procedures with bleeding.

7. What is the half-life of a drug?

The half-life of a drug is the time taken for the drug to achieve a plasma concentration of 50% from the initial concentration.

The clinical significance is half-life is to calculate the drug administration frequency, like doxycycline with a half-life of 20 hours is administered once in 24 hours to achieve target concentration.

Drugs with very short life are administered intravenously.

8. What are the action and indications for bisphosphonates?

Bisphosphonates are effective in inhibiting bone resorption by impairing the blood supply and reducing the action of osteoclasts.

They are indicated in the management of osteoporosis, Paget's disease, multiple myeloma, metastatic cancers and for patients taking long-term corticosteroid therapy.

Their main adverse effect is **osteonecrosis of jaw bones.**

9. Amlexanox.

Amlexanox is a topical anti-inflammatory and antiallergenic drug used for the treatment of aphthous stomatitis. In the concentration of 2–5% application, they reduce the ulcer size and healing period.

Amlexanox is a pyridochromene and monocarboxylic acid derivative.

10. Topical metronidazole.

Metronidazole is an antibiotic effective against gram-negative anaerobic organisms. It acts by inhibiting the synthesis of DNA and by oxidation induced degradation to break the single and double strands of DNA and cell death.

The topical form is available as 25% metronidazole gel and effective in antimicrobial property due to the high concentration at the lesion site. The topical form is indicated in the treatment of dry socket, periodontitis, and peri-implantitis.

11. What is Reye's syndrome.

The administration of aspirin in children at recovery stage of viral infection (like chickenpox or flu) causes a severe condition characterized by a reduction in blood glucose, a rise in blood ammonia level and plasma acidic pH. The symptoms include diarrhea, vomiting, tachypnea, lethargy, seizures, convulsions, and loss of consciousness. It is a serious condition and needs immediate medical care.

BIBLIOGRAPHY

1. Eisen D, Ellis CN. Topical cyclosporine for oral mucosal disorders. J Am Acad Dermatol. 1990;23:(6 Pt 2):1259-63.
2. Ghannoum MA, Rice LB. Antifungal agents: mode of action, mechanisms of resistance, and correlation of these mechanisms with bacterial resistance. Clini Microbiol Revi. 1999;12(4):501-17.
3. Haas DA. Drugs in dentistry. In: Compendium of pharmaceuticals and specialties (CPS). 37th edition. Canadian Pharmaceutical Association. 2002:L26-9.
4. Kahan BD. Cyclosporine. N Engl J Med. 1989;321(25):1725-38.
5. Obermann M. Treatment options in trigeminal neuralgia. Ther Adv Neurol Disord. 2010; 3(2): 107-115.
6. Savage NW, McCulbugh MJ. Topical corticosteroids in dental practice. Aust Dent J. 2005;50(4 supp 12): 540-4.
7. Skaar DD, O'Connor H. Potentially serious drug-drug interactions among community-dwelling older adult dental patients. Oral Surg Oral Med Oral Pathol Oral Radiol Endod. 2011;112(2):153-60.
8. van Rossum HH, de Fijter JW, van Pelt J. Pharmacodynamic monitoring of calcineurin inhibition therapy: principles, performance, and perspectives. Ther Drug Monit. 2010;32(1):3-10.
9. Wynn RL, Meiller TF, Crossley HL, editors. Drug information handbook for dentistry. Lexi-Comp Incorporated; 2015.
10. Zahra M, inventor. Composition and method for treatment of oral inflammation an ulceration. United States patent application. 11/986,129. 2009.

CHAPTER 23

Developmental Disorders of Teeth and Orofacial Structures

HIGHLIGHTS

Developmental disorders involve a sequence of interruption in a single or multiple organs during the formative and growth periods. These conditions may be mild or may be very severed and morbid. Oral manifestations many times help to recognize the serious systemic conditions. The diagnosis depends on unique clinical features of each condition supported by pathognomic radiographic findings. This chapter is the compilation of developmental defects involving craniofacial structures including teeth and oral cavity.

Learners are expected to study:

- Developmental anomalies of tooth
- Developmental abnormalities of oral structures
- Types and clinical patterns of enamel hypoplasia.

ESSAY QUESTIONS

1. Enumerate the developmental malformation affecting the tooth structure and briefly explain each condition. (or) describe enamel hypoplasia. Explain the pathogenesis and clinical features of each condition. (or) enumerate the causes for generalized discoloration of teeth and describe the pathogenesis and clinical characteristic of each condition.

Hypoplasia refers to the defective formation of an organ or structure.

Enamel hypoplasia resulting in generalized discoloration of teeth is of 2 types which are as follows:

1. Environmental: Dental fluorosis
2. Genetic:
   a. Amelogenesis imperfecta
   b. Dentinogenesis imperfecta

Environmental Causes

Dental Fluorosis

It is a condition characterized by mottled enamel resulting from drinking water with increased fluoride content (above 1 ppm) during the formative phase of dentition. The ameloblasts are affected due to the increased fluoride resulting in defective or deficient enamel matrix formation and calcification.

Clinical Features

Fluorosis affects only permanent dentition. The clinical appearance depends on the amount and duration of fluoride intake.

The mottled appearances of enamel include:

- *Questionable change:* Occasional white spots on the enamel
- *Mild change:* Opaque white spots involving more tooth surface
- *Moderate and severe changes:* Pitting and brownish discoloration of the enamel and corroded changes.

Severely affected enamel may show a tendency to chip off and get fractured.

Radiographic findings

No abnormalities noted specifically to fluorosis.

Treatment

Cosmetic, restorative procedures.

Genetic Causes

a. Amelogenesis imperfecta (AI)

- Amelo = enamel
- Genesis = production
- Imperfecta = defective

AI is a developmental defect of enamel resulting in brown discoloration of teeth. It is of 2 types:

1. Hereditary enamel hypoplasia
2. Hereditary enamel hypocalcification.

Pathogenesis

In the primary phase of enamel development, the deposition of the enamel matrix begins at the amelodentinal junction and advances towards the outer surface. The enamel organ matrix is composed of 65% organic material and water and 35% of the inorganic material.

In the second phase of the developmental process, water and organic materials are removed and replaced by mineral salts, composing about 96% in the final structure.

A disturbance occurring in the primary phase results in hypoplasia with an altered shape of teeth. The amount of enamel formed will be small in quantity but fully calcified; hence the hardness of the teeth will be reasonable.

A disturbance occurring in the second phase results in hypocalcification, where the enamel matrix is deposited in normal in quantity, but the calcification will be incomplete. This poor quality of enamel is quickly worn off and exposes the underlying dentin.

Clinical Features

- AI affects both deciduous and permanent teeth.
- Teeth are of abnormal size and shape.
- In hypoplastic type, the teeth are brown-yellow with a smooth and glossy surface. The consistency is hard.
- In hypocalcification type, the teeth are dark brown; the surface will be rough and dull. The abrasion and chipping off of enamel result in loss of structural configuration.

Radiographic Features

In hypoplastic type, the tracing of enamel is difficult as its thickness is being reduced in spite of normal calcification.

In hypocalcification, the density of enamel and dentin are same.

Treatment

- Restorative management
- Veneering
- Crown and bridge.

b. Dentinogenesis imperfecta (DI)

- Dens = tooth
- Genesis = formation
- Imperfecta = defective

DI is a developmental disturbance resulting in poor quality of dentin but normal enamel.

Pathogenesis

The dentin is composed of low organic content and increased water with the normal calcium-phosphorous ratio. The enamel is normal, but pulp chamber and dentinoenamel junction are absent. The loss of scalloping of DEJ which is responsible for fixing the enamel to the dentin results in increased fracture susceptibility of the enamel.

Clinical Features

- The teeth appear normal in size, but there is a decrease in thickness and length of roots.
- The teeth will have blue opalescent hue.
- Exposure of dentin due to fractured enamel results in pulpo-periapical lesions and teeth loss.

Radiographic Findings

- Obliterated pulp chamber and pulp canals
- Smaller roots.

Treatment

- Restorative management
- Veneering
- Crown and bridge.

SHORT NOTES

1. Enumerate the developmental disturbances associated with orofacial changes.

Generalized Developmental Disturbances with Specific Oral Manifestations

- Craniofacial dysostosis
- Cleidocranial dysostosis
- Achondroplasia
- Hereditary ectodermal dysplasia
- Osteogenesis imperfecta
- Albers-Schonberg disease.

Generalized Developmental Disturbances with Secondary Oral Manifestations

- Hereditary intestinal polyposis syndrome (Peutz-Jaggers syndrome)
- Sickle cell anemia
- Cooley's anemia (Thalassemia)
- Hemophilia.

Local Developmental Disturbance of Nonodontogenic Structures

- Benign migratory glossitis
- Fissured tongue
- Cleft lip and palate
- Fordyce's granules
- Leukedema.

Local Developmental Disturbances Affecting Odontogenic Structures

- Amelogenesis imperfecta
- Dentinogenesis imperfecta
- Dens in Dente
- Dentin dysplasia
- Gemination, fusion, and concrescences
- Supernumerary teeth, anodontia, oligodontia.

2. Benign migratory glossitis (geographic tongue).

This condition affects the dorsal and lateral aspects of the tongue as large, red patches with slightly raised, white circinate borders. Usually, multiple lesions occur at a time.

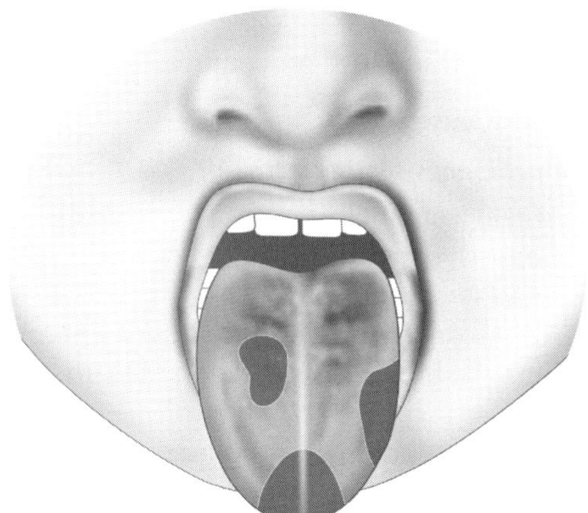

Fig. 1: Migratory glossitis.

The red patches are due to atrophy of filiform papillae, and a white boundary is due to the hypertrophy of papillae.

The lesion resembled the world map and known as geographic tongue.

Usually asymptomatic but occasionally cause burning sensation. The lesions disappear in weeks, and papilla regenerates but new lesion appears at another site which gives a picture of lesion migrating from one area to another and hence known as migratory glossitis (Fig. 1).

Diagnosis is based on the appearance of lesion, location, and recurrence.

Treatment is not needed, but reassurance should be given to the patient about the simple nature. In some conditions, vitamin supplement and topical anesthetics are used.

3. Fissured tongue.

It is a congenital malformation of the dorsal surface of the tongue; otherwise known as a scrotal tongue.

The dorsal surface of tongue shows furrows, grooves, and clefts, directed anteroposteriorly and laterally. The lesions develop over a long period and are asymptomatic. Rarely these grooves and fissures act a source for food debris accumulation and lead to bacterial infection.

Burning sensation may be the related symptom.

Fissured tongue is associated with Melkersson-Rosenthal syndrome and pernicious anemia.

Treatment: Improved oral hygiene with home care irrigation.

4. Macroglossia.

Macroglossia is a larger size tongue that interferes with speech and mastication.

There are two types:

1. ***Primary macroglossia:*** Hereditary condition seen in cretinism and Down syndrome. Hemangioma and lymphangioma are the frequent causes of macroglossia.
2. ***Secondary macroglossia:*** It is an acquired condition to local or systemic factors like untreated malocclusion, prolonged edentulous condition, neurofibroma, amyloidosis, benign or malignant muscle tumors of the tongue.

Underlying cause need to be corrected for the effective management.

5. Lingual varices.

Varices are the varicose vein present at the ventral surface of tongue in some elderly individuals usually above 60 years of age. It appears as a purple-red or bluish black, raised lesion measuring 2–5 mm in size.

Varices are multiple in numbers and appear as black caviar (caviar spot of the tongue).

The varicose veins are dilated, torturous, soft consistency, and blanch on pressure. Sometimes, it occurs at labial and buccal mucosa.

Usually asymptomatic and treatment is not needed.

Clinical significance: Sometimes thrombi develop within varicose veins and appear as a tumor-like growth.

6. Fordyce granules.

Fordyce granules are the sebaceous glands studded with the oral mucosa. They are the normal variant of the oral cavity and commonly seen on the buccal mucosa bilaterally. These granules are yellow-orange in color, small, elevated, and sometimes present in clusters. It is also seen in the labial mucosa. These granules arise during the age of puberty and have a male predilection.

Asymptomatic condition. No treatment is necessary.

7. Leukoedema.

Leukoedema is a developmental condition in which the buccal mucosa is milky white or bluish tinted, folded or striated in appearance. Usually bilateral and symmetrical. Sometimes involve the entire oral mucosa in a diffused pattern.

The edematous condition is due to intracellular edema of epithelial cells of oral mucosa and is responsible for the slightly raised appearance.

When the mucosa is stretched, it assumes a normal pink color and smooth appearance. Smoking may exacerbate the appearance. Asymptomatic and no treatment is required.

Differential diagnosis: White sponge nevus, leukoplakia

8. Supernumerary teeth.

Supernumerary teeth are the extra teeth and are a quite common developmental condition. These extra teeth may completely erupt or impacted. Size and shape may resemble the normal tooth or may be variable.

This condition is associated with aberrant tooth bud formation.

The most common type of supernumerary teeth are:

- ***Mesiodens*** erupts between the maxillary central incisors either in the arch or on the palatal aspect (Fig. 2).
- ***Distomolar*** erupts distal to maxillary 3rd molars and
- ***Paramolar*** erupt adjacent to 1st, or 2nd molars.

If the supernumerary teeth are present in the arch and resemble the adjacent teeth, then it is known as supplementary teeth.

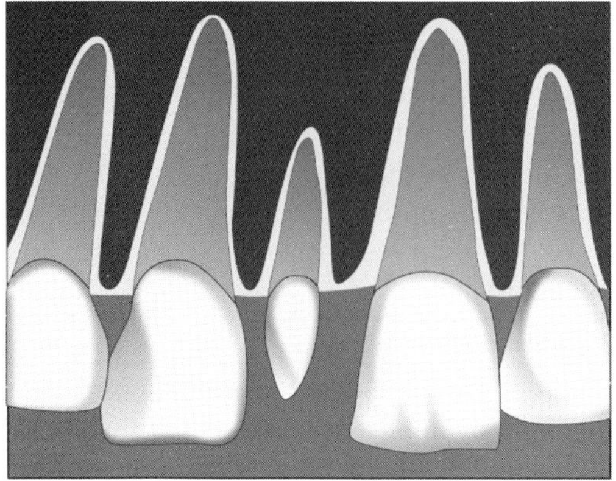

Fig. 2: Mesiodens.

Clinical Significance

- Multiple erupted and impacted supernumerary teeth are common in cleidocranial dysplastic syndrome.
- Malocclusion, food lodgement, dental caries, and gingivitis or periodontitis are the problems associated with erupted teeth.
- Development of odontogenic cysts and tumors are also arising from these extra teeth.

9. Tori (or) exostosis.

Tori are the dense bony prominence develops during the jaw formation and development. They occur both in maxilla and mandible.

In the maxilla, tori occur as a dense bony growth at the hard palate along with the midline. Mandibular tori are usually bilateral, appear as lobular bony nodules, positioned inferior and lingual to premolars.

They are slow growing and asymptomatic. Normal mucosa covers the surface. Larger tori may cause a disturbance in prosthetic placement and requires surgical removal.

Exostoses are developmental bony growth, which occurs as nodules on palate, alveolus or jaw bones. They are hard in consistency and asymptomatic. Infrequent finding and treatment are not required.

10. Tetracycline stain.

Tetracycline therapy is an environmental agent that causes developmental discoloration of teeth *without hypoplasia*.

Tetracycline is a broad-spectrum antibiotic used to treat chronic infectious disease and many childhood infections. When taken by the pregnant mother, the drug can traverse the placental barrier and cause staining of the primary dentition. Children below ten years of age should not be medicated with tetracycline.

The tetracycline gets incorporated into the enamel during development and gives gray to yellow appearance depending on the chemical configuration of the drug, and total dosage. These stains involve teeth in correlation with the chronological pattern of tooth development at the time of administration. The entire dentition may be affected by long-term therapy.

These stains cause an only esthetic disturbance, and hence veneering of teeth is adequate to improve the appearance.

11. Lingual tonsils (or) foliate papillitis (or) papillitis.

The posterior and posterolateral aspect of the dorsal surface of tongue contains aggregates of lymphoid tissues with circumvallate papilla (on the posterior dorsum) and foliates papilla (on the posterolateral tongue surfaces) bilaterally. These natural aggregates occasionally become enlarged, hyperplastic and sometimes inflamed. This condition mimics malignancy.

The enlarged lingual tonsils appear as elevated, yellow colored submucosal swellings on the posterolateral surface of tongue bilaterally (Fig. 3). This may be accompanied by red, inflamed foliate papillae which are often painful.

Lymphoid aggregates commonly occur as movable nodules on the pharyngeal- tonsillar region, uvula, and soft palate. Rarely they may

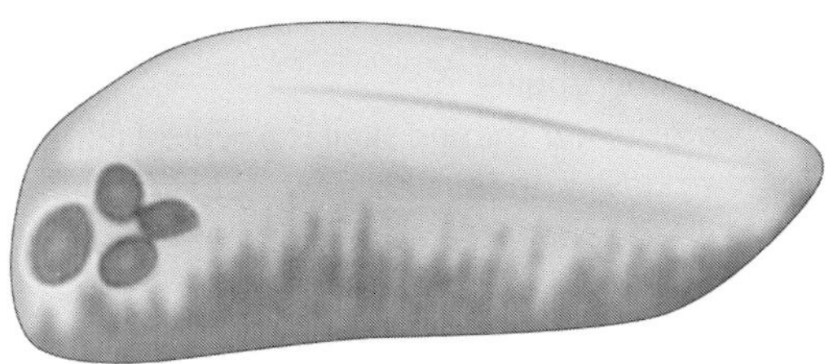

Fig. 3: Lingual tonsils.

be present on the buccal mucosa, floor of the mouth and lingual vestibules.

Upper respiratory tract infections may aggravate these conditions. Diagnosis is based on clinical appearance, site, and duration. There are no severe sequelae of this condition.

12. Linea alba.

Linea alba is a white line occurs on the buccal mucosa parallel to the line of occlusion bilaterally. This extends into the triangular area inside the labial commissure on the respective sides.

This is a normal frictional response and appears distinctive in some individuals.

The habit of taking coarse foods, smoking and other irritants may increase the intensity of frictional cornification.

Variable degree of keratinization in the course of linea alba in the same individual also common.

It is an asymptomatic condition and no need for any treatment.

Differential diagnosis: Lichen planus, lichenoid reaction, leukoplakia.

MULTIPLE CHOICE QUESTIONS

1. The joining of two individual adjacent tooth buds by enamel, dentin and cementum is known as ***fusion***.
   a. Concrescence
   b. Fusion
   c. Gemination
   d. Odontome
   (**Note:** Fusion is the joining of two individual adjacent tooth buds by enamel, dentin and cementum during the developmental stage, resulting in a giant tooth).
2. The fusion of two teeth only by cementum is known as ***concrescence***.
   a. Concrescence
   b. Fusion
   c. Gemination
   d. Odontome
3. The division of single tooth bud resulting in the formation of two teeth called as ***gemination***.
   a. Concrescence
   b. Supplemental
   c. Gemination
   d. Hyperdontia
   (**Note:** Gemination is an attempted division of a **single tooth germ** resulting in complete or incompletely separated crowns with **single root** and root canal. Also known as Siamese twins).
4. The enlarged midroot structure, with large pulp chamber and short apex is known as ***taurodontism***.
   a. Tuberculate
   b. Submerged
   c. Dilaceration
   d. Taurodontism
   (**Note:** Taurodontism is seen in amelogenesis imperfecta, Down syndrome, and Klinefelter syndrome).
5. Dens in Dente is common in ***maxillary lateral incisors.***
   a. Maxillary molars
   b. Mandibular molars
   c. Maxillary lateral incisors
   d. Mandibular canines
6. Harelip denotes ***cleft lip***.
   a. Cleft lip
   b. Angular cheilitis
   c. Double lip
   d. Lip pits
7. Developmental condition of absence of some teeth is denoted as ***oligodontia***.
   a. Anodontia
   b. Oligodontia
   c. Isodontia
   d. Microdontia

8. **Oligodontia** commonly manifests as missing ***maxillary lateral incisors***.
   a. Maxillary lateral incisors
   b. Mandibular lateral incisors
   c. Maxillary canines
   d. Mandibular canines
9. Complete anodontia may be seen in ***rickets***.
   a. Hypophosphatasia
   b. Rickets
   c. Hypothyroidism
   d. Cleidocranial dysplasia
   (**Note:** Complete anodontia may be seen in rickets and ectodermal dysplasia).
10. Multiple supernumerary teeth are seen in ***cleidocranial dysplasia***.
   a. Hyperthyroidism
   b. Hyperparathyroidism
   c. Down's syndrome
   d. Cleidocranial dysplasia
11. A maxillary lateral incisor with a pouch on the crown or root is known as ***dens in dente***.
   a. Dens in dente
   b. Enamel pearl
   c. Peg laterals
   d. Accessory cingulum
12. The consequence of supernumerary tooth is ***adjacent root resorption***.
   a. Esthetic disturbance
   b. Caries progression
   c. Adjacent root resorption
   d. Odontogenic harmatoma
13. Fordyce granules represent ***sebaceous choristoma***.
   a. Salivary gland aberrancy
   b. Sebaceous choristoma
   c. Adipose tissue atrophy
   d. Sweat gland orifice
14. Large head with mangoloid facies is seen in ***thalassemia individuals***.
   a. Hemophilic patients
   b. Thalassemia individuals
   c. Sickle cell patients
   d. Thrombocytopenic individuals
15. Tower shaped skull is a typical feature of ***sickle cell anemia***.
   a. Thalasemia
   b. Sickle cell anemia
   c. Hydrocephaly
   d. Brachycephaly
   (**Note:** Tower shaped skull is a typical feature of sickle cell anemia and oxycephaly).
16. Upper lip cleft occurs at the ***6th and 7th week of intrauterine life***.
   a. 4th and 5th week of intrauterine life
   b. 10th week of intrauterine life
   c. 6th and 7th week of intrauterine life
   d. 14th week of intrauterine life
17. Cleft palate occurs at ***8th week of intrauterine life***.
   a. 4th and 5th week of intrauterine life
   b. 10th week of intrauterine life
   c. 6th and 7th week of intrauterine life
   d. 8th week of intrauterine life
18. **Schizodontia** results in ***one normal and one supernumerary tooth***.
   a. One normal and one supernumerary tooth
   b. Two supernumerary teeth
   c. Two normal teeth
   d. One normal and one impacted tooth
   (**Note: Schizodontia** refers to **twining of a tooth bud** by complete cleavage, resulting in one normal and one supernumerary tooth).
19. **Synodontia** refers to ***fusion of two separate tooth germs***.
   a. Fusion of two crowns
   b. Fusion of two separate tooth germs
   c. Fusion of two teeth roots
   d. Fusion of two deciduous tooth germs
20. Concrescence occurs ***after root completion***.
   a. Before root completion
   b. After root completion
   c. Before crown completion
   d. After crown calcification
21. Sharp curvature on the crown or root of tooth is denoted as ***dilaceration***.
   a. Tuberculate
   b. Dens invaginatous
   c. Dilaceration
   d. Taurodontism
22. If deciduous tooth cause injury to the permanent tooth bud, the permanent tooth will be ***dilacerated***.
   a. Dilacerated
   b. Nonvital

c. Hypoplastic
d. Ankylosed

23. Talon's cusp is an associated finding of ***Rubinstein Taybi syndrome***.
    a. Pierre Robin syndrome
    b. Stickler's syndrome
    c. Velocardiofacial syndrome
    d. Rubinstein Taybi syndrome
    (**Note:** Talon's cusp is an associated finding of Rubinstein Taybi syndrome, Ellis-van Creveld syndrome, and Sturge-Webber syndrome).
24. Leong's premolar denotes the condition of ***dens evaginatous***.
    a. Dens invaginatous
    b. Dens evaginatous
    c. Supernumerary tooth
    d. Supplementary premolar
25. Teeth present at birth are known as ***natal teeth***.
    a. Natal teeth b. Neonatal teeth
    c. Hyperdontia d. Pseudo teeth
    (**Note:** Teeth erupts within 28 days of birth is known as neonatal teeth. Both natal and neonatal teeth are hornified epithelial structures).
26. Turner's hypoplasia frequently involves ***maxillary and mandibular premolars***.
    a. Deciduous mandibular molars
    b. Deciduous canines
    c. Maxillary and mandibular premolars
    d. Mandibular anterior teeth
    (**Note:** Turner's hypoplasia frequently involves maxillary and mandibular premolars and permanent maxillary central incisors).
27. Tulip shape teeth are the finding in ***dentinogenesis imperfecta***.
    a. Amelogenesis imperfecta
    b. Dentinogenesis imperfecta
    c. Regional odontodysplasia
    d. Ectodermal dysplasia
28. Ghost-like teeth in dentinogenesis imperfecta are the result of ***lack of density***.
    a. Loss of structural morphology
    b. Altered pattern of eruption
    c. Lack of density
    d. Dead space in dentin
    (**Note:** Lack of density is due to lack of calcification).

VIVA VOCE

1. What is Melkersson-Rosenthal syndrome.

It is a group of manifestations including cheilitis granulomatosa, fissured tongue, multiple granulomatous swellings, and facial palsy. The proposed etiology is gene mutation.

2. Classification of supernumerary teeth.

Based on morphology and location, the supernumerary teeth are classified into following types:

1. Conical (mesiodens)
2. Tuberculate (barrel-shaped teeth on the palatal aspect of central incisors often in pair)
3. Supplemental (duplication of tooth on the arch)
4. Odontome.

BIBLIOGRAPHY

1. Field A, Longman L. Tyldesley's oral medicine. London: Oxford University Press; 2003.
2. Ghom AG, Ghom SA. Textbook of oral medicine. Jaypee Brothers Medical Publishers; New Delhi; 2014.
3. Greenberg MS. Glick M. Burket's Oral Medicine Diagnosis and Treatment. Orofacial Pain. 10th edition. BC Decker Inc, Elsevier India; 2003:310.
4. Neville BW, Damm DD, Allen CM, et al. Oral and maxillofacial pathology. Elsevier Health Sciences; 2015
5. Rajendran R. Shafer's textbook of oral pathology. Elsevier India; 2009.

CHAPTER 24

Infection Control in Dental Clinics

HIGHLIGHTS

Infection control measures include all the efforts taken to control the spread of infection by disease-causing microbes. It contains a standard set of procedures to minimize the infection spread in healthcare practices. This chapter highlights the strategies to prevent cross-contamination of pathogens and infection control methods to be adopted in dental practice.

Learners are expected to study:

- Infection control protocol for dental clinics.
- Personal protection in dental practice.
- Sterilization and disinfection procedures.

ESSAY QUESTIONS

1. Personal protective barriers in dental practice.

Full Personal protective barriers (PPB) in clinical dentistry includes protective eyewear, masks, gown, and gloves.

Protective Eyewear

Eyewear (goggles with/without shields) protects dental professionals against infectious agents like herpes simplex and hepatitis B virus present in sprays, spatter, and aerosol. It also protects from possible injuries from small restorative materials or tooth fragments from patients mouth during dental procedures.

It protects the eyes during lab procedures like trimming and polishing of dentures.

Protective eyewear also helpful for the use of UV rays irradiation.

Protective eyewear is used by the dentist and dental team should be decontaminated before reuse.

Masks

There are three series of masks with different filter efficiency:

1. N series—95%,
2. R series—99%, and
3. P series—99.97%

The filterability is known as particle filtration efficiency or bacterial filtration efficiency.

Wearing mask by dental professionals protect their mucous membrane of mouth and nose from direct contact with the disease-causing microbes present in aerosol particles of blood and saliva, sprays and spatter of oral fluids from the patient or materials contaminated with oral fluids.

It also reduces the patients from the risk of developing postoperative infection by microorganisms present in the respiratory tract of the dentist and the team.

Wearing mask by the dental team is essentially important when they are performing procedures using headpieces, ultrasonic scalers, air/water syringes, instrument processing, prosthesis placement, and extraction.

The mask should be changed for every patient because the droplets of the previous patient might contaminate the outer surface.

Protective Clothing

Outer protective clothing protects the dental team from taking home the contaminated clothing. Similarly, these clothing protects the patients from the spread of microbes in unsterile dresses with open wounds.

The dentist should remove the protective clothing before leaving the clinical work side.

Protective clothing includes the use of disposable gowns with long sleeves and high neck to cover the regular cloths.

Reusable protective cloths like aprons and lab coats may also be used for regular working but should be removed before leaving the clinical area.

Gloves

Gloves are helpful in preventing the direct contact of dentists' finger in the patient's oral cavity hence protecting patients from microbes present on dentists hand and fingers. The regular habit of wearing gloves will prevent the blood and saliva contamination around the fingernails.

The high incidence of cross-infection among the ungloved dentists and dental team members is the herpes simplex virus infection (herpetic whitlow).

Routine gloving prevent infection spread at three levels:

1. From patient to dentist and dental team members
2. From dentists to patient
3. From patient to patient.

Gloves should never be reused in patient care procedures. Cleaning the gloves with chemical disinfectants or detergents will not be effective because this may cause inherent defects and leads to penetration of fluids.

Also, torn or damaged gloves should be removed immediately.

Different gloves are available (like sterile latex gloves and sterile nonlatex gloves—styrene gloves, polyurethane gloves) in different sizes to provide a better fit.

The order of wearing and removing personal protective barriers:

- Wearing
  - Protective clothing
  - Protective eyewear
  - Mask
  - Gloves
- Removing
  - Protective clothing
  - Gloves
  - Protective eyewear
  - Mask.

2. Describe the routine infection control measures to be performed in a dental clinic (or) describe the functional mode of dental clinics to execute asepsis protocol.

Asepsis protocols need to be followed in every aspect of patient management in a dental clinic.

Before Examining the Patient

- Wear the protective gown, eyewear, mask and gloves
- Clean and disinfect the instruments and dental chair by spraying surface disinfectant
- Remove and discard the used mask and gloves
- Arrange the surface covers and sterile instrument pack
- Cover the headrest, light handles, unit control switches and control buttons
- Remove the items that are not intended for treatment like prescription pads, articulators, etc.

During Patient Examination and Treatment

Immediately after seating the patient:

- Adjust chair and headrest.
- Place napkin.
- Open sterile instrument pack without touching instruments.
- Put on mask and goggles.
- Put on gloves.

During patient treatment:

- Use rubber dam.
- Use high volume evacuation.
- Remove the contaminated gloves and wash hands before handling radiographic unit.
- Do not touch nonsterile surfaces.
- In case of using syringes, insert the needle into the cap using the one-handed scoop

technique after usage to prevent the contact of the needle with any other part of the body.
- ❖ In case of using equipment like light cure apparatus, it should be disinfected before use.
- ❖ Disinfect the impressions/dental prosthesis before sending them to laboratories.
- ❖ Remove the gloves and wash hands before touching case records and prescription or investigation slips.
- ❖ If exposed to patients blood or saliva on bare skin or mucosa, or any injury with contaminated instruments, appropriate postexposure prophylaxis is mandatory.

After Treatment

- ❖ Remove the gloves, mask and discard them in a waste disposal container.
- ❖ Put on new mask and gloves and place all instruments back on tray
- ❖ Place the disposable sharp items and needles directly into the sharp item container.
- ❖ After each patient, flush the air/water syringes, handpiece, and ultrasonic scalars for 30 seconds before removing them from water lines.
- ❖ Remove all surface covers.
- ❖ Disinfect the patient care surfaces that are not covered.
- ❖ Remove gloves, wash, rinse and dry hands

Dental unit water quality: For routine care, the unit water containing below 500 CFU/mL of bacteria should be used.

When multiple dose vial medications are used (e.g. local anesthetic solution), the access diaphragm should be cleaned with 70% alcohol every time before inserting the needle into the vial. Each time, sterile needle and syringe should be used and reusing the needle should never be practiced. Multiple dose vial should always be kept away from the treatment area to maintain the sterile condition.

SHORT NOTES

1. Hand hygiene products in dentistry (or) healthcare set up (or) handwashing agents.

Plain soap without antimicrobial effect is sufficient for removing dirt and transient microorganisms. Alcohol-based hand rubs may be used after using plain soap rinse for effective antisepsis.

Professional handwashing products contain microbial agents, and surgical scrubs contain the highest amount of antimicrobial agents.

Antimicrobial agents used in handwash products include alcohols, chlorhexidine digluconate, idophor, triclosan and quaternary ammonium compounds.

Handwashing should be performed mandatorily in dental clinics:

- ❖ At the beginning of the working hour
- ❖ When hands are soiled
- ❖ After touching contaminated objects or surfaces
- ❖ Before donning and after removing the gloves.
- ❖ Before leaving the working area.
- ❖ At the end of the working hour.

2. Handwashing technique.

Adequate handwashing is a mandate necessary hygienic procedure for dentist and dental team members to reduce the microbial contamination of the hands and fingers.

Handwashing Materials

- ❖ Liquid soap and alcohol-based hand rub
- ❖ Handwashing liquid with antimicrobial agent
- ❖ Hands-free soap dispenser
- ❖ Soft brush for nail cleaning
- ❖ Soft sponge
- ❖ Sterile disposable towels.

Before Starting of Practice

- ❖ Gently clean fingernails (hand and finger jewelery should be removed).

- A liquid antimicrobial product and a soft brush should be used for cleaning the hands, nails, and forearms.
- While rubbing hands simultaneously rinse with water for 15 seconds.
- Hands and forearms should be dried up using sterile towels.

Handwashing During the Practice (To Remove Dirt and Transient Microbes)

- Using a liquid antimicrobial soap, thoroughly wash the hands for 15 seconds.
- Rinse with water for 10 seconds while rubbing hands.
- Dry hands and forearms using sterile paper towels.

Alternate Method: When no Dirt is Visible

- Use alcohol-based hand rub agent to clean the palm of hand.
- Rub hands together to make them dry.

3. Processing of dental instruments.

Dental instrument processing is a series of activities carried out to clean the contaminated instruments. There are seven steps to be followed to prevent the infection spread from a patient to dental team members, to next patient or the environment.

1. Presoaking—to avoid debris from drying.
2. Precleaning—mechanically remove the biological remains saliva and blood. To make the subsequent sterilization effective.
3. Corrosion control, drying, and lubrication—to reduce instrumental damage and to enhance proper functioning.
4. Packaging—to maintain the instrument sterility after sterilization until they are used for next procedure.
5. Sterilization—kills all remnant microbes in the instruments.
6. Sterilization monitoring—measures the effective functioning of sterilizer and completeness of sterilization.
7. Handling the processed instruments—maintaining the sterility of instruments until they are used.

4. Sterilization in dental clinics.

Sterilization is the process of killing all microbes and bacterial endospores (including *Mycobacterium tuberculosis,* fungal spores, hepatitis virus, herpes virus and HIV).

In dentistry, three types of sterilization are followed:

1. **Heat sterilization:** Operates at 250°F to 375°F and the effectiveness is monitored using bacterial spores.
2. **Liquid chemical sterilization:** Chemicals like sterilants, glutaraldehyde, hydrogen peroxide, and periacetic acid solution are the few effective sterilizers at room temperature and used for instruments that cannot withstand high temperature in heat sterilization. Though these agents are sporicidal, their effectiveness cannot be monitored in the dental clinic.
3. **Gas sterilization:** Ethylene oxide gas sterilizes between 72°F and 140°F. Though sporicidal; it is not widely used because it is a high cost technique that requires special handling method and needs a long exposure time.

5. Disinfection in dental clinics.

Disinfection is a process of killing all disease-causing microorganisms but not endospores. Disinfectant is a chemical that is not sporicidal but can kill all other microbes. They cannot provide sterilization.

Commonly used disinfectants in dental clinic are:

- **High-level disinfectants and sterilant:** They kill all microorganisms including bacterial spores on heat-sensitive reusable instruments, e.g. glutaraldehyde, hydrogen peroxide, peracetic acid, hydrogen peroxide with peracetic acid.
- **Intermediate-level disinfectants:** This group of chemicals destroys all vegetative bacteria, most fungi and viruses, and tuberculosis. They are used to disinfect clinical contact surfaces, noncritical surfaces with blood, e.g. chlorine-based

products, phenolics, iodophors, quaternary ammonium compounds with alcohol and bromides.

- **Low-level disinfectants:** They destroy most vegetative bacteria, some fungi, and some viruses. Not effective against tuberculosis. Useful for housekeeping disinfection (floor and walls), and disinfecting noncritical surfaces without blood, e.g. quaternary ammonium compounds.

6. Latex allergy.

Use of productive latex gloves may manifest type I immediate hypersensitivity reactions and a **contact allergic stomatitis** in latex allergic patients.

The affected individuals are allergic to proteins in the latex material. They will become sensitized to this protein antigen within first few (one or two) exposure and antibody production takes place. These antibodies bind to mast cells, and on subsequent exposures to latex antigen, these mast cells get activated, and cause adverse effects. Patients may experience ***burning sensation*** and ***soreness*** accompanied by ***erythema*** and sometimes with *vesicles and ulcers*. These symptoms will occur within 20 minutes of contact.

Once identified, ***latex allergy should be documented*** in patients' record.

Management

- It is advisable for sensitive people to avoid natural rubber latex and use nonlatex gloves.
- Use powder-free gloves to avoid airborne infections.
- Antihistamine medication.
- Get physicians advice if allergic reaction develops.

MULTIPLE CHOICE QUESTIONS

1. Father of infection control is ***Ignaz Semmelweis***.
   a. Antoni van Leeuwenhoek
   b. Louis Pasture
   c. Hippocrates
   d. Ignaz Semmelweis.
2. The high-risk group for acquiring cross-infection among health professionals are ***dentists***.
   a. Lab assistants
   b. Clinical nurses
   c. Dentists
   d. Blood bank technicians
3. Source for prion cross-infection in dentistry is contaminated ***endodontic instruments***.
   a. Handpiece
   b. Endodontic instruments
   c. Ultrasonic scalars
   d. Scalpel
4. Heavy utility gloves should be used during ***disinfecting contaminated surfaces***.
   a. Disinfecting contaminated surfaces
   b. Major surgical procedures
   c. Sterilization procedure
   d. Instrument check-up
   (**Note:** Heavy utility gloves should be used during operatory clean up, handling contaminated instruments, precleaning and disinfecting contaminated surfaces).
5. When unloading sterilizers, one should use ***heat resistant gloves***.
   a. Heavy utility gloves
   b. Heat resistant gloves
   c. Dust-free gloves
   d. Nitrile long gloves
6. Extracted teeth used for educational purpose should be ***heat sterilized***.
   a. Sterilized with hydrogen peroxide
   b. Heat sterilized
   c. Sterilized using infrared waves
   d. Thoroughly rinsed in water
7. Extracted teeth with amalgam restoration should not be disposed by ***incineration***.
   a. Composting
   b. Dumping in
   c. Recycling
   d. Incineration
8. Allergic contact dermatitis to gloves is ***type I and type IV hypersensitivity reactions***.
   a. Type I hypersensitivity reaction
   b. Type I and IV hypersensitivity reaction
   c. Type III hypersensitivity reaction
   d. Type I and III hypersensitivity reaction

9. Powder-free gloves are used to reduce the spread of ***latex protein allergens***.
   a. Latex protein allergens
   b. Nosocomial infection
   c. Aerosol infection
   d. Cross contamination
10. Critical and semicritical dental instruments must be ***cleaned and sterilized***.
    a. Air dried and sterilized
    b. Cleaned and sterilized
    c. Air dried and disinfected
    d. Cleaned and disinfected
11. Heat sensitive semicritical instruments must be cleaned and subjected to ***high-level disinfectant***.
    a. Autoclave
    b. Chemical sterilization
    c. High-level disinfectant
    d. Ultrasonic waves
12. Noncritical dental instruments with blood tint must be cleaned with ***intermediate-level disinfectant***.
    a. High-level disinfectant
    b. Intermediate-level disinfectant
    c. Dry heat sterilization
    d. Cold sterilization
    (**Note:** Noncritical dental instruments must be cleaned and with **intermediate–level disinfectant** (in case of blood tint) or **low-level disinfectant** in case of no blood tint).
13. In dry heat sterilization, spore testing is done with ***Bacillus atrophaeus strips***.
    a. *Bacillus atrophaeus* strips
    b. *Bacillus cereus* strips
    c. *Bacillus anthracis* strips
    d. *Bacillus coagulans strips*
14. In steam autoclave and unsaturated chemical vapor sterilization, ***Geobacillus stearothermophillus*** strips are used for spore testing
    a. *Geobacillus stearothermophillus* strips
    b. *Pyrolobus fumari* strips
    c. *Thermoascus aurantiacus* strips
    d. *Thermus thermophilus* strips
15. Bead sterilizers should not be used for sterilizing instrument to ***reuse for other patients***.
    a. Do invasive procedures
    b. Reuse for other patients
    c. Preserve the instrument
    d. Avoid rusting
    [**Note:** Bead sterilizers are used to sterilize **the tips of endodontic instruments** (endodontic files and broaches) as they provide dry heat up to 425°F].
16. Dental plaque is known as ***oral biofilm***.
    a. Microbial deposit
    b. Oral substrate
    c. Oral biofilm
    d. Dental nidus
17. When there is an accidental chemical exposure to eyes, the immediate safety measure to be followed is ***flushing of eyes with water***.
    a. Close the eyes and take rest
    b. Apply antitode
    c. Copius saline irrigation of eyes
    d. Flushing of eyes with water
    (**Note:** Flushing of eyes with water for 10–15 minutes is the recommended protocol)
18. Information about the handling of hazardous chemicals in dentistry is revealed in ***material safety datasheets***.
    a. Chemical data information sheets
    b. Drugs and chemicals charts
    c. Material safety datasheets
    d. Chemical incident report

VIVA VOCE

1. What is the difference between sterilization and disinfection?

Sterilization is the process of killing all microorganisms and disinfection is the process of killing only disease producing microorganisms but not bacterial endospores.

2. What are the possible adverse reactions that can occur with gloving?

- Irritant contact dermatitis
- Allergic contact dermatitis
- Latex allergy.

3. What are the critical patient care items in dentistry?

Dental surgical instruments that penetrate soft tissues, contacting bone, and bloodstream and other instruments that contact the oral tissues like scalers, dental burs, blades.

4. What are the semicritical patient care items in dentistry?

Dental instruments that contact with oral mucosa but will not penetrate the soft tissues, bone or enter bloodstream. Mouth mirror, tongue depressor, cheek retractor, amalgam condenser, handpiece, impression trays are semicritical dental instruments.

5. What are the noncritical patient care items in dentistry?

Apparatus that contact intact skin are non-critical instruments which include blood pressure cuff, and stethoscope.

6. What are the microorganisms present in dental unit water?

- *Pseudomonas* (opportunistic infective agent in urinary tract infection and wound infections) and can cause infection in medically compromised dental patients.
- *Legionella,* causative agent for legionnaires (a type of pneumonia).
- *Nontuberculous mycobacterium* can cause infection in dialysis patients.

7. What are the three basic principles of infection control proposed by WHO?

- Protect the patient
- Protect the practitioner
- Repeat when necessary.

8. What is biofilm?

Biofilm is a mass of microorganisms attached to the surface exposed to moisture.

BIBLIOGRAPHY

1. Kohli A, Puttaiah R. Dental infection control and occupational safety for oral health professionals. Dental Council of India. 2008.
2. Miller CH. Infection control strategies for the dental office. In Ciancio SG. (editors). ADA guide to dental therapeutics, 3rd edition, Chicago, American Dental Association; 2003, pp 551-66.
3. Miller CH. Hand hygiene above, under and beyond the surface. Dent Prod Rpt. 2007;39:134.
4. Miller CH. Select and protect: Part II Dent Prod Rpt. 2007;41:132-36.
5. Miller CH. Cleaning, sterilization and disinfection: the basics of microbial killing for infection control. J Am Dent Assoc. 1993;124:48-56.

CHAPTER 25

Miscellaneous Topics

SHORT NOTES

1. Enumerate the causes of halitosis.

Halitosis is the abnormal breath odors caused by a variety of underlying factors.

The result of the metabolic activity of oral gram-negative bacteria on degenerated epithelial cells, inflammatory cells, and food particles is the release of volatile sulfur compounds and cause unpleasant breath odor. Bad breath is common on awakening due to the absence of self-cleansing mechanisms like a movement of the tongue and salivary flow. But if it persists during the daytime, then the following factors should be considered:

- ***Oral and nasal***—oral infection like severe gingivitis, periodontitis or abscessed teeth, tonsillitis, nasal and nasopharyngeal discharge.
- ***Respiratory diseases***—lung abscess and bronchitis.
- ***Fever and dehydration***
- ***Diseases of salivary gland***—suppurative parotitis.
- ***GIT disorders***—gastritis, gastric or peptic ulcer, digestive disorders.
- ***Metabolic diseases***—diabetic mellitus (acetone odor), high fat diet, uremia (fishy or ammonia smell), liver failure (mousy odor).
- ***Drugs***—organophosphorus, anticholinergics, sublingual isosorbide, disulfiram
- ***Psychoneurosis***

2. Describe mycosis fungoides.

It is otherwise known as **cutaneous lymphoma**. It is a rare form of chronic skin disease and starts as pruritus. The next is "premycotic" stage is associated with skin eruptions (urticarial or psoriatic like). This stage is followed by a red or purple colored skin tumors (tomato-like) which finally ulcerates and fungates (mycotic stage).

The aggressive form produces ***Sezary syndrome*** characterized by generalized nodular lesions, papules, hair loss, drooping of lower eyelid, lymphadinopathy, anxiety and depression. The prognosis is poor.

3. Angioneurotic edema (or) angioedema.

Angioedema is a deep cutaneous swelling due to the release of inflammatory mediators.

Pathogenesis

The basic reason is the mast cell response with increased release of histamines, serotonin, bradykinins and other inflammatory mediators. These substances cause increased vascular leakage and edema of the deep layers of connective tissue.

Types

Based on etiology:

- The hereditary type (hereditary angioedema) is due to the deficiency of the CI esterase inhibitors which inhibit the action of plasma kallikrein and functions to break the kininogen and for the production of bradykinin. In the absence of CI esterase, there will be excess kininogen and circulating kinins.

- IgE mediated angioedema occurs due to immediate hypersensitivity reaction following the exposure to an antigen like food substances (milk products, eggs, chocolates, peanuts), antibiotics and analgesics.
- It occurs secondary to infection, connective tissue disorders, and insect bites.

Based on duration:

- Acute—presence of symptoms for less than 6 weeks
- Chronic—presence of symptoms for more than 6 weeks

Clinical Findings

- Females are affected more than males and affect individuals above 30 years.
- The affected organs include lips, eyelids, tongue, oral mucosa and extremities. In severe condition, the mucosa of respiratory tract and larynx also affected.
- The boundaries are ill-defined, and there will be no associated pain, burning sensation, and pruritus.
- Urticaria is common in many patients.

Diagnosis

Lab investigations have limited role. The diagnosis is primarily based on history, symptoms and examination findings.

The basic tests include:

- ESR, CBC
- Allergic testing in suspected cases
- C4 level for C1 esterase activity.

Management

In acute conditions, symptomatic relief is achieved with:

- H1 antihistamines like:
  - Cetrizine 5–10 mg once daily
  - Loratadine 10 mg once daily
  - Chorpheniramine 4 mg 6th hourly
  - Diphenhydramine 25–50 mg once daily
- In resistant cases, H2 antihistamines are added with H1 antihistamines.
  - Ranitidine 150 mg two times/day
  - Cimetidine 400 mg two times/day
- IgE mediated angioedema with laryngeal involvement is treated with:
  - Epinephrine 0.3 mg in a solution of 1:1000, subcutaneous route
  - Diphenhydramine 25–50 mg IM or IV
  - Ranitidine 50 mg IV
  - Antihistamine combined with the corticosteroid (prednisone) reduces the severity of attacks in life-threatening episodes.
- For hereditary angioedema, C1-INH concentrate or fresh frozen plasma IV may be used.

4. Explain the dental findings in patients with anorexia nervosa and the treatment plan.

Anorexia nervosa is a disordered eating problem characterized by a hesitation to obesity and the refusal for maintaining normal body weight especially exhibited by young females (age less than 25 years).

Clinical Findings

- Underweight, history of weight reduction primarily due to caloric restriction or self-induced vomiting after eating.
- Perception of weight loss as an achievement.

Dental Findings

- Dental effects are due to gastric acid regurgitation
- Wear facets leads to loss of vertical dimension and development of premature occlusal contact and traumatic occlusion
- Dental erosion particularly on palatal aspect of maxillary incisors
- Notched incisal edges of anterior teeth
- Loss of tooth contour
- Bilateral parotid gland hypertrophy
- Traumatized oral mucosa is seen in patients using objects for inducing vomiting.

Dental Management

- Patient education about diet and oral health
- Advice regular dental examination, oral prophylaxis, and topical fluoride application
- Defer definitive dental treatment like restorations and endodontic therapy until control of eating disorder is established
- Definitive dental treatment depends on the severity of structural loss of tooth and may include composite and glass ionomer restorations, porcelain laminate veneers or full mouth rehabilitation.

5. Describe the features of non-Hodgkin lymphoma. Add a note on the dental management for non-Hodgkin patients.

Non-Hodgkin lymphoma (NHL) is a group of lymphoproliferative tumors with a range of behavioral pattern and treatment response. There are two types:

1. B-cell (most common, 85–90% of cases) and T-cell (10–15%). It originates from lymphoid tissues and spreads to other organs. Extranodal dissemination is also common.
2. NHL affects all age groups but common in patients above 40 years of age, males are affected more.

Classification

- Pattern of distribution: Diffuse and nodular.
- Cell type: Lymphocytic, histiocytic and mixed.
- Degree of cellular differentiation: Well-differentiated, moderately, and poorly differentiated

There are more than 30 types of NHLs. The most common forms are:

- Diffuse large B-cell lymphoma (DLBCL)—active and destructive form
- Follicular lymphoma—indolent lymphoma but may transform into DLBCL
- Mucosa associated lymphoid tissue (MALT) tumor usually develops in the abdomen but may transform in to DLBCL.
- Burkitt's lymphoma—less common type. Clinically aggressive form and seen in immunocompromised individuals like patients undergone for organ or bone marrow transplant. Epstein-Barr virus infection is also a causative factor.

Clinical Features

- Usually, patients present with painless, persistent lymphadenopathy
- Common symptoms are fever, weight loss, night sweats, widespread itching
- If the bone marrow is affected, lymphoma cells predominate and cause anemia
- If the brain is affected, the patient may present with headaches, visual disturbance, and seizures.

Diagnosis

- Lymph node and bone marrow needle biopsy
- Blood smear test, complete blood count, and differential count
- MRI, lymphangiogram.

Complications

Infection is secondary to immunosuppression from chemotherapy, radiotherapy or due to the disease itself.

Dental Consideration

- Patients may present with painless cervical lymphadenopathy.
- Waldeyer's ring is most commonly affected
- Intraoral tumors occur on the cheek and palatal mucosa, gingiva, floor of the mouth, and present as swelling.
- If jaw bones are affected, the mobility of teeth, neurologic disturbance, and jaw fracture may occur.
- Asymptomatic ulcerations present on oral soft tissues.

Dental Management

- Treatment should be provided for the elimination of the potential source of bacteremia like periodontitis, carious teeth, etc. before chemotherapy.

- Nonfunctional, nonrestorable, partially erupted teeth should be extracted before chemotherapy.
- Extraction should be carried out 5 days before initiation of chemotherapy for maxillary teeth and 7 days before for mandibular teeth. For radiotherapy, extraction should be carried out 3 weeks before initiation.
- For patients receiving chemotherapy, before initiating dental procedures, CBC and platelet counts should be evaluated. Routine dental procedures can be performed if total WBC count is above 2,000/mm^3 and platelet count is above 50,000/mm^3. For emergency procedures, platelet replacement therapy with oncologists consent is essential when platelets are below 50,000/mm^3. However, if WBC count is below 2,000/mm^3 and neutrophil count is less the 500–1,000/mm^3, consultation with the oncologist is recommended.
- Management for mucositis following chemo-and radiotherapy.

Treatment Modalities for NHLs

- Radiation and chemotherapy are the two possible modalities
- Bone marrow transplant and monoclonal antibodies against B cell surface antigens.

6. Briefly describe Hodgkin's lymphoma.

It is a curable form of malignancy affecting the lymph nodes, spleen, liver and bone marrow. It occurs in children and young adults. It has bimodal age distribution—early adulthood (15–40 years, commonly around 25–30 years), late adulthood (after 55 years of age).

Etiology

Combination of factors like infection, environmental exposure, and genetic alterations play a role. The Epstein-Barr virus (EBV) is a cofactor. In many cases, the tumor cells are EBV positive. Patients with HIV infections have a higher prevalence of HL.

Clinical Features

- Painless enlargement of lymph nodes
- Asymptomatic lymphadenopathy above diaphragm in 80–90% cases
- Cervical node enlargement
- Unexplained weight loss, fever, and night sweats
- Pruritus is a symptom seen in young women with HL
- Pel-Ebstein fever in some patients (a cyclic pattern of high fever).

Diagnosis

Lymph node biopsy—Reed-Sternberg cells (large sized, bilobular nucleus) confirm diagnosis.

Dental Significance

- Primary jaw lesions are uncommon
- Increased susceptibility to bacterial, viral and fungal infections.

7. Postexposure prophylaxis for a dental professional following occupational exposure to HIV.

Following an accidental exposure to HIV through needle prick or other sharp instrument piercing which are used to treat a patient with a medical history of HIV infection.

- Through washing of injured site with plain water.
- Place a gauze soaked with a disinfectant solution (for example, povidone iodine or 75% alcohol) for 15 minutes at the injured site.
- Chemoprophylaxis should be started immediately following the exposure.
- The serological examination should be carried out to detect the HIV antigen. HIV can be detected after 72 hours of acquiring infection and viremia develops in 5 days.

Postexposure Prophylaxis

Depending on the viral load of the patient two or three antiretroviral drugs are used for prophylaxis. The drugs should be two nucleosides with/without a protease inhibitor. The effect of these retroviral drugs will last for 4 weeks and prevent seroconversion with 80% success rate.

8. What is biofeedback? How it is helpful in dentistry.

Biofeedback is a therapeutic learning mechanism that helps to improve body function by observing electrical signals generated (feedback) from the body (bio).

It is a method of alternative therapy to improve the physical performance by learning and practicing a voluntary control of the autonomous nervous system. It improves the life quality by allowing the subjected individual to "see" or "hear" body activities.

Biofeedback in Dentistry

The commonly used biofeedback method in dentistry is related to muscles. The electrodes attached over your skeletal muscles will display a range of readings on the computer monitor.

Biofeedback Devise and Function

Biofeedback equipment consists of a computer, electrodes, and signaling devices. The electrodes should be attached to the masseter muscle for assessing the temporomandibular joint function or the intensity of the myofascial pain. The electrodes capture the signals when muscles contracts and relaxes. During the contractile phase (like clenching or grinding), an upward arrow or a beep sound will be displayed. In a relaxed state, the arrow goes down, or the sound stops.

Application

In the management of:

- Chronic orofacial pain
- Myofascial pain dysfunction syndrome
- Temporomandibular disorders.

Advantages

- Noninvasive
- It improves quality of life through behavioral modification
- It reduces the need for pharmacological medications
- No adverse effects.

9. Enumerate the types of transcutaneous electric nerve stimulation. State the mode of action and uses of TENS in dental practice.

Transcutaneous electric nerve stimulation (TENS) is an alternative method for pain management. Two theories explains the basic mechanism of TENS in pain control which are as follows:

1. ***Gate control theory of pain:*** Pain is transmitted by small unmyelinated 'C' fibers and the active state of C fibers keeps the gate in relatively open position. The myelinated "A" fibers release inhibitory effect on C fibers and this action closes the gate. TENS act by closing the gate by increasing the input from large fibers and diminishing the input from small fibers.
2. ***Endogenous opioid theory:*** TENS activate local circuits within the spinal cord and release the endogenous opioid to control the pain.

Types

Two types are available:

1. High-frequency TENS—operate by gate control mechanism and pain relief is effective only for a short duration.
2. Low-frequency TENS—operate by releasing endogenous opioid and pain relief will persist for a longer duration.

   The components of TENS device includes TENS unit, lead wires, and electrodes.

Application in Dentistry

- To manage acute and chronic pain:
  - TMJ disorders
  - Trigeminal neuralgia
  - Postherpetic neuralgia.
- To increase salivary secretion in patients with xerostomia.

Advantages

- Noninvasive
- The patient can use on their own to manage the pain after learning the adjustment mechanism.

Contraindications

- Patients with cardiac pacemakers
- Patients with cerebrovascular problems
- Epileptic patients
- Cannot be used in apprehensive patients as it needs patients cooperation.

10. Describe Rumple-Leede test.

Rumple-Leede test is applied in patients with bleeding diathesis. The test measures the capillary wall integrity and quantitative plus qualitative defects of platelets.

Method

- Place the blood pressure cuff on the patient's arm. Record the patient's blood pressure.
- Inflate the cuff to a middle point between systolic and diastolic blood pressure and maintain for 5 minutes.
- Reduce and wait 2 minutes.
- Count petechiae below antecubital fossa.
- The test is positive if 10 or more petechiae appeared per 1 square inch.
- The petechiae formation distal to a tourniquet or sphygmomanometer on releasing the pressure is known as the Rumpel–Leede sign.

Basic Principle of the Test

An inflated blood pressure cuff at a specific pressure, for a specific time will produce an increased pressure and hypoxia in the capillaries distal to the cuff. Decreased capillary resistance ruptures the capillaries, resulting in bleeding and petechiae formation. The result is nonspecific. A positive test in women aged above 40 years may not be pathogenic.

Contraindications

- Platelet count <50,000/mm^3
- Bleeding disorders
- Anticoagulant therapy
- Skin changes due to aging
- Aspirin ingestion within a week before performing the procedure.

11. Write the salient features of Angina bullosa hemorrhagica.

- Angina bullosa hemorrhagica (ABH) is an acute condition of blood-filled bulla on the oral cavity. They are not attributed to any blood disorders, vesiculobullous conditions, systemic diseases or other known causes.
- It is a benign condition. It occurs on the soft palate and is characterized by the sudden appearance in middle aged individuals. Minor trauma, iatrogenic causes and use of steroid inhalers are the few reported causes of onset.
- The widely accepted pathological reason is the low-grade trauma or irritation rupturing the epithelial-connective-tissue junction, causing superficial capillary bleeding, and formation of hemorrhagic bullae.
- Spontaneous rupture of the bulla will lead to ulcer of 1–3 cm in diameter which heals without scar formation is characteristic.
- The bulla frequently develops on the soft palate; however, the buccal mucosa and tongue may also develop such lesions.
- Symptoms of sudden onset, painless nature, and spontaneous rupture of the bulla help in establishing the diagnosis. Histopathological findings are non-specific. Treatment is not required. Topical application of benzydamine hydrochloride will relieve the symptoms.

MULTIPLE CHOICE QUESTIONS

1. Cross bun skull is seen in ***congenital syphilis***.
   a. Congenital syphilis
   b. Fallot's tetrology
   c. Rickets
   d. Acromegaly
   (**Note:** Cross bun skull seen in congenital syphilis is vertical forehead, sunken nasal bridge, and prominence of frontal eminences—frontal bosses).

2. Craniotabes occurs in ***osteogenesis imperfecta***.
   a. Thalassaemia
   b. Osteogenesis imperfecta
   c. Myxoedema
   d. Tetany
   [**Note:** Craniotabes (softening of the skull) occurs in the early stage of rickets, hydrocephalus, congenital syphilis, hyperparathyroidism and osteogenesis imperfecta].
3. Ping-pong ball and egg shell crackling effects of the skull are the first signs of ***rickets***.
   a. Osteomalasia
   b. Rickets
   c. Hydrocephalus
   d. Skull vault fracture
4. Boxy head with the prominence of frontal and parietal eminences seen in ***rickets***.
   a. Osteomalasia
   b. Rickets
   c. Hydrocephalus
   d. Skull vault fracture
   (**Note:** Boxy head or Rachitic head is a condition in which skull appears larger than normal size with the prominence of frontal and parietal eminences, seen in rickets).
5. Bulldog scalp is seen in ***acromegaly***.
   a. Rickets
   b. Congenital syphilis
   c. Pituitary dwarfism
   d. Acromegaly
   (**Note:** Bulldog scalp is seen in acromegaly due to excessive growth of skin and subcutaneous tissues of the scalp).
6. Joffroy's sign is associated with ***hyperthyroidism***.
   a. Bell's palsy
   b. Costen syndrome
   c. Hypocalcemia
   d. Hyperthyroidism
   [**Note:** Joffroy's sign (bilateral absence of wrinkling on looking up) is a sign of hyperthyroidism].
7. Unilateral wrinkling of the forehead and unilateral smile are seen in ***Bell's palsy***.
   a. Bell's palsy
   b. Tetany
   c. Tetanus
   d. Trotter syndrome
8. Ape-like facial appearance is seen in ***acromegaly***.
   a. Rickets
   b. Congenital syphilis
   c. Paget's disease
   d. Acromegaly
9. The face appears pale, puffy with dull and emotionless appearance in ***myxoedema***.
   a. Cretinism b. Myxoedema
   c. Tetanus d. Myasthenia gravis
   [**Note:** In hypothyroidism (myxoedema), the face appears pale, puffy with dull and emotionless appearance; eyelids appear swollen and drooping].
10. A sneering smile is seen in ***myasthenia gravis***.
    a. Risus sardonicus
    b. Scleroderma
    c. Myasthenia gravis
    d. Bell's palsy
    (**Note:** A sneering smile seen in myasthenia gravis and is due to the weakness of zygomatic and risorius muscles).
11. Tobacco pouch mouth is seen in ***scleroderma***.
    a. Scleroderma
    b. Myasthenia gravis
    c. Wegener's granulomatosis
    d. Masseter hypertrophy
    (**Note:** Tobacco pouch mouth is a condition of partially open mouth with protruding teeth, seen in scleroderma).
12. Saddle nose is seen in ***anhidrotic ectodermal dysplasia***.
    a. Le Fort II fracture
    b. Anhidrotic ectodermal dysplasia
    c. Leprosy
    d. Sarcoidosis
    (**Note:** Saddle nose is seen in congenital syphilis, infantile hypothyroidism, anhidrotic ectodermal dysplasia and Wegener's granulomatosis, polychondritis).
13. Chvostek's sign is associated with ***latent tetany***.
    a. Latent tetany
    b. Amyloidosis
    c. Lipoma
    d. Postherpetic neuralgia
    (**Note:** Chvostek's sign is sudden contraction of facial muscles following a light tap over the facial nerve seen in latent tetany).

14. **Carp mouth** is seen in ***tetany***.
    a. Scleroderma
    b. Crohn's disease
    c. Tetany
    d. Scurvy
    (**Note:** Carp mouth is rigid and fixed facial expression due to the facial muscle spasm in tetany).
15. Fixed smile or suppressed smile is seen in ***Wilson's disease***.
    a. Myasthenia gravis
    b. Ehlers-Danlos syndrome
    c. Wilson's disease
    d. Scleroderma
    (**Note: Fixed smile or suppressed smile** is seen in scleroderma and Wilson's disease).
16. Fish mouth is seen in ***Cushing's syndrome***.
    a. Cushing's syndrome
    b. Addison's disease
    c. Guillain-barre syndrome
    d. Sjőgren syndrome
17. Lip-tie is seen in ***Ehlers-Danlos syndrome***.
    a. Ectodermal dysplasia
    b. Ehlers-Danlos syndrome
    c. Cleido-cranial syndrome
    d. Scleroderma
18. Crocodile skin tongue is seen in ***Sjőgren syndrome***.
    a. Mikulicz syndrome
    b. Sjőgren syndrome
    c. Plummer vinson syndrome
    d. Dry beriberi
    (**Note:** Crocodile skin tongue in Sjőgren syndrome is due to the papillary atrophy and furring).
19. Cobblestone tongue is seen in ***ariboflavinosis***.
    a. Crohn's disease
    b. Hyperplastic candidiasis
    c. Ariboflavinosis
    d. Pierre Robin syndrome
20. Peg-shaped teeth are seen in ***ectodermal dysplasia***.
    a. Goltz-gorlin syndrome
    b. Gorlin-goltz syndrome
    c. Generalized relative microdontia
    d. Ectodermal dysplasia
21. Maldon teeth are seen in ***fluorosis***.
    a. Amelogenesis imperfecta
    b. Fluorosis
    c. Turner's hypoplasia
    d. Tetracycline staining
    (**Note:** Maldon teeth are seen in ***endemic fluorosis*** with chalky white appearance).
22. Life protecting hormone is ***cortisol***.
    a. Adrenaline
    b. Cortisol
    c. Insulin
    d. Thyroxine
    (**Note:** Life protecting hormone is cortisol or hydrocortisone).
23. Life-saving hormone is ***aldosterone***.
    a. Epinephrine
    b. Norepinephrine
    c. Aldosterone
    d. Cortisol

VIVA VOCE

1. Name few conditions associated with prominent forehead.

- Acromegaly
- Leontiasis ossium
- Chronic hydrocephalus
- Frontal bossing.

2. In which conditions, macroglossia is seen?

- Congenital macroglossia
- Acromegaly
- Hypothyroidism
- Cretinism
- Hurler's syndrome
- Amyloidosis
- Down's syndrome
- Hemangioma and lymphangioma
- Mucopolysaccharidosis
- Congenital hemihypertrophy.

3. Name the conditions with microglossia.

- Starvation and malnutrition
- Uni-or bilateral hypoglossal nerve palsy
- Facial hemiatrophy
- Myasthenia gravis.

BIBLIOGRAPHY

1. Bang NU, Beller FK, Deutsch E (Eds). Thrombosis and bleeding disorders, theory and methods. Academic Press, New York; 1971.
2. de Moor RG. Eating disorder-induced dental complications: a case report. J Oral Rehabili. 2004;31(7):725-32.
3. Dohrmann RJ, Laskin DM. An evaluation of electromyographic biofeedback in the treatment of myofascial pain-dysfunction syndrome. Journal Am Dent Associ. 1978; 96(4):656-62.
4. Horie N, Kawano R, Inaba J, et al. Angina bullosa hemorrhagica of the soft palate: a clinical study of 16 cases. J Oral Sci. 2008; 50(1):33-6.
5. Little JW, Falace D, Miller C, et al. Dental Management of the Medically Compromised Patient-E-Book. Elsevier Health Sciences; 2017.
6. Maeda S, Miyawaki T, Nomura S, et al. Management of oral surgery in patients with hereditary or acquired angioedemas: review and case report. Oral Surg Oral Med Oral Pathol Oral Radiol Endod. 2003;96(5):540-43.
7. Sluka KA, Walsh D. Transcutaneous electrical nerve stimulation: basic science mechanisms and clinical effectiveness. J Pain. 2003;4(3):109-21
8. Vakil RJ, Golwalla AF, et al. Physical diagnosis, textbook of symptoms and physical signs, 14th edition. Medie Promoters and Publishers Pvt. Ltd; 2012.

2 PART

Part 2 Outline

CHAPTER 26

Radiation Physics

HIGHLIGHTS

X-rays are electromagnetic radiant energy which are capable of penetrating the body and ionize biological atoms. Understanding of this electromagnetic radiation requires basic knowledge about fundamental substances or subatomic particles. The application of x-rays in diagnostic imaging system is inevitable.

Learners are expected to study:

- Nature and types of radiation
- Source of radiation
- Production of X-rays
- Properties of X-rays
- Factors in production of X-rays
- Compton effect
- Photoelectric effect
- Radiation measuring units.

ESSAY QUESTIONS

1. What are X-rays? Write in detail the mechanism of X-ray production. (or) enumerate the parts of X-ray tube and describe about X-ray generation.

X-rays are ionizing, electromagnetic radiation composed of energy packages called photons. X-rays are generated when the high speed electrons collide with target nuclei in a device called Coolidge tube.

X-Ray Machine

The X-ray machine consists of:

- X-ray tube within a tube head
- Power supply components
- Control panel
- Supporting arm mounted on a wall (supports tubehead).

X-ray Tube

It is the basic apparatus for generating X-rays. X-ray tube is placed within a tubehead to which beam indicating device (BID) is attached. X-ray tube is made up of pyrex (leaded glass) and contains two electrodes, cathode and anode in vacuum (Fig. 1).

Cathode (Negative Charged)

Comprises: Spiral tungsten filament; molybdenum focusing cup.

Tungsten filament is the source of electron and is 2 mm in diameter and 1 cm in length. The low-voltage filament electrical circuit allows the flow of current and heat the filament to *glowing hot (incandescence)* and make to emit electrons at a rate proportional to filament temperature.

Focusing cup (molybdenum) is negatively charged and directs the electron beam in a straight line towards the anode focal spot.

The *evacuated X-ray tube* helps:

- To prevent the collision of moving electrons with gas molecules which would reduces their speed.
- To prevent "oxidation" and "burnout" of filament.

Anode (Positive Charged)

Anode is made up of copper and consists of a target made up of tungsten block. The function of the target is to convert the kinetic energy of

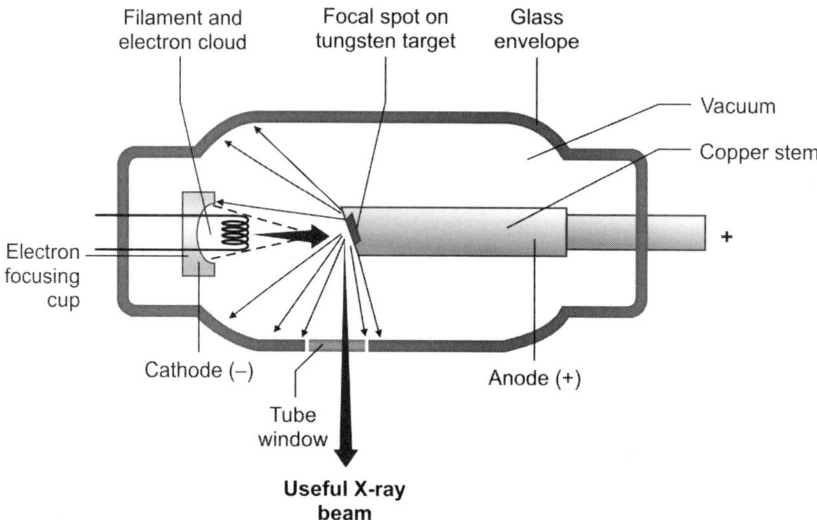

Fig. 1: X-ray tube.

electrons into X-ray photons when they hit the focal spot. Only 1% of kinetic energy is changed to X-ray photons, whereas 99% is transformed as heat.

Power Supply

It provides:

- Low-voltage current to heat the tungsten filament by a step-down transformer.
- High-voltage current to generate a high potential difference between the cathode and anode by a step-up transformer.

Timer

It controls the X-ray production through step down transformer by allowing high current at low voltage supply to heat up the cathode filament. Once the filament temperature reaches the required mA to produce electrons, the timer allows high voltage low current supply to direct the electrons towards the anode.

Steps in X-ray Production

- *Production of high speed electrons—thermionic emission*: When the cathode filament is heated to incandescence, its atoms absorb energy. When the outer orbital electrons acquire high energy, they move away from the surface by a process called thermionic emission. The application of large potential difference across the electrodes accelerates the electrons at high speed from cathode towards anode target.
- *Focusing of electrons*: The focusing cup converge the electron beam towards the focal spot of the target.
- *Stopping of high-speed electrons and production of X-rays*: When the fast moving electrons strike the target, the electrons interact with target and produce X-rays by two processes.
  1. **Bremsstrahlung radiation** (General radiation): Bremse = Brake; strahl = ray. When the high speed traveling electrons are suddenly stopped by hitting the target, X-rays are produced by energy conversion. The energy of the resulting X-ray photons is in a continuous spectrum and dental X-ray machines majorly produces this type of X-rays (Fig. 2).
  2. **Characteristic radiation:** Minor source of radiation in X-ray tube and produced when electrons have sufficient energy to ionize the tungsten atom of target focal spot.

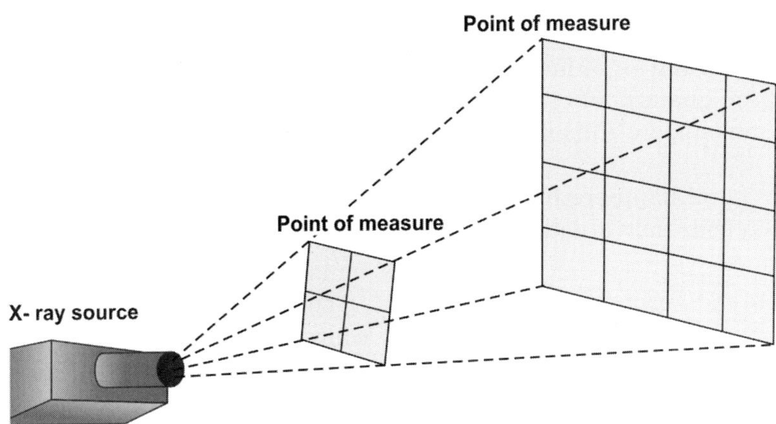

Fig. 2: Inverse square law.

2. Describe the factors controlling the production of X-rays. (or) list the factors that control the quality and quantity of the X-ray beam. (or) enumerate the factors involved in the production of X-rays.

Factors Controlling the Quality of X-ray Beam

Quality describes the mean energy or penetrating ability of the X-ray beam.

Voltage

Voltage refers to the potential difference between two electrical charges.

In X-ray tubehead, voltage is the electrical force that causes electrons to move from cathode to anode.

When voltage is increased, speed and energy of electrons are increased resulting in high penetrating X-ray beam.

↑Voltage → ↑speed and energy of electrons → ↑Penetrating power of X-ray beam.

Voltage is measured in volts and kilovolts. Dental X-ray units operate using kilovolts of 65 to 100 Kv.

Kilovoltage Peak

Kilovoltage peak (kVp) or peak voltage.

kVp regulates the speed and energy of the electrons.

↑kVp → high energy X-ray → highly penetrating X-ray beam.

Density and kVp

Density is the overall darkness of the image.

Adjustment in kVp results in change in the density of the radiograph.

Contrast and kVp

Contrast refers how sharply the dark and light areas are differentiated in an image.

When low kVp settings are used (65–70 kVp), high contrast image results.

kVp adjustment	Density	Contrast
↑kVp	↑(Dark image)	Low
↓kVp	↓(Light image)	High

Exposure Time and kVp

Exposure time is the period when X-rays are produced.

An adjustment in exposure time is needed when kVp is altered to compensate the penetrating power.

↑kVp → ↓Exposure time and vice versa.

Factors Controlling the Quantity of the X-ray

Quantity denotes the number of X-ray photons.

Milliamperage

Regulates the temperature of the cathode filament and so the quantity of X-rays.

↑Milliamperage → ↑cathode filament temperature → ↑number of electrons.

Milliampere-Seconds

Both milliampere and exposure time directly influences the quantity of electrons. The product of milliampere and exposure time, is mA.

Increase in milliampere increases the overall density and results in darker image and vice versa.

↑Milliampere and ↓ exposure seconds or vice versa.

Factors Influencing both Quantity and Quality

Intensity is used to describe both quantity and quality together.

It is the product of quantity and quality/unit of area/unit of time exposure.

$$\frac{\text{Intensity} = \text{kVp} \times \text{mA}}{(\text{Area}) \times (\text{Exposure})}$$

Higher kVp and mA produces an X-ray beam with higher energy.

Inverse Square Law

The intensity of radiation beam is inversely proportional to the square of distance from the source (Fig. 2).

$$\frac{I_1}{I_2} = \frac{D_2^2}{D_1^2}, \text{ Or}$$

$$\frac{\text{Original intensity} = (\text{New distance})^2}{\text{New intensity} = (\text{Original distance})^2}$$

Filtration

Use of 1.5 mm thick aluminium for dental X-ray machines operating at 70 kVp will result in removal of low energy photons and increase in the penetrating energy of the beam.

Collimation

Round and rectangular collimators are used to reduce the X-ray beam size and therefore the amount of tissue irradiated Intraoral radiographic machines collimate the beam size to a circle with 7 cm diameter. This beam size reduction reduces the volume of tissue irradiation and thereby the radiation dose.

3. Describe dosimetry. (or) define the units of radiation measurement.

Dosimetry is the measure amount of radiation exposure or radiation dose. Dose describes the amount of energy absorbed by unit mass of interest. Exposure is a measure of ability of the radiation to produce ionization in air under standard temperature and pressure.

The measurement units are referred as conventional and traditional units, e.g. roentgen, radiation absorbed dose (rad) and roentgen man (rem). To standardize unit to metric system, conventional units are replaced by International System of Units, e.g. coulomb per kilogram (C/Kg), Gray and sievert.

Exposure

The quantity of ionization generated by X-rays in air is described as exposure.

The traditional unit of exposure for X-rays is roentgen.

Roentgen is the quantity of X-radiation that produces an electrical charge of 2.58×10^{-4}

Coulombs in a kilogram of air under standard temperature and pressure.

Roentgen is essentially limited to measurement in air.

No SI unit equal to roentgen exists. Exposure is simply stated in coulombs per kilograms which measures the number of ion pairs in 1 kg of air.

Absorbed Dose

The amount of radiation energy absorbed per unit mass is termed as radiation absorbed dose or rad—the traditional unit.

Rad is a unit that describes the absorbed dose of radiation capable of accumulating 100 ergs of energy in a gram of tissue (100 erg/g)

The SI Unit equivalent to rad is Gray, and 1 rad = 0.01 Gy.

Dose Equivalent

The assessment of biological effects caused by various form of radiation is known as dose equivalent.

Rem (roentgen equivalent man) is the traditional unit.

Rem is the product of absorbed dose and a quality factor specific for the type of radiation.

The SI Unit of the rem is sievert (sv) and 1 sv = 100 rem.

Effective Dose

The effective dose is used to determine the radiation risk in humans. It is the sum of product of equivalent dose to each organ or tissue (H_T) and the tissue weighting factor (W_T)

The unit of effective dose is sievert. The tissue weighing factor for bone marrow is 0.12 and for bone surface and skin is 0.01.

Radioactivity

The measurement of radioactivity describes the decay rate of sample of radioactive material.

The SI unit is becquerel (Bq). 1 Bq equals 1 disintigration/second.

The traditional unit is curie.

Measurements Used in Dental Radiography

In dental radiography, the Gray and Sievert are equal and the roentgen, rad and rem are approximately equal.

The prefix "milli", meaning 1/1,000 allows expressing the small quantities of exposure, dose and dose equivalent. (For example milliard).

SHORT NOTES

1. Describe particulate radiation.

Particulate radiations are atoms or subatomic particles that have mass and travel at high speed to transmit their kinetic energy. They are emitted by radioactive substances called radionuclides.

Four types of particulate radiations are recognized which are as follows:

1. *Electrons*: Based on their origin, electros are subclassified into:
   a. Beta particles: Fast moving electrons emitted by a radioactive nucleus.
   b. Cathode rays: Streams of high speed electrons generated in an X-ray tube.
2. *Alpha particles*: They are emitted by the nuclei of heavy metals. Alpha particles have two protons, two neutrons and no electrons.
3. *Protons*: Accelerated hydrogen nuclei carrying a mass of 1 and charge of +1
4. *Neutrons*: Accelerated neutral particles with mass of 1.

2. What are electromagnetic radiation? (or) what is electromagnetic spectrum?

Electromagnetic energy is defined as the propagation of wave like energy in oscillating electric and magnetic fields that are perpendicular to each other. Electromagnetic spectrum is grouping of waves according to their energy level and speed with which they travel.

Examples of electromagnetic radiation: X-rays, gamma rays, cosmic rays, visible light, infrared rays, ultraviolet rays, microwaves, radio waves and radar waves.

They travel through space either as:

- Particle—possessing bundle of energy called photons or quanta with no mass and travel at speed of light.
- Wave—possessing the properties of wavelength, velocity and frequency.

3. Write the properties of electromagnetic radiations.

- Have no mass, weight or electrical charge.
- Travel at the speed of light = 3 × 1,86,000 miles/second (or) 108 meters/second.
- Travel in both particle and wave form.
- Waves possess different measurable energies like frequencies, wavelength and particles possess quantum energy.
- Propagate in electric and magnetic fields that are perpendicular to each other.

4. Outline the properties of X-rays.

X-rays are weightless particles of pure energy (photons) that have no electrical charge and travel in waves.

- X-rays are invisible and cannot be detected by any senses.
- X-rays possess no mass and no weight
- X-rays travel with speed of light (3×10^{-8} m/s)

- X-rays travel in a wave form with wide range of wavelengths (0.01–0.05 nm) and high frequency.
- X-rays travel in straight line. They can be scattered from the original direction but the new trajectory is linear.
- X-rays cannot be focused to a point.
- X-rays penetrate the materials which absorbs or reflect light.
- X-rays are differently absorbed by matter and this depends on the penetration ability of the X-rays and atomic structure of the material.
- The absorption property of X-rays produce an image on the photographic film which in turn can be made visible by processing.
- X-rays ionize materials.
- X-rays produce biological changes in living tissue and this property is helpful in radiotherapy.
- X-rays cause certain substances to fluoresce in longer wavelength.

5. Briefly describe Bremsstrahlung radiation. (or) describe braking or general radiation.

When electrons from the cathode filament hit the target in the anode, many electrons interact with the tungsten atom undergo *many interactions* within the target. The radiation produced in this manner is known as *general radiation* or *braking radiation (bremsstrahlung radiation).*

Bremse = Brake ; Strahl = Ray

Sudden stopping of high-speed electrons when hit the anode in the tungsten target in the anode X-rays are produced (Fig. 3).

General radiation is produced when an electron hit the nucleus or when passes very close to the nucleus of the tungsten atom.

The electron that misses the nucleus continue to interact many times producing lower energy X-rays before it imparts all of its kinetic energy.

About 70% of the X-ray energy produced in the anode is general radiation and the photons have continuous spectrum of energy.

6. Define scattering and explain about Compton scatter.

The tendency of X-ray photon to deviate from its path when passing through a matter is known as scattering.

When an X-ray photon collides with a loosely bound outer orbital electron of an atom, it gives up part of its energy to eject the electron from its orbit and produces *ionization*. The emitted electron is known as *Compton electron* or *recoil electron* and the atom becomes positive charged ion (Fig. 4).

After ionization, the X-ray photon carries a low energy level and moves in an altered direction (scattering). The low energy X-ray photon keeps interacting with other atoms and completely liberates its energy.

In dental X-ray units, 62% of scatter radiation is Compton scattering.

7. Describe about coherent scatter.

Coherent scatter or unmodified scatter occurs when a low energy X-ray photon interacts with outer orbital electrons. No change in the atom occurs, and scattered photons are produced. The X-ray photon is scattered in different direction from that of incident photon (Fig. 5). There is no loss of energy and no occurrence of ionization and the X-ray photons simply undergo a change in direction hence it is known as *unmodified* rays.

Coherent scatter accounts for 8% of the interactions in dental X-ray beam.

8. What is characteristic radiation and how it is produced?

Characteristic radiation is produced when a high-speed electron hits and removes one of its *inner orbital electrons* of tungsten target. This creates a void in the tungsten atom.

Another *outer orbital electron* is attracted by the void to replace the dislodged electron. This results in the emission of a photon with an energy equivalent to the difference in two orbital binding energies. The X-rays produced by these interactions are known as characteristic radiation.

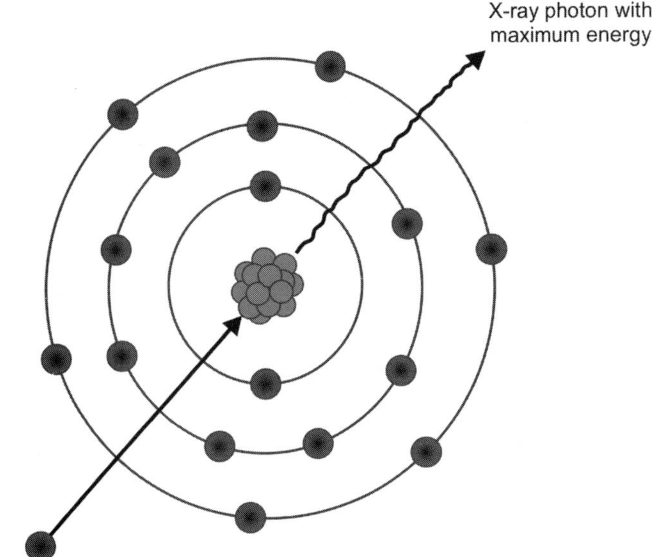

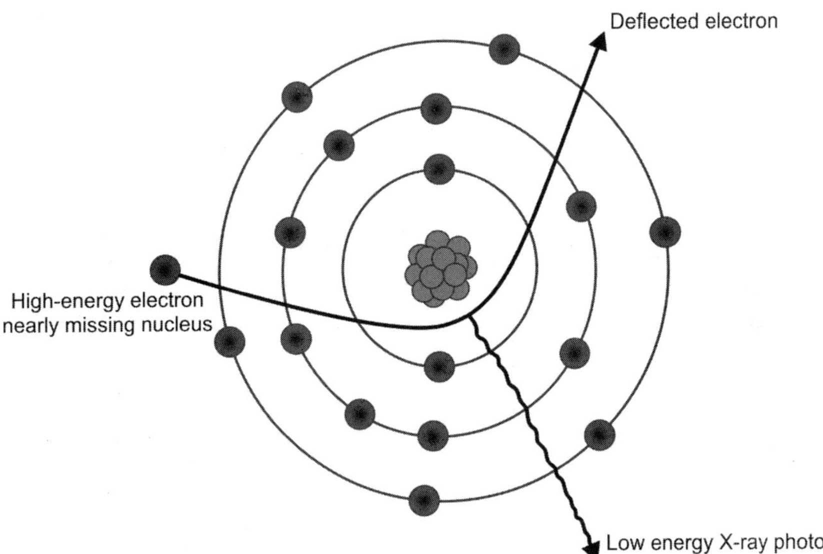

Fig. 3: Bremsstrahlung radiation.

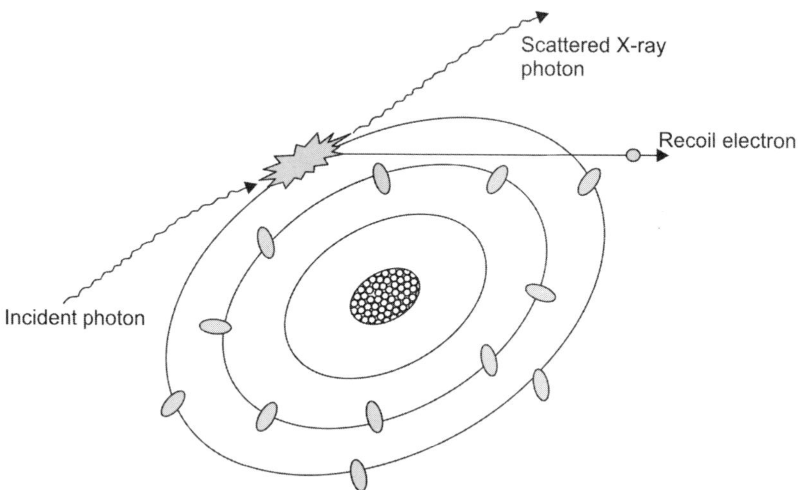

Fig. 4: Compton scatter.

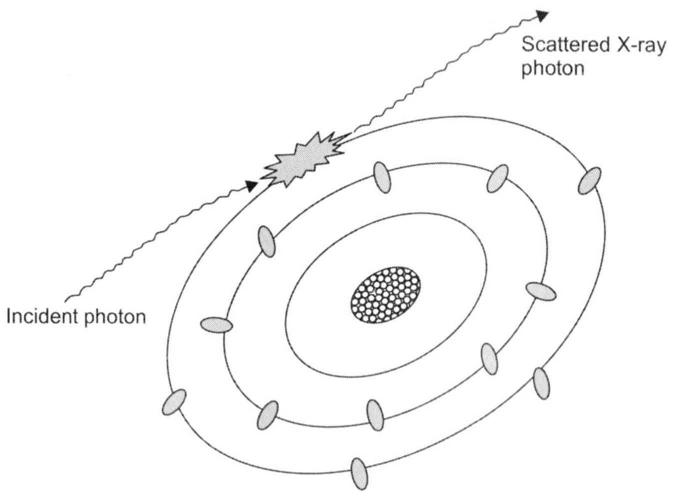

Fig. 5: Coherent scatter.

This type of radiation is very minimal the dental X-ray machine and occurs at 70 kVp or above.

9. Name the types of anode used in X-ray tube.

X-ray machines use stationary and rotating types of anode.

In *stationary anodes, oil* is circulating between the glass envelop and tube housing for the purpose of dissipating the heat from target.

In *rotating anodes*, the tungsten is in the form of bevelled disk that rotates when the tube is in function. As a result, electrons will strike the successive areas of the target and distribute the heat over an extended area.

10. Describe the effects of X-ray photons after they exit the tubehead.

When the diagnostic x-ray photons reaches the patient:

- It may travel through the patient with no interaction

- It may get absorbed by the body structure
- It may be scattered to different direction.

No interaction: About 9% of primary X-ray photons pass through patient tissues without producing any interaction and leaves.

Photoelectric absorption: When the incident photon collides with orbital electrons, it gives up its energy to dislodge the electron from the atom and the process is known as ionization. The electron ejected from the shell is called as *photoelectron or recoil electron* possesses negative charge and the remaining atom hold positive charge and become positive ion. About 30% of dental X-ray photons are absorbed by photoelectric effect.

Thompson scatter (coherent or unmodified scatter): When a low energy incident photon passes near the low energy outer orbital electron, the photon is not absorbed but scattered without a loss of energy (Fig. 5). The incident photon interacts with the electron by vibrating it momentarily and then disappears. The coherent scatters contribute little to film fog.

Compton scatter: The incident photon collides with a loosely bound outer shell electron and looses only part of its energy to eject an electron from its orbit (Fig. 4). This ionization results in a negatively charged. Compton electron, a photon of scattered radiation, and a remaining positively charged atom. About 62% of the photons undergo Compton scattering.

MULTIPLE CHOICE QUESTIONS

1. The fundamental unit of mater is known ***atom***.
   a. Atom
   b. Element
   c. Ion
   d. Particle
2. Atomic number of hydrogen is ***one***.
   a. Zero
   b. One
   c. Two
   d. Four
3. Neutral atom consists of ***equal number of protons and electrons***.
   a. Two protons and two electrons
   b. Equal number of protons and neutrons
   c. Two protons and two neutrons
   d. Equal number of protons and electrons
4. Electrically unbalanced atom is known as ***ion***.
   a. Orbital electron
   b. Orbital shell
   c. Ion
   d. Trace element
5. The electrostatic attraction between nucleus and electrons is known as ***binding energy***.
   a. Electrostatic force
   b. Binding energy
   c. Nuclear affinity
   d. Bond strength
6. Binding energy for K-shell electron is ***70 keV***.
   a. 90 kv
   b. 90 keV
   c. 70 kv
   d. 70 keV
7. The amount of energy required to remove an electron from its orbit is ***equal to greater than its binding energy***.
   a. Equal to outer shell energy
   b. Equal to or less than outer shell energy
   c. Equal to or less than binding energy
   d. Equal to greater than its binding energy
8. One or two atoms joined by chemical bonds is known as ***molecule***.
   a. Atom
   b. Ion
   c. Molecule
   d. Element
9. Atom without nucleus is known as ***ion***.
   a. Neutron
   b. Ion
   c. Molecule
   d. Element
10. The distance between the crests of two waves is defined as ***wavelength***.
    a. Wavelength
    b. Frequency
    c. Amplitude
    d. Intensity
11. The wavelength of radiation determines the ***penetrating power***.
    a. The distance of the wave
    b. Energy
    c. The speed of the wave
    d. Penetrating power

12. Unit of wavelength is ***nanometer***.
    a. Millimeter
    b. Micrometer
    c. Microns
    d. Nanometer
    (**Note:** 1 nm = 10^{-9} m).
13. The energy of electromagnetic radiation is determined by ***wavelength and frequency***.
    a. Wavelength and frequency
    b. Wavelength and intensity
    c. Intensity and frequency
    d. Amplitude and speed
14. Diagnostic X-rays are ***high frequency and short wavelength rays***.
    a. High frequency and long wavelength rays
    b. Low frequency and long wavelength rays
    c. Low frequency and short wavelength rays
    d. High frequency and short wavelength rays
15. The wavelength of X-rays used in dentistry is ***0.01 nm***.
    a. 0.1 nm
    b. 0.01 nm
    c. 0.001 nm
    d. 0.0001 nm
16. The electrical current to the filament of X-ray tube is regulated by ***low voltage circuit***.
    a. High voltage circuit
    b. Low voltage circuit
    c. Low current circuit
    d. High voltage and low current
17. X-rays are produced at ***positive anode***.
    a. Tungsten filament
    b. Positive anode
    c. Negative cathode
    d. Copper target
18. Thermionic emission occurs at ***negative cathode***.
    a. Tungsten filament
    b. Positive anode
    c. Negative cathode
    d. Copper stem
19. Compton scatter accounts for ***62% of X-ray produced at anode***.
    a. 30% of X-ray produced at anode
    b. 8% of X-ray produced at anode
    c. 62% of X-ray produced at anode
    d. 98% of X-ray produced at anode
20. Photoelectric absorption accounts for ***30% of X-ray produced at anode***.
    a. 30% of X-ray produced at anode
    b. 8% of X-ray produced at anode
    c. 62% of X-ray produced at anode
    d. 98% of X-ray produced at anode
21. Coherent scatter accounts for ***8% of X-ray energy produced at anode***.
    a. 30% of X-ray energy produced at anode
    b. 8% of X-ray energy produced at anode
    c. 62% of X-ray energy produced at anode
    d. 98% of X-ray energy produced at anode
22. Coherent or Thompson scatter occurs when ***low energy X-rays interact with matter***.
    a. Low energy X-rays interact with matter
    b. Electrons collide with air
    c. High energy X-rays interact with matter
    d. Electrons collide with each other
23. 70% of X-ray energy produced at anode is ***Bremsstrahlung radiation***.
    a. Characteristic radiation
    b. Bremsstrahlung radiation
    c. Heat waves
    d. Kinetic energy
    (**Note:** General or braking or bremsstrahlung radiation).
24. Characteristic radiation are produced in dental X-ray tube when using kVp of ***70 or above***.
    a. 100 or above
    b. 70 or above
    c. 10 or above
    d. 50 or above
25. Most common type of scatter in X-ray tube is ***compton scatter***.
    a. Coherent scatter
    b. Compton scatter
    c. Selective scatter
    d. Dynamic scatter
26. The quality of X-ray beam is controlled by ***kilovoltage peak***.
    a. Milliampere
    b. Kilovoltage peak
    c. Kilowatt
    d. Electron volt
27. Dental radiographic unit functions at ***65–100 kV***.
    a. 90–120 kV
    b. 90–120 mA
    c. 65–100 kV
    d. 65–100 mA

28. Use of 65–75 kV produce X-rays of ***low energy, less penetrating, longer wavelength***.
    a. Low energy, less penetrating, shorter wavelength
    b. High energy, less penetrating, shorter wavelength
    c. High energy, high penetrating, longer wavelength
    d. Low energy, less penetrating, longer wavelength
29. Higher kilovoltage produces X-rays with ***high energy, high penetrating, short wavelength***.
    a. Low energy, less penetrating, short wavelength
    b. High energy, less penetrating, short wavelength
    c. High energy, high penetrating, longer wavelength
    d. Low energy, less penetrating, longer wavelength
30. The quantity of radiation is controlled by ***milliamperage and exposure time***.
    a. Milliamperage and exposure time
    b. Milliamperage and kilovoltage
    c. Kilovoltage and exposure time
    d. Inverse square law
31. Milliamperage regulates ***cathode temperature and quantity of X-ray photons***.
    a. Cathode temperature and exposure time
    b. Quality of X-ray photons and tube voltage
    c. Cathode temperature and quantity of X-ray photons
    d. Potential difference between cathode and anode
32. Milliamperage preferred for dental X-ray tube is ***7–15 mA***.
    a. 10–15 mA
    b. 7–15 mA
    c. 60–75 mA
    d. 40–55 mA
33. If the length of position indicating device is changed from 16 inches to 8 inches, the resultant beam intensity will be ***four times more intense***.
    a. Two times more intense
    b. Two times less intense
    c. Four times more intense
    d. Four times less intense
34. Roentgen is useful for exposure measure of ***X-rays and gamma rays alone***.
    a. X-rays and alpha rays alone
    b. X-rays alone
    c. X-rays and gamma rays alone
    d. X-rays, alpha and gamma rays alone
35. The heat storage capacity for the dental X-ray tube anode is ***20 kHU***.
    a. 2 kHU
    b. 20 kHU
    c. 120 kHU
    d. 200 kHU

(**Note:** HU = heat unit).

VIVA VOCE

1. What is radiation?

Radiation is the production and transmission of energy through a space or a substance in the form of waves or particles.

2. What is ionizing radiation?

Radiation is capable of producing an ion by removing or adding an electron to an atom is known as ionizing radiation. They can be classified into:

a. Particulate radiation and
b. Electromagnetic radiation.

3. What is primary radiation?

The X-ray beam produced at the target and exits the tube head is referred as primary radiation or useful beam.

4. What is secondary radiation?

The X-radiation that is generated when the primary beam interacts with soft tissues and bones of head and neck region.

5. What are scatter radiation?

Scatter radiation is produced when a X-ray beam interact with matter and get deviated away from the original path. They travel through the patient's body and the X-ray room. In this way, the scattered rays are dangerous for both patient and operator.

6. What is radioactivity?

Radioactivity is spontaneous decay or disintegration of some unstable atoms or elements to attain a more stable state by giving off energy as rays or particles.

7. Name the two types of X-rays produce in X-ray tube.

a. General or braking radiation (or) Bremsstrahlung radiation
b. Characteristic radiation.

8. Why tungsten selected as filament material?

- High atomic number
- High melting point (3370°C)
- Low vapor pressure
- Property of drawing into thin wire.

9. What is the purpose of using copper in anode?

Copper has good thermal conductivity and reduces the risk of target melting by dissipating heat.

10. Give few examples for particulate radiation.

Alpha particles, beta particles and cathode rays (electrons), protons and neutrons.

11. Give few examples for electromagnetic radiation.

Cosmic rays, X-rays, gamma rays, visible light, ultraviolet rays, infrared rays, radio waves and microwaves.

12. What happens when a high voltage circuit is activated in X-ray tube?

- Cathode electrons are accelerated towards the anode
- X-rays travel from filament to target
- Heat is produced.

13. What is half value layer?

Half value layer (HVL) is the thickness of filter material, e.g. aluminium that reduce the beam intensity by half. HVL determines the penetrating power of the beam. Higher the HVL, greater will be the penetrating power.

14. What is tube rating?

Tube rating defines the maximal exposure time for the tube to function without any damage to the target due to overheating. The manufacturer defines the tube rating specification for each X-ray machine.

Tube rating = the range of kVp and mA for the maximal safe intervals (ms).

15. What is duty cycle?

It is the amount of successive exposures that can be made within a particular period (frequency of exposure). The interval between the consecutive exposures must be sufficient to allow the heat dissipation in the anode.

BIBLIOGRAPHY

1. Barratt MR, Pool SL, editors. Principles of clinical medicine for space flight. Springer Science & Business Media; 2008.
2. Karjodkar FR. Essentials of oral and maxillofacial radiology. Jaypee Brothers, Medical Publishers Pvt. Limited; 2014.
3. Keith S, Murray HE, Spoo W. Toxicological profile for ionizing radiation. Atlanta, Georgia, USA. Agency for Toxic Substances and Disease Registry. ATSDR; 1999.
4. Langland OE, Langlais RP, Preece JW. Principles of dental imaging. Lippincott Williams and Wilkins; Baltimore; 2002.
5. Seeram E. Radiation dose in computed tomography. Radiol Technol. 1999;70(6): 534-52.
6. Stoeckl C, Glebov VY, Meyerhofer DD, et al. Hard x-ray detectors for OMEGA and NIF. Review of Scientific Instruments. 2001; 72(1):1197-200.
7. Whaites E, Drage N. Essentials of dental radiography and radiology. Elsevier Health Sciences; 2013.
8. White SC, Pharoah MJ. Principles and interpretation. St Louis. 2014:431-3.

CHAPTER 27

Radiation Biology

HIGHLIGHTS

This section enlightens the effects of *ionizing radiation* on biological molecules, cells, tissues, and organs. The interactions are through the water or organic molecules and resulting in *free radicals* formation which causes cell destruction. There is wide variation among different cells and organs regarding their response and effects that may occur either immediately or progressively over a period.

Learners are expected to study:

- Different effects of radiation
- Radiation effects on biomolecule, cells, tissues, and organs
- Effects of radiation on oral and perioral structures
- Relative radiosensitivity of various tissues and organs.

ESSAY QUESTIONS

1. Describe the effects of radiation on various biological systems. (or) describe the biological changes following radiation exposure. (or) write about the radiation induced changes in different body structures.

Radiation acts on biological system through direct and indirect effects and produces free radicals.

Direct effects: Biological molecules are ionized following radiation. The resulting free radicals alter the original molecules and create biological changes.

RH (original molecule) + X-ray photon $\rightarrow$ R^0 + H^+ + e^-

R^0 = Free radical

Indirect effects: Radiation exposure results in the radiolysis of water leading to the formation of *free radicals and oxidizing toxins* like peroxyl radicals and hydrogen peroxide which in turn causes biological changes and cellular destructions.

These free radicals and toxins affect:

- Biological molecules
- Intercellular structures
- Cell kinetics
- Tissues and organs.

Effects on Biomolecules

Nucleic acids: Radiation targets DNA of nucleic acids and produces:

- Changes or loss of a base
- Disruption of hydrogen bonding
- Breakage of DNA strands
- Cross-linking of DNA strands.

Proteins: Radiation exposure alters the secondary and tertiary structures of proteins leading to denaturation. Enzymes get inactivated and failed to participate in biological reactions. Moderate amount of radiation dose (2–4 Gray) is required to induce protein denaturation.

Effects at Intracellular Level

Chromosomal aberrations: During mitosis, DNA condenses to form chromosomes.

When radiation exposure occurs after DNA synthesis (in G2, mid and late S—late mitosis), *chromatic aberration* (single arm breakage) is the result (Figs. 1 and 2).

Chromosomal aberration (double arm breakage) occurs if exposure happened before DNA synthesis in G1 or early S phase (Figs. 1 and 3).

Chromosomal aberrations are noticeable in peripheral blood lymphocytes and serve as markers to identify the extent of radiation damage.

Cytoplasm

Larger doses of radiation (30–50 Gray) cause mitochondrial damage in rapidly dividing cells.

Changes in Cell Kinetics

A mitotic delay occurs on rapidly dividing cells following irradiation.

A moderate dose causes longer mitotic delay resulting in smaller sized cells and some cell death. Larger doses produce severe mitotic

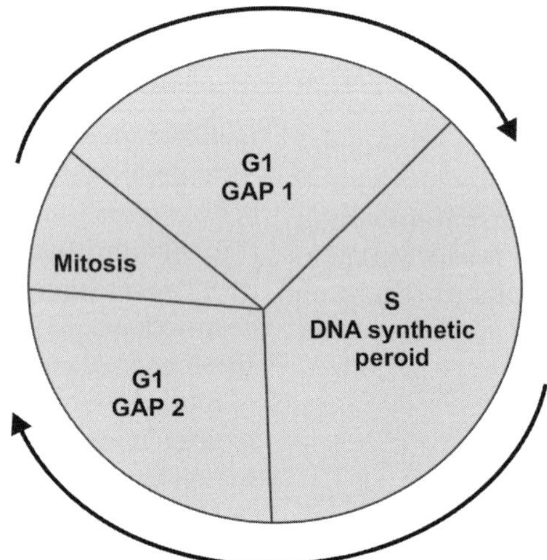

Fig. 1: Cell Cycle: cell moves in the cycle from mitosis to gap 1 (G1) to DNA synthesis *(S) to gap 2 (G2) and again* to the next mitosis.

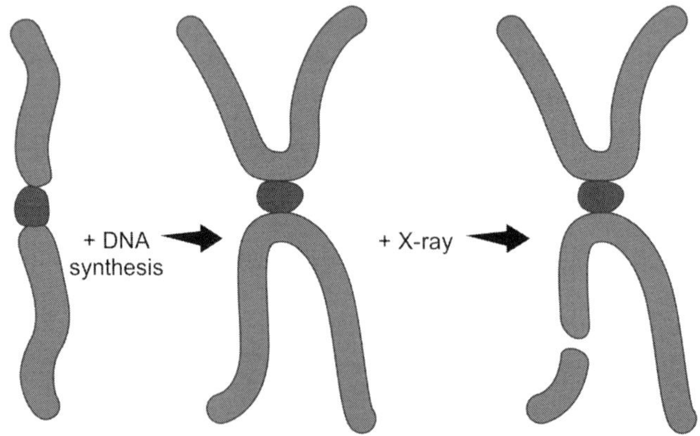

Fig. 2: Irradiation of the cell after DNA synthesis results in a single arm (chromatid) aberration.

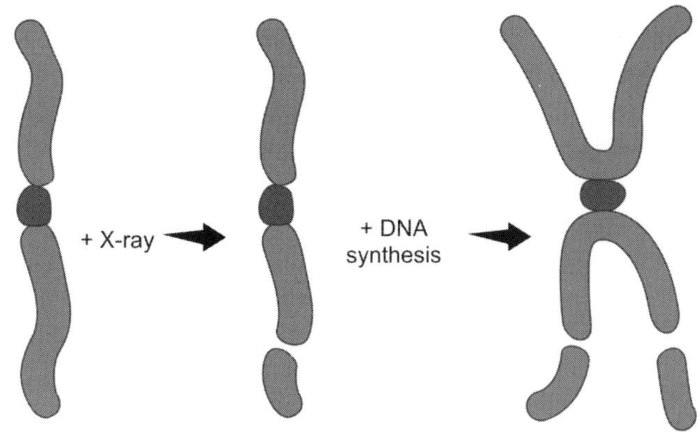

Fig. 3: Irradiation before DNA synthesis results in a double arm (chromosome) aberration.

delay with loss of dividing capacity and cell death.

Effects on Tissues and Organs

Depends on the response to radiation, tissues and organs are classified as radiosensitive and radioresistant. These results further depend on the dose and quantity of cell death.

Tissues and Organs Response to Radiation

Based on their radiation response, various tissues and organs are classified as highly radiosensitive, intermediate radiosensitive, and radioresistant (Table 1).

2. Describe the effects of radiation on oral and paraoral structures. (or) describe the hazards of therapeutic radiation on oral and paraoral structures.

Radiotherapy induces deterministic effects on the oral cavity. The following hazardous effects are expected for the total dose of *50 Gy over 5 weeks.*

Oral Mucosa

Mucositis: After 2 weeks of radiotherapy, oral mucosa becomes *erythematosus* and tender. If therapy is continued, mucous membrane breaks down and form *ulcers*, covered by the yellow pseudomembranous slough.

It is a highly painful condition. Opportunistic local *fungal infection* is common at this stage.

Long-term effects occur due to the gradual obliteration of the blood vessels and fibrosis of the connective tissues. The mucosa becomes *thin, atrophic and avascular.*

Medical Management

Pain can be managed with nonopioid analgesics alone or in combination with opioids.

Topical anesthetic agents like benzydamine hydrochloride and an antifungal lozenge containing polymixin, tobramycin, and amphotericin-b will be effective.

Table 1: Tissues and organs response to radiation.

Highly radiosensitive (exposure dose ≤2,500 rad)	Intermediate radosensitive (exposure dose 2,500–5,000 rad)	Radioresistant (exposure dose >5,000 rad)
▪ Lymphoid organs like spleen and bone marrow ▪ Reproductive organs ▪ The mucous membrane of the intestine and oral cavity	▪ Blood vessels and endothelial cells ▪ Growing bone and cartilage ▪ Salivary glands ▪ Liver ▪ Lungs ▪ Kidney	▪ Optic lens ▪ Mature erythrocytes ▪ Muscles ▪ Nerves

Effects on Oral Mucosa

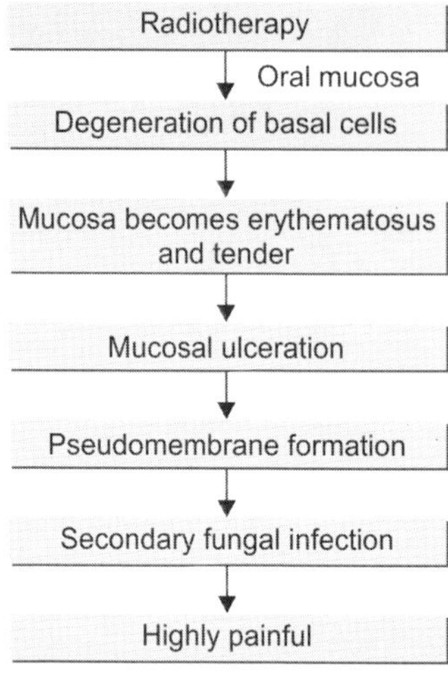

Taste Buds

Radiotherapy causes severe *degeneration of the taste buds.* Patients experience loss of taste sensation at the second or third week.

Taste sensitivity may decrease by 1,000–10,000 times that of normal and may lead to the state of near insensitivity. Taste sensation may regain between 60–120 days.

Effects on Taste Buds

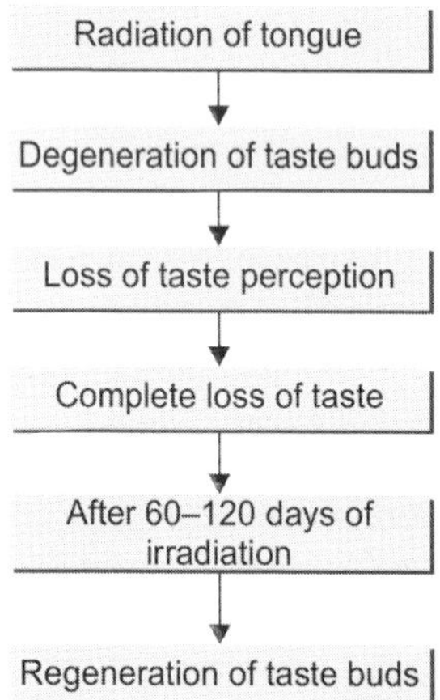

Salivary Glands

- When major salivary glands are exposed to radiation, progressive reduction in salivary secretion occurs.
- The total dose of *6,000 Gy for 5 weeks cause irreversible effects* like necrosis of serous cells, vascular atrophy and progressive fibrosis of gland leading to 50% reduction in total secretion.
- Thick, viscous secretion leads to *dryness of mouth.* Salivary PH is reduced. After 6–12 months of radiotherapy, the salivary flow rate is improved. Xerostomia persisting more than a year has less chance for recovery.

Medical Management

Use of sialagogues like pilocarpine 15 mg/day will stimulate the salivary secretion.

Teeth

Radiation effects on teeth vary according to the developmental stage.

If radiotherapy is indicated.

Before calcification: It may destroy the tooth bud.

After calcification: Dwarfed tooth, retarded root or failure to form one or few teeth.

Adult teeth are resistant to radiotherapy.

Radiation Caries

Definition: Radiation caries develops in patients who have undergone radiotherapy in head and neck region that includes exposure to salivary glands. Salivary changes like reduced flow, decreased PH, reduced buffering capacity and high viscosity initiates a rampant carious lesion.

Classification of Radiation Induced Caries

1. *Widespread superficial form:* Most common type. It affects palatal, lingual, buccal, occlusal and incisal surfaces.
2. *Cervical caries:* Cementum and dentin in the cervical region get affected. The lesion may progress circumferentially around the teeth resulting in loss of crown.
3. *Pigmentation type:* Dark pigmentation of the entire crown. The incisal margin may worn out.

Management

- Avoidance of dietary sucrose

- Daily topical application of 1% neutral sodium fluoride gel.
- Good oral hygiene and restorative procedures.

Bone

Irradiation of mandible causes:
- Obliteration of periosteal vasculatures
- Destruction of osteoblasts and osteoclasts
- Replacement of marrow with fat and fibrous connective tissues.

These changes result in:
- Hypovascular, hypocellular, hypoxic marrow tissues
- Endosteal atrophy
- Empty lacunae of compact bone and brittleness.

Postradiation osteoradionecrosis (PRON): PRON is the severe complication following irradiation.

Management: Hyperbaric oxygen therapy.

Facial Skin

Erythema is the early sign which fads quickly. Later changes cause progressive fibrosis and give a woody consistency.

Summary

Radiation produces adverse effects on oral structures which depends on the duration, frequency, and dose of radiation therapy. The response of different oral structures also varies in severity (Table 2).

Table 2: Effects of radiation on oral and paraoral structures.

Structure	Radiation effect
Oral mucosa	Mucositis ▪ Erythema ▪ Tenderness ▪ Ulceration ▪ Fungal infection ▪ Thin and atrophic
Taste buds	▪ Degeneration of taste buds ▪ Loss of taste perception ▪ Complete loss of taste sensation
Salivary glands	▪ Destruction of acinar cells ▪ Thick scanty viscous saliva ▪ Reduction of salivary pH
Teeth	Before calcification Destruction of tooth bud After calcification ▪ Dwarfed tooth ▪ Retarded root ▪ Absence of few teeth Radiation caries ▪ Widespread superficial form ▪ Cervical caries ▪ Pigmentation type
Bone	Osteoradionecrosis
Facial skin	▪ Erythema ▪ Edema ▪ Denudation ▪ Woody consistency

Contd...

Contd...

SHORT NOTES

1. Describe the deterministic effects of radiation. (or) describe the nonstochastic radiation effects.

The biological effects of ionizing radiation are broadly classified into two forms:
1. Deterministic effects (or) nonstochastic effects
2. Stochastic effects.

Deterministic outcomes are those in which the **radiation dose** determines the *severity of biological effects* and is directionally proportional. The radiation dose has a threshold value.
- The biological effects occur in *all patients* receiving radiation *above the threshold limit.*
- When the patient's radiation *dose is less than the threshold limit,* no response will occur.

Nonstochastic effects require larger doses to cause saviour impairment of health.

Examples:

- Oral changes following radiotherapy.
- Acute radiation syndrome following whole body irradiation.
- Cataract formation.

2. Describe the stochastic effects of radiation.

The biological effects of ionizing radiation are broadly classified into two forms.

a. Deterministic effects
b. Stochastic effects

In stochastic effects, the **radiation dose** determines the *probability for developing a biological effect rather* than the severity of effects.

- The radiation dose determines the adverse incidence
- Stochastic effects follow ***all or none*** law. Following radiation, a person either has or does not have the adverse effects.

Examples:

- Radiation induced cancer
- Increased radiation exposure to a person or population increases only the probability of cancer and not its severity.

3. Classify the cell types based on their response to radiation. (or) write the classification of mammalian cells based on radiosensitivity. (or) categorize the radioresponse of different cells.

Different cells of the same individual respond differently to radiation.

1. **Vegetative intermitotic cells**:
   a. These are most radiosensitive:
      Examples:
      - Early precursor cells like spermatogenic or erythroblastic series
      - Basal cells of the oral mucous membrane

   b. They divide at regular intervals.
   c. They have long mitotic futures.
   d. They do not differentiate between mitoses.
   e. These cells retain their primitive properties and replace themselves.
2. **Differentiating intermitotic cells**:
   a. These cells are radiosensitive but slightly lesser extent than vegetative intermitotic cells:
      Examples:
      - Intermediate dividing and replicating cells of inner enamel epithelium
      - Hematopoietic cells in the intermediate stage of differentiation
      - Spermatocytes and oocytes.

   b. They divide regularly but with less frequency.
   c. These cells undergo some differentiation between mitoses.
3. **Multipotent connective tissue cells:**
   a. These cells have intermediate radiosensitivity:
      Examples:
      - Vascular endothelial cells
      - Fibroblasts
      - Mesenchymal cells.

   b. They divide irregularly and when there is a demand for more cells.
   c. They undergo limited amount of differentiation.
4. **Reverting postmitotic cells:**
   a. These cells are radioresistant:
      Examples:
      - Acinar and ductal cells of salivary glands
      - Parenchymal cells of liver, thyroid, and kidney.

   b. They divide infrequently.
   c. These cells are highly specialized in function.
5. **Fixed postmitotic cells:**
   a. Most resistant type of cells:
      Example: Neurons, striated muscle cells, squamous epithelial cells.
   b. These are highly differentiated cells.
   c. They are incapable of the division following maturation.

4. Classify the radiation response of various tissues. (or) classify the organs and tissues based on their radiation response.

Radiosensitivity of an organ or tissue is measured by its response to irradiation (Table 1). If radiation induces a small amount of cell death in an organ, they undergo repair, and usually, there will not be any clinical effects. If it induces more cell death, there will be a strong clinical damage to the organ.

The severities of the changes are dose dependent.

5. What are the factors that modify the radioresponse of cells? (or) what are the factors that alter the cellular responses to radiation?

The variation in exposure parameters of radiation and cellular environment may alter the radioresponse of cells.

- **Dose:** The deterministic effects of radiation are dose dependent. If the total dose absorbed by an organ is less than the threshold limit, no adverse effects occur. If the total dose exceeds the threshold value, adverse effects occur in proportion to the dose received.
- **Dose rate:** Dose rate indicates the number of exposures in which the total dose is delivered.

  Exposure of a given dose at high rate cause severe biological damage than the same dose if given at lower rate. Lower dose rate allows for repair of damage and thereby less total damage.
- **Oxygen:** When radiation occurs at the hypoxic condition, cellular resistance to radiation increases by two to three times. Presence of oxygen during irradiation leads to the production of toxins and free radicals like hydrogen peroxide and hydroperoxyl radicals.
- **Linear energy transfer (LET):** LET is the amount of radiation energy transferred to tissues per distance traveled in that tissue. If the radiation has high linear energy like alpha particles, they deposit most of their ionizing energy in the small volume of tissues and induce more biological damage.

  The high LET of alpha particles results in greater ionization density and double strand breakage of DNA and so more severe biological damage than X-rays.

6. What is osteoradionecrosis?

Osteoradionecrosis is a pathological process of bone necrosis following a radiation exposure. The bone becomes devitalized (sequestration) and is complicated by pain and infection.

The mandible is affected commonly than maxilla due to its sparse vascularity.

Three etiological factors are recognized: Radiation, trauma, and infection.

Following radiation, the blood vessels are obliterated. The cellular marrow is replaced with fibrous tissues and infiltered by inflammatory cells resulting in **hypoxic, hypovascular, and hypocellular** marrow. The devitalized bone may undergo sequestration.

The hypovascularity increases the risk of infection. Microorganisms reach the bone from radiation-induced breakdown of oral mucosa. This infection causes a nonhealing wound in the irradiated bone.

The other possible cause is given by, "*radiation-induced fibroatrophic theory*,"—the increased formation of fibroblasts and scar tissues at the irradiated bone.

A dose of radiation less than 6,500 rads reduces the risk of osteoradionecrosis and radiation therapy above 7,500 rads will significantly increase the chance.

Preventive Methods

- Avoid irradiation of bone which has subjected to previous surgery or extraction and the healing is incomplete.
- Avoid irradiation of lesion near the bone.
- Avoid high dose of radiation.
- Surgery in the irradiated area.
- Avoid trauma in the irradiated region.

Management

- Good oral hygiene

- Hyperbaric oxygen therapy
- Antibiotics
- Nutritional supplements.

7. What is acute radiation syndrome? (or) Write about the effects of whole body irradiation.

An acute radiation syndrome is a group of signs and symptoms experienced by a person after exposure to the high amount of radiation at a short time like atom bomb blast or radiation accidents.

Prodromal period:

- Whole body irradiation of about 1.2 Gy produces symptoms within minutes to hours.
- Early symptoms include nausea, vomiting, diarrhea, weakness, and fatigue.
- The autonomous nervous system causes these effects.
- The severity and time of onset of the symptoms are dose dependent.

Latent period:

- It is the period between the irradiation and occurrence of biological damage.
- This period extends for hours to days if the dose is above 5 Gy and for few weeks if the dose is less than 2 Gy.

Hematopoietic syndrome: Exposure of 2–7 Gy affects hematopoietic stem cells. There will be rapid reduction in the circulating granulocytes, platelets, and erythrocytes. The clinical findings include infection, bleeding, and anemia.

Periodontitis is the associated dental complication.

Gastrointestinal syndrome: Exposure of 7–15 Gy causes injury to intestinal villi and denudation of mucosal epithelium. This leads to mucosal ulceration, hemorrhaging of the intestine, diarrhea, dehydration, weight loss and septicemia.

Cardiovascular and central nervous syndrome: Exposure of 50 Gy cause death in 1–2 days due to collapse of the circulatory system, fall in blood pressure and necrosis of cardiac muscles. Damage to nervous system causes disorientation and convulsions. The syndrome is irreversible.

8. Write about the direct effects of radiation on living systems.

- Ionization of biomolecules by X-ray photons or secondary electrons is defined as direct effects of radiation.
- When the biological molecules absorb the energy of X-ray photons, ionization begins, and free radical formation takes place by the production of unpaired electrons.
- These free radicals are highly reactive and highly unstable hence quickly reforms into a stable form by dissociation or cross-linkage.
- One-third of biological reactions following radiation is through direct effects.

Example:

When a biomolecule RH absorbs the energy of an X-ray photon, free radicals are produced as follows:

$$RH + \text{X-ray absorption} \rightarrow R^0 + H^+ + e^-$$

Free radical R undergo either:

- Dissociation

$$R^0 \rightarrow X + Y^0$$

- Cross-linking

$$R^0 + Y^0 \rightarrow RY$$

As the altered molecules are differing from the original molecule, there is a biological change in the organism.

9. Write about the indirect effects of radiation on living systems.

During radiation exposure, water molecules of the body absorb energy and undergo ionization. The resulting free radicals react with biomolecules and produce changes. This type of reaction is called indirect effects of radiation. Two-third of radiation-induced biological effects occur with indirect effects.

Radiolysis of water: Interaction of radiation with water causes ionization of water molecules and release of *free radicals* like hydrogen (H^+) and hydroxyl ions (OH^-) (Fig. 4).

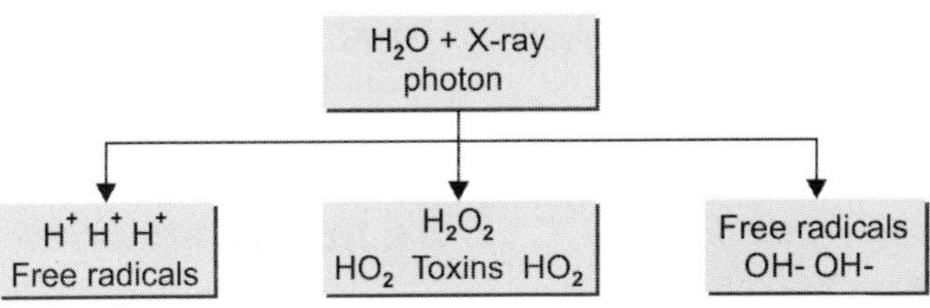

Fig. 4: Radiolysis of water.

These free radicals produce damage to the biological molecules by either directly interacting with them or by producing toxins like peroxyl radicals and hydrogen peroxide. These products alter the chemical and biological properties of the biomolecule resulting either death or malignant transformation of these molecules.

10. Write about radiation-induced cancers.

Radiation-induced cancers occur commonly in a population exposed to high amount of radiation like atomic bomb survivors. Children are approximately twice as radiosensitive for cancer induction as adults.

The role of radiation on cancer induction is likely to be:

- An irritatant that produce changes in the cell differentiation mechanism
- An Inducing agent for gene mutation
- Promoter for cell multiplication.

Susceptibility of Different Organs to Radiation-Induced Cancer

Based on the radiation susceptibility to cancer, the organs are classified as highly susceptible, moderately susceptible, and less susceptible (Table 3).

Table 3: Susceptibility of different organs to radiation-induced cancer.

Highly susceptible	Moderately susceptible	Less susceptible
▪ Colon ▪ Stomach ▪ Lung ▪ Bone marrow	▪ Breast ▪ Esophagus	▪ Bladder, liver ▪ Thyroid, skin ▪ Salivary glands ▪ Brain, bone surface

11. Hyperbaric oxygen therapy.

Hyperbaric oxygen therapy is employed in the treatment of many conditions like gangrene, osteoradionecrosis, necrotizing fasciitis, and infections like actinomycosis that devitalize the cells and tissues. The patient is placed in a treatment chamber (above 1 atmospheric pressure) and allowed to breath 100% oxygen.

The elevated level of oxygen stimulates vasoconstriction and allows the peripheral blood towards the hypoxic tissues. The increased blood supply enhances new angiogenesis and epithelization which in turn prevents infection and support healing.

Side effects: Oxygen toxicity can cause seizures, barotrauma (collapse due to alteration in lung pressure), myopia and fluid leakage from the middle ear.

Contraindications: Diabetes mellitus and thyroid disorders may increase the chances of oxygen toxicity.

MULTIPLE CHOICE QUESTIONS

1. The short-term effects of radiosensitivity are due to the response of ***parenchymal cells***.
   a. Parenchymal cells
   b. Connective tissue
   c. Fine vasculatures
   d. Epithelial cells
2. Long-term effects of radiation are due to the response of damage to ***fine vasculatures***.
   a. Parenchymal cells
   b. Connective tissue
   c. Fine vasculatures
   d. Epithelial cells

3. Long-term effects of radiation in an organ is ***fibroatrophy***.
   a. Fatty necrosis
   b Fibroatrophy
   c. Loss of blood supply
   d. Loss of function
4. Recovery of taste sensation following the radiotherapy will take ***2–4 months***.
   a. 2–4 months
   b. 6–8 months
   c. 12 months
   d. 24 months
5. Predominant cells of adult pulp tissue are ***post mitotic cells***.
   a. Vegetative cells
   b. Intermitotic cells
   c. Multipotent connective tissue cells
   d. Postmitotic cells
   (**Note:** Revert and fixed postmitotic cell).
6. Oral complication associated with acute radiation syndrome is ***periodontitis***.
   a. Periodontitis
   b. Osteoradionecrosis
   c. Radiation mucositis
   d. Oral ulcers
7. The most radiosensitive period for fetus is ***organogenesis***.
   a. Embryogenesis
   b. Organogenesis
   c. Fetal developmental stage
   d. Less than 6 months of age
   (**Note:** Organogenesis period = 8–45 days).
8. Brain is more sensitive to radiation at ***8th–15th week of postconsumption***.
   a. 8th–15th weeks of postconception
   b. 1st–8th weeks of postconsumption
   c. 12th–18th weeks of gestation
   d. 18th–38th weeks of gestation
9. Radiation-induced gene mutation was first explained by ***Muller***.
   a. Mendal
   b. Muller
   c. Eric Van Tschemark
   d. Thomas Morgan
   (**Note:** Muller explained this concept in *drosophila)*.
10. Adverse effect following radiotherapy for ankylosing spondylitis is ***leukemia***.
    a. Fibrosis of vessels b. Leukemia
    c. Bone marrow failure d. Lymphoma
11. Type of Ionizing radiation that produces severe biological damage is ***alpha rays***.
    a. X-rays
    b. Alpha rays
    c. Gamma rays
    d. Beta rays
12. Biological effects of radiation will increase about increasing ***dose rate***.
    a. Exposure time
    b. Cell division
    c. Frequency of exposure
    d. Dose rate
13. Latent effect associated with whole body irradiation is ***leukemia***.
    a. Fibrosis of vessels
    b. Leukemia
    c. Bone marrow failure
    d. Lymphoma
14. The amount of radiation damage will be more for cells at ***G1 and early S phase***.
    a. G1 and early S phase
    b. Before DNA synthesis
    c. G2 and late S phase
    d. After DNA replication
15. Chromosome aberration will result if radiation exposure occurs at ***G1 phase***.
    a. G1 phase
    b. G2 phase
    c. Late S phase
    d. After DNA replication
16. The amount of radiation damage will be minimal for cells at ***G2 phase***.
    a. G1 phase
    b. G2 phase
    c. Early S phase
    d. Before DNA replication
17. Chromatid aberration will result if radiation exposure occurs ***after DNA synthesis***.
    a. After DNA synthesis
    b. Before DNA synthesis
    c. Early S phase
    d. G1 phase

18. Tooth eruption mechanism is ***radioresistant***.
    a. Highly radiosensitive
    b. Moderately radiosensitive
    c. Radioresistant
    d. Radioresponsive
    (**Note:** Eruption rate is not affected by radiotherapy).

VIVA VOCE

1. What is threshold dose?

Amount of radiation that produces visible biological damage is known as threshold dose.

2. What is doubling dose?

This is the amount of radiation required by a population to produce many spontaneous additional mutations in the next generation.

Doubling dose helps to measure the genetic exposure risk of radiation.

3. Define radiation caries.

It is a rampant form of caries with widespread attack and rapid onset. Salivary changes following radiotherapy like reduced flow, decreased pH, increased viscosity and less cleansing action induce caries.

4. What are accumulative effects of radiation?

Whenever biological tissues are exposed to radiation, there is some injury and is followed by repair. But residual injury may remain within DNA or cytoplasm and each succeeding radiation injury adds a small amount to this residual damage and is known as the accumulative effect of radiation and lead to future health problems.

5. What are the host factors that influence radiation effects?

Intrinsic resistance, type and sensitivity of tissues exposed, rate of cell division, and phase of cell cycle.

6. Why radiotherapy is indicated for malignancy.

The rate of cell division determines the biological effects of radiation. Hence, malignant cells that divide rapidly are destroyed by radiation.

BIBLIOGRAPHY

1. Attix FH, Tochilin E, (Eds). Sources, fields, measurements, and applications: radiation dosimetry. Academic Press; 2016.
2. Reuther T, Schuster T, Mende U, et al. Osteoradionecrosis of the jaws as a side effect of radiotherapy of head and neck tumour patients—a report of a thirty year retrospective review. Int J Oral Maxillofac Surg. 2003;32(3):289-95.
3. Whaites E, Drage N. Essentials of dental radiography and radiology. Elsevier Health Sciences; 2013.
4. White SC, Pharoah MJ. Principles and interpretation. St Louis. 2014:431-3.
5. White SC. 1992 assessment of radiation risk from dental radiography. Dentomaxillofac Radiology. 1992;21(3):118-26.

CHAPTER 28

Radiation Protection

HIGHLIGHTS

The radiation protection describes all measures that need to be applied in the radiology centers to protect patients from the harmful effects of radiation without compromising the quality of diagnostic images. The protective measures are applicable both to the patients and the professionals. This chapter deals with radiation safety measures before, during and after exposure to dental X-rays.

Learners are expected to study:

- As low as reasonably achievable (ALARA) concept
- Different types of filtration used in dental radiology
- Collimator in dental radiology
- Patient protection and operator protection
- Personal and equipment monitoring devices
- Radiation exposure guidelines.

ESSAY QUESTIONS

1. Describe in detail the basics of patient protection from X-ray exposure.

(or)

Mention the key rules to be followed while taking radiographs to reduce patient exposure.

Radiation protection measures should be followed before, during and after the dental X-ray exposure to reduce the adverse effects of radiation on a dental patient.

Patient Protection Before Exposure

1. ***Prescribing dental radiographs:*** *Radiographic selection criteria* (or) *high yield* (or) *referral criteria* states that diagnostic radiographs should be advised after examining the patient clinically and confirming that the radiographic information is essential to substantiate the diagnosis, treatment, and prognosis.

   Professional judgment should be used to decide the type, number, and frequency of dental radiographs.
2. **Proper equipment:**
   Filtration: The X-ray beam is polychromatic containing both high and low energy X-ray photons. The low energy X-ray photons have less penetrating power and absorbed by the patient tissue rather carrying diagnostic information to the film. Thus low energy photons increases patient's exposure dose. With the use of filters, these low energy X-ray photons are removed from reaching the patient.

Inherent filtration: Occurs when the primary beam travels through the insulating oil, the tube head seal, and the glass window.

Added filtration: The aluminum disc placed between the collimator and the tube head seal filters the X-ray beam.

X-ray machine requires 1.5 mm thickness of aluminum disk when it operates at or below 70 kVp and 2.5 mm thick disk when operates above 70 kVp.

Total filtration (Inherent and added filtration)

Collimation: Collimation reduces the size of X-ray beam so that the area of tissue exposed to primary X-ray beam is minimal to fulfil the diagnostic requirements.

Use of collimators should restrict the beam size to a diameter of not more than 2.75 inches or 7 cm when it reaches the patient's skin for an X-ray machine operating above 50 kVp. The size reduction improves the image quality by decreasing the scatter radiation and thereby film fog in addition to reducing the patient exposure dose. The use of rectangular collimation results in 71–80% dose reduction (Fig. 1).

Position indicating device(PID): PID is used to focus the X-ray beam without deviating from the path so that limiting the occurrence of scatter radiation. Precision instrument and Rinn XCP film holding devise with rectangular collimation are example (Fig. 2).

Patient Protection During Exposure

- **Thyroid collar:** Is an adjustable lead safeguard used to wrap around the patient's neck for preventing the scatter radiation reaching the thyroid gland.
- **Lead apron:** Is a pliable lead protector to cover the patient's chest and abdomen for stopping the scatter radiation from reaching the reproductive and blood forming organs.
- **Fast film:** F-speed film or insight and E - speed or ektaspeed film are the fastest intraoral films available.
- **Beam alignment devices:** Aids in the stabilization of the film intraorally and

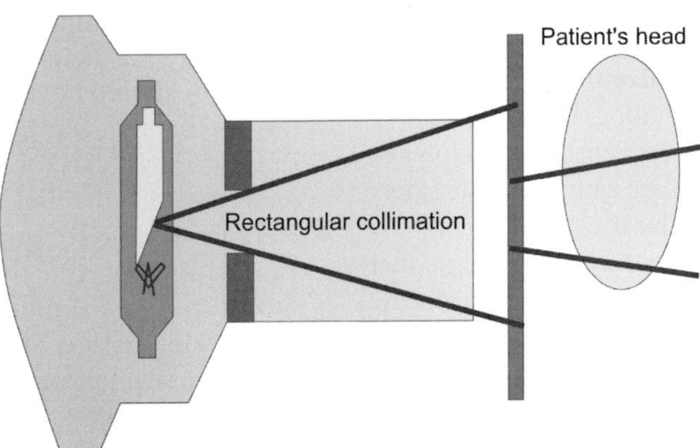

Fig. 1: The X-rays are less divergent on using rectangular collimator.

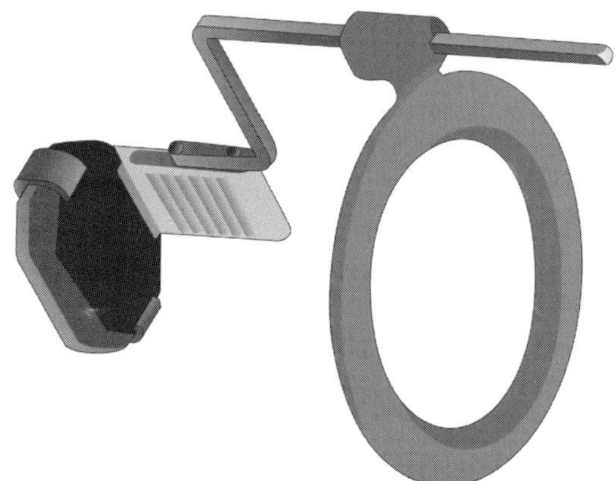

Fig. 2: Film holding instrument with position indicating device.

reduces the chances of slipping thereby reduces the patient's exposure.
- **Exposure factor selection:** A setting of 70–90 kVp is ideal for dental X-ray units.
- **Appropriate technique:** Enhances the quality of images and avoid retakes.

After Exposure

- **Proper film handling**: Artifacts caused by improper handling results in a non-diagnostic image which must be retaken and exposes patients to radiation.
- **Proper film processing**: Film processing is a step to convert the latent image to visible image.

2. Discuss operator protection in dental radiography. (or) discuss personal protection in dental radiography.

The application of standard operator protection principles can minimize the radiation dose received by a dental radiographer.

Protection guidelines: Provide guidelines to the dental radiographer with the basic safety information. It includes the following:

- ***Distance recommendations:*** Radiographer must stand at least 6 feet away from the X-ray tube head during exposure (Fig. 3). If this distance is not possible, a protective barrier must be used.
- ***Position recommendation:*** To avoid primary beam, the radiographer should stand perpendicular to the primary X-ray beam, or at 90°–135° angle to the beam (Fig. 3).
  Also, the dental radiographer should:
  - **Not keep the film** in place during exposure.
  - **Not hold the tube head** during exposure.
- ***Shielding recommendations:*** A protective barrier that can absorb the primary beam will protect the operator from primary and scatter radiation. Dental radiographer should stand behind the protective lead barrier or drywall during exposure.
- ***Radiation monitoring:*** Radiation monitoring can identify excessive occupational exposure.
- ***Equipment monitoring:*** Dental X-ray machine should be examined for any radiation leak. Any radiation other than the primary beam emitted from the tube head is known as leakage radiation. Leakage radiation should be monitored by using a film device that can be obtained through the state health sector or from the dental X-ray machine manufacturers.
- ***Personal monitoring:*** The amount of radiation received by the operator is monitored by "film badge" or radiation monitoring badge. Film badge holds an X-ray film segment or radiosensitive crystal within a plastic case. This should be clasped at the waist level of the operator while taking the radiographs. When the badges are not worn, they should be stored in a

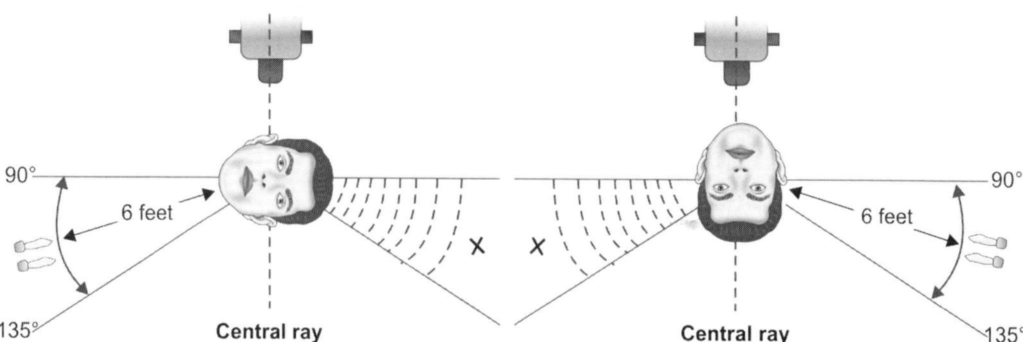

Fig. 3: Position and distance rule.

radiation safe area. The badges should be submitted to the radiation monitoring authorities in the scheduled period (e.g. once in 3 months or semiannually) to detect the amount radiation exposure.

3. Discuss radiation exposure guidelines.

Radiation exposure guidelines have been established to safeguard the radiation professionals and patients. The guiding strategies include radiation safety legislation and exposure limits for the public and occupationally exposed personals.

Radiation safety legislation: Has been established to protect the patient, radiographers, and public from the harmful effects of radiation.

These include:

- ***Radiation Control for Health and Safety Act:*** To standardize the operation of equipment.
- ***The Federal Consumer-Patient Radiation Health and Safety Act:*** This rule is responsible for education and official recognition of professionals operating radiographic equipment.

Maximum permissible Dose (MPD): It is defined as the maximum dose equivalent that a body is permitted to receive within a specific period. MPD is the radiation dose that can be tolerated by the body with minimal or no damage.

As per *NCRP guidelines,* the MPD for radiology professionals is 5 rem/year, and for nonoccupational individuals, the MPD is 0.1 rem/year.

Maximum accumulated dose (MAD): States that the radiology workers must not exceed an accumulated lifetime radiation dose.

MAD is calculated using formula based on the persons age.

MAD = (N – 18) × 5 rems/year

N = Person's age in years.

18 = Refers to the minimum age of a person permitted to work with radiation.

ALARA Concept

ALARA = As low as reasonably achievable concept states that all exposure to radiation must be kept to a minimum.

All possible measures need to be taken in radio diagnostic centers to reduce the adverse effects of radiation.

SHORT NOTES

1. What is ALARA concept?

As low as reasonably achievable concept declares that *all exposure to radiation must be minimum.*

ALARA concept: *Every probable method of minimizing the radiation dose should be employed to avoid the radiation induced hazards.* Strict adherence to this principle will protect both patients and operators.

This concept is not specifically mentioning any radiation dose as reasonable amount.

2. Discuss different types of filtration.

Use of filtration selectively removes soft, low energy, long wavelength X-ray photons from the primary beam and permits photons with sufficient energy to carry diagnostic information to the film.

In dental X-ray machine, two types of filtration are used:

- **Inherent filtration:** Occurs when the primary beam travels through the insulating oil, tube head, and the glass window. Inherent filtration of dental X-ray machine is approximately equal to the filtering effect of 0.5 to 1 mm of aluminum.
- **Added filtration:** Takes place when the X-ray beam travels through an aluminum disk placed between the collimator and tube head. 1.5 mm aluminium filters are used in dental X-ray machines operating at or below 70 kVp and 2.5 mm aluminium is required when above 70 kVp is used.

The use of rare earth elements like samarium, erbium, etc. in combination with aluminum filtration reduces overall patient exposure by 20–80%.

Total filtration: Inherent plus added filtration. The X-ray machine operating at 70 kVp require a minimum total of 1.5 mm aluminum filtration and machine operating above 70 kVp require a minimum total of 2.5 mm aluminum filtration.

3. Describe collimator. (or) what is collimation ?

Collimation is the process of reducing the X-ray beam size and shape before reaching the patient's skin to reduce the exposure dose. The collimator is an apparatus that restricts the size and shape of X-ray beam as it leaves the tube head. These devices are made up of lead diaphragm with a circular aperture.

Principle: The amount of scatter radiation produced is proportional to the area exposed.

Purpose of Collimation

- Significant reduction in patient exposure
- Decreased amount of scatter radiation reduces film fog and increases image quality
- A decrease in beam size reduces penumbra and increases image sharpness.

For intraoral radiographs, the beam size is reduced to match with film size. The beam is collimated to a circle having a diameter of 7 cm at the patient's skin surface when the tube is operating above 50 kVp.

Types of Collimators

- Round position indicating device
- Rectangular position indicating device
- Use of rectangular collimation results in 71–80% dose reduction
- Film holders with rectangular collimators and round position indicating device (PID)
- Precision instrument with rectangular collimation
- XCP with rectangular collimation.

4. Define half-value layer.

Half-value layer (HVL) is the thickness of the specified material required to reduce the beam intensity by half when placed on the path of X-ray beam.

Aluminum filters are used to remove the low energy, less penetrating, long wavelength X-ray photons and increases the mean penetrating quality of the beam by reducing its intensity. HVL determines the penetrating ability of the beam.

For example, if a dental X-ray beam has a half-value layer of 2 mm, it requires 2 mm thickness of aluminum to reduce its intensity by half (50%).

Measurement of HVL requires a dosimeter. The HVL should be at least 1.5 mm aluminum at 70 kVp and 2.5 mm aluminum at 90 kVp.

5. Describe personal monitoring devices to detect dental radiation. (or) explain about film badges. (or) write about thermoluminescent dosimeter.

Refer Essay Question 2—personal monitoring.

6. What is pocket dosimeter?

A pocket dosimeter is a device used to check the *quantity of X-ray beam* to verify whether the machine output is changed over time.

The number of X-ray photons is determined by the mA and exposure time. So, to determine the machine output, the exposure parameters need to be standardized, e.g. 0.25 seconds, 7 or 10 mA, and 65 or 70 kVp and quantity of radiation is measured using pocket dosimeter. For this setup, the baseline reading is always be 180 milliroentgen.

When a new reading is taken to check the machine output it should be same as the baseline value, then no further testing of beam quantity is necessary.

7. Describe source to film distance concept. (or) describe the effect of focal spot to film distance in exposure dose.

Principle: Extended radiation source—patient distance (focal spot to film distance) will reduce the amount of radiation to the patient.

Inverse square law: States that the beam intensity is inversely proportional to the square of the Source to film distence (SFD).

The distance between the focal spot and the film should be as great as is technically acceptable.

Two standard focal spot to film distances (FSFDs) used in intraoral radiography are *20 cm* (8 inches) and *41 cm* (16 inches).

When X-ray tube operates above 50 kVp, the x-ray source-skin distance should not be less than 18 cm.

Application: The use of longer FSFD (or) SFD results in 32% dose reduction in exposed tissue volume. This is because at the great distance the beam is less divergent.

Smaller focal spot size thereby increases the radiographic resolution.

8. Source of radiation exposure in daily life.

Radiation from a natural source is composed of radon, cosmic radiation, terrestrial radiation and internal radiation.

Decay process of natural radon produces *radon gas* which is taken into lungs. It remains as same until it undergoes subsequent decay process and in this way leads to chronic radiation exposure.

Cosmic radiation: Originates in outer space. Altitude, latitude, and solar activity modify the cosmic rays reaching earth.

Terrestrial radiation: Originates from soil nuclides of radium, uranium, thorium and their decay products.

The internal source of radiation is dependent on inhalation and ingestion of radionuclides.

9. Describe radiation risk estimation for dental radiography.

Risk estimates can be explained as two types:

1. **Absolute risk:** It is defined as the difference between risk in an irradiated population compared to that in a normal population. Absolute risk is calculated as a probability for a cancer free person to develop cancer after getting exposure to a risk factor.
2. **Relative risk (r):** It is the ratio of the risks in irradiated and nonirradiated populations.

When r is:

≤1, there is no cancer risk after exposure.

≥1, there is increased cancer risk after exposure.

In dental radiology, risk estimation is measured by absolute risk.

10. Discuss patient education regarding radiation protection.

The dental radiographer should explain how patients are protected from radiation exposure during the entire procedure:

- Before get started the procedure, all possible protective measures were taken to reduce the unnecessary exposure.
- The X-ray equipment we use is frequently tested for its integrity to follow the safety guidelines.
- During X-ray exposure, we use thyroid collar and a lead apron to protect your body from X-ray radiation.
- We use the fastest film available.
- We use the effective technique to avoid making mistakes that require re-exposure.

MULTIPLE CHOICE QUESTIONS

1. The annual maximum permissible dose (MPD) limit for dentists and radiation workers is ***50 mSv***
   a. 50 R
   b. 50 mSv
   c. 35 R
   d. 35 mSv
2. The lifetime cumulative exposure limit for radiation workers is calculated by the formula ***10 × age in years***.
   a. 1.5 × age in years
   b. 10 × age in years
   c. 1.5 × working hours/year
   d. 10 × working hours/year
3. The maximum permissible dose for pregnant women is ***5 mSv***.
   a. 1 mSv
   b. 5 mSv
   c. Zero
   d. 10 mSv

4. Collimators are made up of ***lead***.
   a. Aluminium
   b. Tungsten
   c. Phosphorus
   d. Lead
5. Filter is made up of ***aluminium***.
   a. Aluminium
   b. Tungsten
   c. Phosphorus
   d. Lead
6. Aluminum filters are used to remove X-rays with ***long wavelength***.
   a. High penetration power
   b. High energy
   c. Poly chromatic waves
   d. Long wavelength
   (**Note:** Aluminum filters remove the low energy, less penetrating, long wavelength X- rays).
7. To filter extreme high energy X-ray photons ***rare earth elements*** are used.
   a. Intrinsic filters
   b. Aluminium foils
   c. Rare earth elements
   d. Step wedges
8. Device used to measure the quantity of X-ray beam is ***pocket dosimeter***.
   a. Collimators
   b. Pocket dosimeter
   c. Film badges
   d. Image densitometer
   (**Note:** Pocket dosimeter and ionization chamber measures the quantity of X-ray beam).
9. Exposure to cosmic ray is higher at ***altitude***.
   a. Plateau
   b. Valley
   c. Altitude
   d. Ocean
10. Use of rectangular collimation reduced patient exposure by ***60%***.
    a. 30%
    b. 60%
    c. 10%
    d. 90%
11. Use of thyroid collar is recommended for ***intra-oral radiography***.
    a. Intraoral radiography
    b. Orthopantomography
    c. Computed tomography
    d. Cephalography
12. Thyroid collar is not recommended for extraoral radiography because it ***obscures diagnostic information***.
    a. Reduces the quantity of X-rays reaching the patient
    b. Increases the amount of scattered radiation
    c. Obscures diagnostic information
    d. Obstructs cassette positioning
13. MPD for occupationally exposed pregnant women is ***0.1 rem/year***.
    a. 1.0 rem/year
    b. 0.1 rem/year
    c. 10 rem/year
    d. 100 rem/year
    (**Note:** 0.1 rem/year (or) same that for a non-occupationally exposed individual).
14. The effective energy range of X-ray photons to produce image is ***35 and 55 keV***.
    a. 60 and 70 keV
    b. 35 and 55 keV
    c. 10 and 15 keV
    d. 50 and 80 keV
15. The use of thyroid collars reduces the radiation exposure to thyroid gland by ***92%***.
    a. 98%
    b. 100%
    c. 92%
    d. 96%

VIVA VOCE

1. What is deterministic effect.

Any somatic effect that increases in severity in direct proportion to radiation dose after reaching the threshold limit is defined as a deterministic effect.

These effects occur soon after or months to a year later from relatively large exposure. *Examples:* Skin or mucosal erythema, cataracts, fibrosis, abnormal growth and development following the uterine exposure.

2. What is stochastic effect.

The probability of radiation effects and not its severity is dose depended. There is no threshold limit below which cancer will not occur. The probability for developing cancer increases as the exposure increases.

3. What is MPD.

Maximum permissible dose is the highest amount of radiation approved to receive by an individual in a specific period.

4. What is filtration?

X-rays are polychromatic beam containing both low and high energy photons, but only photons having energies between 35 and 55 keV are more efficient in producing diagnostic images.

Filtration is the process by which selective removal of both low and high energy photons from the beam thereby allowing only photons with *sufficient penetrating energy* to reach the patient. Thus the use of filter reduces patient's exposure dose.

5. Name the filter material used in dental X-ray machine.

About 1.5 mm thick aluminum is commonly used as a filter in dental radiographic machines operating at or below 70 kVp, whereas 2.3 mm aluminum is used when above 70 kVp is used. **Selective filtration:** *Rare earth elements* like samarium, erbium, niobium, gadolinium, terbium activated gadolinium oxysulfide and thulium activated lanthanum oxybromide are used with aluminum to further reduce the patient exposure by selectively removing both extremely low and high energy photons. The use of rare earth filters increases the exposure time (and hence increases the X-ray machine workload. and reduces the image quality by decreasing contrast, sharpness and resolution).

6. What are the benefits of using collimator?

- Significant reduction in patient exposure
- Decreased amount of scatter radiation reduces film fog and increases image quality
- The decrease in beam size reduces penumbra and increases image sharpness.

7. What is distance-position rule?

The radiographer should stand 6 feet away from the tube head at an angle of 90–135° to the primary beam direction during film exposure.

This rule will protect the dental radiographer from the occupational radiation exposure by avoiding primary beam reaching him.

8. What is ALARA stands for?

As low as reasonably achievable.

9. What is the function of NCRP?

National Council on Radiation Protection and Measurement: Identifyes the adverse effects of radiation and the risk associated with its use.

10. What is the role of ICRP?

International Commission on Radiology Protection: Establishes the guidelines to restrict the radiation dose received by Public and occupationally exposed individuals.

BIBLIOGRAPHY

1. Dowsett D, Kenny PA, Johnston RE. The physics of diagnostic imaging. CRC Press; 2006.
2. Langland OE, Langlais RP, Preece JW. Principles of Dental Imaging, 2nd edition. Philadelphia: Lippincott Williams and Wilkins, 2002.p.57
3. Weissleder R, Wittenberg J, Harisinghani MG. Primer of Diagnostic Imaging, 5th edition. St. Louis: Mosby; 2011.
4. Whaites E, Drage N. Essentials of dental radiography and radiology. 5th edition, Chuchill Livingstone. Edingburgh, Scotland, 2013
5. White SC, Pharoah MJ. Oral radiology E-Book: Principles and interpretation. Elsevier Health Sciences; 2014.

CHAPTER 29

Image Receptors, X-ray Film, Intensifying Screens, and Grids and Image Characteristics

HIGHLIGHTS

Image receptors are materials used to capture and store images in radiography. In dentistry, film, filmscreen combinations are widely used. However, electronic sensors are used in the digital imaging system.

Radiographic films are comparable to photographic films that are adapted for dental use. Dental radiology uses nonscreen films for intraoral purposes and screened films for extraoral radiography.

Learners are expected to study:

- Composition of intraoral film
- Contents of intraoral film packet
- Types, sizes, and speed of intraoral film
- Film storage and protection
- Composition and uses of intensifying screens
- Composition and uses of grids.

ESSAY QUESTIONS

1. Describe the major imaging characteristics of an X-ray film. (or) enumerate the factors that determine image quality.

Radiographic image characteristics include both visual and geometric characteristics. An ideal radiograph is a diagnostic one which provides more significant information.

Visual characteristics: Density and contrast influences the diagnostic quality.

Density: The overall degree of *darkness or blackness* of an exposed film is known as radiographic density.

Processing of unexposed film shows some density known as, *the inherent density* of the base. This minimal density is called as *gross fog* or *base plus fog.*

Factors Influencing the Radiographic Density

- ***Exposure:*** Increasing the milliamperage (mA), peak kilovoltage (kVp), or exposure time *increases the number of photons* reaching the film and increases the image density.

  Reducing the focal spot-film distance increases the image density.
- ***Subject thickness and density:*** When the subject is thicker, more beam will be attenuated, and the resultant image will appear lighter. Exposure factors (kVp or time) should be adjusted to suit for subject density.

  Dense objects (well absorbs the radiation) appear as a light image in the radiograph—*radiopaque*. Less dense objects absorb less radiation while allowing most of the X-rays to pass through it and appear as a dark image on radiograph—*radiolucent.*
- **Contrast:** Contrast is the difference in densities between adjacent light and dark areas in a radiograph. An image showing *both dark and the light regions* has *high contrast or short gray scale of contrast.* An image composed of only *light gray and dark gray areas* has *low contrast or long gray scale of contrast.*

Factors Influencing the Radiographic Contrast

- ***Subject contrast:*** Refer to the characteristics like thickness, density and composition of the subject that influence the image contrast. It can be altered by altering kVp. When high kVp is used, (above 90 kVp) low contrast image results with many shades of gray. When low kVp (65–70 kVp) is used, high contrast image results with areas of black and white.
- ***Film contrast:*** High contrast film reveals areas of small difference in subject contrast more clearly than low contrast film. Inherent qualities of the film, processing time and temperature of developer will influences film contrast.
- ***Geometric characteristics:*** The formation of an accurate radiographic image is dependent on minimizing specific geometric characteristics that are present to a certain degree in every radiograph.
- ***Image or geometric unsharpness (penumbra):*** Penumbra refers to the diffusion of detail and appears as a fuzzy, unsharp margin surrounding the teeth and osseous structures. In dental radiographs, penumbra can be minimized by:
  - Reducing the focal spot size
  - Increasing the source—object distance
  - Reducing the film object distance.
- ***Image magnification:*** Magnification is the equal enlargement of the actual size of the object on the radiograph. It is possible to minimize magnification by:
  - Increasing source film distance
  - Reducing object film distance.
- ***Image shape distortion:*** Refer to the uneven development of the same object in different parts.

It can be minimized by using paralleling technique where the central beam is perpendicular to the tooth and film which are parallel to each other.

SHORT NOTES

1. Describe the composition of dental X-ray film.

X-ray film is an image receptor and has four basic components (Fig. 1):

1. Base
2. Adhesive layer
3. Emulsion
4. Protective layer

Base: Film base is *0.2 mm thick* and is made up of flexible plastic (polyethylene terephthalate). It is transparent and exhibits slight bluish tint to emphasize contrast and increase image quality. The base *supports the emulsion and increases the strength.* It also serves to tolerate

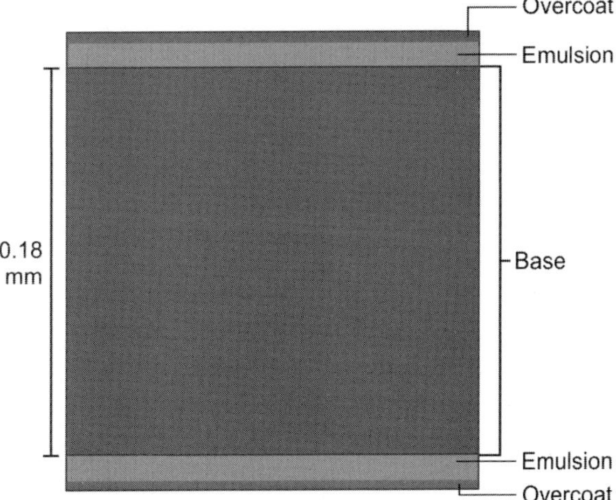

Fig. 1: Composition of an X-ray film.

the heat, moisture and chemical changes during processing.

Adhesive layer: A thin, transparent adhesive is added on the film base before the application of emulsion and functions to attach the emulsion on either side of the base.

Film emulsion: The emulsion is a coating attached by an adhesive layer on either side of the film. It is a homogenous blend of gelatine and silver halide crystals.

Gelatine: It is used to suspend and disperse silver halide crystals over the film base. During film processing, gelatine absorbs the processing solutions and allows the chemicals to react with silver halide crystals.

Silver halide crystals: Silver halide crystals are sensitive to X-rays and visible light. They are composed *primarily of silver bromide* and a lesser amount of silver iodide. Size of iodide crystals are larger than bromide hence their addition disturbs the regularity of bromide crystal structure and increases its sensitivity to X-ray rediation.

The photosensitivity of silver halide crystals is further increased by the addition of small amounts of *trace materials* like sulfur or gold.

The silver halide grains are flat, tabular with a mean diameter of 1.6 μm in E speed film and are globular with 1 μm size in D speed film.

Protective layer: It is a thin, transparent coating placed over the emulsion. It protects the surface from manipulation, mechanical and processing damage.

2. List and explain different types of intra-oral film. (or) list and explain different types of nonscreen films.

Intraoral film otherwise called the nonscreen film is used to capture the image of teeth and supporting structures. Three types of film are available which are as follows:.

1. **Periapical film:** Peri = "around", apex = "terminal end of a tooth root."

   This film image is used to see the entire tooth and the supporting structures.

   Three sizes are available:
   1. **Size 0:** Smallest available size and is used for children. (22 × 35 mm)
   2. **Size 1:** To examine the anterior teeth in adults. (24 × 40 mm)
   3. **Size 2:** *"Standard size adult film"*—to examine anterior and posterior teeth in adults. (31 × 41 mm)
2. **Bitewing film:** It is used to examine the mandibular and maxillary posterior teeth crowns in one film. It has a "wing" or "tab." The patients bite on the wing to stabilize the film.

   Indication for bitewing film is: To examine
   - Interproximal surfaces (proximal caries)
   - Crestal bone pattern and height.

   Three sizes are available:
   1. **Size 0:** For posterior teeth in small children
   2. **Size 2:** For posterior teeth in adults and is commonly used type
   3. **Size 3:** *Used only for bitewing images.* This film shows all the posterior teeth on one side of the arch in one film.
3. **Occlusal film:** The film is so named because the patient occludes or bites on the entire film during exposure. It is used to examine the larger areas of maxilla or mandible. The film size is 57 × 76 mm.

3. Intraoral film packet.

The intraoral radiographic films are placed in a packet with ancillary materials to protect it from light and moisture. The film with its surrounding packaging is referred to as a "film packet" and is made up of four separate items:

1. **X-ray film:** The dental radiographic film is a double emulsion film. A small, raised dot known as *identification dot* is located on one corner of the film which is used to determine film orientation (right and left sides of the patient) after processing.

2. **Paper film wrapper:** It is a protective sheet that covers the film and shields the film from light.
3. **Lead foil sheet:** A single piece of lead foil is located *behind the film* in the packet. This sheet shields the film from backscattered radiation and prevents film fog.
4. **Outer wrapping:** Soft vinyl or paper wrapper seals the film, protective paper and lead foil sheet. This wrapper protects the film from exposure to light and saliva.

Outer wrapper of the film packet has two sides:

1. ***Tube side:*** Tube side is white with a raised dot on one corner that corresponds to the identification dot on film.
2. ***Label side:*** Label side is color coded and contains a clinch. The packet should be unsealed only in the darkroom.

4. Describe film sensitivity. (or) briefly explain film speed.

Film sensitivity or film speed determines the amount of radiation and exposure time to produce an image on the film with standard density. The silver halide crystals size, emulsion thickness, and the radiosensitive dyes decide the film speed.

Film speed is expressed as a reciprocal of the exposure needed to produce an optical density of 1. A fast film requires less exposure to produce a density of 1.

Fast film: More sensitive films require less mAs and have greater film speed hence called fast films. The larger the silver halide crystals, the faster will be the film. Currently, group E film (Ektaspeed) and group F film are in use.

Slow film: A film that requires more mAs are less sensitive to radiation and are called as slow films. Slow films are not in manufacture today. Film speed is slightly increased by increasing the temperature of the processing solution, but this may cause fog and graininess on film. Depleted processing solution slows down the effective speed.

5. Write briefly about extraoral film. (or) write in brief about screen film.

Majority of extraoral films are screen films. A screen film is one that uses the indirect exposure. The energy of the X-ray beam is converted into light by *intensifying screens.* Intensifying screens reduces the X-ray dose to the patient.

- The film is sandwiched between the two intensifying screens in a cassette.
- When the cassette is exposed to X-rays, the screens convert the X-ray energy to light, which in turn expose the film. The film is sensitive to fluorescent light rather than radiation.
- Silver halide crystals are sensitive to ultraviolet and blue light hence they are sensitive to screens that emit UV light, green, and blue light (300–500 nm). The appropriate screen film combination is mandatory.
- High contrast medium speed films are suitable for skull view, and less contrast wider latitude films are used for cephalometric radiography.

6. Discuss the differences between screen and nonscreen films. (or) discuss the differences between intraoral and extraoral films.

The properties of intraoral and extraoral X-ray films differ in terms of sensitivity and shape of the silver halide crystals, type of package, film speed, and exposure (Table 1).

7. Describe the composition and uses of intensifying screens.

Intensifying screen is a device to convert X-ray energy to light energy.

Principle: X-rays cause certain materials like phosphors to fluoresce (emit UV or visible light radiation). This ability of phosphors to fluoresce when excited by X-rays makes the intensifying screens possible.

Composition: Base, phosphor layer, and protective plastic coat (Fig. 2).

Table 1: Comparison between intraoral and extraoral X-ray films.

Property	Intraoral (or) nonscreen (or) direct films	Extraoral (or) screen (or) indirect films
Silver halide crystals	Sensitive to X-rays	Silver halide crystals are coated with sensitizing dyes that are sensitive to UV light, green, or blue (300–500 nm)
Package	Film is inserted in a vinyl cover between black papers and a lead foil behind the film	The film is inserted between two intensifying screens on either side in a cassette
Types of film	1. High contrast-medium speed (skull view) 2. Low contrast—High speed (OPG) 3. Low contrast—wider latitude (cephalometric)	Based on usage: 1. Periapical films 2. Bitewing films 3. Occlusal films Based on speed: 1. D - speed film 2. F - speed film 3. E + speed film
Silver halide grain shape	Flat or triangular	Tubular
Film exposure	By X-rays	By sum of the effects of X-rays and visible light emitted by screen phosphors

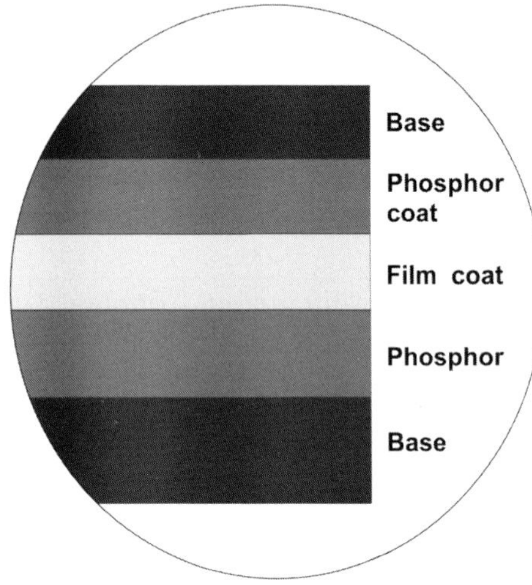

Fig. 2: Intensifying screen layout.

Base

- About 0.25 mm thick polyester plastic
- Provides mechanical support for the film
- It may also serve as a reflecting layer—reflects light emitted by screen back to film.

Phosphor Layer

- Composed of radiation sensitive phosphorescent crystals supported in a plastic material.
- Phosphor crystals are made up of rare earth elements like lanthanum and gadolinium with the addition of trace amounts of niobium, thulium or terbium to increase the fluorescence (rare earth screens).
- Most dental extraoral radiography uses screen-film combination having a speed of 250 or faster.

Coat

Up to 8 μm thick plastic is coated over phosphor to protect the phosphor layer and provide a surface that can be cleaned.

Function

- Presence of intensifying screens makes films 10–60 times more sensitive to X-rays than when they used alone.
- Significant reduction in radiation dose to patient.

8. Describe the composition and functions of grid.

A grid is a material that *reduces the scatter radiation* from reaching radiographic film during exposure. It is employed in extraoral radiographic procedures to *minimize the film fog* caused by scatter rays and to *increase the image contrast.*

Composition

A grid is composed of alternating strips of radiopaque (*lead*) and radiolucent (plastic) material (Fig. 3).

Types of Grid

- Focused grid
- Moving or Bucky grid
- Criss-cross grid
- Parallel grid

The grid is placed between the patient and film. During exposure, the grid permits the passage of X-rays only between two lead stripes. Secondary photons generated in the subject are scattered toward the film, are absorbed by the radiopaque material of the grid.

Focused grid: In *focused grid,* the lead strips are inclined gradually as they move from the center. Lines through each of these strips converge to a point and hense known as focused grid.

Moving grid: Moves perpendicular to the direction of the grid lines during exposure.

Criss-cross grid: Criss-cross grid is the one in which two grids are sandwiched together so that the strips are both parallel and right angle to the long axis of the grid. Crossed grid removes more scattered radiation.

Parallel grid: In *parallel (or) linear grid* all strips are vertical and arranged parallel to each other and also to the X-ray tube. Use of parallel grid is recommended when tilted tube technique is used.

Grid lines: Grids are manufactured with varying number of line pairs of lead and plastic materials per inch. Grids with *80 or more line pairs* are preferred because they do not show the grid lines on image.

Grid ratio: It is the ratio of heights of the lead strips to the width of radiolucent spacer. Higher the grid ratio more effective will be the removal of secondary photons. The various grid ratios available are 5:1, 6:1, 8:1, 10:1, and 12:1. Grid ratio of 8 or 10 is preferred.

9. Describe Bucky grid. (or) Potter-Bucky grid.

The grid is an apparatus used in extraoral radiographic procedures to minimize the scatter rays and thereby *decrease the film fog and enhance the image contrast.* A grid is made

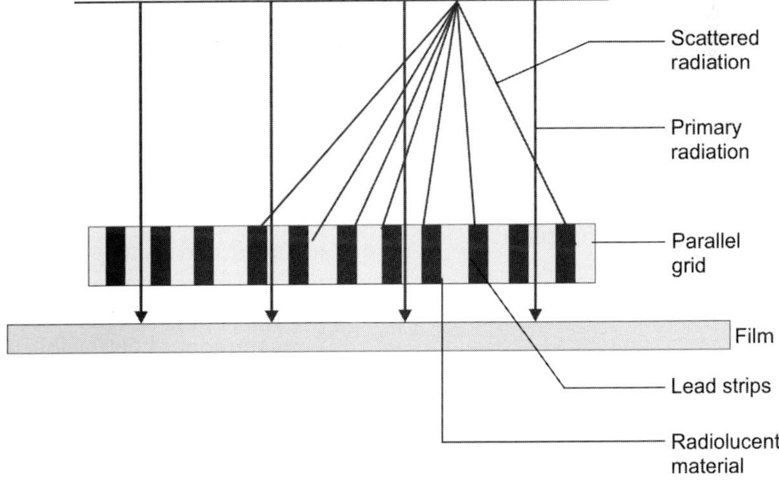

Fig. 3: Structure of a grid.

by placing alternating strips of radiopaque (*lead*) and radiolucent (*plastic*) material. It is placed between the patient and film. During exposure, the grid permits the passage of X-rays only through the radiolucent stripes. When secondary photons generated in the subject are scattered toward the film, they are absorbed by the radiopaque material of the grid. But the image of the *radiolucent* grid lines may be visible on the processed radiograph and interfere with diagnostic quality.

To prevent the formation of radiolucent grid line image, a special type of *moving grid* is used. The grid moves perpendicular to the direction of the grid lines during exposure and this movement has the *blurring out effect on radiolucent lines* and does not interfere with absorption of scattered photons. The apparatus used for moving the grid is called as bucky and hence the name Bucky grid.

10. Describe the label side of the film packet.

The label of the packet contains a color coded clinch that should be unsealed in the darkroom. When film is placed in mouth, the color coded side of the packet must face the tongue or palate.

The information carried by the label side includes:

- A circle that corresponds to the raised identification dot on the film
- The film speed
- The number of the films enclosed.

11. Describe the film duplication procedure.

Armamentarium

- Film duplicator—commercially available light source which provides diffuse light that in turn evenly exposes the duplicating film
- Duplicating film
- Films to be duplicated
- Darkroom.

Procedure

Dental radiographs to be duplicated (original image) is placed on the light screen of film duplicator by using film organizers.

- On the top of these radiographs, duplicating films should be arranged with their emulsion side facing the image. To avoid blurring, good contact should be established between the original and duplicating film.
- Film duplicator lid should be closed properly without disturbing the film position.
- After selecting the exposure time, the light source is activated to expose the duplicating film.
- The exposed film is then processed either by manual or automatic processing technique.
- The processed duplicate radiograph is then labeled with patient's name, right or left side and date.

12. What is characteristic cure? (or) explain H and D curve.

Hunter and Driffield introduced characteristic curves. They are constructed by taking a series of exposures of certain film type, developing the film and reading the density by use of densitometer and plotting the density reading against a known exposure.

In a typical H and D curve, there will be great variations in exposure at high and low level which results in small change in density.

The characteristic curve will give useful information about *speed, contrast, and latitude* of the film.

13. Describe how intensifying screens reduce radiation dose.

- A pair of intensifying screens absorbs 60% of X-ray photons that reach the cassette after exposing patient.
- The phosphor in the screen is efficient in converting X-ray photons to visible light.
- Each absorbed X-ray photon is converted into 4,000 low energy, visible light (blue or green) photons which then expose the film. 1 X-ray photon = 4,000 visible light photon.

14. What are intraoral measurement grids?

Intraoral measurement grids are used to *quantify and evaluate bone levels.* They are commercially available that superimpose thin radiopaque or radiolucent lines in the vertical or horizontal planes in 1-mm gradations. The marking grid incorporated into the film packet or it is placed in front of the film packet during exposure. No increase in exposure is necessary, and the films are processed without changing the parameters. The measurement or marking grid should not be confused with grids used in extraoral radiography to absorb object scatter.

15. What is radiographic noise?

Radiographic noise is the *appearance of the uneven density* of the uniformly exposed film.

It is seen in small areas of the film as localized variation in density. The primary causes of noise are radiographic mottle and radiographic artifact.

Radiographic mottle: Uneven densities resulting from the physical structure of the film and intensifying screens.

Radiographic artifacts: Defects caused by errors in film handling, e.g. fingerprints, bends on film, marks, or scratches.

In intraoral films, mottle may be seen as *film graininess* that is caused by the visibility of silver grains on the image when high temperature processing solution is used.

MULTIPLE CHOICE QUESTIONS

1. Silver bromide in the emulsion influences the ***film speed***.
   a. Base adhesion
   b. Sensitive spikes
   c. Film speed
   d. Image quality
2. Spectral sensitivity is film's response to ***various colors***.
   a. Different radiation
   b. Various colors
   c. Light exposure
   d. Intensifying screens
3. To make intensifying screen base as reflective, manufacturer adds ***titanium dioxide***.
   a. Terbium bromide
   b. Lanthanum sulfide
   c. Neodymium oxide
   d. Titanium dioxide
4. Image details in films using intensifying screens with reflective layer will be ***less sharp***.
   a. High contrast
   b. Low contrast
   c. More sharp
   d. Less sharp
5. Grids are commonly used in dentistry for ***cephalometry***.
   a. Orthopantomography
   b. Cephalometry
   c. Lateral oblique
   d. PA mandible
   (**Note:** Grids are used in dentistry for cephalometric and TMJ radiographs).
6. Step wedge is made up of ***aluminum***.
   a. Lead
   b. Copper
   c. Tungsten
   d. Aluminium
7. Step wedge is used to monitor the ***qualities of film***.
   a. Qualities of film
   b. Exposure parameters
   c. Dark room integrity
   d. Processing technique
   (**Note:** Step wedge is used to monitor the *densities and contrast*).
8. Image shape distortion is minimal on using ***paralleling technique***.
   a. Bisecting technique
   b. Bitewing technique
   d. Paralleling technique
   d. Tube shift technique
9. Fog in film results in ***increased film density***.
   a. Increased image contrast
   b. Increased film density
   c. Image distortion
   d. Image unsharpness
   (**Note:** Fog results in increased film density and decreased contrast).
10. Image sharpness is the ability of radiograph to define ***the edges precisely***.
    a. Closely placed structures
    b. Boundaries of lesion
    c. Morphological features
    d. The edges precisely

11. Resolution is the property of the radiograph that allows the detection of ***different structures that are close together***.
    a. Different structures that are close together
    b. Structures in different shades of gray
    c. Different structures with same density
    d. Structures that reflects radiation
12. A radiograph displaying many shades of gray is said to have ***long scale contrast***.
    a. Short scale contrast
    b. High contrast
    c. Long scale contrast
    d. High density
    (**Note:** Low contrast or long scale contrast).
13. Variation in true size or shape of radiographic image is known as ***distortion***.
    a. Elongation
    b. Unsharpness
    c. Haziness
    d. Distortion
14. Moisture resistant barrier for the film is ***paper wrapper***.
    a. Lead foil
    b. Paper wrapper
    c. Adhesive coat
    d. Base
15. The ideal grid ratio is ***8:1***.
    a. 5:1
    b. 8:1
    c. 10:1
    d. 12:1

VIVA VOCE

1. Define radiograph.

A radiograph is a two-dimensional representation of a three-dimensional object. In conventional mode, a radiograph is an image produced by exposing the radiographic film to X-rays and then processing it get a visible image. Radiopaque and radiolucent are the terms used to describe the appearance of all structures seen on a radiograph.

2. What is a duplicate radiograph?

A duplicate radiograph is one that is identical to the original X-ray film and is mainly used for patient's referrals to specialists, for insurance claims, and for teaching-learning purposes.

3. What is duplicating film?

It is a type of photographic film used to make an identical copy of a radiograph (both intraoral and extraoral).

The *key differences* between X-ray film and duplicating film:

- The duplicating film should not be exposed to X-rays and have to be used in darkroom setting.
- The duplicating film should contain emulsion on one side only.
- When exposed for a longer period of light, duplicating film appears lighter in contrast to X-ray film which appears darker on prolonged exposure to radiation.
- The emulsion coated side seems dull and the other side appears shiny.

Duplicating films are available in three sizes: 5 × 12 inch, 6 × 12 inch, and 8 × 10 inch.

4. What is two film packet in dental radiology?

An intraoral X-ray film packet may contain two films and produces two indistinguishable radiographs when exposed using the same exposure parameters required producing a single radiograph. The two film pocket is used when a duplicate record of a radiographic image is required (patient referral, insurance claims, etc.).

5. What is film latitude?

Film latitude is the ability to distinguish different densities on a film. It refers to the range of exposures (mAs) to which an X-ray film will respond with a diagnostically acceptable range of densities (range from 0.5 to 2.5).

Wide latitude film record wide range of subject contrast but have lower contrast (long grayscale). High kVp produces an image with wide latitude and low contrast.

6. What is radiographic noise?

Radiographic noise is the appearance of uneven densities on a uniformly exposed film.

7. What is the purpose of using lead foil in intraoral films?

- The lead foil placed in the back of the film, prevent the radiation backscattered by the tissues reaching the film and reduces film fog.
- It absorbs some of the radiation after they pass they penetrate the tissues and expose the film hence reduces secondary radiation to an extent.
- Lead foil contributes to the rigidity of the packet.

8. Why intensifying screens are used in intraoral films?

Use of intensifying screens reduces the "resolution" of the image. So, we cannot get fine details.

9. Why grids are not used in intraoral and panoramic radiography?

The function of the grid is to reduce the amount of scattered radiation originating in the object and thereby improves the contrast.

In intraoral radiography, secondary radiation does not lower the image quality due to small field size, hence do not require grids.

In panoramic radiography, the usage of a small exposure field size does not require grid.

10. What is radiographic blurring?

It is image unsharpness caused by:

- **Image receptor blurring:** Slow speed films have fine silver grains hence fine sharpness. Faster films have larger grains and less sharp images.
- **Motion blurring:** Image unsharpness is due to movement of the film, subject or X-ray source during exposure.
- **Geometric blurring:** Loss of image sharpness occur due to larger focal spot size, reduced the distance between the focal spot and an object and increased distance between the film and object.

11. What is parallax?

The image on each side of the double emulsion film will cause some loss of image unsharpness. Dental films are double side emulsion coated, and beam is divergent hence some unsharpness occur when the image is recorded.

Parallax is the *apparent change in position or size of the subject* when it is viewed from different side of the film. In intraoral images, the effect of parallax is *more apparent when wet films are viewed.*

BIBLIOGRAPHY

1. Bailoor DM, Nagesh KS. Fundamentals of oral medicine and radiology. 1st edition. Jaypee Brothers Medical Publishers;New Delhi; 2005.
2. Langland OE, Langlais RP, Preece JW. Principles of dental imaging. Lippincott Williams & Wilkins; Baltimore, 2002.
3. Whaites E, Drage N. Essentials of dental radiography and radiology. Elsevier Health Sciences; 2013.
4. White SC, Pharoah MJ. Oral radiology: principles and interpretation. St. Louis: Mosby.
5. Zietlow MH, inventor; Eastman Kodak Co, assignee. Dental X-ray films. United States patent US 5,370,977; 1994.

CHAPTER 30

X-Ray Film Processing and Faulty Radiographs

HIGHLIGHTS

Photographic film is adapted for dental imaging purposes and on exposure to X-radiation which has passed through orofacial structures; latent image is formed on the film. The subsequent chemical processing in darkroom leads to conversion of the dormant image into a visible image for the diagnostic purpose. This chapter highlights the different types of dental X-ray film, the composition of the film, proper film processing techniques with a detailed description of image formation. This knowledge will help to enhance the film handling capability and reduces film related errors.

Learners are expected to study:

- Definition and formation of latent image
- Description of processing
- Manual and automatic processing
- Darkroom set up
- Composition and function of processing solution
- Processing errors
- Faulty radiographs.

ESSAY QUESTIONS

1. Describe in detail film composition and explain latent image formation.

X-ray film has four basic components:

1. Base
2. Adhesive layer
3. Emulsion
4. Protective layer

Base

Film base is *0.2 mm thick* and is made up of flexible, polyester (polyethylene terephthalate). It is transparent and exhibits slight bluish tint to emphasize the contrast. The base increases the strength of the film and also supports the emulsion.

Adhesive Layer

The thin adhesive layer is added on both sides of the film base before the application of emulsion and functions to attach the emulsion to the base.

Film Emulsion

Emulsion is a coating attached by an adhesive layer on either side of the film. The emulsion is a homogenous mixture of gelatine and silver halide crystals.

Gelatin: It is used to suspend and disperse silver halide crystals over the film base. During processing, gelatine absorbs the processing solutions and allows the chemicals to react with silver halide crystals.

Silver halide crystals: These crystals are sensitive to X-rays and visible light. They are composed *primarily of silver bromide* and a lesser amount of silver iodide. The photosensitivity of silver halide crystals is further increased by the addition of small amounts of *trace materials* like sulfur or gold.

The silver halide grains are flat, tabular with a mean diameter of 1.6 μm in E speed film and are globular with 1 μm size in D speed film.

Protective Layer

It is a thin, transparent coating placed over the emulsion. It protects the surface from manipulation, mechanical and processing damage.

Latent Image

The latent image is the *dormant or invisible image* that is formed after exposure of the film and before processing.

When the film is exposed to X-ray radiation, silver halide crystals especially bromide ions are energized by the X-ray beam through Compton and photoelectric interaction. These crystals are then ionized by removal of an electron from the bromide resulting in separation of silver and bromine atoms.

Irregularities in the lattice structure known as *sensitive specks* draw the free electrons and become negatively charged. Now, this negative charged sensitive speck attracts the positively charged silver and forms neutral aggregates of metallic silver known as *latent image centers.* This process occurs many times at a single site within a crystal.

The metallic silver at each latent image site makes the crystals sensitive to chemical developing and image formation. Developer solution converts metallic silver sites into black, solid silver grains that can be visualized. Fixer solution takes away the underdeveloped halide crystals and makes the film appear plain in unexposed regions.

2. Describe in detail the conversion of a latent image to visible image. (or) reveal the detailed outline of visible radiographic image formation. (or) explain in detail about film processing.

When x-rays strike the silver halides (AgIBr) film emulsion, the energy is stored in the form of latent image.

"Processing the film completes what the exposure started". The latent image becomes visible after the film is immersed in processing chemical solutions that change the exposed silver halide salts into metallic silver. Processing is the common procedure that converts an invisible image to visible, can be carried out either manually or automatically.

Purpose of Film Processing

- To transfer the invisible image into visible.
- To preserve the visible image without distortion.

Film Processing

Manual processing should proceeded in the dark-room.

During processing, the exposed film is subjected to series of a chemical reaction. The initial step in film processing is, "*selective reduction*"—the reduction of energized, exposed silver halide crystals into metallic silver, while the unexposed silver halide crystals are removed from the film (Fig. 1).

- The film is placed in a chemical solution called *"developer"* for a specific period and at a specific temperature. The developer recognizes the exposed and unexposed halide crystals, and then reduces the exposed silver halide crystals into black metallic silver, producing dark or black areas on the film (Flowchart 1).
- Unexposed silver halide crystals remain unaffected.
- The film is immersed in water to clean the remnants of developer solution.
- The film is next placed in *"fixer"* solution for the specific time. It takes out the unexposed silver halide crystals and produces bright areas on the film.

The black metallic silver remains on the film.

After fixing, the film is thoroughly cleaned in tap water. This removes the remnant chemical solutions and then dried.

Visible Image

The visible image is made up of dark, bright, and shades of gray areas.

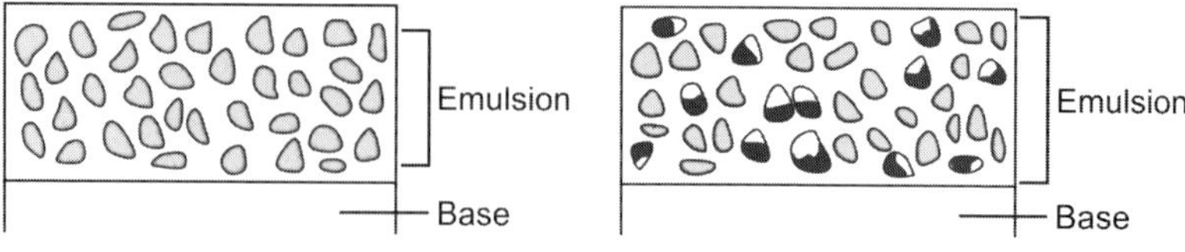

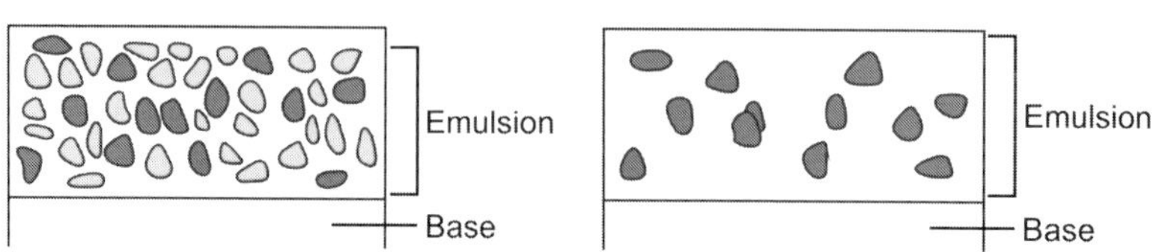

Fig. 1: Changes occurring on emulsion during film development process.

Flowchart 1: Formation of latent and visible images.

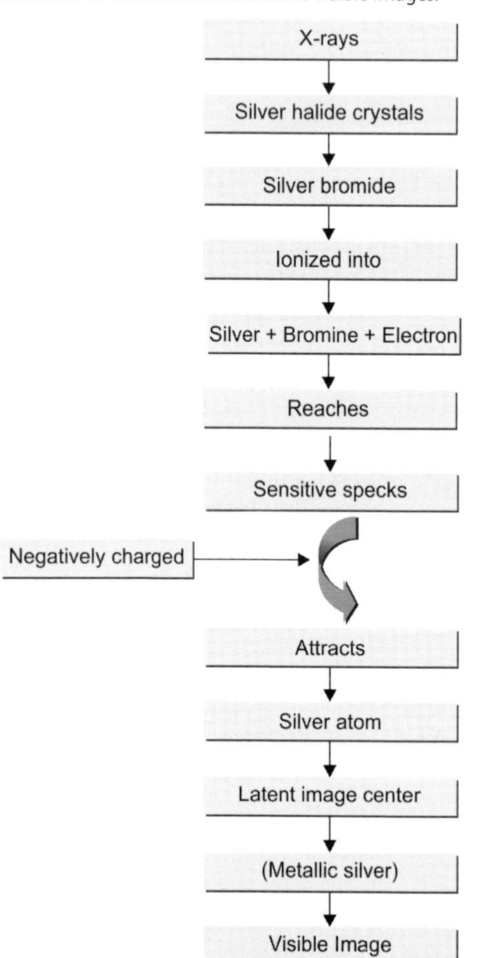

Black areas = Deposits of black metallic silver. The amount of the metallic silver varies in proportion to the properties of the structures exposed to diagnostic radiation.

White areas = Removal of unexposed silver halide crystals.

Structures that *permit the passage of X-ray beam* appear black or *radiolucent.*

Structures that *resist the passage of X-ray beam* appear *white or radiopaque.*

3. What are film processing solutions? Write the composition of two chemical solutions required for film processing.

The film processing solutions are the chemicals required to convert latent image to a visible image. They are available in three forms:

1. Powder
2. Ready to use liquid
3. Liquid concentrate (most commonly used type because it is easy to mix and container occupies less storage space)

   Both powder and liquid concentrate forms should be mixed with distilled water. *Developer* and *fixer* are the two chemicals used as processing solution.

Composition of Developer Solution

The four basic ingredients are (Table 1):

1. Developing agent
2. Preservative

3. Accelerator and
4. Restrainer.

Composition of Fixer Solution

The four basic ingredients are (Table 2):

1. Fixing agent
2. Preservative
3. Hardening agent
4. Acidifier.

4. Describe the problems encountered in film processing and state the feasible solution for each. (or) state the possible processing errors and the remedial measures to overcome.

Processing errors affects the diagnostic quality of the image by resulting in a partial or complete loss of images or unclear images of structures that are captured. Many errors are attributed to one or several causes.

Table 1: Composition and function of developer solution.

Ingredient	Chemical	Function
Developing agent (or) reducing agent	▪ *Hydroquinone* (paradihydroxybenzene) This is temperature sensitive—inactive below 60°F and highly active above 80°F. Optimal temperature is 68°F for the developing solution ▪ *Elon or Metol* (monomethyl-para-aminophenol sulfate)	▪ Converts the exposed silver halide crystals to *black metallic silver* ▪ Slowly imparts gray tones and contrast in the image ▪ Reduces the exposed halide crystals to *black metallic silver* ▪ Quickly transmits gray tones in the image
Preservative	*Sodium sulfite*	▪ Prevents rapid oxidation of the developing agents ▪ Increases the half-life of hydroquinone and elon
Accelerator (or) activator	*Sodium carbonate*	▪ Activates the developer agents ▪ Provides the *alkaline*. pH for developing agents ▪ Softens the gelatin of the film emulsion and allows the chemicals to reach silver halide crystals
Restrainer	*Potassium bromide*	▪ Prevents the action of developer on unexposed silver halide crystals ▪ Prevents image fogging

Table 2: Composition and function of fixer solution.

Ingredient	Chemical	Function
Fixing agent (or) clearing agent	Hypo = *Ammonium thiosulfate*	▪ Removes all the undeveloped and underdeveloped silver halide crystals from the emulsion by forming stable, water soluble complexes with silver ions ▪ The black image produced by the developer becomes readily distinguished
Preservative	*Sodium sulfite (or) ammonium sulfite*	▪ Reduces the chemical disintegration of the fixer solution ▪ Prevents developer staining from binding with oxidized developer that is carried over into fixing solution
Acidifier	*Acetic acid pH 4–4.5*	▪ Neutralizes the alkaline developer and prevents further developing. ▪ Allows diffusion of thiosulfate into emulsion and silver thiosulfate complexes out of emulsion
Hardening agent	Aluminium salts	▪ Aluminium complexes with gelatin and prevents the damage to the gelatine on subsequent handling ▪ Shrinks and hardens the gelatin in the emulsion

Processing errors are grouped into four possible categories:
1. Time and temperature errors
2. Chemical contamination errors
3. Film handling errors
4. Static electricity errors.

Time and Temperature Errors

The errors due to processing time and due to temperature of the processing solutions are underdeveloped film, overdeveloped film, and reticulation of emulsion (Table 3).

Chemical Contamination Errors

Developer spots, fixer spots and yellow or brown stains are the errors that occur due to chemical contamination of the processing solution (Table 4).

Table 3: Time and temperature errors.

Errors	Film appearance	Reason	Solution
Underdeveloped film	*Light image*	▪ Inadequate developing time ▪ Low temperature of developing solution ▪ Inaccurate timer or thermometer ▪ Depleted or contaminated developer solution	▪ Check development time ▪ Check developer temperature ▪ Replace faulty timer or thermometer ▪ Replenish developer with fresh solutions as needed.
Overdeveloped film	*Dark image*	▪ Excessive developing time ▪ Too hot developer solution ▪ Inaccurate timer or thermometer ▪ Concentrated developer solution ▪ Inadequate fixation ▪ Improper safe lighting	▪ Check the development time ▪ Check the developer temperature ▪ Replace the faulty timer or thermometer ▪ Correct the developer strength using distilled water ▪ Check for safe light integrity
Reticulation of emulsion	Cracked appearance	Sudden temperature change between developer and water bath	Avoid drastic temperature differences

Table 4: Chemical contaminations errors.

Error	Film appearance	Reason	Solution
Developer spots	*Dark or black spots*	▪ Film contaminated with developer before processing ▪ Black wrapping paper sticking to film surface ▪ Film in contact with another film or tank *during fixation* ▪ Excessive roller pressure during automatic processing ▪ Dirty rollers in automatic processing	▪ Care in the removal of the film from the pocket ▪ Careful fixing ▪ Check the cleanliness and functional status of the automatic processer
Fixer spots	*White or light spots*	▪ Film contaminated with fixer before processing ▪ Film in contact with another film or tank *during development*	▪ Careful removal of film from the pocket and expose to processing solutions with utmost care
Yellow or brown stain	Yellow or brown color	▪ Depleted developer ▪ Depleted fixer ▪ Contaminated solutions ▪ Insufficient fixation time ▪ Insufficient washing	▪ Replenish chemicals with fresh solutions as needed ▪ Adequate fixation time ▪ Rinse for a minimum of 20 minutes

Table 5: Film handling errors.

Error	Film appearance	Reason	Solutions
Developer cut-off	*Straight white border*	Undeveloped portion of the film due to low level of developer	Check developer level before processing and add if needed
Fixer cut-off	*Straight black border*	Unfixed portion of the film due to the low level of fixer	Check fixer level before processing and add if needed
Overlapped films	*White or dark areas appear on film where overlapped*	Two films contacting each other during processing	Separate films during processing so that no contact takes place
Air bubbles	*White spots*	Air trapped on the film surface after being placed in the processing solutions	Gently agitate film racks after placing in processing solutions
Fingerprint artifact	*Black fingerprint*	Film touched by fingers that are contaminated with developer	Gently hold the film only at the edges
Static electricity	*Thin, black branching lines*	▪ Opening the film pocket quickly ▪ Opening the film pack before touching the conductive object.	Touch the conductive object before unwrapping the film
Scratched film	*White lines*	Soft emulsion removed from the film by a sharp object	Careful handling of films and film racks
Fingernail artifact	*Black crescent-shaped marks*	Film emulsion damaged by operators fingernail	Gently handle the film and hold at the edges alone

Film Handling Errors

Improper handling of the X-ray film before and during exposure and at the time of film processing results in number of errors (Table 5).

Static Electricity Errors

Lightning marks occur on the processed radiographs either due to forcible removal of the film from the pocket or due to the excess bending of the film.

5. List the possible errors that can occur due to improper film exposure and the appropriate steps to overcome such errors. (or) state the exposure errors that result in faulty radiograph.

When taking the radiograph, the improper exposure parameters may results in different types of errors (Table 6). It is necessary to avoid such exposure errors to avoid the incidents of faulty radiographs.

6. What is faulty radiograph? Enumerate the common causes of faulty radiographs. (or) mention the types of intraoral radiographic errors.

A faulty radiograph is one in which the diagnostic quality of the image is suboptimal or unacceptable in contrast to typical radiographic image with appropriate contrast, density, sharp outlines.

The causes of faulty radiographs are due to (Table 7):

- Developing errors
- Processing errors.

7. Discuss darkroom requirements and add a note to safe lighting.

The darkroom is the place in radiology unit where the exposed films can be handled and processed to produce diagnostic radiographs. An ideal darkroom should have:

- Convenient location
- Adequate size

Table 6: The exposure errors.

Error	Film appearance	Reason	Solution
Cone cut (or) collimator cut-off	*A curved or straight radiopaque border representing the unexposed region*	X-ray beam is not centered on the film	▪ Central ray should be aligned with the center of the film ▪ Use of localizing ring with a film holding device ▪ Patient position should not be changed after the position indicating device (PID) is arranged
Film reversal effect (or) herring bone pattern (or) tire track appearance	*Light film with the geometric pattern of the lead foil embossed on it*	Film packet is placed backward in the mouth	The uncolored surface of the film packet should contact the lingual aspect of the teeth
Improper film placement	*The image of the desired structures do not appear completely on the film*	The center of the film is not aligned with the center of the appropriate tooth	Align the center of the film with the center of the area being radiographed
Horizontal overlapping	*The interproximal areas of the teeth appear to be overlapped when the teeth are not overlapped*	▪ The central ray is not aligned at a right angle to the film ▪ The film is not parallel to the tooth in the horizontal plane	▪ The central ray should pass through the contact points ▪ Place the film parallel to the teeth in the horizontal plane
Overexposed film	*Dark in appearance*	Excessive exposure	Exposure parameters should be checked
Underexposed film	*Light in appearance*	Inadequate exposure	Exposure parameters should be checked
Foreshortened image	*Images of teeth appear too short with blunted roots*	▪ Excessive vertical angulation ▪ The central ray should be at the right angle to the film surface but not to the imaginary bisector	Use appropriate vertical angulation. ▪ The central ray should be at right angle to the imaginary bisector
Elongated image	*Images of teeth appear too long*	▪ Insufficient vertical angulation ▪ The central ray should be at the right angle to the long axis of the tooth rather than to the imaginary bisector	▪ Use of appropriate vertical angulation ▪ The occlusal plane should be parallel to the floor ▪ The film should be placed near the tooth as much possible in the bisecting angle technique and should be placed parallel to the tooth in paralleling technique
Double exposure	*Two images appear on the same film*	More than one exposure to the same film packet	Exposed films should be separated immediately from the unexposed film
Blurred images	*Wavy or fuzzy image*	Movement of patient, film or tube head during exposure	▪ Ask the patient "not to move" before exposing the film ▪ Check for the integrity of the tube head before exposing.

Contd...

Contd...

Error	Film appearance	Reason	Solution
Crescent marks	*Black marks or artifacts appear on the film*	Excessive bending of the film packet that result in a cracked emulsion	Overbending of the film packet should be avoided
Failure to remove dental appliances and facial jewelery	*Superimposition of radiopaque images*	Failure to ask the patient to remove the metallic objects in the mouth or face	Remove any obstructive intraoral appliances, and facial jewelry

Table 7: Causes of faulty radiographs.

Errors	Causes
▪ Radiopaque artifacts	Leaving dental appliances in mouth and jewelry in face
▪ Blurred image	Movement of film, patient or tube head during exposure
▪ Cone-cut	Partial coverage of film by Beam indicating device (BID) ▪ Too steep vertical angulation ▪ Faulty film placement
▪ Herringbone pattern or Ping-pong ball effect	Film reversal—back side of the film is placed toward the beam indicating device
▪ Black dot in apical area	The film side identification dot is placed towards the apical part of the teeth
▪ Double image	Film exposed twice to radiation
▪ Overlapping of teeth	▪ Plane of the film is not parallel to the teeth ▪ Incorrect horizontal angulation
▪ Foreshortening of image	▪ Increased vertical angulation ▪ The central ray is perpendicular to the plane of the film but not to the imaginary bisector
▪ Elongation of image	▪ Decreased vertical angulation ▪ Central ray is directed perpendicular to the long axis of the tooth rather than to the imaginary bisector
▪ Dimensional distortion of image	Elongation of palatal root and foreshortening of two buccal roots on maxillary molars
▪ Phalangioma—image of the patients finger bone	When the patient is holding the film; sometimes the finger is positioned in front of the film instead of behind the film
▪ Light image	▪ Inadequate developing time ▪ Low temperature of developing solution ▪ Inadequate exposure due to increased FFD or insufficient kVp, mA, or exposure time
▪ Dark image	▪ Excessive exposure due to decreased FFD or excessive kVp, mA, or exposure time ▪ Excessive developing time ▪ Increased temperature of the developer solution
▪ Yellow or brown stain	▪ Depleted developer ▪ Depleted fixer ▪ Contaminated solutions ▪ Insufficient fixation time ▪ Inadequate washing
▪ Film fog	▪ Improper safe lighting ▪ Prolonged exposure to safe light ▪ Light leaks ▪ Contaminated solutions ▪ Deteriorated film

- Correct lighting
- Adequate workspace and storage space
- Temperature and humidity control.

Location and Size

The darkroom should be in the area close to X-ray units. It should be at least 4 × 5 feet (1.2 × 1.5 m) and should be based on the following requirements:

- Volume of radiographs processed
- Number of persons using the room
- Type of processing equipment used
- Space required for film storage.

The room should have light proof and good ventilation.

Lighting

The term ''darkroom" or "light-tight room" suggests that the room might be completely dark, exclude all visible light, and no light leaks can be present. This is because the X-ray films are susceptible to visible light.

Room Lighting

Overhead white light providing adequate illumination is required to perform procedures like cleaning, mixing chemicals and stocking materials.

Safelight

The purpose is to provide illumination in the darkroom to carry out processing activities safely without exposing or damaging the film. It is a low intensity illumination of relatively long wavelength in the orange-red portion of the visible light spectrum.

Safelight consists of a lamp with a low-wattage (71/2–15 watt) bulb and a universal red GBX-2 filter for handling both intra- and extraoral films. The filter removes the blue-green portion of visible light and permits the passage of light only in orange-red portion.

The safelight must be fixed at 4 feet above the working area on the wall behind the processing tank.

Processing Tanks

The equipment required for manual processing is called processing tank (Fig. 2) and its recommended size for dental radiology unit is 20 × 25 cm (8 × 10 inches).

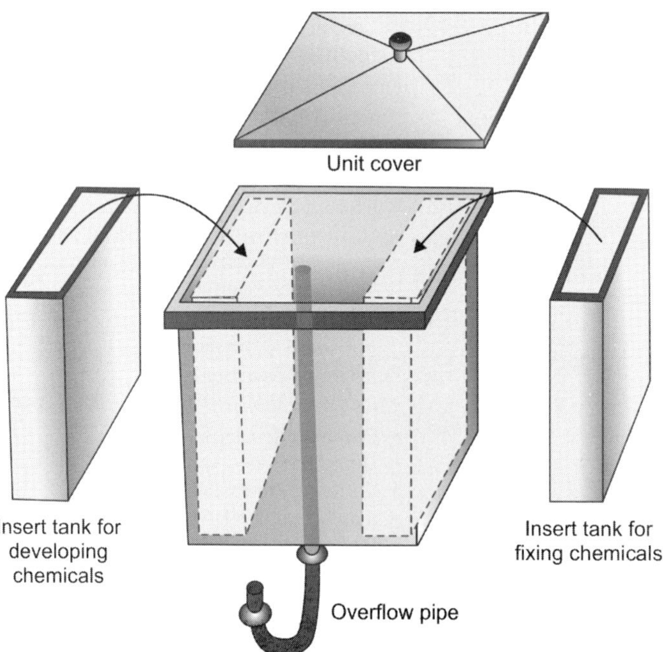

Fig. 2: Manual film processing tank.

Master Tank

Consists of two insert tanks and is filled with circulating water.

Insert Tank

The master tank holds two removable, one gallon insert tanks to hold the developer and fixer. The developer is always placed on the left side and fixer on the right side of the master tank. The water in the master tank separates the two insert tanks.

Thermometer

A nonmercury thermometer is clipped to the side of the developer solution and is used to determine the temperature of the developer solution. The optimum recommended temperature is 68°F, and below 60°F, the chemicals work too slowly and result in underdevelopment, whereas over 80°F, the chemicals work too rapidly and produce film fog.

Timer

A timer is used to indicate how long film should be placed in the developer, rinse water, fixer, and wash water.

Drying Racks

Two or three drying racks can be mounted on a wall for film hangers. Drip trays must be placed underneath the racks. An electronic fan can be used to circulate air and speed the drying. Cabinet dryers that circulate warm air around the film can also be used.

SHORT NOTES

1. Outline the steps of manual film processing.

Manual film processing (hand processing, tank processing) is a step-by-step procedure of developing, rinsing, fixing, washing and drying dental X-ray films to view the image.

Developing

The first step is introducing the exposed film to the developer which softens the film emulsion and allows the other chemicals to reach the film. The developer converts *the exposed silver halide crystals* into *black metallic silver.* The optimum temperature used for developer solution is 68°F with developing time of 5 minutes (between 68 and 70°F)

Rinsing

Rinsing the film in water for 20–30 seconds removes the residual developer that clings to the film and stop development process.

Fixing

The rinsed film is then introduced to fixer solution to *remove the unexposed silver halide crystals* and *harden the film emulsion.* The fixation time should be two times of the developing time.

Washing

The film is washed in a water bath for a minimum of 20 minutes to remove all the excess chemicals from the emulsion thoroughly.

Drying

Finally, the film is air dried at room temperature in a dust free environment or in a heated drying cabinet (temperature should not exceed 120°F).

2. List and describe the steps for automatic film processing. (or) discuss the mechanism of automatic film processer with its parts.

Automatic processing is a simpler way of processing both intraoral and extraoral films.

The automatic processor (Fig. 3) consists of an in-line arrangement and transport mechanism that receives the unwrapped film and transfers it through the *developing, fixing, washing and drying* sections.

The transport system is a series of rollers driven by a constant-speed motor. The roller functions to:

- Move the film through the developing solutions
- Agitate the solution through their motion
- Press the film emulsion and force some solution out of the emulsion so that the emulsions rapidly fill again with solutions.

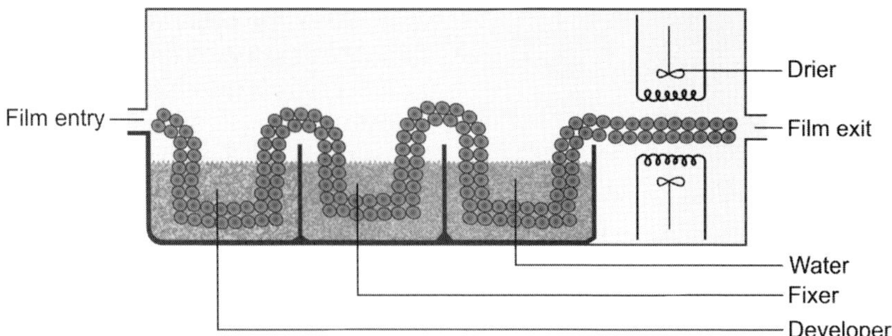

Fig. 3: Automatic film processor.

- Minimize the carryover of developer solution into fixer tank.

The *Developer compartment* holds the *highly concentrated*, developer solution that reacts at temperatures between 80 and 95°F. This high temperature aids in rapid development in contrast to manual processing developer solution. The film is then directly transported to *fixer compartment* without rinsing. Fixer solution is also highly concentrated and contains additional hardening agents. Here the film is rapidly cleared and then hardened.

Water compartment: Holds circulating water to wash the film after fixation.

After washing, the film is transported to *drying chamber* that dry the wet film using heated air.

The whole process takes 4–6 minutes, and processed radiographs are retrieved through the film recovery slot.

3. Describe film mounting methods.

A mounting technique is required to transfer the radiographic interpretative findings to patient's record.

Labial mounting method: Orientation is "from the lips"—as the dentist is looking at the patient.

The *raised or convex side* of the embossed dot should face the dentist who is interpreting. By this method of viewing the film, the *patient's right is on the dentist's left side,* and the *patient's left is on the dentist's right side.*

Lingual mounting method: Orientation is "from the tongue"—as the dentist is looking out from a position inside the oral cavity.

The *depressed or concave side* of the embossed dot should face the dentist who is interpreting. In this method, the *patient's right is on the dentist's right side* and the *patient's left is on the dentist's left side.*

MULTIPLE CHOICE QUESTIONS

1. The temperature sensitive chemical in the developing solution is ***hydroquinone***.
   a. Elon
   b. Sodium sulphite
   c. Hydroquinone
   d. Sodium corbonate
2. "Cone-cut" in a radiographic film is otherwise called as ***collimator cut-off***.
   a. Partial image
   b. Collimator cut-off
   c. Filter cut-off
   d. Unexposed part
3. Herringbone effect is the result of ***film reversal***.
   a. Light leak
   b. Old film
   c. Contaminated processing solution
   d. Film reversal
4. To record the root lengths of maxillary molars, the preferred radiographic technique is ***paralleling technique***.
   a. Paralleling technique
   b. Bisecting angle technique
   c. Bitewing radiograph
   d. SLOB technique
5. X-ray films are highly sensitive to ***short wavelength***.
   a. Long wavelength
   b. Short wavelength

c. Orange spectrum
d. Red spectrum
(**Note:** X-ray films are *less sensitive* to long wavelength, Orange-red region of the light spectrum and are *highly sensitive* to short wavelength, a blue-green region of the light spectrum).

6. Thermometer used in processing tank should contain ***alcohol or metal***.
   a. Mercury
   b. Hydrogen
   c. Water
   d. Alcohol
   (**Note:** Thermometer used in processing tank should contain alcohol or metal).

VIVA VOCE

1. What are rapid processing chemicals?

These are chemicals similar in composition with the film processing solution but are highly concentrated.

They normally develop films in 15 seconds and fix them in 15 seconds at room temperature.

2. Will you refer fast processing solution in your practice?

I will prefer conventional solutions for routine use and prefer rapid processing solutions *only in emergency situations.*

3. What is the problem in using rapid processing solution and tell the possible solution to correct it.

The image obtained using rapid processing solution will be acceptable for immediate assessment but discolor over time. Also, the contrast will not be the same degree of conventionally processed films.

To overcome this, rapidly processed films should be placed in conventional fixing solution for 4 minutes and washed for 10 minutes to improve the contrast and keep them stable in storage.

4. How to check for depleted processing solution (or) when to change the processing solution?

Immediately after preparing the new solution, a double film pocket is exposed to the first radiographed patient. These pocket films are processed in the newer solution, and one film is handed over to the patient, and another one should be mounted on the corner of a view box as reference film. As successive films are processed, they should be compared with the reference film.

When the solution become deteriorates, contrast and density of the image will become inferior to that of the reference film image and is the indication for changing the solution (both developer and fixer).

5. What is phalangioma?

Image of the distal phalanx (bone finger) seen in the radiographic image is known as phalangioma. This is commonly associated with bisecting technique when the patient is asked to hold the film. They may keep the finger in front of the film instead of holding at the back.

6. What is replenishment?

With the usage of processing solutions, the activity of developer and fixer become slow down gradually, and their effect on the film also diminishes. To compensate for this loss of activity, replenishment of solution is done by adding a fresh developer and fresh fixer to the respective insert tank depending on the workload.

For example, in manual processing with a average work load of 30 intraoral or 5 extraoral films per/day, 8 ounces of each developer and fixer should be added freshly per/gallon of solution per/day.

Insufficient replenishment of developer results in loss of image contrast and that of fixer causes inadequate hardening of the emulsion.

7. Why mercury containing thermometers are not used in processing tanks?

Mercury is a toxic substance, and if the thermometer breaks, the mercury will spill out and contaminate the processing solutions.

8. What is a latent image?

The pattern of stored energy on an exposed film is known as latent image. This image remains invisible until the film undergoes processing.

9. What is dimensional distortion?

When maxillary molars are radiographed using *bisecting angle* technique, distortion in the length of the roots of molar may take place as elongation of palatal root and foreshortening of the two buccal roots. Both buccal and palatal roots do not lie in the bisecting plane.

Using paralleling technique will avoid distortion.

10. What are advantages of using automatic film processing?

Automatic processor is preferred for the following reasons:

- Less processing time
- Automatically controlled time and temperatures
- Less equipment
- Less space.

The major advantages include:

- The requirement of only 4–6 minutes for the entire processing.
- Consistency in density and contrast properties.

BIBLIOGRAPHY

1. Hardman PK, Tilmon MF, Taylor TS. Radiographic solution contamination. Oral Surg Oral Med Oral Pathol.1987;63(6):733-7.
2. Langland OE, Langlais RP, Preece JW. Principles of dental imaging. Lippincott Williams & Wilkins;Baltimore, 2002.
3. Whaites E, Drage N. Essentials of dental radiography and radiology. 5th edition. Chuchill Livingstone. Edingburgh, Scotland, 2013.
4. White SC, Pharoah MJ. Oral radiology: Principles and interpretation. Elsevier Health Sciences; 2014.
5. White SC, Pharoah MJ. Principles and interpretation. St Louis. 2014:431-3.

CHAPTER 31

Projection Geometry

HIGHLIGHTS

Certain qualities of radiograph are defined by the geometric description like exposure factors, focal spot size and its relation to object and film. These related factors, in turn, describe the sharpness, magnification, and distortion features of the image.

Learners are expected to study:

- Three geometric characteristics of the image
- Factors helping to improve the quality of radiographs
- Causes for geometric unsharpness, magnification and distortion
- Radiographic localization of foreign object or impacted tooth within the jaw.

ESSAY QUESTIONS

1. Explain object localization techniques (or) describe the methods to obtain three-dimensional radiographic information of an object. (or) briefly write the technique to decide the location of an impacted tooth.

Purpose

- Adds a third dimension to two-dimensional radiographs.
- Determines the buccal or lingual position of an object.
- Identifies the object's relative position.

Uses

Localization is needed to determine the position of foreign bodies, broken needles, broken instruments, restorative materials, retained roots, impacted tooth, supernumerary tooth, nonerupted tooth or fracture of alveolus or condyle.

Two techniques are used:

1. Tube shift method (Clark's technique)
2. Buccal object rule (Richard's technique)

Tube Shift Method

Clark invented tube shift method and hence known as Clark's rule.

It determines the **buccolingual relationship** of the impacted tooth or foreign objects within the jaws by taking two periapical radiographs at different angles.

The first radiograph is taken in a usual method, whereas the second radiograph should be taken with different horizontal angulation by shifting the tube about 20° either mesially or distally. The point of entry, film position and vertical angulation should remain same as the previous exposure.

Comparison of the Two Images—SLOB Rule

If the **object travels on the same side of the reference point**, when **the tube head** is shifted horizontally, it indicates that the object is located on the **lingual side** (Figs. 1A and B).

When the **object shifts in opposite direction of the reference point**, when **the tube head** is moved in mesial direction (horizontally), it indicated that the object is placed on the **buccal/labial side** (Figs. 2A and B).

The localization (of impacted tooth, pathosis or foreign object) is made concerning a reference object.

Buccal-Object Rule Method

This method was proposed by Richards.

In this technique, the horizontal angulation of the central beam should be changed to locate vertically positioned structures like root canals, and the vertical angulation of the central beam should be changed to locate horizontally positioned structures like a mandibular canal. The technique requires two different radiographs on the same region to locate the position of the hidden

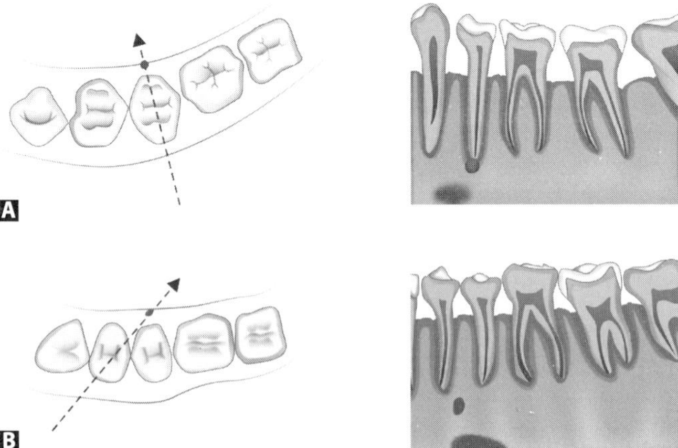

Figs. 1A and B: Same side lingual: (A) The object is seen on the apex of the second premolar when the radiograph was taken with routine bisecting angle principle; (B) The object is moved mesial to the second premolar when the radiograph was taken by shfiting the tube mesial to the reference tooth second premolar.

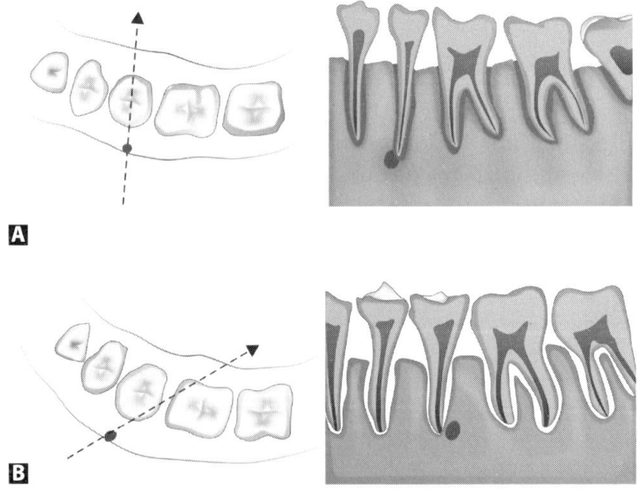

Figs. 2A and B: Opposite side buccal: (A) The object is located in the apex of second premolar when the radiograph was taken with routine bisecting angle technique; (B) The *object is distal* to the second premolar when the radiograph was taken by *shfiting the tube mesial* to the reference tooth second premolar.

object in relation to the known object. In second radiograph, the horizontal or vertical angulation of the beam needs to be altered. When the second radiograph compared with the first, the buccal object appears to move in the same direction as the beam.

If buccal and lingual objects are superimposed, the two may be separated and identified by applying this rule.

Right Angle Technique

In this method, two radiographs are taken perpendicular to each other to locate an object in the maxilla. Usually, a **periapical view and then an occlusal view** of the same region should be taken. The position of the object on each radiograph is interpreted with anatomic landmarks.

For example, if a radiopaque structure (impacted canine) is noted on the apical region of root of lateral incisor, its mediolateral position is identified by occlusal projection.

Definitive Evaluation Method of Localization

Least reliable method of localization.

Based on ***shadow cast principle:*** The closer the object to the film, the sharper the image definition and hence the location of the object in search can be identified.

Only one film exposure is required. As the film is positioned lingually in the patient's mouth, an object located lingually will appear more sharply defined than an object situated buccally.

SHORT NOTES

1. List the three geometric characteristics of an image.

The three geometric characters for a high quality radiograph are image clarity, magnification, and distortion.

To enhance the radiographic quality, the image clarity should be maximized with high image sharpness and resolution.

Image Sharpness

Sharpness denotes the well demarcated boundaries of two adjacent but different density objects in a radiograph. Unsharpness refers to a hazy shadow surrounding the image. This image unsharpness is called as penumbra or edge gradient.

Image Resolution

Image spatial resolution is the property of a radiograph in revealing the smaller objects that are closely placed.

Image Magnification

Equal enlargement of the image is known as magnification. All objects on the radiograph are larger than the real size.

Image Shape Distortion

Unequal enlargement of the different parts of the same object is known as image distortion. The amount of distortion depends on the thickness, position, and shape (thick objects are more distorted than thin).

2. Enumerate the steps required to improve the quality of radiographs. (or) write the measures needed to produce an accurate image. (or) describe the methods to minimize the loss of image clarity.

The diagnostic quality of the image is enhanced by taking measures to maximize the clarity and minimize the magnification and distortion.

To Maximize the Clarity

Use of smaller, effective focal spot: The preferred focal spot size for a dental X-ray machine is 1.0 mm or less. The size of the effective focal spot is a function of an angle in the face of the target with respect to the long axis of the electron beam.

Small angle results in a smaller, effective focal spot that reduces the penumbra and increases image sharpness and resolution. But small focal spot has greater wear effect on the target. The preferred angle for the effective focal spot is between 10 and 20°.

Use of long, open ended cylinder: The use of long cylinder with open end increases the focal spot object distance thereby lessens the divergence of X-ray beam and reduces image blurring. Longer focal spot-object distance allows photons that travel in a parallel direction to expose the object.

Reducing the object and the film distance: The closer the object and film, minimal will be the divergence of X-ray photons, and greater will be the image clarity.

3. Define image distortion. Explain how to reduce image distortion.

Image distortion is defined as deformation in image details like ***size and shape*** due to magnification compared to the facts.

Image Size Distortion

Image size distortion or image magnification is the increase in the size of the image on radiograph compared with the real size of the object.

Reason

The divergent path of photons in an X-ray beam cause enlargement of the image on the radiograph.

Steps to Avoid Image Size Distortion

1. Increase the distance between focal spot and film
2. Decrease the distance between object and film
3. Use of long, open-ended cylinder as an aiming apparatus in X-ray machine.

Image Shape Distortion

Image shape distortion is due to different enlargement in different parts of the same object.

Reason

- Not all parts of the object are at the same focal spot-to-object distance.
- Physical shape of the object may also prevent its optimal orientation with film.

Steps to Minimize Image Shape Distortion

The long axis of the film must be parallel to the long axis of the object, and the central x-ray beam should be perpendicular to both film and object.

Types of Image Distortion

- **Foreshortening:** This type of error occurs if the central X-ray is focused at right angle to the film, but **not to the tooth**—image is shorter than the real size. This distortion occurs because different parts of the object are at unequal distance from the film.
- **Elongation:** It is the error that results if the central X-ray is perpendicular to the object but **not to the film.** The concomitant radiographic image will be relatively too larger for the real size of the tooth.

Uneven Root Height

When the film is placed parallel to the object (tooth) but if the direction of the central beam is not perpendicular to both the film and object, the resultant radiograph reveals a distorted image with uneven root lengths. This type of image distortion is quite common in maxillary molar region and the palatal root appears relatively larger than the actual size.

4. Describe peripheral egg shell effect.

Photons traveling through the periphery of a curved surface are more attenuated than the photons that travel at right angles to the surface. The reason for more attenuation is because the photons have to travel longer path of distance at the periphery. This effect is more pronounced on hard tissue structures composed of dense layer surrounding a more lucent inner structure like the border of the maxillary sinus, nasal fossa, lamina dura, and pathological cysts with corticated boundaries than soft tissue masses, such as tongue which is uniformly dense.

MULTIPLE CHOICE QUESTIONS

1. In bisecting angle technique, if the central ray is positive to the bisector, the likely error is ***foreshortening***.
   a. Partial image
   b. Image distortion
   c. Foreshortening
   d. Elongation
2. In bisecting angle technique, if the central ray is negative to the bisector, the likely error on image is ***elongation***.
   a. Cone-cut
   b. Image overlapping
   c. Foreshortening
   d. Elongation
3. Film placement parallel to the long axis of tooth will result in ***minimal distortion***.
   a. Accurate image
   b. Minimal distortion
   c. Radiographic noise
   d. Horizontal overlapping
4. Penumbra is ***image unsharpness***.
   a. Double image
   b. Image unsharpness
   c. Wet film
   d. Emulsion peal
   (**Note:** Penumbra is the unsharpness or blurring that surrounds the edge of the radiographic image).
5. The focal spot blur is ***smaller at the cathode side and larger at the anode side***.
   a. Larger at the cathode side and smaller at the anode side
   b. Smaller on both cathode and anode side
   c. Smaller at the cathode side and larger at the anode side
   d. Larger on both cathode and anode side

VIVA VOCE

1. What are the prime exposure factors?

Kilovoltage peak (kVp), current (mA), exposure time milleampere seconds (mAs), and source - to image distance (SOI) are the four prime exposure factors.

2. What is image sharpness?

It is the property that clearly differentiate the margins of different radiodensity structures on a radiograph.

3. What is image resolution?

It is the property of the radiograph to illustrate the small structures that are closely placed.

4. What is the reason for blurred image?

The X-ray photons originating from different points on the focal spot travel in a straight line to reach the object but do not reach precisely at the same site on the film. The resultant image reveals the blurred edges of the object with loss of sharpness and clarity. The larger the focal spot size, there are more chance for image blurring.

5. What are the factors that improves the image quality (or) how to reduce the loss of image clarity?

- Using small focal spot size within the feasible limits to increase the image sharpness and clarity.
- Using long, open-ended cone to increase the focal spot-to-object distance and minimize the blurring by decreasing the ray beam divergence.
- Decreasing the object to film distance to minimize the image unshrpness.

6. How to minimize the image shape distortion?

Image shape distortion denotes the unequal magnification of the different sites within the same object. This can be minimized by:

- The long axis of the tooth should be parallel to the long axis of the film.
- The central ray should be perpendicular to both the film and tooth.

7. What is image foreshortening?

In bisecting angle technique, if the central ray is more positive to the bisector instead of being perpendicular, the image will appear smaller than the real size and is known as foreshortened image.

8. What is elongated image?

In bisecting angle technique, if the central ray is more negative to the bisector instead of being perpendicular, the image will appear larger than the real size and is known as image elongation.

BIBLIOGRAPHY

1. Cherryman G. Clark's positioning in radiography. British Dental Journal. 2005 199(11): 752.
2. Forsberg J, Halse A. Radiographic simulation of a periapical lesion comparing the paralleling and the bisecting-angle techniques. International Endodontic Journal. 1994;27(3):133-8
3. Forsberg J. Radiographic reproduction of endodontic "working length" comparing the paralleling and the bisecting-angle techniques. Oral Surg, Oral Med Oral Pathol.1987;64(3):353-60
4. Legg LM. Dental radiography: an overview. Radiologic technology. 2003;75(1):15-37.
5. Thali J, Viner MD, Brogdon BG, editors. Brogdon's forensic radiology. Boca Ration. CRC Press, 2010.p.43
6. Verhoeven JW, Ruijter J, Cune MS, et al. Oblique lateral cephalometric radiographs of the mandible in implantology: usefulness and reproducibility of the technique in quantitative densitometric measurements of the mandible in vivo. Clinical Oral Implants Research. 2000;11(5):476-86.
7. Whaites E, Drage N. Essentials of dental radiography and radiology. Elsevier Health Sciences; 2013.
8. White SC, Pharoah MJ. Oral radiology: Principles and interpretation. Elsevier Health Sciences; 2014.

CHAPTER 32

Quality Assurance in Dental Radiography

HIGHLIGHTS

Radiographic quality assurance refers to the measures taken to ensure that high quality diagnostic radiographs are produced constantly at the smallest exposure to both the patient and radiographer. A quality assurance plan includes both quality control tests and quality administration procedures.

Learners are expected to study

- ❖ Quality control tests for dental X-ray equipment and film processing
- ❖ Quality administration procedure
- ❖ Tests used to check for fresh film, film screen contact and frequency of testing
- ❖ Tests used to check proper safe lighting
- ❖ Tests used to check the strengths of developer and fixer solutions
- ❖ Preparation of reference radiographs and standard stepwedge radiographs.

ESSAY QUESTIONS

1. List and briefly explain the tests used to check the strength of the developer solution.

To check the strength of the developer solution any one of the three following tests can be used:

1. Reference radiograph
2. Stepwedge radiographs
3. Normalizing device

Reference Radiograph

A reference radiograph is one that is taken with accurate exposure parameters and processed by applying the typical standards and then used to compare the film densities of radiographs that are processed daily.

Steps to prepare a reference radiograph:

1. ***Film preparation:*** Fresh film is used to make reference radiograph.
2. ***Film exposure:*** Correct exposure factors are mandatory for film exposure.
3. ***Film processing:*** Fresh chemicals are used and recommended time and temperature should be followed.

Viewing the reference radiograph and the daily radiographs side by side on a view box: Once the processing solution is freshly prepared, a properly taken radiograph by applying the right techniques and exposure parameters should be processed by following the exact time-temperature principles. The resulting image will display the optimal density and contrast and should be taken as a reference film. It is mounted at the corner of view box for daily referral purpose.

Comparison of the daily radiographs with the reference radiograph can be interpreted as:

- ❖ **Matched densities:** If the densities seen on the reference radiograph match the densities of the daily radiographs, the developer strength is adequate.
- ❖ **Unmatched densities:** If the densities on the daily radiographs appear lighter than the reference radiograph, the developer solution is either weak or cold. If the densities on the daily radiographs appear darker than the reference radiograph, the developer solution is either too concentrated or warm.

Stepwedge Radiographs

A stepwedge is a tool used to check the accurateness of the processing solution. It predicts the speed and contrast of the image. It is made by layers of lead foil steps or aluminium sheets in 2 mm increments.

When a stepwedge is kept on the top of the test film and then expose this set up to X-rays, then the layers will absorb the varying amount of X-rays. When processed, different film densities are seen on the radiograph.

Test Procedure

- *Film preparation:* A stepwedge is made from lead foils in the film packet. Five lead sheets should be placed together and stapled at one corner. Then, the top layer should be cut at 4/5th level, the second layer at 3/5th level, a third layer at 2/5th level and the fourth layer at 1/5th level. This creates a step-like pattern.
- *Film exposure:* Exposure parameters are checked and the stepwedge is kept over the film and then exposed.
- Using fresh chemicals, the exposed film should be processed. The resulting radiograph will exhibit different densities as a result of the stepwedge and is known as the standard stepwedge radiograph.
- On daily basis, after replenishing the processing solution, process an exposed stepwedge films to get the standard or stepwedge radiograph.
- View the standard radiograph and the daily radiograph side by side on a view box and compare the densities on the daily radiographs with the densities on the step-wedge film.

Result Interpretation

The density at the mid-layer level of the step-wedge radiograph is used for comparison.

- **Matched densities:** If the densities seen on the stepwedge film match the densities seen on the daily radiographs, the developer solution strength is adequate.
- **Unmatched densities:** If the densities on the daily radiographs differ from that of stepwedge radiograph by more than two steps the developer solution is depleted.

Normalizing Device

A commercially available dental radiographic normalizing and monitoring device can be used to monitor the developer strength and film density.

SHORT NOTES

1. Discuss the schedule of radiographic quality assurance plan.

Quality assurance plan includes quality control tests and quality administration procedures.

Daily Procedures

- Comparing radiographs with reference film
- Enter findings in a retake log
- Replenishing processing solutions
- Temperature check for processing solutions
- Stepwedge test.

Weekly Procedures

- Replacement of processing solutions
- Cleaning manual and automatic processing units
- Check and clean view boxes
- Review of retake log to implement corrective actions.

Monthly Procedures

- Check for darkroom safelight and light leaks
- Check and clean intensifying screens
- Check the presence of exposure charts on each X-ray machine.

Yearly procedures: Machine calibration

- Collimation-beam alignment test
- Focal spot size test
- Halfvalue layer test
- Kilovoltage test
- Milliamperage test
- Timer test
- Tube head stability test
- X-ray output test.

2. Describe the test used to check safe lighting. (or) explain coin test (or) write about Penny test.

To test the effectiveness of safelight, coin test or penny test should be carried out on a monthly basis.

Procedure

- *Preparation of the darkroom*: All the lights including safelight should be turned off in the darkroom.
- *Film preparation:* An unexposed film should be unwrapped and placed on a flat surface at least 4 feet away from the safelight and a coin should be placed on the top of the film.
- *Turn* on *the safelight:* The coin and the film are allowed to get exposed to the safelight for 3–4 minutes. Remove the coin and process the film.

Result Interpretation

- *Proper safe lighting:* If no visible image of the coin is seen on the processed radiograph, the integrity of safelighting is correct.
- *Improper safe lighting:* If the image of the coin and a fogged appearance is noted on the processed film, the safelight is not secure (Fig. 1).

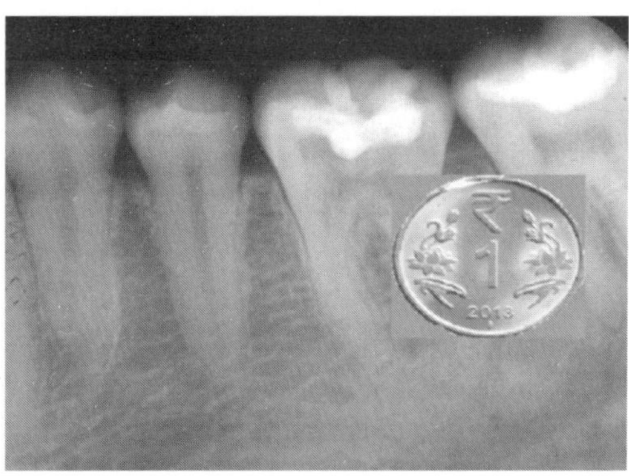

Fig. 1: Penny test (or) Coin test.

3. Describe half-value layer test. (or) discuss the test performed to check the penetrating quality of x-ray beam.

The quality of X-ray photons is a function of **kVp** that determine its wavelength and penetrating power.

Half-value Layer

50% of the X-ray photons should penetrate through a standardized thickness of aluminum depending on kVp.

- If the X-ray machine has a ***maximum of 69 or less kVp***, 50% of the X-ray output must pass through at least ***1.5 mm of aluminum.***
- If the X-ray machine delivers a maximum of ***70 or more kVp***, then 50% of the X-ray output must pass through at least ***2.5 mm of aluminum.***

To test HVL, the operator should place discs of 1.5 or 2.5 mm aluminum above a pocket dosimeter. The X-ray machine is set at maximum kVp setting. The operator then compares output readings in mR with and without aluminum discs in place, by keeping all exposure parameters constant.

Example: If the machine is set at 65 kVp, the reading without aluminum is 200 mR, then 100 mR of X-ray radiation should pass through the 1.5 mm aluminum disc which is placed between the beam indicating device and pocket dosimeter. If the machine fails, it must be repaired.

4. Describe the infection control procedures to be followed for radiography.

The purpose of infection control procedures is to avoid cross-contamination between patients and between patient and radiographers.

The sequence is as follows:

- *Prepackage X-ray films and sterilize X-ray holding instruments:* To prevent contamination of bulk supplies, they should be dispensed in procedure quantity. Prepackage of a required number of films in a container and dispensing them with sterile film holding instrument will prevent cross-contamination.
- *Disinfection of PID, X-ray tube head, working surfaces, dental chair, thyroid collar, and apron:* Surface disinfectants like iodophors, chlorines, and phenolic compounds can

be used. To clean surfaces, spray-wipe-spray technique is recommended. Surface with electronic controls need special care hence well moistened, disinfectant, folded double paper towel should be used for wiping.

Radiographic Exposure

After seating the patient, the radiographer should wash his/her hands and wear disposable gloves and place the film in position and expose it. The exposed film should be set in a container and carried to the darkroom

- *Film processing:* The radiographer should remove the gloves, and take the container to the darkroom. The film packet should be opened and the film is removed from the protective plastic envelope. This film is then subjected to processing.
- *Remove all barriers and spry all working surfaces and apron with disinfectant:* After completing exposure, all the working surface, and apron should be disinfected and prepared for next patient.

5. Discuss the test used to check the fixer solution strength.

Fixer solution removes the unexposed silver halide crystals resulting in clear areas on the processed radiograph. When the fixer solution is at full strength, it takes 2 minutes to clear the film, whereas it takes longer time if the strength is lost.

To check the fixer strength, ***clearing test*** with the following test should be performed.

- Film should be unwrapped and immediately immerse it in the fixer solution.
- The time taken by the film for clearing should be noted.

Interpretation

Fast clearing: If the film clears in 2 minutes, the fixer is of adequate strength.

Slow clearing: If the film is not completely cleared after 2 minutes, it should again be immersed in the fixer solution. If the film is not cleared in 3 to 4 minutes, the fixer solution is depleted. The solution should be replaced.

6. Describe the test used to check for fresh film.

When each box of film is opened, it should be tested for freshness.

One film from the newly opened film box should be unwrapped and processed using freshly prepared chemicals.

Interpretation

- *Fresh film:* If the processed film appears clear with a slight blue tint, the film is fresh and has been stored properly.
- *Fogged film:* An expired film or an improperly stored film will appear fogged.

7. Discuss the basic steps in quality administration procedure.

Quality administration procedure refers to all the efforts to be taken by the dental radiology unit or clinic to maintain the high-quality in technique and equipment care which include the following steps:

- Description of plan
- Assignment of duties
- Monitoring schedule
- Maintenance schedule
- Record-keeping log
- Method for evaluation and revision
- In-service training.

8. What are the basic infection control steps to be followed in radiology?

- Following the universal precaution to avoid contamination through body fluids like blood and saliva and to protect the radiographers and other healthcare personals from acquiring cross infections like herpes simplex, HIV, hepatitis B, and tuberculosis.
- Wearing protective apparels like gloves, mask, and apron.
- Maintaining sterile working environment by disinfecting the working surface including

the processing area, X-ray machine, dental chair, and other accessory instruments. The effective surface disinfectants to be used are iodophors, phenol, and chlorine compounds.

- Nondisposable instruments like film holding device need to be thoroughly cleaned with soap and running water followed by ethylene dioxide sterilization.
- Disposable containers should be used for film handling.
- Disposable barriers should be used to cover the sensors during exposure.

9. What are the guidelines to prescribe a dental radiograph?

To minimize the radiation exposure to patients, the following guidelines should be followed before advising a dental radiograph:

- Dentist should advise radiograph only after completing the clinical examination to support the treatment procedure. Patients without any evidence of dental disease do not require a radiograph.
- For ***new patients with permanent dentition*** (adolescence and adults), a combination of posterior bitewing radiographs and orthopantomogram or posterior bitewing radiographs and selected periapical radiographs based on the symptoms is preferred.
- ***Full mouth intraoral radiographs*** should be advised only when there is a generalized dental problem like multiple carious teeth/generalized periodontitis or history of multipledental treatment.
- ***For children with mixed dentition,*** a combination of orthopantomogram and posterior bitewing radiographs or posterior bitewing radiographs and selective periapical radiographs based on the symptoms is required for radiographic examination.
- ***For kids with deciduous dentition***, selective periapical radiographs based on symptoms and occlusal radiographs or posterior bitewings is preferred.
- ***Recall visits:*** The radiographic examination ***for adult patients with increased caries risk*** include posterior bitewings at 6–18 months intervals and ***for patients with deciduous and mixed dentition*** with closed contact points, posterior bitewings are preferred at 6 to 12 months intervals.
- ***For patients with periodontal disease***, the recall radiograph is limited to selective periapical and/or bitewings based on symptoms and disease status.
- ***For screening the growth and development of children and adolescent patients***, radiographs are selected based on clinical evaluation.
- Selective radiographs should be advised for the following clinical conditions:
  - Periodontal disease
  - Deep carious lesions or large restorations, teeth with severe attrition, abrasion, or erosion
  - Malpositioned tooth or clinically missing/partially impacted teeth
  - Tooth with soft tissue swelling/sinus tract
  - Dental trauma/injury
  - Growth abnormalities, facial asymmetry and dental abnormalities
  - To check the oral manifestation of diagnosed or suspected systemic disease
  - To diagnose foreign objects
  - Temporomandibular joint disorders
  - To evaluate the abutment teeth for prosthesis
  - Unexplained bleeding/sensitivity of teeth.

MULTIPLE CHOICE QUESTIONS

1. Wire mesh test is used for testing the ***film-to-screen contact***.
   a. Cassette integrity
   b. Film-to-screen contact
   c. Object-source distance
   d. Quantity of X-ray photons

2. The equipment used to test the quality of viewbox lighting is the ***photographic light meter***.
   a. Photographic light meter
   b. Fluorescent bulb tester
   c. Stepwedge test
   d. Penny test
3. Light source used in viewbox is ***fluorescent bulbs***.
   a. Halogen bulbs
   b. Incandescent bulbs
   c. Ultraviolet bulbs
   d. Fluorescent bulbs
4. To perform coin test ***exposed film is used***.
   a. Unexposed film is used
   b. Exposed film is used
   c. Double exposed film is used
   d. Processed film is used
5. The penetrating power of the X-ray beam is measured by ***half-value layer***.
   a. Filtration test
   b. Half-value layer
   c. Photometer
   d. Densitometer
6. The interval for taking bitewing radiographs to check occult carious lesion in children is ***6–12 months***.
   a. 3–6 months
   b. 6–12 months
   c. 12–18 months
   d. 18–24 months
7. For adolescent patients with no increased caries risk, the recommended recall interval for taking posterior bitewings is ***18–36 months***.
   a. 6 –12 months
   b. 12–16 months
   c. 14–18 months
   d. 18–36 months
8. For the adult patients with high caries risk, the recommended interval for taking bitewings is ***6–18 months***.
   a. 3–6 months
   b. 6–18 months
   c. 18–20 months
   d. 20–24 months
9. For children in deciduous dentition stage and are not at high-risk for caries, the recommended interval to take bitewing radiographs is ***12–24 months***.
   a. 12–16 months
   b. 12–24 months
   c. 18–36 months
   d. 24–36 months
10. For adults who are not at high risk for caries, the recommended interval to take bitewing radiographs is ***24–36 months***.
    a. 12–16 months
    b. 12–24 months
    c. 18–36 months
    d. 24–36 months
11. For a fractured incisor tooth with normal vitality response ***no radiograph is required***.
    a. Periapical radiograph is required
    b. Anterior bitewing radiograph is required
    c. Radiograph is essential only if restoration is planned
    d. No radiograph is required

VIVA VOCE

1. What are administrative radiographs?

Administrative radiographs are one taken for the purposes of claiming medical reimbursement or insurance claim, and submitting for legal issues/examination boards. Administrative radiographs are not intended for diagnostic or treatment purpose.

2. What are the factors associated with increased caries risk?

- Poor oral hygiene
- Increased occurrence of caries
- Occurrence of rampant caries
- Broken/poor quality restorations
- Conditions like enamel hypoplasia due to amelogenesis/dentinogenesis imperfecta
- Family history of increased caries incidence
- Systemic conditions associated with dry mouth and hypocalcified dentition
- Dietary habits like frequent sugar intake.

3. What is quality assurance in dental radiology?

Quality assurance in dental radiology include all the efforts taken in the dental radiology unit to provide a consistent high quality diagnostic radiographs.

4. What are the parameters to be checked during X-ray machine calibrations?

- The intensity and reproducibility of X-ray output is checked with radiation dosimeter.
- Check for the size and alignment of the X-ray beam
- Check for beam energy by using either kVp or half-value layer measurement
- Accuracy and reproducibility of the timer in the X-ray machine.
- Verifying the mA settings
- Check for tube stability
- Check for focal spot size.

5. How the X-ray beam alignment is checked?

The size alignment of the X-ray beam is checked by making a cross pattern using pinholes on the films and then centering the aiming cylinder to make exposure; if all the processed films show the exposed area inside the holes, then indicate good alignment.

6. What is the optimal temperature of the processing solutions?

The optimal temperature for the manual processing solution is 20° or 68°C. For automatic processor, it is 28° or 82°C.

7. What is reference film?

It is the diagnostic image taken with optimal exposure parameters and processed when the processing solutions are freshly prepared by maintaining the time-temperature guidelines. This film is used to compare the images taken in the radiology unit to monitor the quality on daily basis.

BIBLIOGRAPHY

1. Akdeniz BG, Lomcali G. Densitometric evaluation of four radiographic processing solutions. Dentomaxillofac Radiol. 1998; 27(2):102-6.
2. American Dental Association Council on Scientific Affairs.The use of radiographs: update and recommendations. J Am Dent Assoc. 2006;137(9)1304-12.
3. Langland OE, Sippy FH, Langlais RP. Textbook of Dental Radiology. 2nd edition. Charles C Thomas Pub Limited; 1984.
4. Whaites E, Drage N. Essentials of dental radiography and radiology. Elsevier Health Sciences; 2013.
5. White SC, Pharoah MJ. Principles and interpretation. St Louis. 2014:431-3.

CHAPTER 33

Intraoral Radiographic Techniques

HIGHLIGHTS

Dental radiographs demand adequate information for accurate diagnosis. Film based radiographic images require the use of particular technique and precautions to maximize the diagnostic and interpretative value of the radiograph. Minimizing the patient exposure to radiation and obtaining high-quality radiographs depends on applying the precise techniques in film placement, central ray angulation, maintaining the film-object-central beam orientation, exposure parameters, and film processing.

Learners are expected to study:

- Types of Intraoral radiographs (periapical, bitewing, occlusal)
- Intraoral radiographic techniques (Bisecting angle technique and paralleling technique)
- Indications for different techniques
- Advantages of different techniques.

ESSAY QUESTIONS

1. Discuss in detail the principle and technique of paralleling periapical radiography. (or) describe in detail about long cone technique.

Principle of Paralleling Technique

It is based on the rule of parallelism such that long axis of the film is placed parallel to long axis of the tooth (Fig. 1).

The central beam is directed perpendicular to both film and tooth hence also called right angle technique. Thus the image of tooth seen in radiograph is the actual size of the tooth.

X-ray source to object distance is more to achieve the parallelism hence also called long cone technique.

Intraoral X-ray machine—exposure parameters: 8 mA or 10 mA, 60–70 kVp.

Patient positioning: The patient must be protected with lead aprons with thyroid collars and instructed to remove the ornaments.

The occlusal plane should be aligned parallel to plane of the floor.

The median sagittal plane should be perpendicular to the floor.

Maxillary projections: Patient is instructed to sit erect with back straight such that ala-tragus plane is parallel to maxillary occlusal plane

Mandibular projections: Patient's head is tilted slightly backward to align the occlusal plane parallel to the floor.

Film placement:

- The film holder is essential to align the long axis of the film and long axis of the teeth in parallel plane.
- Exposure side of the film is placed facing the teeth surface.
- The identification dot should face occlusal or incisal surface.
- Vertical film positioning for anterior teeth.
- Horizontal film positioning for posterior teeth.
- Teeth under examination should be in the center.

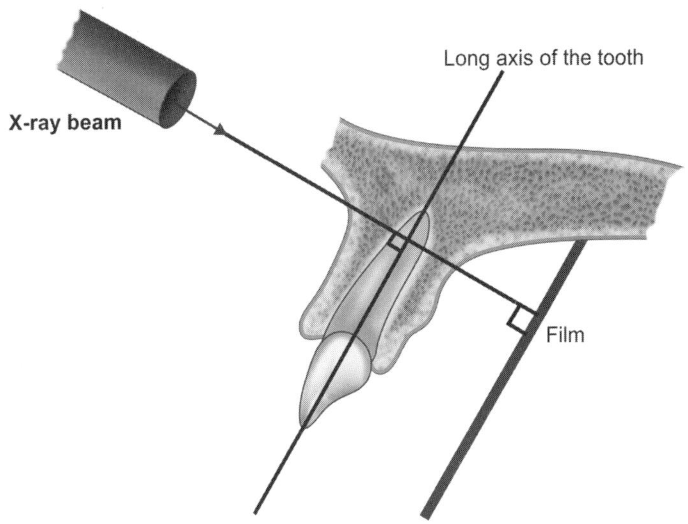

Fig. 1: Paralleling technique principle.

Cone Placement

Maxillary projections (Figs. 2 to 5)

Teeth	Anatomical landmarks [center of the position indicating device (PID) is aligned]
Incisors	Tip of the nose
Canine	Ala of the nose
Premolars	Point of intersection of ala-tragus plane and vertical line dropped from the pupil of eye
Molars	The point of intersection of the ala-tragus plane and vertical line dropped from outer canthus of orbit.

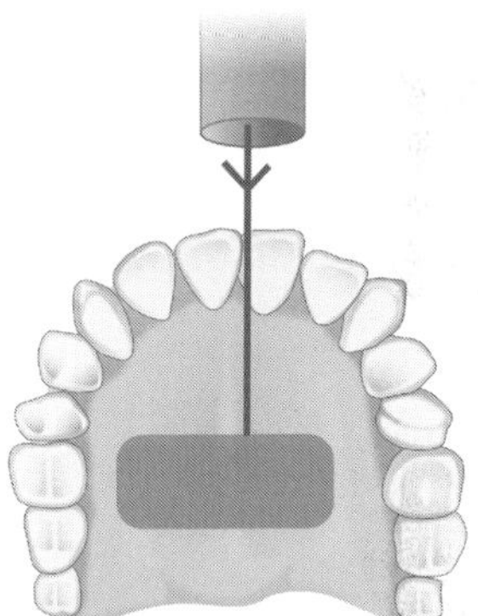

Fig. 2: Maxillary incisor projection: Paralleling angle technique.

Mandibular projections (Figs. 6 to 9)

Teeth	Anatomical landmarks [center of the position indicating device (PID) is aligned]
Incisors	3 cm above the inferior border of the mandible in the midline
Canine	3 cm above the inferior border of the mandible over the canine
Premolars	Below the pupil of eye about 3 cm above the inferior border of mandible
Molars	Below the outer canthus of eye about 3 cm above the inferior border of mandible

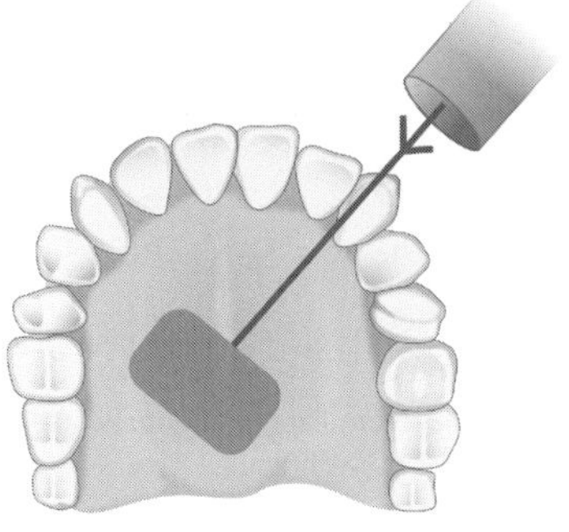

Fig. 3: Maxillary canine projection: Paralleling angle technique.

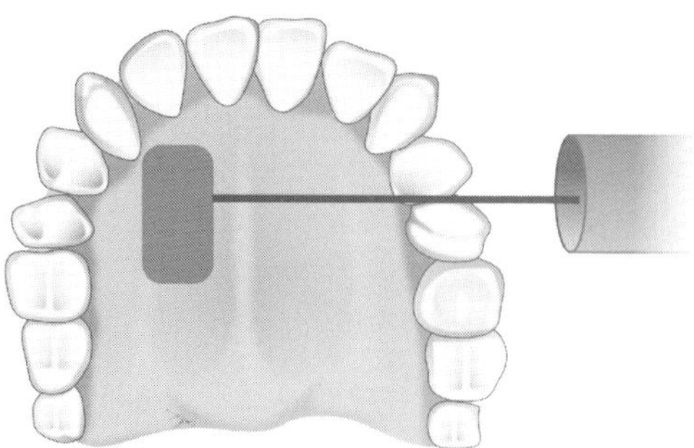

Fig. 4: Maxillary premolar projection: Paralleling angle technique.

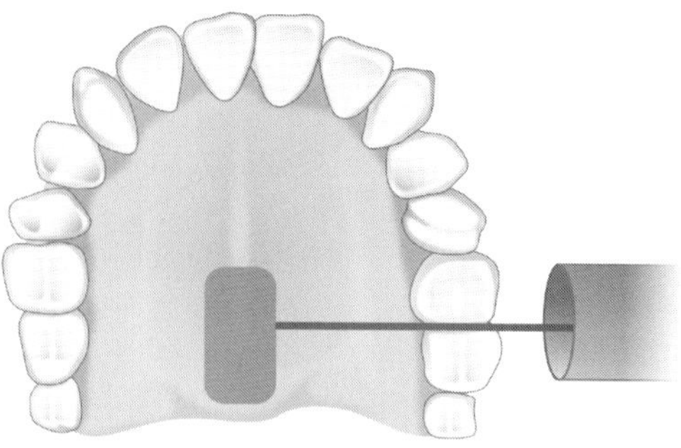

Fig. 5: Maxillary molar projection: Paralleling angle technique.

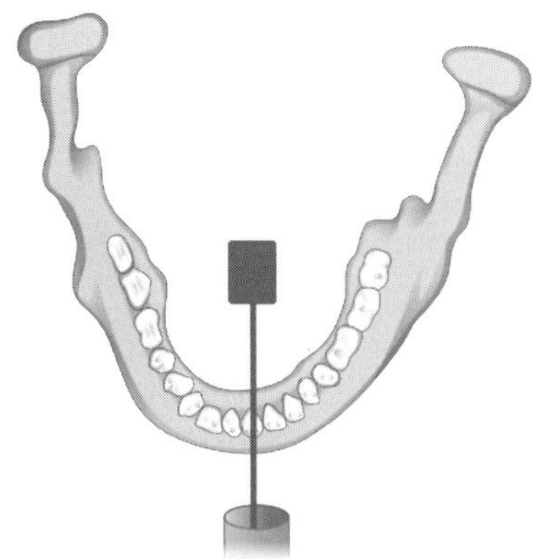

Fig. 6: Mandibular incisor projection: Paralleling angle technique.

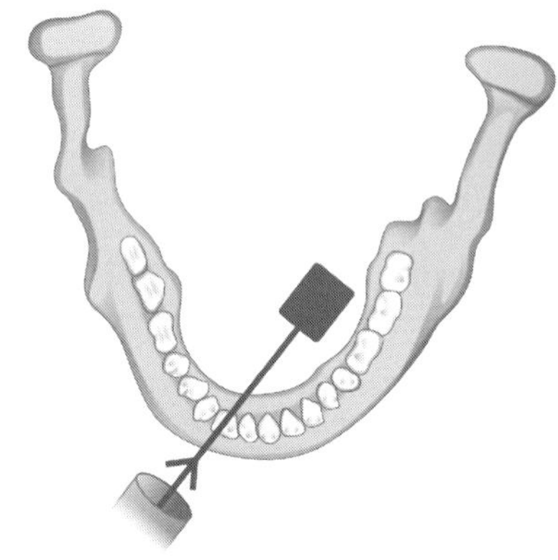

Fig. 7: Mandibular canine projection: Paralleling angle technique.

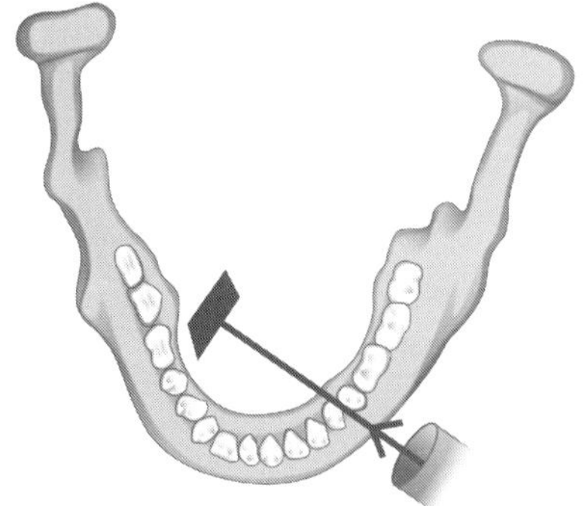

Fig. 8: Mandibular premolar projection: Paralleling angle technique.

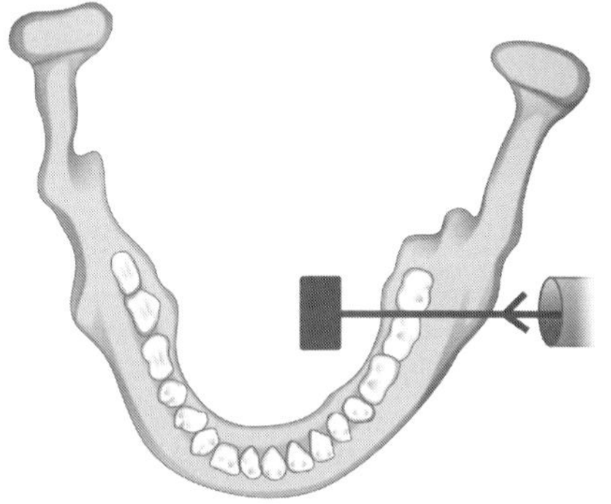

Fig. 9: Mandibular molar projection: Paralleling angle technique.

Indications

To detect:

- Pulpal lesions [Dental caries (DC), fracture, attrition, abrasion, erosion, pulp calcification, and pulp stones]
- Traumatic injuries in teeth and jaws
- Periapical lesions (apical periodontitis, periapical abscess, periapical granuloma, dental cyst and radiopaque lesions like odontoma, condensing osteitis, etc.)
- Periodontal lesions (horizontal and vertical bone loss).
- Pericoronal lesions like dentigerous cyst
- Impacted or unerupted teeth and supernumerary teeth.
- Dental anomalies like dens invaginatus, dentin dysplasia, ghost teeth, etc.
- Structural alterations of teeth like amelogenesis and dentinogenesis imperfecta.
- In endodontics to determine pulp involvement and to identify the root length in the root canal treatment.
- Age estimation in forensic odontology.

Advantages

Accuracy is more with less chance for image distortion. The image is very representative of actual tooth size with maximum details and definition.

Disadvantages

The film holder is mandatory, and these devices in some cases cause lot of discomfort by impinging on oral tissues.

Film placement is difficult in child patients or adults with a shallow palate and small mouth.

2. Explain in detail the bisecting angle technique. (or) describe in detail about short cone technique.

Principle of Bisecting Angle (Short Cone) Technique

Bisecting angle technique is based on the Cieszynski's rule of isometry which states that two triangles are equal when they share a common side and have two equal angles.

The film is placed as close to the lingual surface of the tooth such that the plane of the film and long axis of tooth forms an angle at the apex.

An imaginary bisector bisects this angle and represents the common side of the two triangles.

Central beam is directed perpendicular to the bisector and forms the third side of both the triangles (Fig. 10).

Short Cone Technique

Intraoral X-ray machine—exposure parameters: 8 mA or 10 mA , 60-70 kVp .

Patient positioning: Patients are instructed to remove ornaments and wear lead aprons with thyroid collars for radiation protection.

Maxillary projections: Patient is instructed to sit erect with back straight such that ala-tragus plane is parallel to maxillary occlusal plane

Mandibular projections: Patient's head is tilted slightly backward to align the occlusal plane parallel to the floor.

Film placement (general guidelines): Exposure side of the film is placed facing the teeth surface with the identification dot facing occlusal or incisal aspects.

The film is placed vertically for anterior teeth and horizontal for posterior teeth.

Position or Beam Indicating Device Placement (Pid or Bid)

In bisecting angle technique, the ***vertical angulation*** is the angle that directs the central

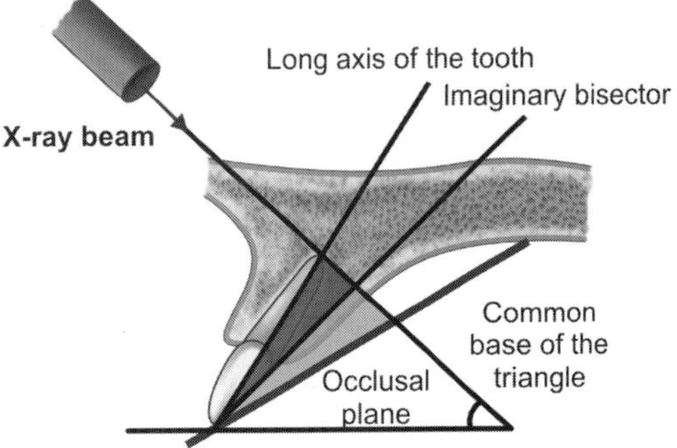

Fig. 10: Bisecting angle technique principle.

beam perpendicular to the imaginary bisector and is different for different teeth (Tables 1 and 2).

Horizontal angulation is formed when the central beam is directed through the contact points of teeth to be examined, and it is usually at right angles to the buccal or facial surface of teeth in each region.

Maxillary Projections (Table 1)

Table 1: Maxillary projections.

Teeth	Vertical angulation	Anatomical landmarks	Central ray is perpendicular to bisector and is directed through
Incisors (Fig. 11)	+40°	Tip of the nose	The contact point of the central incisors
Canine (Fig. 12)	+45°	Ala of the nose	Canine eminence
Premolars (Fig. 13)	+30°	Point of intersection of ala-tragus plane and vertical line dropped from the pupil of eye	Interproximal area between first and second premolar
Molars	+20°	Point of intersection of ala-tragus plane and vertical line dropped from outer canthus of orbit	Interproximal area between first and second molar

Mandibular Projections (Table 2)

Table 2: Mandibular projections.

Teeth	Vertical angulation	Anatomical landmarks	Central ray is perpendicular to bisector and is directed through
Incisors (Fig. 14)	–15°	3 cm above the inferior border of the mandible in the midline	Contact area of central incisors
Canine (Fig. 15)	–20°	3 cm above the inferior border of the mandible over the canine	Middle of canine
Premolars (Fig. 16)	–10°	Below the pupil of eye about 3 cm above the inferior border of mandible	Interproximal area between first and second premolar
Molars	–5°	Below the outer canthus of eye about 3 cm above the inferior border of mandible	Interproximal area between first and second molar

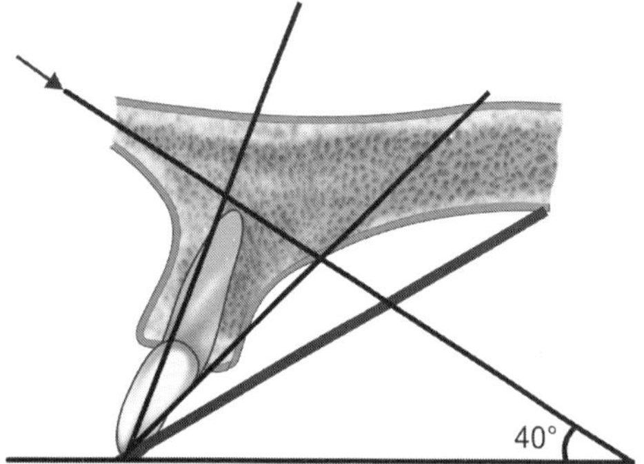

Fig. 11: Maxillary incisor projection: Bisecting angle.

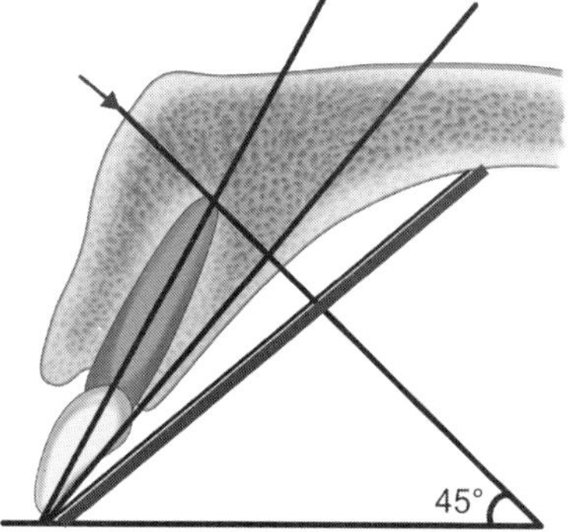

Fig. 12: Maxillary canine projection: Bisecting angle technique.

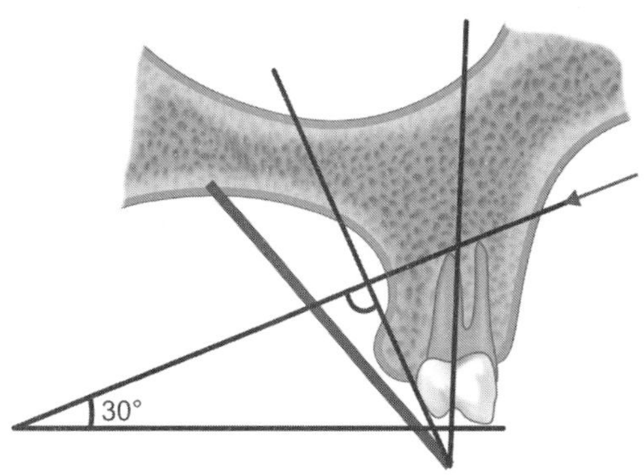

Fig. 13: Maxillary premolar projection: Bisecting angle technique.

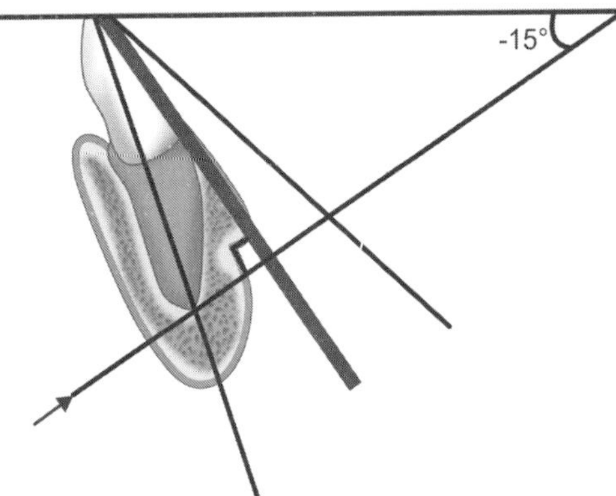

Fig. 14: Mandibular incisor projection: Bisecting angle technique.

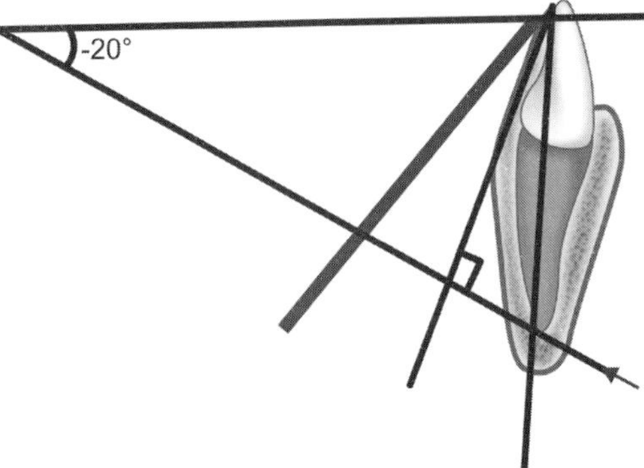

Fig. 15: Mandibular canine projection: Bisecting angle technique.

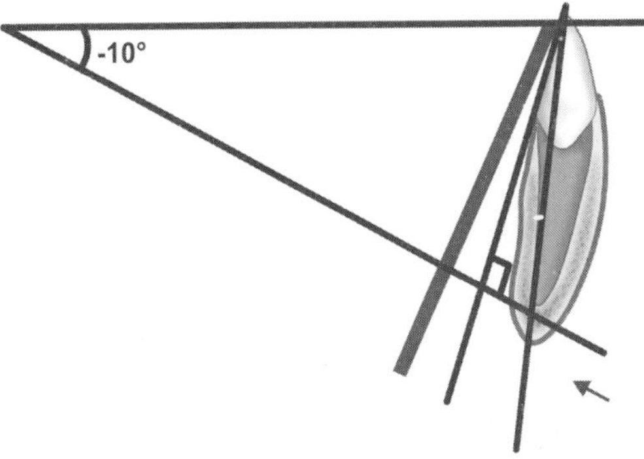

Fig. 16: Mandibular premolar projection: Bisecting angle technique.

Indications

To detect

- Pulpal, periapical and periodontal lesions.
- Dentoalveolar fracture.
- Impacted or unerupted teeth and supernumerary teeth.
- Dental anomalies like dens invaginatus, dentin dysplasia, ghost teeth, and structural alterations of teeth like amelogenesis, and dentinogenesis imperfecta.
- Some systemic diseases (loss of lamina dura in hyperparathyroidism, symmetric widening of PDL space in scleroderma)
- Dental age estimation in forensic odontology.

Advantages

- The film holder is not essential.
- Radiation exposure is less due to the use of short PID.

Disadvantages

Image distortion and cone cut.

3. Differences between paralleling and bisecting angle techniques.
(or)
Describe in detail principle, technique, advantages and disadvantages of the long cone and short cone technique.

Paralleling technique	Bisecting angle technique
Based on the principle of parallelism	Based on Cieszynski rule of isometry
Also called right-angle or long cone technique	Short cone technique
Object-film distance is more	Object-film distance is less.
The long axis of the teeth and the film are parallel with the central beam directed perpendicular to both	The film is placed as close as possible to the tooth, and the central beam is directed perpendicular to the imaginary bisector (bisects the angle formed between the film and teeth)
The film holder is mandatory to hold the film parallel to long axis of teeth	Film holder is not essential, and finger holding method can be used to stabilize the film
Less image distortion as the use of film holder avoids the need for vertical angulation	Image distortion is more in case of improper vertical angulation
Source to object distance is more (16 inches)	Source to object distance is less (8 inches)
Radiation exposure is more	Radiation exposure is less
Simple technique and easy to learn	More techniques sensitive
Can be accurately duplicated or repeated and is easy to standardize.	Comparison and standardization of serial radiographs have less validity than paralleling technique
It is difficult to place the film parallel to the tooth especially in child patients or adults with a shallow palate and a small mouth	The film placement is easier and causes less discomfort than paralleling technique
Less image magnification due to the use of a long cone	Image magnification is more when compared to paralleling technique

4. Explain in detail the various projections in bitewing radiography.

Bitewing Radiography

It is also called interproximal technique used to examine the crowns of both maxillary and mandibular teeth, the interproximal areas and crestal bone on the same radiograph.

Bitewing Film

An intra-oral periapical film with a bitewing tab attached becomes a bitewing film.

- ❖ Size 1: Intra-oral periapical film is used for anterior bitewing
- ❖ Size 2: Intraoral periapical film is commonly used
- ❖ Size 3: Intraoral periapical film is used when premolar and molar bitewing taken in one film.

Bitewing Film Holder

Rinn XCP bitewing film holder with collimator is recommended.

Projections

Premolar Bitewing

Patient Preparation

- ❖ Instructed to remove ornaments like nose studs
- ❖ Patient's occlusal plane should be made parallel to the floor.

Film Placement

The film is placed between the tongue and teeth, and the patient is instructed to bite on the tab with the anterior end of the film aligned to the middle of the mandibular canine, and the film is centered on the second premolar.

Cone Placement

- ❖ Middle of position indicating device at the level of occlusal plane
- ❖ Vertical angulation: +5°
- ❖ Horizontal angulation: Central beam is directed center of the film through the premolar contact areas.

Molar Bitewing

Patient Preparation

- Instructed to remove the ornaments
- The patient occlusal plane should be made parallel to the floor.

Film Placement

The film is placed between the tongue and teeth and the patient is instructed to bite on the tab with the distal end of the film aligned 2 mm beyond the most posterior erupted molar.

Cone Placement

- Middle of position indicating device at the level of occlusal plane
- Vertical angulation: +10°
- Horizontal angulation: Central beam is directed center of the film through the first and second molars below the lateral canthus of the eye at the level of the occlusal plane.

Vertical Bitewing

- Long axis of the film is placed in a vertical direction
- Film is centered vertically (Fig. 17).
- Longer bitewing tab is used, and the patient is instructed to bite such that the teeth meet the tab in end-end position.
- Vertical angulation: +10°
- Horizontal angulation: Central beam is directed through the interproximal surfaces of the teeth.
- It is used mainly to assess the bone loss in post-treatment cases.

Full Mouth Bitewing

In case of anterior bitewing, totally three projections are taken (two for canines on both the sides and one for incisor region).

In case of posteriors: One premolar and one molar projection for the right side. One premolar and one molar projection for the left side.

Indications of Bitewing Radiography

- To detect proximal caries
- To detect secondary caries below restoration
- To identify the height of the alveolar crest
- To check the interproximal areas for calculus deposition..

Advantages

- Less radiation exposure when compared to full mouth intraoral periapical films (half the radiation exposure).
- Good perspective of alveolar bone crest than IOPA

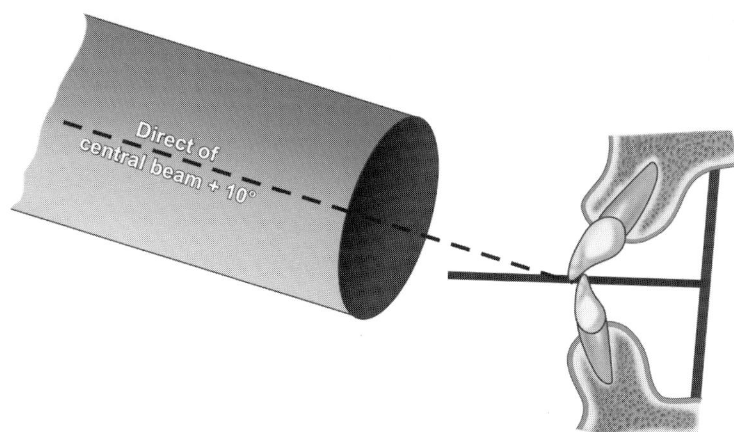

Fig. 17: Vertical bitewing technique.

- Bitewing radiography assures accurate assessment of changes in bone height.

Disadvantage

Periapical lesions cannot be seen.

5. Discuss in detail about occlusal radiography.

Occlusal Radiography

Intraoral radiography used to display large segment of upper and lower dental arch which cannot be covered in periapical radiography.

Occlusal Film

- Film size: 5.7 × 7.6 cm or 3 × 2.3 inches.
- The white side of the film should be positioned towards the jaw to be examined between the occlusal surface of the maxillary and mandibular teeth.
- The film is stabilized by patient biting the surface of the film.

Maxillary Occlusal Projection (Table 3)

Patient preparation: The patient is positioned upright in the dental chair such that the occlusal plane is parallel to the floor and the midsagittal plane is perpendicular to the floor. *Equipment preparation:* 65 kVp, 10 mA, 15 impulses are the exposure parameters and 8 or 16 inches PID can be used.

Mandibular Occlusal Projection (Table 4)

Patient preparation: The patient head is reclined and positioned such that ala-tragus line is 45° above horizontal and occlusal plane is perpendicular to the floor.
Equipment preparation: 65 kVp, 10 mA, 15 impulses are the exposure parameters and 8 or 16 inch PID is recommended.

Indications

- To get a larger view than periapical radiographs as it includes a larger segment of the dental arch and in trismus cases where periapical radiograph cannot be taken.
- Used along with periapical radiography in Miller's technique for object localization in three dimensions.
- To locate roots, supernumerary teeth, unerupted and impacted teeth. Foreign bodies and calculus in ducts of submandibular and sublingual glands.
- Evaluation of:
  - Anterior, medial and lateral outline of the maxillary sinus.
  - Extent and displacement of fracture in the maxilla or mandible.
  - The buccolingual extent of osteomyelitis, cysts, and malignancies of jaws.

Table 3: Maxillary occlusal projection.

Projection	Film placement	Image field	Cone/PID placement	Vertical angulation
Anterior maxillary occlusal	The long axis of the film is perpendicular to the midsagittal plane of the patient and such that the posterior most borders of the film touching the rami	Dentition from canine to canine	Centre of PID is oriented to the tip of the nose	+45°
Cross-sectional (Fig. 18)	Same as anterior maxillary occlusal	(Dentition from the second molar to second molar)	Centre of PID is oriented to bridge of the nose	+65°
Lateral topographical	The long axis of the film is positioned parallel with a sagittal plane on one side of interest with a white side of the film facing the side of the maxillary arch to be covered and is gently pushed to touch the ramus	Teeth from lateral incisor to contralateral 3rd molar. (side of interest)	Centre of PID is oriented to a point 2 cm below the lateral canthus of the eye	+60°

Table 7: Mandibular occlusal projection.

Projection	Film placement	Image field	Cone/PID placement	Vertical angulation
Anterior mandibular occlusal	The long axis of the film is perpendicular to the midsagittal plane of the patient and such that the posterior most borders of the film touching the rami	Dentition from canine to canine and inferior cortical border.	Centre of PID is oriented to tip of the chin	–55°
Cross-sectional (Fig. 19)	Same as anterior mandibular occlusal	Dentition from the second molar to the second molar. *Best indicated for revealing sialolith in Wharton's duct*	Central beam is directed to the center of film through the floor of mouth is 3 cm below the tip of the chin	90°
Lateral topographical view	Long axis of film is positioned parallel with the sagittal plane on the side of interest and is gently pushed to touch the ramus	Teeth from lateral incisor to contralateral 3rd molar.	Central beam directed through a point 3 cm posterior and 3 cm lateral to midline	–55°

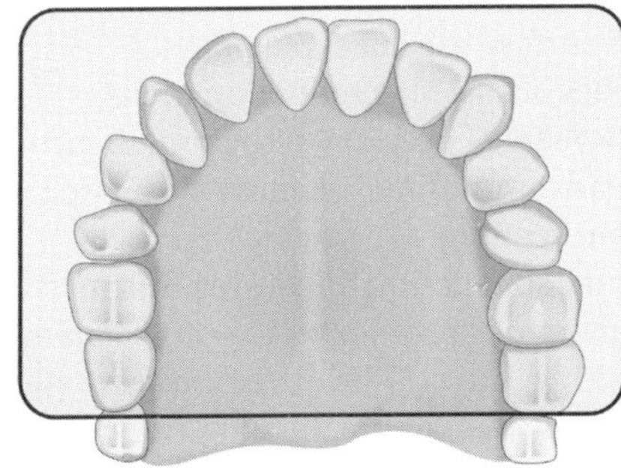

Fig. 18: Cross-sectional maxillary occlusal projection.

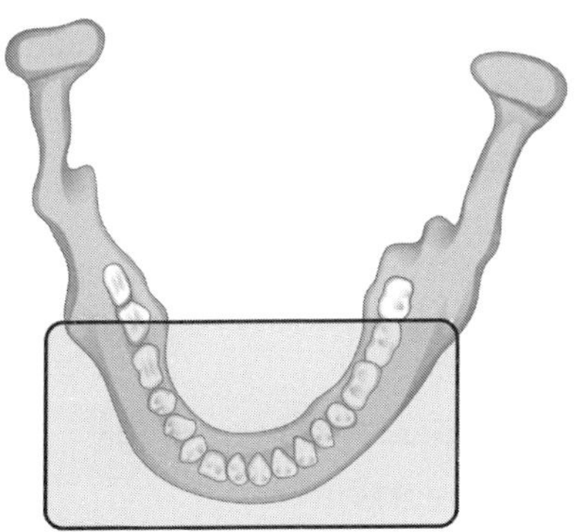

Fig. 19: Cross-sectional mandibular occlusal projection.

SHORT NOTES

1. Enumerate the various intraoral projections.

Periapical Radiography

- Bisecting angle technique
- Paralleling technique

Bitewing Radiography

- Premolar bitewing
- Molar bitewing
- Vertical bitewing (anteriors)

Occlusal Radiography

Maxillary Projections

- Anterior maxillary cross-sectional
- Cross-sectional
- Lateral topographical view

Mandibuar Projections

- Anterior mandibular cross-sectional
- Cross-sectional
- Lateral topographical view.

2. Indications of periapical radiography.

- To detect pulpal lesions (DC, fracture, attrition, abrasion, erosion, pulp calcification and pulp stones).
- In endodontics (to determine pulp involvement and to determine root length in root canal treatment).
- To determine traumatic injuries in teeth and jaws (dentoalveolar fracture).
- To evaluate periapical lesions (apical periodontitis, periapical abscess, periapical granuloma, dental cyst, and radiopaque lesions like odontome, condensing osteitis, etc.).
- To assess periodontal lesions (horizontal and vertical bone loss).
- To assess pericoronal lesions like dentigerous cyst.
- Age estimation: Intraoral periapical radiographs help in dental age and in personal identification in forensic odontology.
- To detect impacted or unerupted teeth and supernumerary teeth.
- To detect dental anomalies like dens invaginatus, dentin dysplasia, ghost teeth, etc.
- To determine structural alterations of teeth like amelogenesis-and dentinogenesis imperfecta.
- Intraoral periapical radiographs also help in revealing many hidden systemic diseases.

Examples: Loss of lamina dura in hyperparathyroidism, and symmetric widening of PDL space in scleroderma.

3. Indications of occlusal radiography.

- To get a larger view than periapical radiographs as it includes a larger segment of the dental arch.
- Used along with periapical radiography in Miller's technique for object localization in three dimensions.
- To locate roots, supernumerary teeth, unerupted-and impacted teeth.
- To locate foreign bodies and calculus in ducts of submandibular and sublingual glands.
- Evaluation of anterior, medial and lateral outline of the maxillary sinus.
- In patients with trismus where periapical radiograph cannot be taken due to limited mouth opening.
- Evaluation of location, extent, and displacement of fracture in maxilla or mandible.
- Evaluation of the buccolingual extension of osteomyelitis, cysts, and malignancies of the jaws and their extent in palate in case of maxillary lesion and floor of the mouth in the mandibular lesion.

4. Discuss pediatric intraoral radiography.

General Considerations

Shallow palate and floor of the mouth in children cause difficulty in film placement.

Children are apprehensive and can be allayed by familiarising the procedure by briefly explaining.

Reduce the exposure parameters due to the small surface area of exposure.

10 years of age: 50% reduction in mA

10–15 years of age: 25% reduction in mA

Lead aprons and fast films to ensure radiation protection.

Small size mouth can also result in increased incidence of gag reflex which can be managed by asking the child to breathe through the nose or by distracting their attention.

Intraoral Periapical Radiography

- Principle technique is same as adults.
- Pediatric precision or XCP film holder can be used.

3–6 Years of Age

- IOPA film Size: 0 is used
- A total number of IOPA taken for full mouth survey is 4 (two in each maxilla and mandible).

Mixed Dentition: 7–12 years of age

IOPA film size: 1 is used.

- Full mouth survey: Two incisors (one for maxilla and one for mandible)

- Four canine (right and left maxilla and right and left mandible)
- Four posteriors (right and left maxilla and right and left mandible)
- Total: **10.**

Bitewing Radiography

Principle and techniques are same as the adult procedure.

Vertical angulation is +5–10° and horizontal angulation is through the interproximal surface.

3–6 Years of Age

IOPA film size: 0 with paper loop is used.

Total number of posterior bitewing taken for full mouth survey is 2 (one on each side).

Mixed Dentition: 7–12 Years of Age

Size 2 IOPA film is used with a bitewing tab attached.

Total number of posterior bitewing is 2–4

Occlusal Radiography

The procedure is similar to adult except for the film size and exposure parameters.

Exposure parameters: 65 kVp, 10 mA, 10 impulses or 90 kVp, 10 mA, three impulses are recommended.

Size 2 IOPA film is used.

The exposure side should face the jaw of interest with the patient biting the film in end-end bite relation.

The long axis of the film should be positioned on side to side direction with the PID device directed to the middle of the film through the midline of the arch. For maxillary projection the central beam is directed through the tip of the nose.

For mandibular occlusal radiography, the patient is instructed to tip the head back so that the occlusal plane is 25° above the plane of the floor. The central beam is directed through the tip of the chin to the midline of the film.

Projection	Maxilla	Mandible
Vertical angulation	+ 60°	– 30°

5. Discuss the vertical occlusal radiography.

Vertex occlusal projection: Plan view of tooth-bearing portion of maxilla from above.

Indication

Mainly used for assessment of the buccopalatal position of unerupted canine.

Procedure

The patient is seated with head supported, and the occlusal plane parallels to the floor.

The film is placed such that the long axis of the film is placed anteroposteriorly and the patient is asked to bite on it.

X-ray tube head is positioned above the patient head in the midline aiming downwards through the vertex of skull such that X-ray beam is directed down the long axis of root canals of upper incisors.

Disadvantages

- Long exposure time
- Radiation exposure to the eye.
- Superimposition of a shadow of the frontal bones may obscure the anterior part of the maxilla.

6. Vertical angulation used for various intraoral radiographic techniques.

Vertical angulation in bisecting angle technique.

Teeth	Maxilla	Mandible
Incisors	+40°	–15°
Canine	+45°	–20°
Premolars	+30°	–10°
Molars	+20°	–5°

Vertical Angulation in Bitewing Technique

Teeth	Maxilla or Mandible
Premolar	+5°
Molar	+10°
Vertical	+10°

Vertical Angulation in Occlusal Technique

Projection	Maxilla	Mandible
Anterior cross-sectional	+45°	–55°
Cross-sectional	+65°	90°
Lateral topographical	+60°	–55°
Pediatric	+60°	–30°

MULTIPLE CHOICE QUESTIONS

1. Cieszynski's principle of isometry is followed in ***bisecting angle technique***.
   a. Bisecting angle technique
   b. Long cone technique
   c. Paralleling technique
   d. SLOB technique
2. The film is placed as close as possible to the lingual surface of the teeth in ***short cone technique***.
   a. Short cone technique
   b. Long cone technique
   c. Paralleling technique
   d. SLOB technique
3. The imaginary bisector in short cone technique forms the ***common side of the equal triangles***.
   a. Apex of triangle
   b. Longest side of the equal triangles
   c. Common base of the equal triangles
   d. Common side of the equal triangles
4. Central beam perpendicular to the imaginary bisector forms the ***common base for the equal triangles***.
   a. Apex of triangle
   b. Longest side of the equal triangles
   c. Common base of the equal triangles
   d. Common side of the equal triangles
5. The overlapping of tooth images at the interproximal spaces is caused due to ***improper horizontal angulation***.
   a. Improper film placement
   b. Patient movement
   c. Improper vertical angulation
   d. Improper horizontal angulation
6. Elongation and foreshortening of images occur due to ***Improper vertical angulations***:
   a. Improper film placement
   b. Patient movement
   c. Improper vertical angulation
   d. Improper horizontal angulation
7. Use of the film holding device, such as XCP along with rectangular collimator helps in ***reducing the patient exposure***.
   a. Film placement
   b. Enhancing the object-film orientation
   c. Reducing the patient exposure
   d. Controlling the X-ray beam size
8. Positioning of tube head such that central beam is directed downward from the horizontal in the vertical plane is described as ***positive vertical angulation***.
   a. Zero horihontal angulation
   b. Positive vertical angulation
   c. Negative vertical angulation
   d. Neutral zone
9. Positioning of tube head such that central beam is directed upward from the horizontal in the vertical plane is described as ***negative vertical angulation***.
   a. Zero horihontal angulation
   b. Positive vertical angulation
   c. Negative vertical angulation
   d. Neutral zone
10. Maxillary distal oblique molar projection in periapical radiography is usually indicated for evaluation of ***impacted teeth***.
    a. Maxillary sinus
    b. Zygomatic arch
    c. Impacted teeth
    d. Coronoid process
11. Central beam directed 3 cm above the external maxillary notch on the inferior border of mandible in ***mandibular distal oblique molar projection***.
    a. Lateral topographic occlusal projection
    b. Mandibular distal oblique molar projection
    c. Postero-anterior mandible projection
    d. Vertex occlusal projection
12. Proximal caries are best diagnosed with ***bitewing radiographs***.
    a. Periapical radiographs
    b. Bitewing radiographs
    c. Orthopantomogram
    d. Occlusal radiographs

13. The use of film holder in bitewing technique reduces the incidence of ***cone-cut images***.
    a. Cone-cut images
    b. Film fog
    c. Unwanted patient exposure
    d. Image noise
14. Intraoral technique in which both maxillary and mandibular teeth are seen is ***bitewing radiograph***.
    a. Vertical occlusal radiograph
    b. Cross-sectional occlusal radiograph
    c. Bitewing radiograph
    d. Orthopantamograph
15. The following IOPA size film is recommended for bitewing projection of both premolar and molar in one film is ***size 3***.
    a. Size 2
    b. Size 3
    c. Size 4
    d. Size 5
16. In pediatric bitewing projection to cover both premolar and molar of each side the following film size is recommended ***size 2***.
    a. Size 2
    b. Size 3
    c. Size 4
    d. Size 5
17. Which of the following radiographic technique is indicated to evaluate the buccolingual extent of a lesion in the jaw is bone ***occlusal radiography***.
    a. Occlusal radiography
    b. Orthopantomography
    c. Bitewing radiography
    d. Lateral oblique view
18. Which mandibular occlusal projection is best indicated to detect stones in the duct of submandibular gland is ***cross-sectional view***.
    a. Horizontal view
    b. Cross-sectional view
    c. Paralleling view
    d. Lateral view
19. Intraoral radiographic technique best indicated in case of trismus is ***occlusal view***.
    a. Paralleling technique periapical view
    b. Bitewing view
    c. Occlusal view
    d. Bisecting angle technique periapical view
20. Exposure required for the edentulous patients is approximately ***25% less than edentulous ridge***.
    a. 50% more than dentulous ridge
    b. 50% less than edentulous ridge
    c. 25% more than dentulous ridge
    d. 25% less than dentulous ridge
21. A total number of film required for full mouth survey of edentulous patients is ***14***.
    a. 8
    b. 14
    c. 10
    d. 16
22. In which occlusal projection zygomatic process of maxilla superimposes over the tooth of molar teeth in ***lateral maxillary occlusal***.
    a. Cross-sectional maxillary occlusal
    b. Lateral maxillary occlusal
    c. Cross-sectional mandibular occlusal
    d. Lateral mandibular occlusal

VIVA VOCE

1. Indications of bitewing radiography.

- To detect proximal caries
- To detect secondary caries below restoration
- To detect the height of alveolar crest
- To detect calculus deposits in interproximal areas.

2. Advantages of bisecting angle technique.

- The film holder is not essential.
- Less radiation exposure due to the use of a short cone.
- Film placement is simple and comfortable for the patients.

3. What is vertical angulation in periapical radiography?

- In bisecting angle technique, the central beam is directed perpendicular to the imaginary bisector (bisects the angle formed between the film and teeth).
- It is the angle formed between the central beam passing through the apex of teeth with that of the occlusal plane.
- The vertical angulation is the angle that directs the central beam perpendicular to

the imaginary bisector and is different for different teeth.
- It is positive for the maxilla and negative for the mandible.

4. What is horizontal angulation in periapical radiography?

- Horizontal angulation is formed when the central beam is directed through the contact points of teeth to be examined.
- It is usually at right angles to the buccal or facial surface of teeth in each region.

5. Enumerate the film holders used in the paralleling technique.

- Extension cone paralleling (XCP) instruments.
- Precision rectangular collimating device.
- Snap-A-ray intraoral film holder.
- Hemostat and rubber bite blocks.
- Stabe disposable film holder.

6. Reason for less image magnification and increase definition in paralleling technique.

- Long source-object distance with a reduction in the size of the apparent focal spot.
- Central beam is directed perpendicular to both film and tooth.

7. Disadvantages of the finger-holding method of film placement in bisecting angle technique.

- Radiation exposure to the patient's finger.
- Overbending of the film is due to excessive force exerted by some patients to stabilize the film.
- The film may slip without patient's knowledge resulting in an improper image field.
- Increased incidence of a cone-cut as there is a possibility for misalignment of the cone to that of the film in the absence of external guide.

8. Special considerations to avoid gag reflex during intraoral radiography.

- Ask the patient to breathe through the nose.
- Deviate the attention of the patient as when their concentration is not about the procedure as it helps in reducing the gag reflex.
- Avoid film placement such that the borders touching the soft palate as it may trigger the gag reflex.
- Instruct the patient that during film placement that tongue should be relaxed and positioned well to the floor of the mouth.
- In extreme cases, topical anesthetic mouthwashes/sprays can be used to produce temporary numbness of tongue and palate.

9. Special consideration for stabilizing the film in edentulous patients.

- Placement of film becomes complicated due to its tipping into the voids due to missing teeth.
- Cotton rolls are placed between the ridge and film holder to support the film holder and prevent its tipping.

10. Special considerations for periapical radiography in endodontic practice.

Problems faced in endodontic practice: Film placement is difficult due to the presence of rubber dam and clamps.

Root canal assessment become problematic in a distorted image like foreshortened and elongated images.

Identification and separation of root canals in multirooted teeth becomes difficult.

Possible remedies:

- Tapping the intraoral film packet to one end of a wooden tongue spatula and is held in place by the patient.
- Specialized endodontic film holder like endoray (a small basket is present in the bite platform area to accommodate the handles of all endodontic instruments and still maintaining parallelism between the teeth and film).

BIBLIOGRAPHY

1. Fava LR, Dummer PM. Periapical radiographic techniques during endodontic

diagnosis and treatment. International Endodontic Journal.1997;30(4):250-61.
2. Foss OA, Klaksvik J, Benum P, et al. The rotation ratios method: a method to describe altered pelvic orientation in sequential radiographs. Acta Radiologica. 2007; 48(9):1011-9.
3. Forsberg J, Halse A. Radiographic simulation of a periapieal lesion comparing the paralleling and the bisecting-angle techniques. International Endodontic Journal. 1994;27(3):133-8.
4. Gupta A, Devi P, Srivastava R, et al . Intra oral periapical radiography-basics yet intrigue: A review. Bangladesh Journal of Dental Research and Education. 2014;4(2):83-7.
5. Langland OE, Langlais RP, Preece JW. Principles of dental imaging. Lippincott Williams and Wilkins; 2002.
6. Whaites E, Drage N. Essentials of dental radiography and radiology. Elsevier Health Sciences; 2013
7. Wenzel A. Bitewing and digital bitewing radiography for detection of caries lesions. Journal of Dental Research. 2004;83: C72-5.
8. Whitley AS, Jefferson G, Holmes K, et al. Clark's Positioning in Radiography 13E. Thirteenth edition. CRC Press; 2015.
9. White SC, Pharoah MJ. Principles of radiographic interpretation. Oral radiology principles and interpretation. St Louis (MO): Mosby Elsevier. 2009:256-69.

CHAPTER 34

Extraoral Radiographic Techniques

HIGHLIGHTS

Extraoral radiograph techniques refer to methods of obtaining skull and maxilla-mandibular images. The film is placed in a cassette and used in pair with intensifying screens. The single film provides greater diagnostic details and helps the dentist to precisely localize the extent of bony lesions and also to predict the generalized osseous deformities in association with dental structures. There are many types of extraoral radiographs. Some types are used to view the entire skull, whereas other types are focused on the maxilla and mandible.

Learners are expected to study:

- Various types of extraoral radiographs.
- Extraoral radiography units.
- Indications for different techniques.
- Errors and artifacts in OPG.

ESSAY QUESTIONS

1. Discuss panoramic radiography in detail. (or) explain in detail principle, technique, indications, advantages, and disadvantages of panoramic imaging. Add a note to the positioning errors of the technique.

Panoramic Imaging

It is an extraoral radiographic technique that allows the examination of all four-quadrant teeth and supporting structures of the jaws in a single image.

Principle of Tomography

The cassette and the tube head rotate about the patient's head in opposite directions (Fig. 1).

Rotation Center or Pivotal Point

It is around which the cassette and X-ray tube head are connected and rotated around the patient during exposure.

Three Centers of Rotation

These are double-center rotation, triple-center rotation, and moving-center rotation.

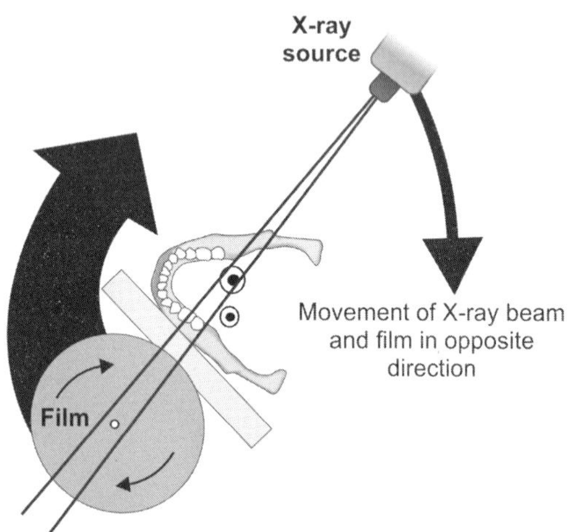

Fig. 1: Orthopantomograph principle.

Armamentarium

- *X-ray tube head:* Narrow fan-shaped X-ray beam.
- *Positioning apparatus:* Beam marker, chin-rest, and lateral head supports and bite block.
- *Exposure parameters:*
  - *kVp* = 70–100
  - *mA* = 4–12.
  - *Time:* 18 seconds approximately.

Focal trough or image layer: Three-dimensions curved zone within which structures are demonstrated. Objects placed anterior or posterior to it appears blurred.

Patient positioning: Explain the procedure to the patient which are as follows:

- Patient is asked to remove all objects from head and neck as they appear as ghost images.
- Sit or stand with the back straight and erect to prevent spine shadow bite on the disposable bite block.
- A lead apron is placed for radiation protection.
- Frankfort plane should be parallel to the floor with the midsagittal plane perpendicular to the floor. The patient should remain still during exposure.

Film placement: A screen film is placed between two intensifying screens in a cassette. Cassette is placed in the cassette holder which moves around the patient.

Interpretation

Ideal Orthopantomogram (Fig. 2)

Teeth should be arranged with a smile, like an upward curve posteriorly and be separated from each other. Posterior teeth should be uniform on both the sides. Apices of anterior should not be cut-off. Crown must not appear fractured.

Mandible: Condylar and coronoid process, TMJ, ramus, body, and angle of the mandible, teeth and supporting structures.

Mid-facial region: Maxillary sinus, zygomatic complex, nasal cavity and maxillary dentition

Soft tissue shadows: Earlobe, Soft palate, uvula, tonsils, tongue, posterior wall of pharynx, lip, cheek, nasolabial fold and nose.

Air shadows: Oropharynx, nasopharynx, maxillary sinus, nasal fossa.

Positioning Errors

- *Patient's head too far forward from the focal trough.*
  - Narrowing of anterior teeth.
  - Cervical spine superimposition on rami.

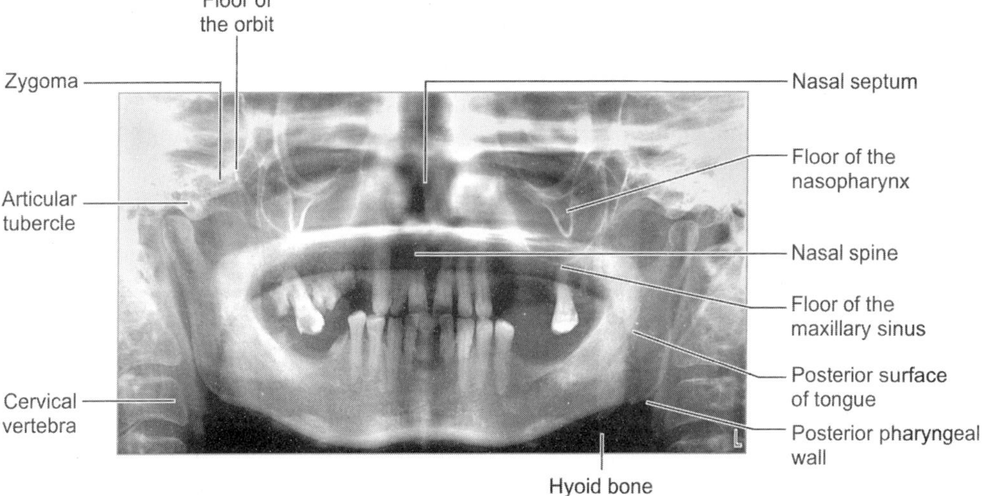

Fig. 2: Interpretation of anatomical structures in orthopantomogram.

- *The patient head is backward from the focal trough.*
  - Widening of the anterior teeth.
  - TMJ is not clear.

Midsagittal plane positioning errors

- *Patient is tilted in the machine.*
  - A widened gap between upper and lower posterior teeth on one side.
  - Condyle enlarged on one side.
  - Enlarged mandible.
  - Bony details appear fuzzy.

Occlusal plane positioning errors

- *Chin tipped too low: (Frankfort plane downward).*
  - Smile line is exaggerated.
  - Apices of mandibular anterior are cut off.
- *Chin tipped too high: (Frankfort plane upward).*
  - Reverse smile line.
  - Hard palate and floor of the nasal cavity superimpose over the maxillary teeth roots.
  - Blurred maxillary incisors.

Artifacts

- *Ghost image:* Objects located between the X-ray source and behind the center of rotation produce ghost images, e.g. spine, neck chains and horns of hyoid produces ghost images.
- *Double image:* Midline structures like turbinate of the nose, the body of hyoid and spine produce a double image.

Indications

To examine:

- The extent of lesions.
- The eruption pattern, growth, and developments.
- Multiple impacted teeth.
- Cysts and tumors.
- Jaw fracture.

Contraindications

- Routine screening.
- Periodontal assessment of pocket less than 5 mm.
- As an alternative to intraoral radiographs.

Advantages

- Radiation dosage is about 1/3rd of dose from full mouth survey.
- Large area is imaged.
- Preorthodontic assessment of periodontal status.
- For the record and reference purposes.

Disadvantages

- Structures located outside the focal trough cannot be assessed accurately.
- Shadow of soft-tissues superimpose the hard tissue and reduces the accuracy.
- The overall magnification in panoramic radiograph is 15–20%.
- Resolution, sharpness, contrast is low compared to intraoral radiographs.

2. Enumerate the various skull radiographic projections and explain in detail the PA skull projection.

Skull Projections

They are PA skull projection, lateral skull projection, Waters' projection and submentovertex projection.

Equipment: Skull projections are taken in an extraoral radiographic machine called craniostat or cephalostat. X-ray source, grid, and cassette must be labeled R or L before exposure (screen film is used). Patient positioning table with exposure parameters (kVp and mA) is different for each projection.

PA Skull Projection

X-ray beam passes in posterior to the anterior direction through the skull.

Equipment Preparation

The radiographic machine used is cephalostat with the grid. Cassette must be labeled R or L prior to exposure. Exposure parameters: 70 kVp and 30–50 mA are commonly preferred.

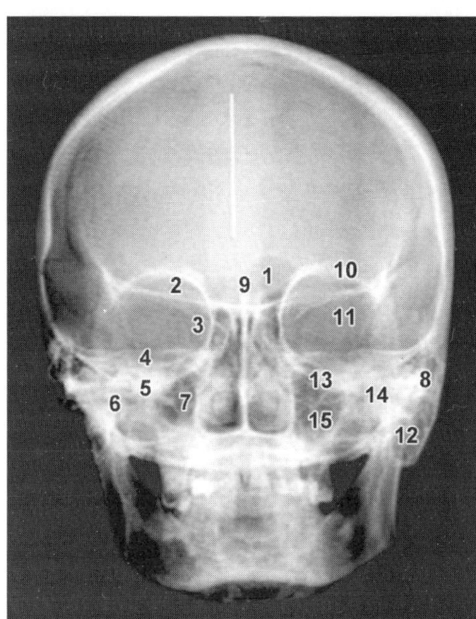

1. Frontal sinus
2. Superior orbital fissure
3. Ethmoidal air cells
4. Superior part of petrous bone
5. Anterior ethmoidal septum
6. Inferior orbital canal
7. Inferior lateral recess of sphenoid sinu
8. Coronoid process
9. Floor of sella turcica
10. Superior rim of orbit
11. Lesser wing of sphenoid
12. Mastoid process
13. Foramen rotundum
14. Base of the skull
15. Maxillary antrum

Fig. 3: Identification of anatomical structures in the posteroanterior skull view.

Patient Positioning

The patient is positioned to face the cassette such that forehead and nose touch the cassette. Head is centered over the cassette such that the midsagittal plane perpendicular to floor and Frankfort plane parallel to floor and perpendicular to film.

Film Placement

A screen film size of 8 × 10 inches or 20 × 25 cm is used. Cassette placed perpendicular to the floor in the cassette-holding device. The long axis of the cassette is positioned vertically facing the patient.

Projection of Central Beam

Central beam is directed perpendicular to the film plane coincident with the midsagittal plane of the patient at the level of the bridge of the nose. The distance between the X-ray source and midsagittal plane should be approximately 5 feet (60 inches) and the film is placed 15 cm away from the midsagittal plane.

Indications

- Examination of the skull for growth and development, trauma, disease and developmental abnormalities.
- For evaluation of facial structures including frontal and ethmoidal sinuses, nasal fossa and orbits (Fig. 3).

3. Discuss mandibular lateral oblique projection in detail. (or) describe extraoral radiographic technique that is best indicated to view the large lesions in the mandible. Explain the technique and indications of the various views of the same projection in detail.

Mandibular Lateral Oblique Projection

It is used to examine large lesions in mandible which cannot be covered in the periapical radiograph and when higher resolution is required than panoramic projection. Two projections are depending upon the region of the lesion.

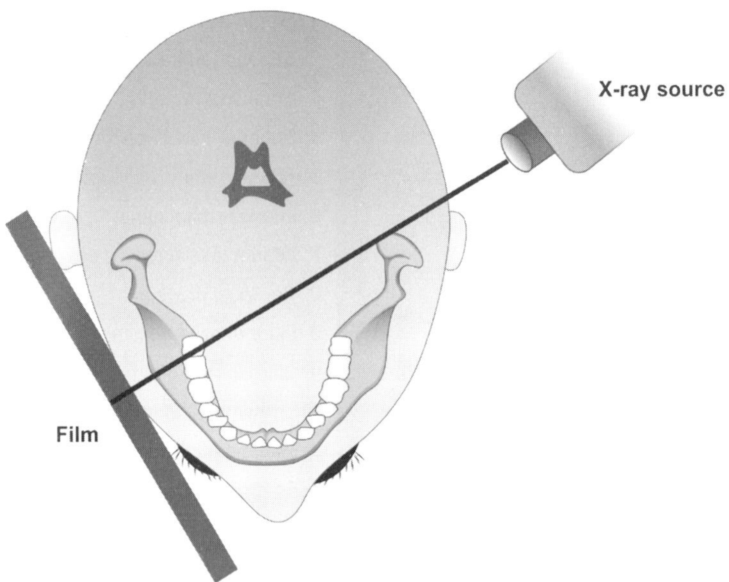

Fig. 4: Lateral oblique projection of the mandibular body.

Body of the mandible projection: It demonstrates premolar and molar region and inferior border of the mandible.

Equipment preparation: Exposure parameters: 65 kVp, 10 mA and ¼ seconds. It can be taken in the intraoral radiographic machine. If cephalostat is used, open-ended aiming cylinder is used.

Patient positioning: The head is tilted to the side of examination, and the mandible is protruded to avoid spine superimposition.

Film placement: Around 5 × 7" screen film is used. The patient should position the cassette on the cheek region centered over the lower first molar. The lower border of the cassette should be in the plane of the inferior border of the mandible and extend 2 cm below the inferior border.

Projection of central beam: Central beam is perpendicular to film directed from a point 2 cm below the angle of mandible on the tube side towards the first molar region (Fig. 4).

Indications

- To view the mediolateral extent of large lesions like cyst and tumors in the mandibular body region.
- To examine fractures in the body of the mandible.
- For evaluation of sialolith in submandibular gland duct.

Ramus Projection

It demonstrates ramus from the angle of the mandible to the condyle and third molar region of both maxilla and mandible (Fig. 5).

Equipment preparation: Exposure parameters: 65 kVp, 10 mA and 1/4 seconds. It can be taken in the intraoral radiographic machine. If cephalostat is used, open-ended aiming cylinder is used.

Patient positioning: Head is tilted towards the side being examined, and the mandible is protruded to avoid spine superimposition.

Film placement: 5 × 7 inches (13 × 18 cm) screen film is used. Patient should keep the cassette on the cheek region centered over the ramus and far enough posteriorly to include condyle. Lower border is parallel and extends 2 cm beneath the lower border of the mandible.

Projection of central beam: Central beam is perpendicular to film and directed from a point 2 cm beneath the lower border of the

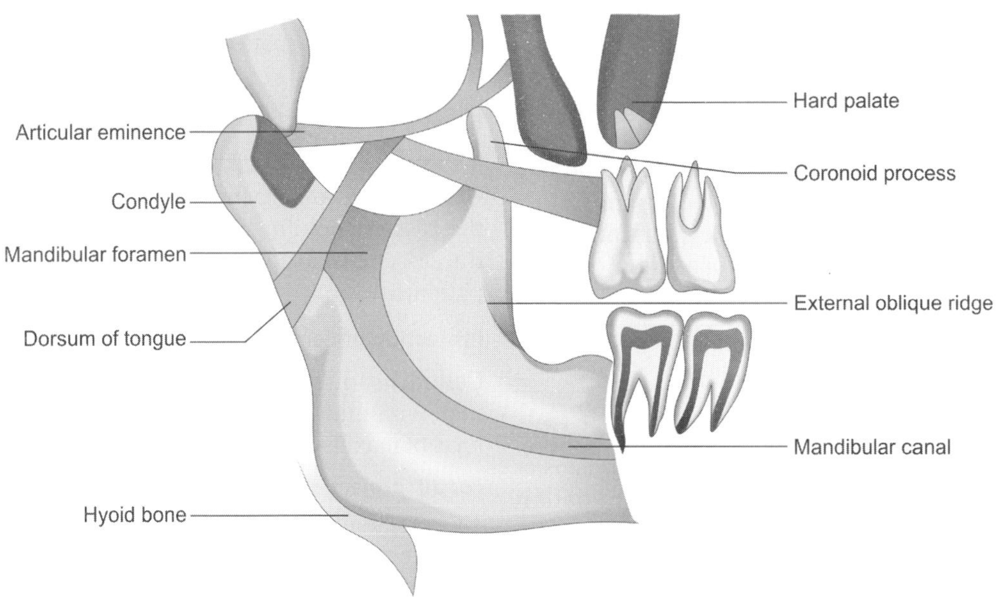

Fig. 5: Identification of anatomical landmarks in lateral oblique projection of the mandibular ramus.

mandible in the first molar region on the tube side towards the ramus region on the side of interest.

Indications

- To view the mediolateral extent of large lesions like cyst and tumor in ramus and posterior most region of the mandible.
- To evaluate fractures in ramus of the mandible.
- For evaluation of sialolith.
- Assessment of the presence and position of impacted teeth.

SHORT NOTES

1. Indications of OPG.

Refer Essay Question 1.

2. Discuss the merits and demerits of OPG.

Advantages

- Radiation dosage is about 1/3rd of dose from full mouth survey.
- Provide diagnostic details of teeth and supporting structures of both jaws.
- Simplicity: Minimal amount of time and training for the dental radiographer.
- Accurate assessment of dimension of lesions involving a posterior region of the mandible when margins are well-defined.
- Bilateral condyle lesions and other parts of mandible seen in one film facilitate comparative study.
- Preorthodontic, presurgical assessment and for initial evaluation of generalized periodontal status.
- For documentation, record and reference purpose.

Disadvantages

- Structures present outside the focal trough may not be evident.
- Soft tissue shadow overlies the required hard tissue structures and reduces the accuracy.
- The overall magnification obtained in panoramic radiograph is 15–20%.
- Resolution, sharpness, contrast are low as compared to intraoral radiographs.
- Some patients do not conform to the shape of the focal trough, and as a result, some structures are out of focus.

- Intensifying screens result in loss of image quality.
  - Dental caries, periodontal status, bone loss, periapical pathosis are not seen with clarity.
  - Technique sensitive, hence positioning errors result in faulty radiographs.
  - Cannot be used for evaluation of the buccolingual extent of a lesion.

3. Describe Waters' projection.

- Occipitomental projection (0° and 30°)
- Variation of PA projection.

Equipment Preparation (0° and 30°)

The radiographic machine used is cephalostat with a grid to prevent scattered radiation and improve contrast. Cassette: It must be labeled R or L before exposure. Exposure parameters: Usually 70 kVp and 100 mA are the recommended parameters.

Patient Positioning (0° and 30°)

Head is positioned such that midsagittal plane is perpendicular to film plane. The patient should be positioned to face the film and in a head tilted back direction so that the canthomeatal line is at 45° to the cassette with the nose and chin touching the cassette. If sphenoidal sinus should be projected onto the film plane, the patient is instructed to open the mouth.

Film Placement

8 × 10 inch (20 × 25 cm) screen film is used. Cassette placed perpendicular to the floor in the cassette holding device. The long axis of the cassette is positioned vertically facing the patient.

Projection of Central Beam (0° projection)

Central beam is directed horizontal 0° coincident with midsagittal plane of patient at the level of maxillary sinus through the occipit.

For 30° projection

The direction of the central beam is downward from above the head and at 30° horizontal to the lower border of orbit.

Indications

For 0° projection

- This projection is mainly for the investigation of the maxillary antrum and facial skeleton (Fig. 6).
- For the detection of midfacial fractures:
  - Le Fort I
  - Le Fort II

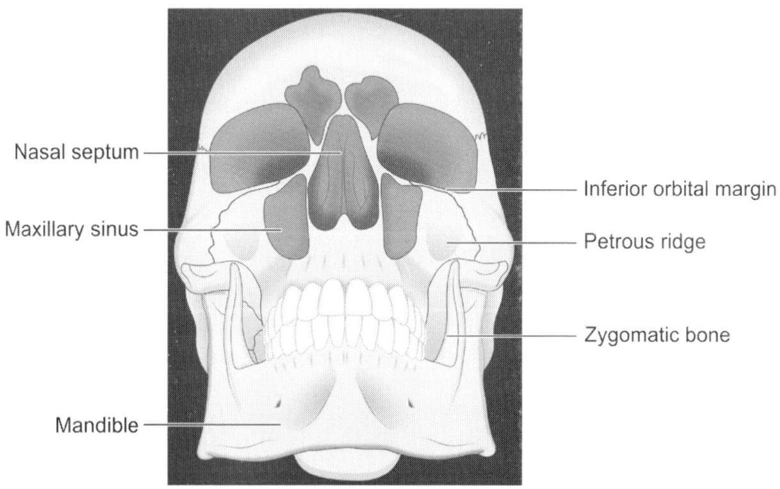

Fig. 6: Waters projection revealing the anatomical structures.

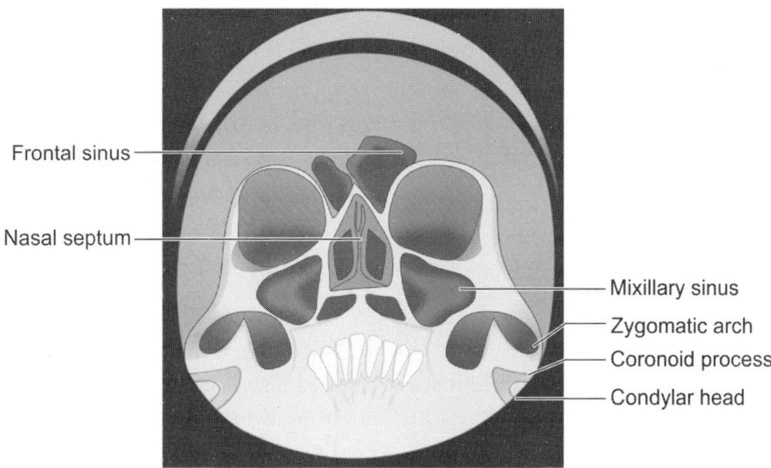

Fig. 7: Modified Waters' projection revealing anatomical structures.

- Le Fort III
- Zygomatic complex
- Nasoethmoidal complex
- Orbital blow-out.

For 30° projection (Fig. 7)

- This projection enables the diagnosis of certain bony displacements.
- For the detection of midfacial fractures:
  - Le Fort I
  - Le Fort II
  - Le Fort III
- Coronoid process fractures.

Both (0°-and 30° projections) are indicated to diagnose the suspected facial fracture but at different angles.

4. Explain submentovertex projection.

This view reveals structures including the base of the skull, sphenoidal sinuses and the facial bones from below. Also called base or full axial projection and it is an anteroposterior projection.

Equipment Preparation

The radiographic machine used is cephalostat with a grid. Cassette: It must be labeled R or L before exposure. Exposure parameters: 70 kVp and 100 mA.

Patient Positioning

Head and neck extended backward as possible such that vertex of the skull touches the center of the cassette. Patient's midsagittal plane is perpendicular to floor and Frankfort plane vertical and parallel to floor with canthomeatal line should extend 10° past vertical.

Film Placement

8 × 10 inch (20 × 25 cm) screen film is used. The film cassette is placed in the vertical direction behind the patient's head and should be centered over the skull vertex.

Projection of Central Beam

Central beam is directed from below the mandible upward towards the vertex of the skull and is positioned far enough anterior to pass about 2 cm in front of a line connecting right and left condyles.

Indications

- Bony lesions involving the palate, pterygoid region, and the base of the skull.
- Examination of the sphenoidal sinus.
- Evaluation of the lateral wall of maxillary antrum.

- Assessment of the thickness of the posterior mandible in mediolateral direction before surgical procedures.
- The less exposure parameters used in submentovertex view reveals the fracture of the thin zygomatic arches accurately. The SMV taken with reduced exposure factors is called jughandle view.

5. Explain lateral skull projection.

Equipment Preparation

The radiographic machine used is cephalostat with a grid. Exposure parameters: 70 kVp and 100 mA.

Patient Positioning

The side of interest (right or left) of patient's head is positioned and centered over the cassette. Midsagittal plane of the patient is parallel to the cassette and perpendicular to floor.

Film Placement

8 × 10 inch (20 × 25 cm) screen film is used. Placed in the cassette holding device adjacent to side of interest perpendicular to the floor.

Projection of Central Beam

The central beam is directed through the external auditory meatus to the center of the cassette from the opposite side perpendicular to it.

Indications

- Fractures of the cranium and the skull base.
- Midfacial fractures and the downward and backward displacement of the maxilla.
- Investigation of the frontal, sphenoidal and maxillary sinuses.
- Conditions affecting the skull vault, like:
  - Paget's disease
  - Multiple myeloma
  - Hyperparathyroidism
- **To examine sella turcica for:**
  - Pituitary gland tumor in acromegaly.
  - Enlargement or ballooning of the sella.

6. Explain cephalometric projection.

Cephalometric radiography is an extraoral radiographic technique that applies standardized landmarks to predict the maxilla-mandibular jaw relations with the base of the skull and the occlusal relation of teeth for orthodontic assessment.

Indications

- In orthodontics: Initial diagnosis and pre-operative evaluation, treatment planning and monitoring of treatment and appraisal of treatment results.
- Before orthognathic surgery:
  - Preoperative skeletal and soft-tissue evaluation.
  - Postoperative assessment and term follow-up.

Equipment

The equipment consists of cephalostat with head positioners and ear rods, cassette with screen film of 18 × 24 cm. Aluminum-wedge filter between patient and cassette for attenuation of X-ray beam in soft tissues. X-ray source to film distance is 60 inch. The X-ray beam is collimated.

Projections

PA Cephalometric

Technique and positioning: The head stabilizing device of the cephalostat is rotated through 90°. The patient is positioned in the radiographic unit with the head tilted in a forward direction. The head is immobilized by positioning the ear rods into the external auditory meatus. The central ray is horizontally directed through the cervical spine at the level of the rami of the mandible.

Lateral Cephalometric

Technique and positioning: The patient is positioned within the cephalostat. The sagittal plane of the head should be vertical and parallel to the film and the Frankfort horizontal plane. Teeth should be in the maximum intercuspal position. The head is immobilized with the help of ear rods. The aluminium wedge is placed between the patient and the anterior part of the cassette to attenuate the X-ray beam selectively in the region of the soft tissues. This allows the soft tissue profile on the radiograph.

Cephalometric Planes, Angles and Points

Planes: Frankfort horizontal plane, mandibular plane, maxillary plane and SN plane.

Angles: SNA, SNB, ANB, maxillary incisal inclination and mandibular incisal inclination.

Cephalometric points: Orbitale (Or), nasion (N), sella (S), anterior nasal spine (ANS), subspinale or point A, prosthion (Pr), infradentale (Id), supramental or point B, pogonion (Pog), gnathon (Gn), menton (Me), gonion (Go), posterior nasal spine (PNS), articulare (Au), and porion (Po).

7. Describe reverse Towne's projection.

Towne's projection is AP skull projection. Reverse Towne's is opposite of Towne's view and is a PA skull projection mainly indicated to examine condylar neck fractures.

Equipment Preparation

The radiographic machine used is cephalostat with grid. Exposure parameters: 70 kVp and 100 mA.

Patient Positioning

Head centered in front of the cassette with canthomeatal line oriented downward 25–30°. The patient is instructed to open the mouth as wide as possible to visualize the condyles.

Film Placement

Cassette is held on the holding device in front of the patient with the patient's forehead touching the cassette.

Projection of Central Beam

The central beam directed towards the film in the sagittal plane through the occipital bone from the opposite side of the cassette.

Indications

- High fractures of the condylar necks.
- Intracapsular fracture of the TMJ.
- Condylar hypoplasia and hyperplasia.
- To examine the articular surfaces of the condylar head.
- To reveal a medially displaced condyle.
- Pathology related to the posterolateral wall of the maxillary sinus.

8. Briefly explain about PA view of the mandible.

This projection shows the mandibular posterior structures. It is a variant of PA skull view but is not indicated for skull details as it allows the overlapping of the base of the skull and nasal bones.

Equipment Preparation

The radiographic machine used is cephalostat with the grid. Cassette must be labeled R or L before exposure. Exposure parameters: 70 KVp and 30–50 mA.

Patient Positioning

The patient is positioned to face the cassette such that forehead and nose touch the cassette. Head is centered over the cassette with the midsagittal plane perpendicular to floor and Frankfort plane parallel to the floor and perpendicular to film.

Film Placement

8 × 10 inch (20 × 25 cm) screen film is used. Cassette placed perpendicular to the floor in the cassette holding device. The long axis of the cassette is positioned vertically facing the patient.

Projection of Central Beam

Central beam is directed perpendicular to the cassette and through the cervical spine at the level of the ramus.

Indications

- Mandibular fractures involving the following:
  - Posterior body

- Angle and rami of the mandible
- Lower condylar neck

- Cysts and tumors mainly in the posterior third of body or rami to see the mediolateral expansion.
- Mandibular hypoplasia or hyperplasia.
- Maxillofacial deformities.

9. Describe rotated PA view of the mandible.

It reveals details of the parotid gland and ramus of the mandible on one side of the face.

Technique

The patient is positioned facing the film such that tip of the nose is touching the film with occlusal plane horizontal. Head is then rotated 10° to the side of interest to avoid the superimposition of the skull base. Central beam is projected in horizontal (0°) direction on the side of interest.

Indications

- To view sialolith in parotid glands.
- To see the mediolateral expansion of cysts or tumors in the ramus.
- To ensure new bone formation in submasseteric space infection.

MULTIPLE CHOICE QUESTIONS

1. Panoramic radiography is based on the principle of ***tomography***.
   a. Rotation
   b. Focal trough
   c. Tomography
   d. Image slicing
2. Which of the following moves around the patient head in panaromic radiography? ***X-ray tube head and cassete***.
   a. Film
   b. Film and X-ray machine
   c. X-ray tube head
   d. X-ray tube head and cassette
3. Three-dimensional zone in which structures are demonstrated in panoramic radiography is called ***focal trough.***
   a. Cross sectional image
   b. Focal trough
   c. Tomographic layer
   d. Image band width
   (**Note:** Focal trough or image layer).
4. Radiopaque artifact seen on the panoramic film produced by a radiopaque object that is penetrated twice by the X-ray beam is called ***ghost image***.
   a. Double image
   b. Image superimposition
   c. Ghost image
   d. Image distortion
5. Reverse smile line in panoramic film appears when patient's chin is positioned ***too high***.
   a. Too low
   b. Too high
   c. Too close to source
   d. Away from the source.
   (**Note:** Patient's chin is positioned too high or Frankfort plane is placed upward).
6. Exaggerated smile line in the panoramic film appears when patient's chin is positioned ***too low***.
   a. Too low
   b. Too high
   c. Too close to source
   d. Away from the source.
   (**Note:** Patient's chin is positioned too low or Frankfort plane is placed downward).
7. In panoramic radiography, when the patient is positioned too far-forward on the bite block, anterior teeth appear ***narrowed and blurred***.
   a. Widened and elongated
   b. Narrowed and foreshortened
   c. Spaced and blurred
   d. Narrowed and blurred
8. In panoramic radiography, when the patient is positioned too far back on the bite block, anterior teeth appear ***widened and blurred***.
   a. Widened and elongated
   b. Narrowed and foreshortened
   c. Widened and blurred
   d. Narrowed and blurred
9. Which of the following projection is best indicated to view maxillary sinus? ***Water's view***.
   a. Jughandle view
   b. Water's view
   c. Reverse Towne's view
   d. Posteroanterior skull view

10. Which view is best indicated to view zygomatic arch fracture? ***jughandle view***.
    a. Jughandle view
    b. Waters' projection
    c. Reverse Towne's view
    d. Posteroanterior skull view
    (**Note:** Jughandle view or submentovertex view).
11. Which view is best indicated to view condylar neck fracture? ***reverse Towne's view***.
    a. Jughandle view
    b. Waters' projection
    c. Reverse Towne's view
    d. Posteroanterior skull view
12. Which extraoral view is indicated to view fracture of body of mandible is? ***lateral oblique view***.
    a. Jughandle view
    b. Waters' projection
    c. Reverse Towne's view
    d. Lateral oblique view
13. Which of the following projection is best for examination of soft tissue profile of face is? ***lateral cephalometric view***.
    a. Jughandle view
    b. Waters' projection
    c. Reverse Towne's view
    d. Lateral cephalometric view.
14. Base or full axial projection is named as. ***submentovertex view***.
    a. Jughandle view
    b. Submentovertex view
    c. Reverse Towne's view
    d. Posteroanterior skull view

VIVA VOCE

1. What is focal trough?

- Three-dimensional zone in which structures are demonstrated in panoramic radiography is called focal trough or image layer.
- Structures positioned anterior or posterior to the focal trough appears blurred.
- Closer the rotation centers to the teeth, narrower the focal trough.
- The focal trough is narrower in the anterior region and wider in the posterior region.

2. What is jughandle view and when it is mainly indicated?

- It is submentovertex projection with reduced exposure time, and it is mainly indicated to view zygomatic arch fractures.
- Exposure time is reduced to one-third that used to visualize the skull.

3. What is PA projection?

X-ray source placed behind the patient such that central beam is passed from structures posterior to anterior.

4. What is AP projection?

X-ray source placed behind the patient such that central beam is passed from structures anterior to posterior.

5. What is ghost image?

Objects located between the X-ray source and behind the center of rotation produce ghost images.

Examples:

- Ghost image of the palate superimpose on apices of maxillary teeth as a wide radiopaque line.
- Spine, neck chains and horns of hyoid bone produces ghost images.

Ghost images have the same shape as its counterpart and it appears on opposite side. It appears higher up and is blurred.

6. What is the reason for double images in OPG?

- Double images occur in the central portion of the OPG where objects are intercepted twice by the beam.
- Midline objects like turbinate of nose, body of hyoid and spine produce double image.

7. What are the extraoral film sizes available?

Extraoral film size	Extraoral projection
5 × 7" (13 × 18 cm)	Lateral oblique view of mandible
8 × 10" (20 × 25 cm)	Skull projections or cephalometric projections

8. Why is thyroid collar not recommended for panoramic imaging?

Thyroid collar absorbs the central rays and obscures the diagnostic information.

9. What happens when the patient is not instructed about lip and tongue position during panoramic exposure?

The patient should close the lips and position the tongue on the palate during exposure. Failure to follow this step will lead to:

- Dark radiolucent band will be seen above the apices of maxillary teeth.
- Diagnostic information of the periapical region of maxillary teeth will be obscured.

10. What happens when the patient is not standing perfectly straight in panoramic radiography?

Radiopaque shadow of the spine is seen in the midline of the film.

11. What are the different AP projections of the skull?

- Submentovertex projection.
- Towne's projection.

12. What is Towne's projection?

- The Towne's view is AP projection and is often of value in assessing the status of the condyles, condylar neck and rami because superimposition of the mastoid and zygoma over the condylar neck region in the straight posteroanterior projection often makes interpretation difficult.
- The Towne's view eliminates this superimposition and ensures better visualization of the condylar area and rami.
- The patient lies on his back with the film under his head. The X-ray source is from the front, but rotated 30% from the Frankfort plane and is directed right at the condyles.

BIBLIOGRAPHY

1. Ardran GM, Crooks HE. A comparison of radiographic techniques with special reference to dosage. Br J Radiol. 1953;26:352-7.
2. Karjodkar FR. Essentials of oral and maxillofacial radiology. Second edition. Jaypee Brothers Medical Publishers Pvt Limited. New Delhi. 2014.
3. White SC, Pharoah MJ. Oral radiology: principles and interpretation. 5th edition. St. Louis Mosby; 2004. pp.255-63.
4. Whaites E, Drage N. Essentials of dental radiography and radiology. Elsevier Health Sciences; 2013.

CHAPTER 35

Temporomandibular Joint Projections

TEMPOROMANDIBULAR JOINT PROJECTION

Learners are expected to know about:

- ❖ Transcranial projection
- ❖ Transpharyngeal projection
- ❖ Transorbital projection
- ❖ Temporomandibular joint (TMJ) tomography

SHORT NOTES

1. Describe transcranial projection with its indications.

Transcranial projection is otherwise known as **Lindblom projection.**

This view is used **for evaluation** of:

- ❖ The superior surface of condyle
- ❖ The translation of the condylar processes
- ❖ The surface of the articular eminence.

Technique

The cassette should be placed parallel to the patient's midsagittal plane, centering the condyle of interest.

The central ray is directed downward from opposite side. It enters ½ inch posterior to the external auditory meatus and 2 inches above the external auditory meatus.

Vertical angulation: + 25°

Average horizontal angulation: 20°.

Series of right and left TMJ in the closed and maximal open positions should be taken.

Indications

To diagnose:

- ❖ Displaced condylar fractures
- ❖ Range of condylar motion
- ❖ Disc position
- ❖ Gross osseous changes on the lateral aspect of jaw.

Limitations

Condyle, temporal component, and joint spaces are shattered on the image.

2. Describe transpharyngeal projection. (or) describe parma projection.

This view is indicated for:

- ❖ Visualization of the superior surface of the condyle
- ❖ Screening arthritic changes.

Techniques

- ❖ Patient is asked to held the cassette against the head and turn 7° to 10° away from the side of interest. The cassette should be parallel to midsagittal plane.
- ❖ The central ray is directed through the coronoid notch on the opposite from 0° to –5° perpendicular to the cassette.
- ❖ Patient should be instructed to widely open the mouth when the exposure is made.
- ❖ Exposure factors must be 70 kV, 10 mA, and 0.1 seconds. The exposure time is greatly reduced because no bony structures are superposed.

Limitation

Temporal component cannot be imaged accurately.

3. Describe transorbital projection. (or) describe Zimmer projection.

This view is indicated for:
- Visualization of the superior surface of the condyle from the lateral to medial poles
- Condylar neck fracture.

Techniques

- Cassette should be placed behind the patients head.
- Patient should open the mouth at maximal level or protrude the mandible to position to avoid the superimposition of the articular eminence or skull base over the condyle.
- Central ray should be directed downward at + 35° through the patient's medial canthus, centering the condyle within the orbit. The patient's head is rotated approximately 20° toward the side of interest to avoid superimposition of the mastoid process over the structures of interest.
- Exposure factors must be 75 kV, 15 mA, and 0.1 seconds.

4. Discuss about temporomandibular joint tomography. (or) describe the panoramic projection of temporomandibular joint.

Panoramic TMJ view is principally used for screening the morphology of condyle and initial assessment of condylar translation. It also used to detect the early changes associated with rheumatoid arthritis or degenerative joint disorders.

TMJ tomography is a technique used to examine structures located within a selected plane of tissues while blurring the structures outside the plane. TMJ tomography provides the most definitive imaging of the bony components of TMJ and the glenoid fossa. It also used to examine the joint space and evaluate the movement of condyle in open mouth position.

This view has limited application and provides distorted image of the joint due to its thick image layers.

Limitations

- Condylar position and movements cannot be interpreted.
- Not ideal for early diagnosis of mild osseous changes.

5. Role of computed tomography in the diagnosis of temporomandibular joint disorders.

Computed tomography (CT) is helpful in providing the detailed information about the internal joint structures both osseous and soft tissues in a three dimensional shape. It produces multiple image slices in axial and coronal planes which are manipulated and form images in sagittal plane.

Applications

Computed tomography images are valuable in the diagnosis of:
- Ankylosis
- Neoplasm
- Bone involvement in TMJ arthritis
- Complex joint fractures.

Limitations

Articular disc changes cannot be studied precisely.

6. Temporomandibular arthrography.

Arthrography is useful in viewing the TMJ disc pathology. It is taken by injecting the radiopaque iodine dye as a contrast agent into the joint space under fluoroscopic guidance through the preauricular or transmeatal portal. In this way, this image is helpful in detecting the disc perforation and adhesion by the way the contrast agent filling the joint space.

Applications

To study the:
- Disc position, structure and function
- Disc attachments.

7. Radiographic features of TMJ ankylosis.

TMJ ankylosis is of two types: True (bony) or false (fibrous).

1. True ankylosis results from condyle or ramus attachment with temporal bone.
2. Fibrous ankylosis results from the soft tissue union of the joint components
   - Coronal CT images are the best to diagnose ankylosis.

Bony Ankylosis

- The joint space is either partially or completely obliterated by an osseous bridge
- There is fusion of the condyle to the cranial base
- Elongation of the coronoid process and deepening of the antegoinal notch on the affected side.

Fibrous Ankylosis

- The articular surfaces are eroded and appear irregular.
- The joint space appear narrow.
- Two irregular joint space may appear to fit one another and gives the appearance of characteristic jigsaw puzzle.

VIVA VOCE

1. What is the use of submentovertex projection in the diagnosis of temporomandibular joint disorders.

The submentovertex (SMV) or basal projection is useful in the evaluation of facial symmetries, condylar displacement, and to detect the horizontal rotation of mandible following trauma or orthognathic surgeries.

2. What are Ely cysts?

Ely cysts are the pseudo cysts seen in degenerative joint disorders (TMJ osteoarthritis). In radiographs, they appear as small, round radiolucent lesions surrounded by radiopaque boundaries below the articulating surfaces. These cysts denote the presence of fibrous tissues, granulation tissues, and osteoid structures as a degenerative change.

MULTIPLE CHOICE QUESTIONS

1. Articular disc is best viewed in ***magnetic resonance imaging***.
   a. Arthrography
   b. Computed tomography
   c. Magnetic resonance imaging
   d. Panoramic tomography
2. Joint inflammation and effusion are studied in ***T2—weighted magnetic resonance images.***
   a. T2—weighted magnetic resonance images
   b. T1—weighted magnetic resonance images
   c. Proton—weighted magnetic resonance images
   d. Motion magnetic resonance studies
3. In unilateral internal derangements, the mandible deviates to the ***affected side on opening***.
   a. Normal side on opening
   b. Affected side on opening
   c. Normal side on closing
   d. Affected side on closing
4. Disc perforation is best studied in ***arthrography***.
   a. Arthrography
   b. Computed tomography
   c. Magnetic resonance imaging
   d. Panoramic tomography
5. Resistance to injection of contrast agent in the joint space indicates ***adhesions***.
   a. Adhesion
   b. Perforation
   c. Reduction
   d. Displacement
6. Joint mice denotes ***broken osteophytes***.
   a. Fibrous tissues
   b. Granulation tissues
   c. Broken osteophytes
   d. Ely cysts
7. Sharpened pencil appearance of condyle is seen in ***rheumatoid arthritis***.
   a. Osteoarthritis
   b. Rheumatoid arthritis
   c. Fibrous ankylosis
   d. Osseous ankylosis
8. Sharpened pencil appearance of condyle denotes the ***condylar erosion***.
   a. Condylar hyperplasia
   b. Condylar hypoplasia

c. Condylar erosion
d. Condylar effusion

9. Joint effusion denotes ***influx of fluid into the joint***.
a. Soft tissue calcifications
b. influx of fluid into the joint
c. Crystalline structures in the joint spaces
d. Hyaline metaplasia

10. Jigsaw puzzle appearance is seen in ***fibrous ankylosis***.
a. Bony ankylosis
b. Fibrous ankylosis
c. Osteoarthritis
d. Rheumatoid arthritis

11. Nonspecific condylar destruction denotes ***metastatic tumors***.
a. Metastatic tumors
b. Osteoma
c. Osteochondroma
d. Osteogenic sarcoma

12. Bone formation is a feature of ***osteogenic sarcoma***.
a. Chodrosarcoma
b. Osteogenic sarcoma
c. Malignant primary tumors
d. Malignant metastatic tumors

BIBLIOGRAPHY

1. Karjodkar FR. Essentials of oral and maxillofacial radiology. Second edition. Jaypee Brothers Medical Publishers; 2014.
2. Koch BL, Hamilton BE, Hudgins PA, et al. Diagnostic Imaging: Head and Neck. 3rd edition. Amirsys Publishing Inc; 2016.
3. Mongini F. The importance of radiography in the diagnosis of TMJ dysfunctions. A comparative evaluation of transcranial radiographs and serial tomography. J Prosthet Dent. 1981;45(2):186-98.
4. Petrikowski CG. Diagnostic imaging of the temporomandibular Joint. White SC, Pharoah MJ. Oral radiology, principles and interpretation. 5th edition. St Louis Mosby; 2004. pp 255-63.
5. White SC, Pharoah MJ. Oral radiology: Principles and interpretation. Elsevier Health Sciences; 2014.

CHAPTER 36

Advanced Imaging Modalities

HIGHLIGHTS

Advances in radiographic technology substituted film mages with a filmless radiographic system known as digital imaging in 1987. Similarly, two-dimensional images are complemented by the development of three-dimensional digital imaging which allows the viewing of oral and maxillofacial structures to provide accurate diagnostic information. Nonionizing imaging techniques that use ultrasound and magnetic field are also playing a great role in this era. Also, to enhance the structural and functional details, the use of radioisotopes and contrast agents plays a considerable role.

Learners are expected to know about the basic concepts of:

- Digital imaging
- Three-dimensional digital imaging—CT, CBCT
- Magnetic renosonce imaging (MRI)
- Nuclear scintigraphy
- Contrast radiography

ESSAY QUESTIONS

1. Define digital radiography. Briefly, describe the components of an intraoral digital radiography unit (RVG) and its image reconstruction technique.

Definition

Digital radiography (DR) is defined as a diagnostic imaging technique that uses an image receptor called sensors to convert the image to digital analog that can be analyzed and stored in a computer.

Principle

When an X-ray beam strikes the sensor, an electronic charge is produced on the surface of the sensor which is then digitized. The data received by the sensor in are translated to the analog form and transferred to the computer where it is transformed to digital form by an analog-to-digital converter (ADC).

The image is displayed within 0.5–120 seconds and can be manipulated to enhance the appearance of interpretation.

Components

A **sensor** is used to capture the image. Charge-coupled devices (CCDs) and the complementary metal oxide semiconductor (CMOS) are used in dentistry for intraoral imaging.

A pixel (picture element) is a term used to describe a two-dimensional square area or cell on the silicon detector (sensor) that stores the electrons released radiation. The pixel corresponds to the silver halide grains in X-ray film.

The **computer** digitizes, processes and stores information received from the sensor. The software stores the information in electronic format.

It converts the electronic signals from the sensor into a range of gray shades to visualize on the monitor. The computer recognizes the pixels in a numerical form. The array of numbers for each pixel is between 0 and 255 (a total of 226 shades) that constructs the pixel grayscale resolution.

The software manipulates the pixels to enhance contrast and density without additional radiation exposure.

Procedure

- ***Sensor preparation:*** Sterile sensor should be placed intraorally similar to the conventional film placement. The sensors need to be wrapped with a disposable sleeve for infection control as they cannot withstand heat sterilization.
- ***Sensor placement:*** The sensor with a bite blocks attachments is placed in the oral cavity to aim the beam and sensors accurately. Paralleling or bisecting technique is used for exposure.

Advantages

- Low radiation dose for patient
- Image reconstruction capabilities
- Wider latitude
- Elimination of processing
- High signal-to-noise ratio.

Disadvantages

- Higher initial cost
- Unknown lifespan of the detector.

Application in Dentistry

- 3-D display of periodontal bone defects
- 3-D reconstruction of pulp canals to visualize.
  - Lateral canals and
  - Canal shapes
- To detect arthritic changes in condyle by surface reconstruction of TMJ
- A 2-D and 3-D visualization of anatomic structures for presurgical determination of implant sites.

2. Discuss the principle, technique, indications, advantages, and disadvantages of computed Tomography in detail.

Introduction

Computed tomography is a method of body-section radiography by which images of a layer within the structure is produced, while the images of structures above or below the plane of interest appear blurred.

Sir Godfrey Hounsfield demonstrated the first computed tomography (CT) unit, in 1970.

Principle

A collimated X-ray is focussed on the patient, the resultant rays are received and measured by a detector which transmits this information to a computer. The computer analyzes the signal and displays it on a monitor. For three-dimensional image construction, a three-dimensional array called voxel (volume element) is used. Each voxel has height, width, and depth.

Components

CT unit consists of an X-ray detector made up of crystalline cesium iodide (CsI) or cadmium tungstate ($CdWO_4$). Thousands of these detectors are placed at 360° around the patient. The X-ray generator (**gantry**) revolves around the patient, and the detector is stable. Each detector is separated from the next by an interspace material.

Image Quality

Spatial resolution is the ability to detect separate objects spaced very closely together. CT has a spatial resolution of about 15 line pairs/centimeter which is equivalent to an object size of 0.3 mm.

CT has an excellent low contrast resolution, and even slight differences in tissue density can be detected.

Computed Tomography Interpretations

- Hyperdense dense lesions appear white
- Hypodense—low density lesions appear dark
- Destructive and nondestructive nature of the lesions.

Advantages

- CT allows image visualization in all dimensions—coronal, sagittal, or axial.

- CT is noninvasive, accurate and painless.
- CT is helpful in revealing a detailed view of osseous structures.
- In traumatic cases, it is useful in revealing internal injuries.
- Eliminates superimposition seen in conventional extraoral radiography.

Disadvantages

- Radiation dosage is very high → 10 msv
- In TMJ disorders like articular disc derangements, articular discs are not seen clearly
- Very fine soft tissue details are obscured by bony structures in CT
- Beam scattering caused by metallic objects including implants will produce streak artifacts.

3. What is contrast radiography? Explain sialography in detail.

Contrast Radiography

Contrast radiography is a technique in which radiopaque substances namely the ***contrast media*** is used to enhance the absorption or transmission of the X-rays to increase the contrast and density of the subject of interest to meet specific diagnostic needs.

Different types of contrast radiography are:

- Sialography
- Lymphangiography
- Arthrography
- Angiography
- Urography

Sialography

Definition

Sialography is a contrast radiographic procedure which involves the use of retrograde filling of the radiopaque contrast media, performed for detection of disorders of the major salivary glands.

Contrast Agents

Ideal requirements:

- Safe to use and handle
- Nontoxic
- Easily excreted from body
- No residual side effects
- No penetration through the cell membrane or blood-brain barrier
- Limited transfer of breast milk and placental passage
- Low viscosity to ensure rapid injection and avoid microcirculatory problems.

Contrast Agents Used In Sialography

- ***Iodized, lipid soluble contrast media:***
  - Ethiodal
  - Lipoidal

Advantages

- Satisfactory degree of radiographic opacification
- Good resolution of peripheral ducts.

Disadvantages

- Discomfort to patients
- Retention in case of overfilling
- Inflammation, granuloma, and fibrosis
- ***Water soluble organic iodine compounds:***
  - Hypaque 50, 73
  - Omnipaque
  - Conray 420

Advantages

- Permits filling of finer duct system
- Rapidly removed from tissues.

Disadvantages

- Radiographic contrast is low
- Immediate radiographs after instillation of the medium is needed.

Equipment

- Polyethylene tubing
- 5–10 mL syringe
- Lacrimal dilator
- Contrast medium
- Lemon slices (sialogogue).

Procedure

- Identification of duct orifices
- Exploration of the duct with a lacrimal probe

- Cannulation of the duct:
  - Duct orifice is enlarged to insert salivary cannula
- Introduction of radiographic dye.

Slow injection with the quantity assessed by fluoroscopic observation and is stopped when the patient feels fullness.

0.76–1 mL dye for the parotid gland and 0.5–0.75 mL dye for the submandibular gland.

Three Stages of the Procedure

1. **Ductal phase:** The duct orifice is dilated and cannulated to inject the contrast agent. A radiograph is taken to assess the major duct.
2. **Acinar phase:** Both the duct and the gland parenchyma are filled with the contrast agent.
3. **Evacuation phase:** The cannula need to be removed, and the patient should thoroughly rinse for 2–3 minutes. A radiograph should be taken.

Radiographic View

Parotid gland	Submandibular gland
Lateral view	AP view
AP view	Lateral oblique
Puffed AP view	Occlusal
CT, MRI	CT, MRI

Interpretation

- *Normal parotid gland:* Leafless tree or tree in winter appearance.
- *Normal submandibular gland:* Bush in winter
- *Sjögren's syndrome:* "Cherry blossom" or "branchless—fruit-laden tree."
- *Chronic Inflammation:* Punctate sialactasis
- *Tumor:* Ball in hand appearance.

Indications

To detect:

- Sialolith or foreign bodies are seen as filling defects.
- Fistula, diverticuli, strictures, stenosis of the duct.
- Recurrent swelling and inflammatory processes.
- Tumor location, size, and origin.
- Extent of the glandular destruction.
- Ductal architecture and to detect ductal pathology.

Contraindications

- Salivary gland inflammation
- Patients allergic to iodine
- Salivary calculus closer to duct orifice.

4. Discuss the principle and clinical application of ultrasonography in oral diseases.

Ultrasonography (USG) is a specialized imaging technique where **sound waves** with vibratory **frequencies of 1–20 MHz** are used for the diagnostic purpose.

A high frequency transducer (7.5–10 MHz) is used for the diagnosis of oral lesions.

Types

B-mode ultrasonography reveals the lesion and their borders as a black and white image.

Color duplex ultrasonography reveals the tissue movements and blood flow.

Doppler ultrasonography differentiates the vessels.

Principle

Scanners used in USG generate electrical impulses that are converted into high frequency sound waves by a **transducer** and subsequently transmitted into tissues. Some waves penetrate the tissues, and some are reflected back to the transducer depending on the acoustic impedance of the tissues. Only the reflected waves (echoes) are reconverted to electrical energy, amplified, processed and presented on a screen.

USG Reading

Reading is based on echogenicity (the ability of a surface to echo or return a signal).

Hyperechoic structures "brighter" than their surroundings.

Hypoechoic structures are less "bright" than their surroundings.

Anechoic structures appear black. (No echoes).

Isoechoic structures have the same densities as its surroundings.

Calcified masses appear hyperechoic whereas clear fluid, and blood appear as anechoic

Role of USG in the diagnosis of oral and maxillofacial regions:

- To analyze the normal and abnormal anatomical structures
- To diagnose:
  - Salivary gland diseases
  - Lymphadenopathy and lymphadenitis
  - Subcutaneous diseases
  - Tongue lesions
- Fine needle aspiration biopsy (FNA).

Advantages

- Noninvasive, nonionizing
- No known deleterious bio effects
- Rapid procedure
- Less expensive and easily reproducible
- Real-time guidance for needle aspiration
- Unaffected by metal artifacts such as dental restorations
- May be repeated as often as necessary.

5. Discuss the principle, technique, indications, merits and demerits of MRI in detail.

Principle

The technique is based on magnetic properties of an atom.

MRI uses nonionizing radiation from radiofrequency (RF) band of electromagnetic (EM) spectrum. RF pulses transmitted through the patient are stimulating the atoms in tissue to produce a signal.

Atoms consist of nucleus and electrons. In the nucleus, there are positively charged protons are rotating around an axis, i.e. possess a spin. In natural state magnetic dipoles are randomly oriented resulting in net magnetization of zero. When the patient is placed in EMF, protons align with it. They do this in two ways: Spin up in lower energy state and spin down in a high-energy state.

MRI Terms

Resonance: Transition of nuclei from one energy state to another.

Precession: Oscillation of spinning protons with aslight tilt from parallel.

- **Larmor frequency:** Rate or frequency of precession of protons
- **T1weighted image**
- **T2 weighted image**.

Basic Steps

- External magnetic field applied which causes alignment of protons.
- Radiofrequency pulse sent.
- RF pulse switched off, and protons realign.
- During realignment, a signal can be detected.
- A signal used for image reconstruction in the computer.

MRI Interpretations

- Hyperintense
- Hypointense

Units of Magnetic Field

- Tesla
- The magnetic field of MR imaging: 0.1–4.0 T.

Indications of MRI in Head and Neck

- Assessment of intracranial lesions
- Tumor staging
- TMJ investigations to show bony and soft tissue component-internal derangement of disc, disc perforation
- Diagnosis of salivary gland diseases.

Contraindications

- Cardiac pacemakers
- Ear prosthesis, cerebral aneurysm clips
- Metallic implant and dental filling relative contraindication
- Pregnancy

Advantages

- Ionizing radiation is not used
- Noninvasive
- High contrast sensitivity and is an excellent soft tissue imaging modality.
- Images in all planes obtained without repositioning the patient
- Exposure of patient to the magnetic field of less than 2.5 T has no adverse effects.

Disadvantages

- Expensive
- Long scanning time
- Equipment tends to be claustrophobic, noisy
- Needs trained staff
- Hard tissue like bone does not give an MR signal and the signal is obtained only from the bone marrow.

SHORT NOTES

1. Image detectors used in intraoral digital radiography.
(or)
Intraoral sensors.

In intraoral digital radiography, a small **sensor** is used for recording the image instead of radiographic film. (CCDs) and (CMOS) are the two detectors used for intraoral imaging.

Charge-coupled Devices

Charged coupled devices is a solid state detector comprising a radiosensitive silicon chip. The silicon CCD is divided into picture elements called pixels. The pixel is a small repository pack where the electrons released from the radiation exposure are stored. Pixel is the digital substitute for halide crystals in the X-ray film. The CCD is 640 × 480 individual pixels in size. When X-ray photons strikes the CCD, an electronic latent image is produced which is transferred to the computer and displayed as a visible image on the screen.

Complementary Metal Oxide Semiconductor

They consist of metal oxide semiconductor structure (silicon or silicon coated with phosphors).

The CMOS differ from CCD in the way that:

- The pixels are read
- It has 25% greater resolution
- Low cost and greater durability.

2. Describe the types of digital imaging.

Types of Digital Images

Direct digital imaging: A sensor with a fiber-optic cable linked to the computer is placed into patient's mouth and exposed to X-radiation. The sensor receives the image and then transmits it to the computer. Within seconds of exposure, an image appears on the screen. The software is then used to enhance and store the mage.

Indirect Digital Imaging

Scanning the conventional radiographs: Uses a CCD camera and a computer. The CCD camera scans the available manual radiograph, digitizes and then presents it on the computer monitor.

Storage phosphor imaging: It is a wireless imaging system and is also referred to as photostimulable phosphor imaging (PSP). A flexible, reusable phosphor-coated plate is placed into the mouth and exposed to x-radiation. After exposure, the PSP plate is removed and positioned in an electronic processor where a laser scans the plate. An image is generated and transferred to the computer.

The laser scanning takes 30 seconds to 5 minutes hence this type of digital imaging is less rapid.

3. Discuss the advantages and disadvantages of intraoral digital imaging.

Advantages

- **Superior grayscale resolution:** Digital imaging uses up to 256 gray shades with the comparison of 16–25 gray shades of conventional imaging. So the density and contrast enhancement is an important advantage.

- **Reduced exposure to X-ray:** The sensitivity of CCD reduces the radiation exposure from 50–90% than that required for conventional e-film.
- **Image viewing:** Chairside viewing of the image on the computer monitor within a moment after exposure.
- **Elimination of film and darkroom**
- **Effective patient education tool:** Patients can view the images along with dentist which facilitates the rapport and increases patient's understanding of diseases.
- **Increased effectiveness:** The image storage and professional communication are easier.

Disadvantages

- Initial set up cost
- **Sensor size and thickness:** May cause discomfort or elicit the gag reflex.
- **Infection control:** The sensors are vulnerable heat sterilization hence require disposable plastic sleeves for infection control. These sleeves need to be changed between patients every time.
- **Wear and tear:** The PSP receptors are prone to wear and tear and hence limited longevity.
- **Legal issues:** The use of digital images as evidence in lawsuits is questionable.

4. Describe subtraction radiography.

Digital radiography allows taking away information between two images so that a low contrast object or detail can be easily visualized.

Two subtraction techniques are in use:

1. Temporal subtraction: Information is taken from two images formed at different times.
2. Energy subtraction: Information is taken from two images formed at the same time but with using different X-ray energies.

In dentistry, to detect small changes at the bone level like an interproximal bone loss in periodontal diseases, temporal subtraction is used.

5. Scintigraphy (or) nuclear medicine (or) radionuclide scan.

Nuclear medicine or scintigraphy is a technique that uses a carrier molecule to deliver a *radionuclide or radiopharmaceutical agent* or isotopes to target tissue to ***measure the function*** of that tissue.

Radionuclide or isotope in an organism behaves identically to their stable counterparts because both are indistinguishable.

It is the only technique that can detect and quantities the biologic activity of cells in a tissue or organ. The common nuclide agent used is technetium (Tc).

For bone studies, such as scan for metastatic tumor lesions, ^{99m}TcMDP are used.

For salivary tissues, ^{67}Ga, ^{125}I, ^{18}F are used.

Patients are imaged at various times after the radionuclide injection.

Salivary glands are imaged after 30 minutes while bone scans are carried out after 2 hours waiting period. This waiting period allows the cessation of normal metabolic activity before the isotope scans abnormal activity.

6. Describe the equipment and technique in cone-beam computed tomography.

Cone-beam computed tomography (CBCT) is specially developed to evaluate maxilla-facial complex in three-dimensional imaging.

Principle

A pyramidal or cone shaped X-ray beam is directed towards an X-ray detector on the other side of the patient's head. Multiple 2D projection images are captured in the selected field of view (FOV) according to the region of interest (ROI).

Since one exposure completely covers the entire FOV, only one rotational motion of the gantry is adequate to capture the required information for image reconstruction.

Mechanism of CBCT:
- Production of X-rays
- Image detection
- Image reconstruction
- Image display.

Technique

During CBCT rotation, a single exposure is made at specific intervals and provides projection images, called ***basis* or *projection images.*** The entire image series is known as the ***projection data***. Reconstruction software programs introduce the algorithms to these projection data to create a three-dimensional (3D) ***volumetric data set*** that provides the ***secondary reconstruction images*** in three orthogonal planes (axial, sagittal and coronal).

7. What are the advantages of using CBCT in dentistry?

- CBCT equipment is low-priced than the CT machine.
- It provides high-contrast images and hence useful in the imaging of the craniofacial bones.
- Rapid scan time leads to reduced artifacts.
- Produces images with high resolution in the range of 0.09 mm–0.4 mm.
- Radiation dose is less when compared to conventional CT.

MULTIPLE CHOICE QUESTIONS

1. The number of possible grayscale combination/pixel is known as ***bit depth of image***.
   a. Voxel
   b. Gradient measure of image
   c. Sequence depth of image
   d. Bit depth of image
2. The formula used to detect the number of possible grayscale combination per pixel is $\boldsymbol{2^N}$.
   a. N^2
   b. $2N^2$
   c. 2^N
   d. N^2
3. A transducer in ultrasonography is made up of ***piezoelectric crystals***.
   a. Quartz crystal
   b. Monoclinic crystals
   c. Electron crystallography
   d. Piezoelectric crystals
   (**Note:** A transducer in ultrasonography is made up of piezoelectric crystals like lead zirconate titanate).
4. The smallest element of three-dimensional image is ***voxel***.
   a. Voxel
   b. Pixel
   c. Tesla
   d. Polygons

VIVA VOCE

1. What is an analog image?

When X-ray photons hit the radiographic film, the details registered on the film is known as an analog image.

Analog images consist ***continuous spectrum of gray shades*** between the extremes of white and black.

2. What is a digital image?

A sensor collects the analog details and converts it to a digital image in the computer processing unit. When X-ray beam strikes the sensor, an electronic charge is produced on the surface of the sensor, which is digitized.

The digital image is composed of picture elements called pixels. Each pixel has a ***discrete gray value***.

3. What is a sensor?

A sensor is a small detector placed in the mouth instead of radiographic film, to capture an image in digital radiography.

4. Name few image techniques that do not use radiation.

Ultrasonography, MRI, thermography.

5. What is split-screen technology.

It is a unique feature on digital radiography system that allows the operator to view and compare multiple images on the same screen. This feature is helpful for comparison and evaluation of progression of caries or periodontal diseases.

6. MR or MRI contrast materials.

- Ferromagnetic
- Paramagnetic [Lanthamide-Gadolinium diethylenetriamine pantothenic acid (Gd-DTPA)]
- Super magnetic.

7. What is thermography?

It is a diagnostic method in which small electronic probes called thermistors, liquid crystals or infrared scanners are used to record temperatures in various structures and detect abnormal conditions.

Abnormal conditions like inflammation or malignant tumors are associated with abnormal blood flow and result in different temperature patterns.

8. What is real-time imaging?

Imaging techniques that allow the perception of motion are known as real-time imaging.

9. Name few radionuclide tracers. (or) name some radioisotopes used in nuclear medicine.

Iodine (^{131}I), gallium (^{67}G), Technetium 99m (^{99m}Tc), selenium (^{74}Se).

10. What is coronal axis?

It is an imaginary vertical plane that separates the body into anterior and posterior halves and runs perpendicular to the ground.

11. What is sagittal axis?

It is an imaginary axis that divides the body into right and left half, and runs perpendicular to the ground and through the middle of the body.

12. What is an axial plane?

It is an imaginary horizontal axis that divides the body into superior and inferior aspects and runs parallel to the ground.

13. What is DICOM.

The acronym DICOM refers to **Digital imaging and communication in medicine.** The universal format for handling, storing and transmitting three-dimensional images is called as DICOM **data.**

14. State few differences between CT and CBCT.

Computed tomography	Cone-beam computed tomography
The X-ray beam is fan-shaped	Cone shape X-ray beam is used
The FOV is imaged in many slices, and then the slices are compiled into a 3D representation. Each slice needs a separate scan and separate 2D reconstruction	Single exposure completely covers the FOV and hence one rotational movement of the gantry is sufficient to capture the necessary information for image reconstruction
Less radiation exposure	More exposure
Low cost	High cost factor

BIBLIOGRAPHY

1. Diederich S, Wernecke K, Peters PE. Sialographic and sonographic diagnosis of salivary gland diseases. Radiologe. 1987; 27(6):255-61.
2. Frederiksen NL. Specialized radiographic techniques In White SC, Phanoah MJ, editors. Oral radiology: Principles and interpretation. 5th edition. St Louis Mosby. 2004. pp.255-63.
3. Goldberg BB, Raichlen JS, Forsberg F. Ultrasound contrast agents: basic principles and clinical applications. second edition; Martin Dunitz Ltd; 2001. pp 239-52.
4. Hizi U, inventor; Samsung Electronics Co Ltd, assignee. Anti-blooming shutter control in image sensors. United States patent US 9,100,600. 2015.
5. Kumar M, Shanavas M, Sidappa A, et al. Cone beam computed tomography-know its secrets. Journal of international oral health, JIOH. 2015;7(2):64.

6. Scarfe WC, Farman AG, Sukovic P. Clinical applications of cone-beam computed tomography in dental practice. J Can Dent Assoc. 2006;72(1):75-80.
7. Seeram E. Computed Tomography-E-Book: Physical Principles, Clinical Applications, and Quality Control. Elsevier Health Sciences; 2015.
8. Versteeg CH, Sanderink GC, van der Stelt PF. Efficacy of digital intra-oral radiography in clinical dentistry. J dent. 1997;25(3-4):215-24.
9. White SC, Pharoah MJ. The evolution and application of dental maxillofacial imaging modalities. Dent Clin North Am. 2008;52(4):689-705.

CHAPTER 37

Dental Anomalies, Dental Caries, Pulp, Periapical, and Periodontal Lesions

HIGHLIGHTS

Radiographic examination of the tooth and their supporting structures are essential to confirm the clinical diagnosis and precede the treatment plan. In some conditions, radiographs may serve as an only tool to diagnose the problem involving pulpal, periapical and periodontal tissues. A complete knowledge about various radiopaque and radiolucent lesions involving these structures is essential for successful dental practice.

Learners are expected to study:

- Radiopaque and radiolucent conditions involving pulp
- Radiodiagnosis of periapical lesions
- Radiographic interpretation of periodontal status
- Internal and external root resorption.

ESSAY QUESTIONS

1. Discuss in detail the radiodiagnosis of periapical lesions.

Periapical lesions are classified into periapical radiolucencies and radiopacities.

Peripaical Radiolucencies

- Peripaical periodontitis
- Periapical granuloma
- Periapical abscess
- Periapical cyst
- Residual cyst
- Periapical scar
- Surgical defect.

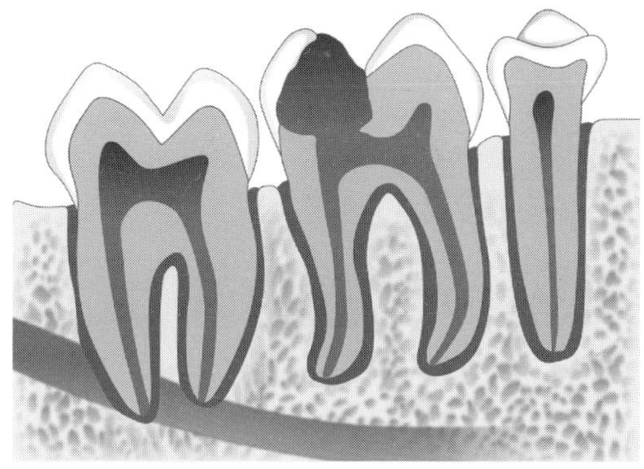

Fig. 1: Periapical periodontitis.

Periapical Periodontitis

Inflammation of periodontal ligament space due to the exit of the toxic products from the necrotic pulp. Discontinuity of lamina dura at the root apex and widened periodontal ligament space are the findings (Fig. 1).

Periapical Granuloma

Granulation tissue formation in the periapical region to neutralize the toxic products from the root canal. It is the ***most common*** periapical radiolucency. Seen as mixed radiopaque and radiolucent but predominantly radiolucent lesion measuring less than 1 cm in size (Fig. 2).

Periapical Abscess

Localized collection of pus in the periapical region as a result of pulpal death results ill-defined periapical radiolucency (Fig. 3).

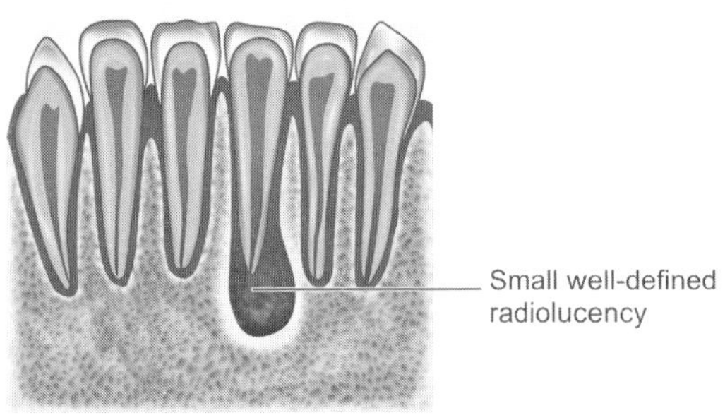

Fig. 2: Periapical granuloma.

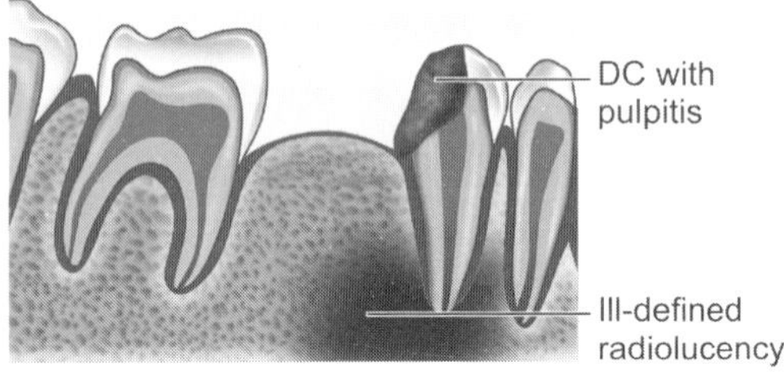

Fig. 3: Periapical abscess.

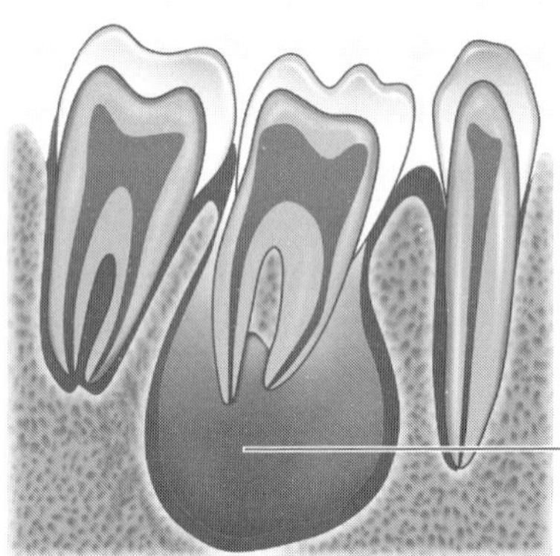

Fig. 4: Periapical cyst.

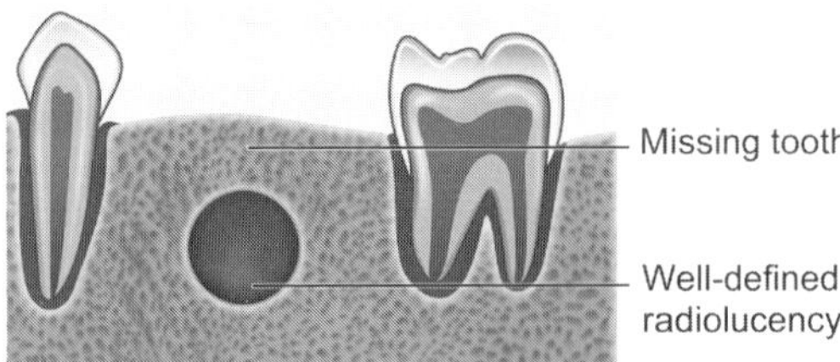

Fig. 5: Residual cyst.

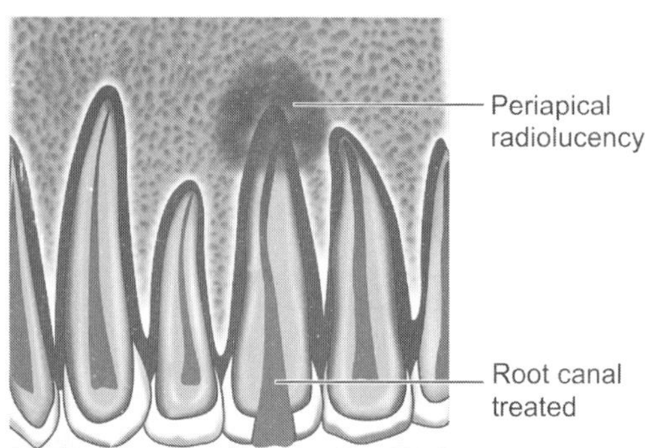

Fig. 6: Periapical scar in a root canal filled tooth.

Periapical Cyst/Radicular Cyst/Dental Cyst

Inflammatory odontogenic cyst, resulting from periapical granuloma.

It is the second most common periapical infection. Well-defined radiolucency is measuring more than 2.5 cm in diameter surrounded by a thin radiopaque border (Fig. 4).

Residual Cyst

Cyst develops after incomplete removal of the infected materials in the periapical region of a tooth. The body reacts to the remnant infection by forming granulation tissue. When there is more proliferation of granulation tissues, the central region will be devoid of nutrient supply and undergoes liquefaction necrosis. It appears as well-defined radiolucency surrounded by a thin radiopaque border (Fig. 5).

Periapical Scar

A thick fibrous tissue mass in the apex of root canal treated tooth.

Appear as a well-circumscribed radiolucency resembling periapical granuloma or cyst (smaller than both). Anterior region of the maxilla is the common site (Fig. 6).

Surgical Defect

Following surgery, there is a defect in the normal healing process by bone deposition. The surgical site is devoid of bone following sufficient period of healing. It is seen as a round radiolucent lesion with a well defined corticated border (Fig. 7).

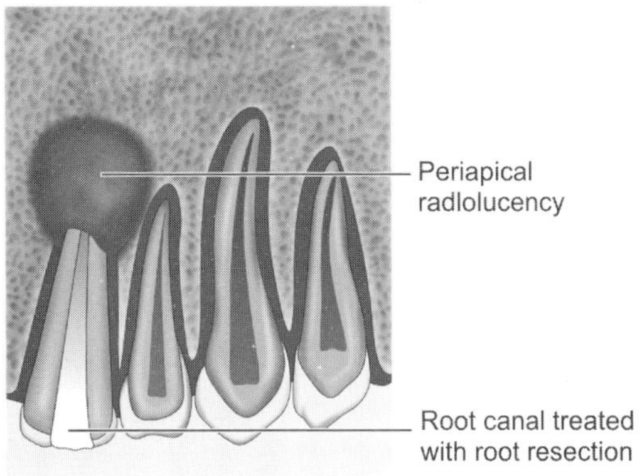

Fig. 7: Surgical defect.

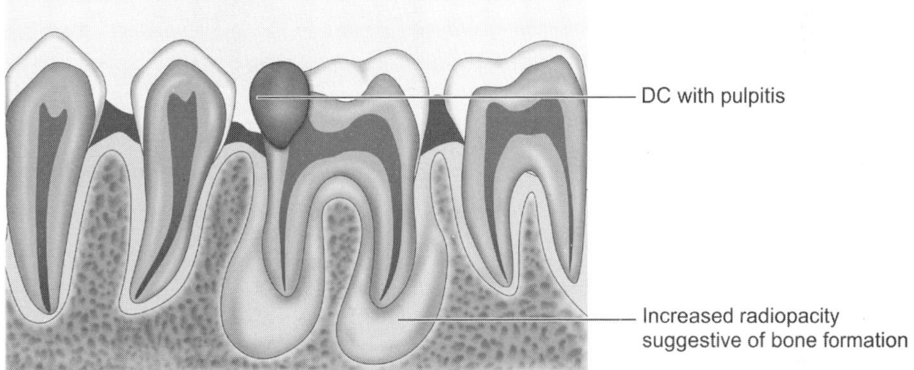

Fig. 8: Condensing osteitis.

Periapical Radiopacities

True radiopacities: Radiopaque structures present in the periapical region.

- Condensing osteitis
- Periapical idiopathic osteosclerosis
- Periapical cementosseous dysplasia
- Hypercementosis
- Odontome
- Foreign bodies

Condensing Osteitis (Focal Sclerosing Osteomyelitis)

Sclerosis of bone induced by inflammation or infection. It is seen in the mandibular first molar region as a dense diffuse radiopacity near the periapical region (Fig. 8).

Peiapical Idiopathic Osteosclerosis (Enostosis)

Localized growth of the cortical bone. Few mm to-2 cm diameters in size.

Appear as a dense, small, isolated, well-defined radiopacities, not contacting the tooth and there is no radiolucent halo at the periphery (Fig. 9)

Periapical Cementosseous Dysplasia

Reactive fibro-osseous lesion derived from periodontal ligament. The mature stage reveals dense radiopacity surrounded by a radiolucent halo in the mandibular anterior region (Fig. 10). The associated teeth are vital.

Hypercementosis

Excessive cementum deposition occurs at the entire root or the root apex because of periapical inflammation. It appears as bulbous root with intact periodontal ligament space and lamina dura (Fig. 11).

Odontome

Developmental hamartoma.

Compound composite odontome present as a many small teeth like structures surrounded by a radiolucent halo (Fig. 12). It has a preference for the maxillary anterior region.

Complex composite odontome is seen as an irregular calcified mass. It is seen as dense radiopacity surrounded by a radiolucent halo in the mandibular posterior region (Fig. 13). Do not resemble the tooth.

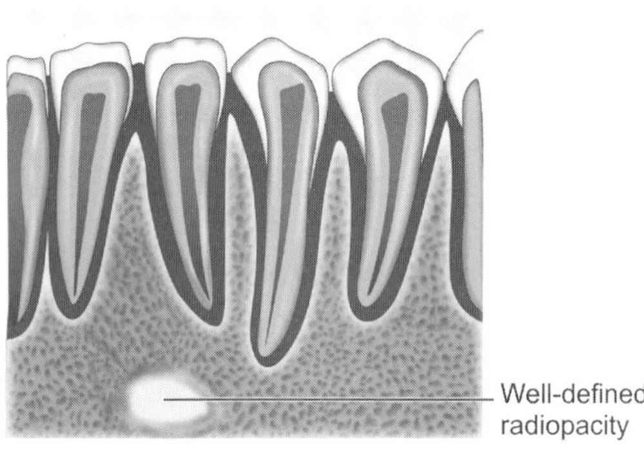

Fig. 9: Peiapical idiopathic osteosclerosis.

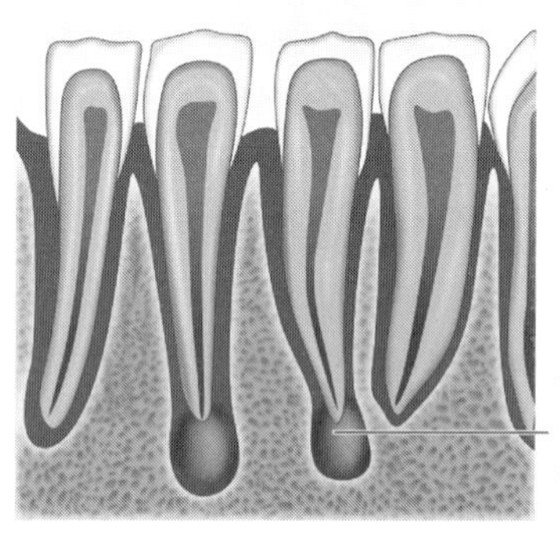

Fig. 10: Periapical cementosseous dysplasia.

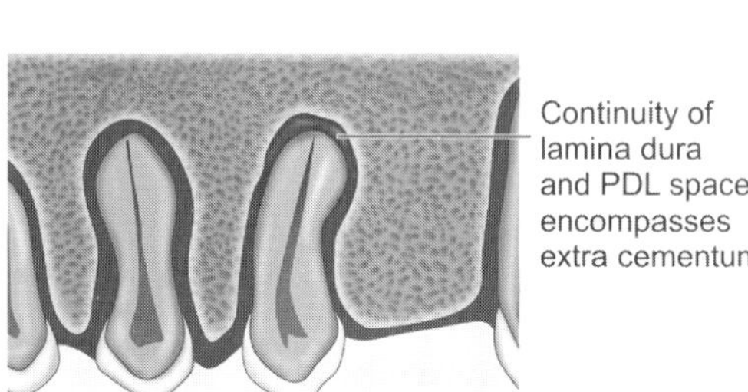

Fig. 11: Hypercementosis.

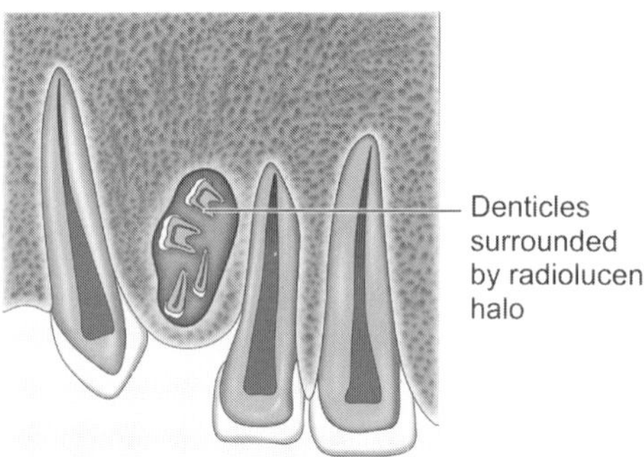

Fig. 12: Compund composite odontome.

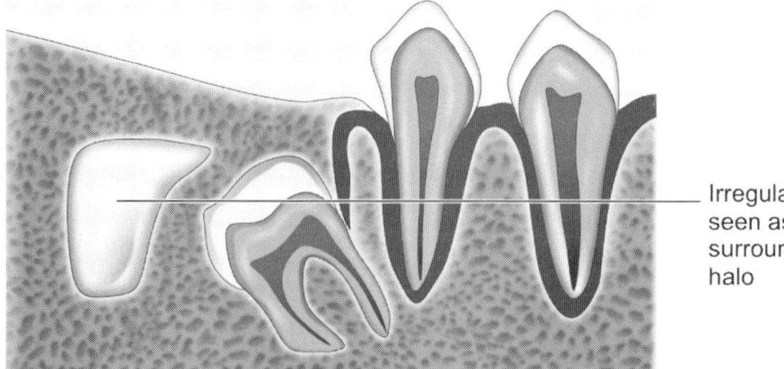

Fig. 13: Complex composite odontome.

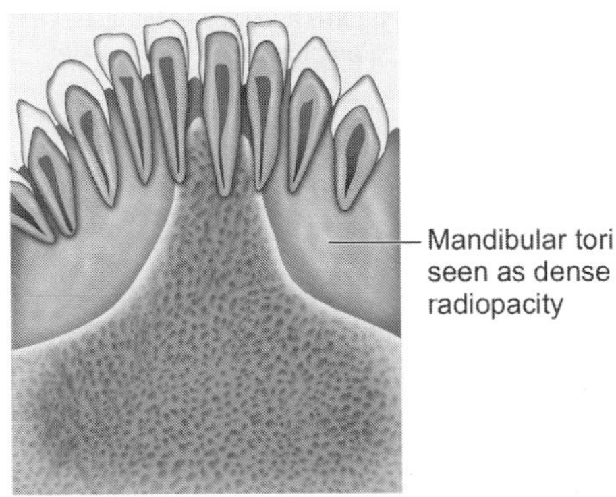

Fig. 14: Mandibular tori.

Foreign Bodies

Restorative materials extruded from the root canal treated teeth seen as radiopaque specks.

False Periapical Radiopacities

Structures not present in the periapical region of the teeth but the image is projected in the periapical region.

Unerupted, Impacted, Supernumerary Teeth

Cause radiopacity with central radiolucency representing the pulp chamber.

Exostosis: Cortical bone protrusion appears as **dense radiopaque** shadow.

- **Torus palatines:** Bony protuberance superimposed over the apical area of roots of maxillary molar teeth.
- **Torus mandibularis:** Superimposed bilaterally over the apical area of roots of mandibular canines, premolars teeth (Fig. 14).

2. Mixed radiolucent and radiopaque periapical lesion.

- **Retained roots:** Linear shaped radiopacity with radiolucency in the center representing the root canal can be seen in the periapical region.
- **Rarefying osteitis and condensing osteitis:** It is associated with the pulpoperipical lesion and seen as coronal radiolucency involving the pulp. Chronic inflammation from pulp serves as an irritating factor for bone resorption seen as diffuse periapical radiolucency (rarefying osteitis) and bone deposition in response to destruction seen as radiopacity surrounding the radiolucency (condensing osteitis).
- **Intermediate stage of periapical cemental dysplasia:** Reactive fibro-osseous lesion derived from periodontal ligament. Three stages with different radiographic appearance:
  1. Radiolucency suggestive of osteolytic stage
  2. Mixed radiolucent radiopaque stage
  3. Radiopaque stage representing the bone deposition.
- **Cemento-ossifying fibroma:** It is a benign fibro-osseous neoplasm. Three stages are seen same as periapical cemental dysplasia. Mixed radiolucent and radiopaque lesion seen in the intermediate stage.
- **Intermediate stage of Paget's disease and fibrous dysplasia:** Paget's disease also called osteitis deformans is an osteodystrophy of unknown cause where physiological bone remodeling is affected due to excess bone deposition and resorption. Fibrous dysplasia is a localized developmental disturbance in bone forming mesenchyme in which the fibrous tissue fails to produce bone matrix and fails to calcify. There is attempted bone formation in the fibrous tissue hence it is a fibro-osseous lesion.
  - Three stages of radiographic appearances in both Paget's disease and fibrous dysplasia are:
    1. Radiolucency suggestive of osteolytic stage
    2. Mixed radiolucent radiopaque stage
    3. Radiopaque stage representing the bone deposition
- **Pyogenic osteomyelitis:** Moth-eaten radiographic appearance representing bone resorption (sequestrum) seen as radiolucency and involucrum (new bone) seen as radiopacity.

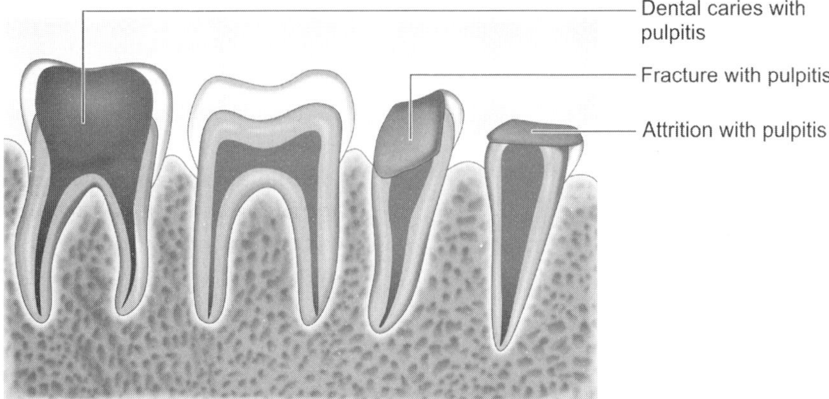

Fig. 15: Pulpal radiolucency due to attrition, caries and fractured crown.

SHORT NOTES

1. Enumerate the various conditions causing radiolucencies involving pulp.

- Dental caries involving pulp (Fig. 15).
- Fracture with pulp exposure
- Attrition with pulp exposure
- Internal resorption—round or ovoid radiolucency in the pulp canal (Fig. 16).
- A developmental disturbance like taurodontism causes enlargement of the pulp chamber appearing as larger radiolucent pulp cavity (Fig. 17).
- Recurrent caries—increased radiolucency at the margin of restoration.

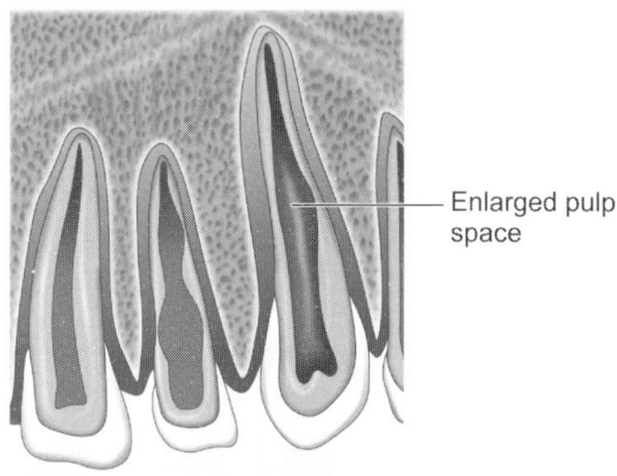

Fig. 16: Internal resorption evident as round and ovoid radiolucencies.

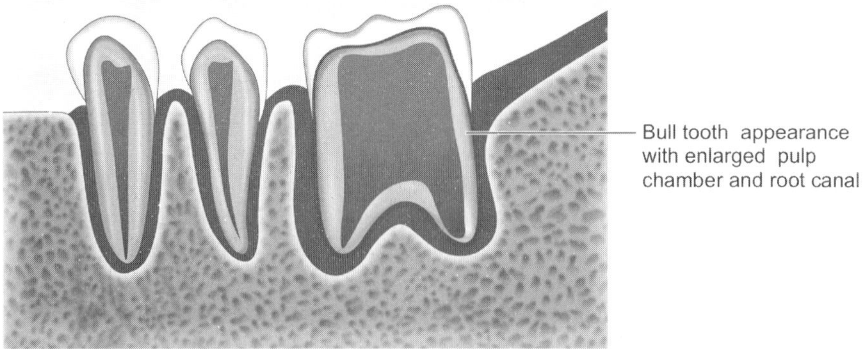

Fig. 17: Bull tooth appearance with enlarged pulp cavity.

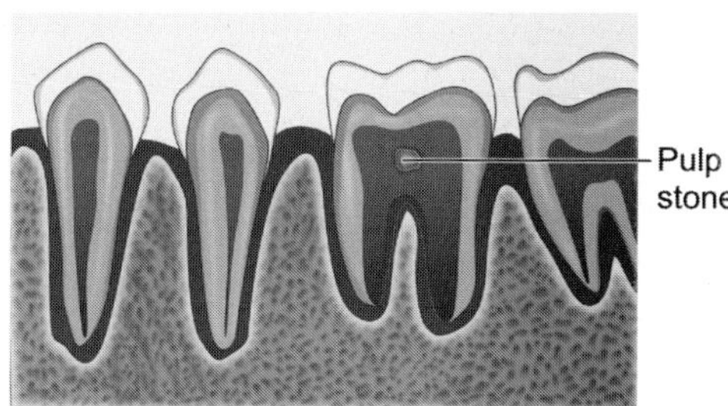

Fig. 18: Pulp stone.

- Radiation caries—dark radiolucency seen near the necks of the teeth following radiotherapy.
- Root caries—ill-defined saucer-shaped defect on a mesial and distal aspect of the root.
- Few restorative materials like composite, plastic, silicate without radiopaque materials like barium, lead or zinc.

2. Enumerate the various conditions causing radiopacities involving pulp.

- **Pulp stone**: Foci of calcification in the pulp chamber seen as round or ovoid radiopacity occupying the pulp chamber (Fig. 18).
- **Restorative materials** which appear radiopaque:
  - Silver amalgam (Fig. 19)
  - Gutta-percha
  - Gold
  - Stainless steel pins
  - Silver points
  - Calcium hydroxide
  - Orthodontic appliances.
- **Talon's cusp**: Hyperplasia of cingulum of maxillary or mandibular incisors. Radiopaque image of Talon's cusp is superimposed on the crown of the involved incisor.

3. Role of radiographs in diagnosis of periodontal lesions.

Intraoral Periapical Radiographs

Horizontal bone loss:
- Alveolar bone height is reduced (Fig. 20)
- Bone margin remains perpendicular to the tooth surface
- Most common pattern of bone loss is: Bone loss may be mild, moderate or severe.
  - Mild: 1–2 mm loss
  - Moderate: 2–3 mm loss
  - Severe: Greater than 3 mm.
- Interdental radiolucency is suggestive of resorption of buccal and lingual cortical plates.

Vertical bone loss:
- Angular bone defect
- Bone loss occurring in oblique direction along the side of the root (Fig. 21).

Furcation involvement:
- Bone destruction is seen as radiolucency of the bifurcation or trifurcation of multirooted teeth
- Based on the severity it is graded from I to IV

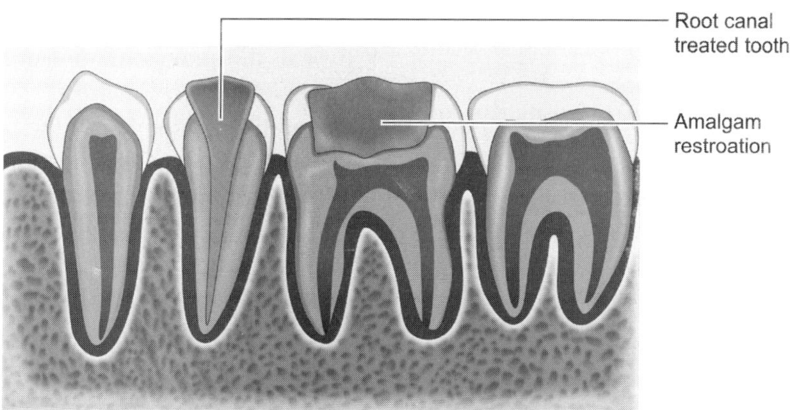

Fig. 19: Radiopaque gutta percha and amalgam restoration.

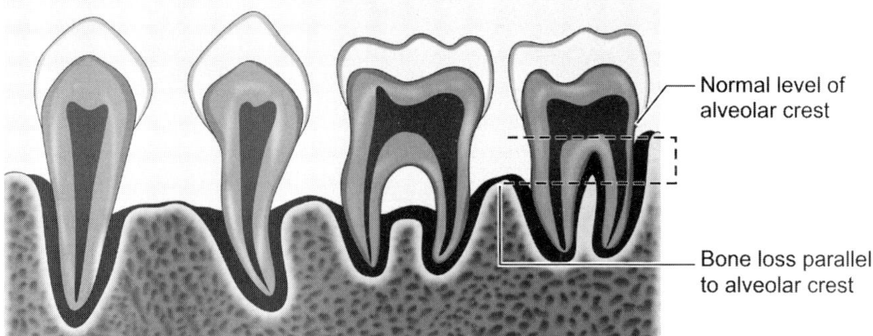

Fig. 20: Horizontal bone loss.

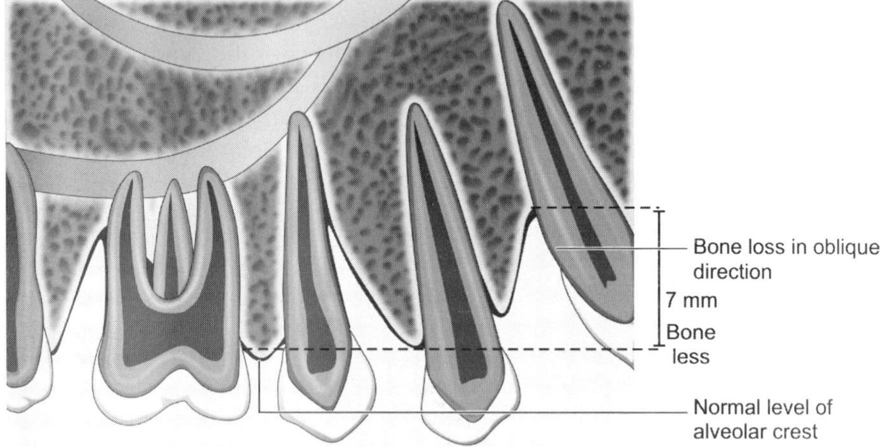

Fig. 21: Vertical bone loss.

Periodontal abscess:

- Localised pus collection in the periodontium associated with a deep pocket and severe bone loss.
- Radiolucent lesion surrounding the root portion of teeth.

Bitewing radiographs:

- To detect the height of alveolar crest
- Early periodontitis—roundening of the alveolar crest
- Open contact points.

Orthopantomogram

Generalized crestal bone loss.

4. Radiographic assessment of periodontal lesions.

- Reveals the amount of bone present.
- The height of alveolar crest.
- Generalized widening of the periodontal ligament space around the tooth.
- Bone loss in furcation area.
- Calculus or overhanging restorations evident as radiopacity helps in the identification of cause for periodontal lesions.
- Open contact areas between the teeth are revealed better in bitewing radiographs
- Root resorption.

5. Differentiate external and internal root resorption based on the radiographic image.

External root resorption	Internal root resorption
Occurs along the periphery of root	Occurs within the crown or root and involves the pulp chamber, pulp canal, and surrounding dentin
Causes: ▪ Chronic inflammation ▪ Cyst and tumors ▪ Impacted tooth ▪ Trauma ▪ Abnormal mechanical forces ▪ Idiopathic	*Causes:* ▪ Pulp polyp ▪ Pulp capping ▪ Trauma
The apical region appears blunted, and root appears shorter than the normal length. Lamina dura and alveolar bone appear normal around the blunted apex	Round to ovoid radiolucency in the midcrown or midroot portion that gives rise to "ballooning" appearance
Asymptomatic and no effective treatment is available	Asymptomatic. Endodontic management or extraction depending on the extent of resorption

6. Enumerate the steps to overcome the limitation of radiodiagnosis of periodontal lesions.

SLOB technique: To assess whether cortical plate destruction has occurred in buccal or lingual aspect. Fine wire grids of 1mm square size can be superimposed in radiographs during exposing radiograph to get the quantitative assessment of alveolar bone.

Digital subtraction radiography:

❖ Two images of the same object are recorded at the different time, and then the intensities of the resultant pixels are deduced to obtain a new image.

❖ This method is used to evaluate dental caries and periodontal changes in the radiographs overtime.

❖ It is not possible for the routine dental radiograph to predict a difference of 0.85 mm in cortical bone thickness but subtraction technique can detect as small as 0.12 mm difference.

7. Describe the radiographic diagnosis of amelogenesis imperfecta.

Three types of amelogenesis imperfecta are:

1. Hypoplasia
2. Hypomaturation
3. Hypocalcification.

1. ***Radiographic appearance of hypoplasia type:***
   - Square shape crown
   - Thin opaque enamel
   - Absence of faint cuspal outline
   - The enamel density is normal except for pitted crown in which well-defined mottled opacity appear.
2. ***Radiographic appearance of hypomaturation type:*** Enamel appears normal in thickness but cannot be distinguished from dentin as its density is almost equal to that of dentin.
3. ***Radiographic appearance of hypocalcification type:*** Enamel appears normal in thickness but more radiolucent.

8. Describe the radiographic diagnosis of dentinogenesis imperfecta.

There are 2 types:

Type I: Dentingenesis imperfecta with osteogenesis imperfect.

Type II: Dentingenesis imperfecta without skeletal deformities. The dental radiographic findings in both types include:

❖ Partial or complete obliteration of pulp chambers

❖ Absence or "threadlike" root canals

❖ Periapical radiolucensies without pulpal involvement.

- Normal alveolar bone attern in both the types.

MULTIPLE CHOICE QUESTIONS

1. The most common periapical radiolucency is ***periapical granuloma***.
   a. Periapical cyst
   b. Periapical abscess
   c. Periapical scar
   d. Periapical granuloma
2. Well-defined periapical radiolucency with opaque boundary measuring above 2 cm associated with nonvital tooth is ***radicular cyst***.
   a. Radicular cyst
   b. Periapical abscess
   c. Periapical scar
   d. Periapical granuloma
   (**Note:** Radicular cyst (or) periapical cyst).
3. Well-defined, round radiolucency seen over the apex of the resected root of endodontically treated teeth is ***periapical scar***.
   a. Periapical cyst
   b. Periapical abscess
   c. Periapical scar
   d. Periapical granuloma
4. Bone disease associated with distinct or denser lamina dura is ***osteopetrosis***.
   a. Paget's disease
   b. Osteopetrosis
   c. Osteomalasia
   d. Myelosclerosis
   (**Note:** Osteopetrosis/marble bone disease/ Albers-Schonberg disease).
5. Dental caries in first molar with pain on percussion clinically and associated with diffuse periapical radiolucency in a intraoral periapical radiograph is more likely to be a ***periapical abscess***.
   a. Periapical cyst
   b. Periapical abscess
   c. Periapical scar
   d. Periapical granuloma
6. Well circumscribed periapical radiolucency surrounded by radiopaque border seen in the periapical radiograph of the edentulous region is more likely to be ***residual cyst***.
   a. Radicular cyst
   b. Periapical abscess
   c. Periapical scar
   d. Periapical granuloma
7. Dental anomaly is most commonly associated with a pulpoperiapical lesion in ***dens in dente/dens Invaginatus***.
   a. Microdontia/peg laterals
   b. Supernumerary tooth/mesiodent
   c. Dens in dente/dens invaginatus
   d. Pulp stones/denticles
8. Enostosis is otherwise called ***peripheral idiopathic osteosclerosis***.
   a. Hypercementosis
   b. Peripheral idiopathic osteosclerosis
   c. Condensing osteitis
   d. Periapical cemental dysplasia
   (**Note:** Dense bone island/peripheral idiopathic osteosclerosis).
9. Most common site for enostosis is ***mandibular first molar***.
   a. Mandibular incisor
   b. Maxillary canine
   c. Mandibular first molar
   d. Maxillary third molar
10. Dense radiopacity seen in the periapical region of a tooth associated with a coronal radiolucency involving the pulp is most likely to be a ***condensing osteitis***.
    a. Hypercementosis
    b. Peripheral idiopathic osteosclerosis
    c. Condensing osteitis
    d. Periapical cemental dysplasia
11. Cyst-like radiolucency of the mandible below the inferior dental canal is ***Stafne's bone cavity***.
    a. Traumatic bone cyst
    b. Stafne's bone cavity
    c. Klestadt cyst
    d. Idiopathic bone cavity
12. Cyst-like radiolucency measuring above 2 cm present at the apex of a vital maxillary incisor is ***incisive canal cyst***.
    a. Midpalatine cyst
    b. Nasolabial cyst
    c. Incisive canal cyst
    d. Globulomaxillary cyst
    (**Note:** Incisive canal cyst moves away from the apex when the horizontal angulation is changed).

13. Cyst-like radiolucency seen in the periapical region of a vital maxillary first molar is most likely a ***midpalatine cyst***.
    a. Midpalatine cyst
    b. Nasolabial cyst
    c. Pseudo cyst
    d. Globulomaxillary cyst
14. Well-defined round or ovoid radiolucency seen above the mandibular canal with scalloped margins is most likely a ***traumatic bone cyst***.
    a. Traumatic bone cyst
    b. Stafne's bone cavity
    c. Klestadt cyst
    d. Idiopathic bone cavity
15. Well defined periapical radiolucency at the apex of the mandibular canine tooth with no pathology is ***anterior lingual mandibular bony cavity***.
    a. Hemorrhagic bone cyst
    b. Canine depression
    c. Y line of Ennis
    d. Anterior lingual mandibular bony cavity
16. Any abnormal displacement of tooth is called as ***luxation***.
    a. Luxation
    b. Intrusion
    c. Extrusion
    d. Avulsion
17. Abnormal displacement of teeth into bone is called as ***intrusion***.
    a. Luxation b. Intrusion
    c. Extrusion d. Avulsion
18. Abnormal displacement of teeth out of bone is called as ***extrusion***.
    a. Luxation b. Intrusion
    c. Extrusion d. Avulsion
19. Ideal image is used to examine the interdental bone loss is ***vertical bitewing image***.
    a. Vertical bitewing image
    b. Horizontal bitewing
    c. Periapical view
    d. Orthopantomogram
20. The radiographic diagnosis of enamel carries is possible when the demineralization is ***30–40%***.
    a. 100% b. 70–80%
    c. 30–40% d. 10%
21. The radiographic depth of proximal carious lesion is ***less than the original clinical depth***.
    a. More than the actual clinical depth
    b. Less than the actual clinical depth
    c. As same as the actual clinical depth
    d. Always magnified and distorted
22. In germination, the pulp chamber appears as ***single and enlarged***.
    a. Single and enlarged
    b. Two separate pulp chamber of normal size
    c. Two separate pulp chamber of smaller size
    d. Single and normal size
23. Root dilaceration is most common in ***maxillary premolars***.
    a. Maxillary incisors
    b. Maxillary premolars
    c. Mandibular canines
    d. Mandibular molars
24. Leong's premolar is the synonym for ***dens evaginatus***.
    a. Dens invaginatous
    b. Dilated odontome
    c. Gestant premolar
    d. Dens evaginatus
25. The common cause for open apical foramen is ***cessation of root development***.
    a. Root resorption
    b. Trauma and crown fracture before root completion
    c. Cessation of root development
    d. Pulpotomy done in young permanent tooth

    (**Note:** Pulpal death leads to cessation of root development).
26. Flame shaped pulp chamber present in ***dentin dysplasia***.
    a. Dentin dysplasia
    b. Odontodysplasia
    c. Turner's hypoplasia
    d. Syphilis
27. Multiple pulp stones is a feature of ***dentin dysplasia***.
    a. Dens invaginatous b. Dens evaginatous
    c. Dentin dysplasia d. Odontodyspalsia
28. The semilunar radiolucency in the cervico proximal region of a tooth denotes ***dental floss injury***.
    a. Tooth brush injury b. Dental floss injury
    c. Abrasion d. Erosion

VIVA VOCE

1. Anatomical radiolucent-radiopaque [mixed] lesions.

- **Developing tooth:** The calcifying crown of developing tooth within the tooth crypt seen as cyst like radiolucency with radiopaque foci.
- **Normal alveolar bone:** Trabeculations seen as radiopaque lines with marrow spaces in between seen as radiolucency.

2. Limitations of radiographic diagnosis of periodontal lesions.

- A radiograph does not reveal the total amount of bone destruction.
- Difficult to differentiate between buccal and lingual crestal bone levels.
- The early stage of bone loss is not evident.
- Depth of the pocket cannot be assessed
- Two-dimensional view of three-dimensional structure (bony defects overlapped by higher bony walls).

3. Conditions associated with loss of lamina dura.

- Fibrous dysplasia
- Vitamin D deficiency: Rickets in children and osteomalacia in adults
- Hyperparathyroidism
- Osteoporosis.

4. Name the lesions with well-defined periapical radiopacity surrounded by radiolucent halo.

- Odontome (compound and complex)
- Mature stage of periapical cemental dysplasia
- Mature stage of cemento-ossifying fibroma
- Benign cementoblastoma.

5. Name the lesions with noncorticated well-defined periapical radiopacity and not surrounded by radiolucent halo.

- Enostosis
- Condensing osteitis
- Exostosis.

6. Mention the names of rare periapical radiolucencies.

- Giant cell granuloma
- Ameloblastoma
- Langerhan's cell disease
- Multiple myeloma.

7. Name few malignant peripical radiolucent lesions.

Radiolucency with diffused margins and band like widening of periodontal ligament space.

- Chondrosarcoma
- Osteosarcoma
- Metastatic carcinoma
- Adenoid cystic carcinoma (posterior hard palate)
- Hemangiosarcoma.

8. What is horizontal and vertical bone loss?

The alveolar bone loss that occurs in a plane parallel to the cemento enamel junction (CEJ) of adjacent teeth is called as a horizontal bone loss.

If the crestal bone loss is not parallel to the plane of CEJ, it is called as vertical or angular bone loss.

9. Describe the radiographic appearance of calculus.

Calculus appears radiopaque in a dental mage. It may be:

- Pointed or irregular radiopaque projections extending from proximal root surfaces.
- Ringlike radiopacity encircling the cervical region.
- Nodular or smooth radiopaque projection from root.

10. What is the false positive outcome in radiograph?

False positive outcome is the appearance of lesion on radiograph when the object of interest is not really affected.

Example: Hypoplastic tooth surface and wear facet concavities resembles the appearance of carious lesion on radiograph.

11. What is the false negative outcome in a radiograph?

False negative outcome is the radiographically unpredictable lesions whereas it is clinically predictable.

Example: Proximal enamel caries are unpredictable in radiographs until the demineralization reaches 30–40%.

12. What is mach band effect?

Mach band effect denotes the optical illusion (false positive) in a radiograph due to difference in density between two adjacent structures like enamel and dentin or between cementum and interdental alveolar crest.

13. What is cervical burnout phenomenon?

Cervical burnout is the optical phenomenon occurring as a radiolucent lesion in the cervical margin of the tooth resembling proimal caries. The cervical burnout occurs near the cervical margin of the tooth whereas the proximal caries occurs near the contact point. They occur more frequently in maxillary radiographs.

Types of cervical burnout: Circular type, wedge type, trapezoid type, and diffused type.

14. What is ghost-like appearance of tooth?

Ghost-like tooth is the radiographic appearance of odontodysplasia or osteogenesis imperfecta. This is because both enamel and dentin are hypoplastic and hypocalcified.

The tooth contains larger pulp chambers, wide root canals, short and poorly outlined roots, absence of enamel or thin, less dense enamel, and the overall appearance is a thin shell of enamel and dentin.

15. How to differentiate internal and external root resorption?

Internal Root Resorption

Irregular widening of pulp chamber and canals that appears homogeneously radiolucent, either round, ovoid or elongated in shape with smooth or slight scalloped outline.

External Root Resorption

If the resorption starts at the root apex:

- The apex appears blunted.
- The lamina dura and the alveolar bone tracks the resorption and appear normal surrounding the shortened root. The loss of lamina dura is common if periapical inflammation is associated with resorption.
- The pulp canal is abnormally widened in the apex

  If the resorption starts at the lateral root surface:
- The buccal and/or the lateral surface of the tooth reveals sharply defined radiolucencies confined to the root surface.
- Alveolar bone sometimes may replace the resorbed lateral surface of the rooth and the condition is known as "***inostosis***".

BIBLIOGRAPHY

1. Bender IB. Factors influencing the radiographic appearance of bony lesions. J Endol. 1997;23(1):5-14.
2. Gröndahl HG, Gröndahl K, Webber RL. A digital subtraction technique for dental radiography. Oral Surg, Oral Med, Oral Pathol. 1983;55(1):96-102.
3. Gelfand M, Sunderman EJ, Goldman M. Reliability of radiographical interpretations. J Endod.1983;9(2):71- 5.
4. Goaz PW, White SC. Oral radiology: principles and interpretation. Louis: Mosby; 1994.
5. Kaffe I, Gratt BM. Variations in the radiographic interpretation of the periapical dental region. J Endod. 1988;14(7):330-5.
6. Mortazavi H, Baharvand M. Review of common conditions associated with periodontal ligament widening. Imaging science in dentistry. 2016;46(4):229-37.
7. Langland OE, Langlais RP, Preece JW. Principles of dental imaging. Lippincott Williams & Wilkins; 2002.
8. White SC, Pharoah MJ. Oral radiology: Principles and interpretation. Elsevier Health Sciences; 2014.

CHAPTER 38

Radiolucent Lesions

HIGHLIGHTS

Radiolucent refers to the portion of processed radiograph that appears dark or black. A dental image appears radiolucent where the tissues are less dense. Lack of density permits the passage of X-ray beam with little or no resistance. Consequently, most of the beam energy reaches the receptor resulting in a dark or radiolucent area. A lesion that appears radiolucent permits the passage of X-ray beam and represents the destruction of bone or space within the bone. Radiolucent jaw lesions are explained based on their appearance and location. Causes include inflammation, cysts, and odontogenic tumors.

Learners are expected to study:

- Anatomical radiolucencies of maxilla and mandible
- Unilocular radiolucent lesion of jaw
- Multilocular radiolucent lesion of jaw
- Moth-eaten radiolucencies
- Periapical, periodontal and inter-radicular radiolucencies.

ESSAY QUESTIONS

1. Discuss in detail the differential diagnosis of unilocular radiolucencies of the jaw.

Unilocular Radiolucencies of the Jaw

- Periapical radiolucencies
- Fissural cysts
- Odontogenic tumors.

Periapical Radiolucencies

- Periapical periodontitis
- Periapical granuloma
- Periapical abscess
- Periapical cyst
- Residual cyst
- Periapical scar
- Surgical defect.

Periapical Periodontitis

Inflammation of periodontal ligament space is caused due to the exit of toxic products from the necrotic pulp at the root apex. It is seen as a widening of periodontal ligament space and loss of lamina dura at the root apex.

Periapical Granuloma

A periapical granuloma is the formation of granulation tissue in the periapical region as a result of host response to neutralize the toxic products from the root canal into periapical tissue. It is the frequently occurring periapical radiolucency presenting as a well-circumscribed radiolucency surrounded by a thin radiopaque border.

Periapical Abscess

It is a localized accumulation of pus in the periapical region as a result of pulpal death. It is seen as ill-defined peripaical radiolucency with no peripheral cortication.

Periapical Cyst

It is an inflammatory odontogenic cyst resulting from the periapical granuloma. It is the second most common pulpo-periapical infection and presenting with a well-defined radiolucency measuring more than 2.5 cm in diameter and is usually surrounded by a thin radiopaque border.

Residual Cyst

The cyst present after removal of the infected tooth. It is seen as a well-defined radiolucency (ovoid or circular) surrounded by a thin radiopaque border

Periapical Scar

A mass of fibrous tissue at the periapical region of a nonvital tooth which is root canal filled. Round, well-circumscribed radiolucency resembling periapical granuloma or cyst (smaller than both). Anterior region of the maxilla is the more common site.

Surgical Defect

The surgical defect is seen as round radiolucency with a well-defined border. It is due to the defective healing process characterized by the absence of bone formation in an area following surgery.

Fissural Cysts

Globulomaxillary Cyst

It is a developmental nonodontogenic cyst along the fusion line between the maxillary process and globular process of the frontonasal process in embryonic life. It is seen as an inverted pear-shaped or tear-shaped radiolucency between the roots of lateral incisor and canine (Fig. 1).

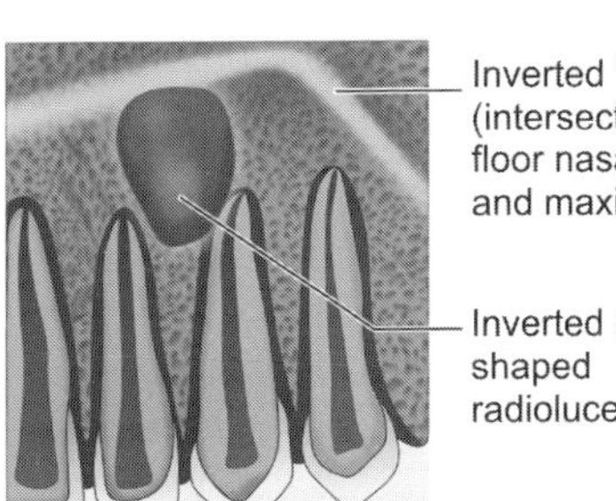

Fig. 1: Globulomaxillary cyst.

Nasopalatine Cyst

A fissural cyst originating from the nests of epithelium that remains after the disintegration of nasopalatine duct early epithelial fetal structure present within the incisive canal. It appears as a heart-shaped radiolucency with a radiopaque border between the maxillary central incisors (Fig. 2)

Median Palatine Cyst

A developmental, nonodontogenic cyst arising from the epithelium entrapped between the two shelves of the palatine bone. It appears as a well-defined radiolucency with a distinct border seen along the midline of palate (Fig. 3).

Median Mandibular Cyst

It is a true fissural cyst originating from epithelial trapping during the fusion process or from the merging of the paired mandibular process at the fourth week of embryonic life. A radiolucent line is seen in the symphyseal region.

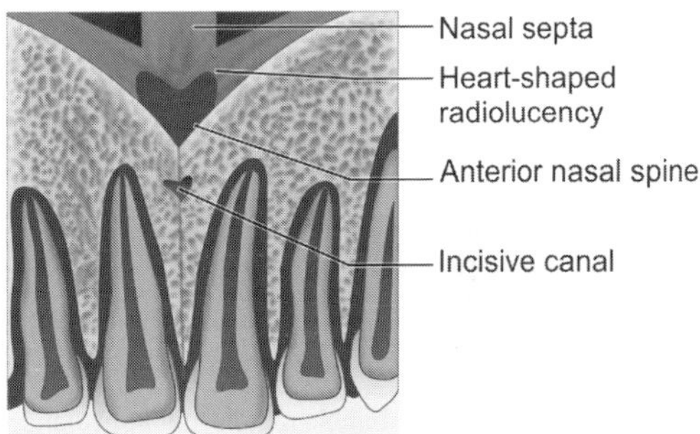

Fig. 2: Nasopalatine cyst.

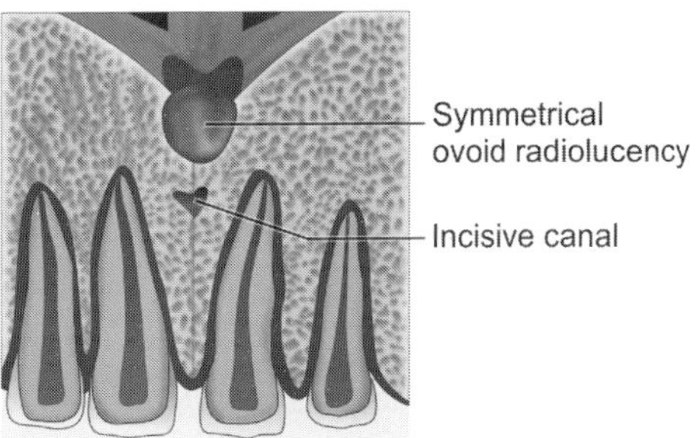

Fig. 3: Median palatine cyst.

Odontogenic Tumors

Unicystic ameloblastoma or mural ameloblastoma: It is an odontogenic tumor arising from the wall of the dentigerous cyst. The frequent site of occurrence is the mandibular third molar region. It presents as pericoronal radiolucency with hyperostotic radiopaque border due to the localized thinning of bone.

2. Discuss in detail about multilocular radiolucencies.

Multilocular radiolucencies are produced by multiple adjacent pathological chambers partially separated by bony septa.

Types

- **Soap-bubble** appearance—radiolucency in which locules are larger (Fig. 4).
- **Honeycomb** appearance—radiolucency in which smaller compartments resembling a honeycomb (Fig. 5).
- **Tennis-racket** appearance—angular compartments resulting from the development of straight septa.

Anatomical Multilocular Radiolucencies

- **Maxillary sinus:** Soap-bubble type radiolucent appearance
- **Bone marrow spaces and trabecular patterns** especially in the mandible (Fig. 6).

Multilocular Radiolucent Lesions

I. Tumors

- Keratocystic odontogenic tumor
- Ameloblastoma
- Odontogenic fibromyxoma
- Metastatic tumors to jaw.

II. Reactive Lesions

- Aneurysymal bone cyst
- Central giant cell granuloma
- Hyperparathyroidism

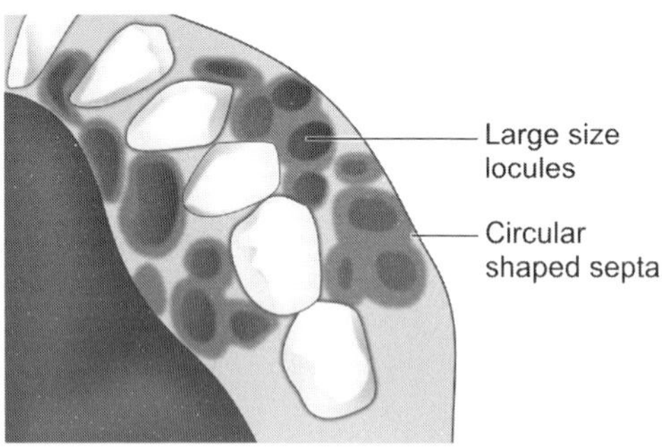

Fig. 4: Multilocular soap-bubble radiolucent appearance.

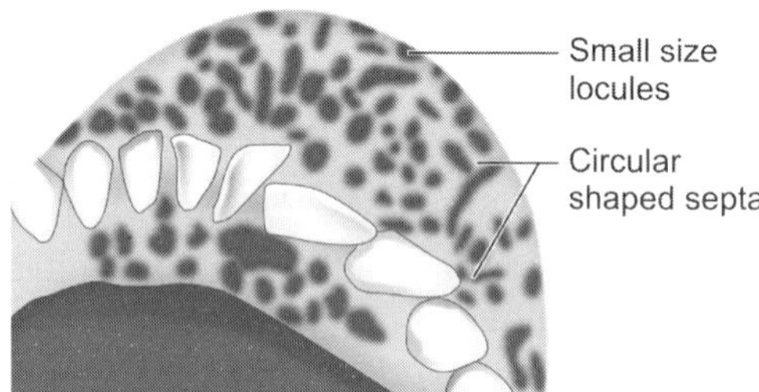

Fig. 5: Multilocular honeycomb radiolucent appearance.

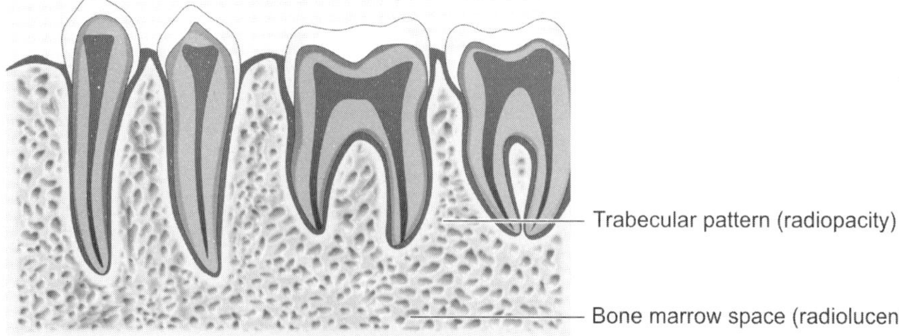

Fig. 6: Radiolucent appearance of bone marrow space.

- Central hemangioma
- Cherubism.

Keratocystic Odontogenic Tumor

WHO (2005) classified the odontogenic keratocystic lesion into unicystic and multicystic odontogenic tumor.

- ***Location:*** Posterior body of the mandible is the common site
- ***Periphery:*** Corticated, scalloped border.
- ***Internal structure:*** Internal septae within the radiolucency giving a ***soap-bubble*** pattern.
- ***Effects on surrounding structures***:
  - Cortical expansion can be seen in occlusal radiograph
  - Associated teeth may show displacement, and in chronic cases, root resorption is present.
  - In the maxilla, it may invaginate the maxillary sinus.

Ameloblastoma

Benign aggressive tumor of odontogenic epithelium which is clinically persistent, and locally invasive. It is a slow growing tumor, common in 20–50 years of age.

- ***Location:*** Mandible molar—ramus region is the common site
- ***Periphery:*** Well-defined, corticated border. Maxillary lesions are ill-defined.
- ***Internal structure:*** Curved internal septae within the radiolucency giving a ***soap-bubble*** or ***honeycomb*** pattern.
- ***Effects on surrounding structures***:
  - The bicortical expansion is seen in the occlusal radiographs.
  - Associated teeth show displacement and root resorption.
  - The maxillary lesions may invaginate the paranasal sinus, orbit, and nasopharynx.

Odontogenic Fibromyxoma

Benign intraosseous neoplasm.

- Mandible premolar-molar regions are the frequent site of occurrence.
- Well defined.
- Straight thin internal septae gives ***tennis-racket*** or ***stepladder appearance.***
  - A large tumor causes cortical expansion
  - Displacement and loosening of the associated teeth are common, but root resorption is rare.

Metastatic Tumors of Jaw

Multiple separated poorly defined radiolucencies is evident when several foci of malignant nests are present and growing separately.

Aneurysmal Bone Cyst

It arises due to the localized proliferative response of the vascular tissues in the bone.

- Mandible molar—ramus region is the common site. Located above the mandibular canal.
- Well-defined.
- Wispy ill-defined septa within the radiolucency giving a ***soap-bubble or honeycomb*** pattern.
- Associated teeth show displacement and root resorption.

Central Giant Cell Granuloma

- It is a reactive lesion of the jaw.
- Mandible (anterior to first molar) is affected twice as common as maxilla (anterior to cuspid).
- Well-defined.
- Wispy ill-defined septa within the radiolucency giving a ***soap-bubble or honeycomb*** pattern.
- Associated teeth show displacement and root resorption.

Hyperparathyroidism

Intraoral periapical radiographs reveals: Partial or complete loss of lamina dura.

Tapered appearance of roots due to loss of lamina dura.

Ground glass appearance is given by the numerous, small, randomly arranged trabeculations.

OPG features: Osteitis fibrosa cystica (localized cystic cavities due to the bone destruction as a result of excess osteoclastic activity).

Central Hemangioma

The abnormal tangle of vascular channels gives rise to a tumor-like mass.

- Mandible (molar ramus region) is twice as common as maxilla
- Well defined
- Multilocular radiolucency with coarse, dense, well-defined trabeculations resembling ***soap-bubble or honeycomb*** pattern.
- Expanding lesions may show a **sunray** or ***sunburst*** appearance.
- Associated teeth show root resorption.
- Mandibular and mental foramen may be enlarged.

  Pathological fractures occur in severe cases.

Thinning of the cortical boundaries is present.

Cherubism

- Bilateral angle of the mandible
- Well-defined by cortical border
- Wispy fine septa within the radiolucency giving a multilocular pattern
- Teeth are floating in cyst like spaces.

SHORT NOTES

1. Radiographic features of metastatic carcinoma.

Malignant tumors that most commonly metastasize to the jaw bones are from breast, adrenal gland, colorectal, genital and thyroid in women and from lung, prostate, kidney, bone and adrenal gland in men. It accounts for about 1–3% of all metastasis.

Radiographic Features

There are multiple varied radiographic appearances in metastatic tumors to the jaw.

- ***Solitary well-defined cysts like radiolucency***—slowly growing tumor or a tumor under successful treatment.
- ***Solitary poorly defined radiolucency***—it is the common pattern of metastatic carcinoma appearance in the posterior mandible. In the initial stage it may appear as multilocular pattern but later they coalesce to single radiolucent lesion.
- ***Multiple, separated, poorly defined radiolucencies*** is evident when several foci of malignant nests are present and growing separately.
- ***Multiple punched out radiolucencies***—several nests of slowly growing tumor cells located close to each other in the bone.
- ***Radiopaque pattern with any of the preceding radiolucent appearance***—osteoblastic activity is induced by the tumor
- ***Salt and pepper*** appearance-widely disseminated tumor with malignant nests appearing as radiolucency (pepper) and sclerotic areas seen as radiopacities (salt)
- ***Dense solitary radiopaque area***: Osteoblastic activity is more.

2. Describe the radiographic features of hyperparathyroidism.

It is an endocrine abnormality characterized by excess secretion of the parathyroid hormone, which helps in calcium homeostasis.

- **Primary hyperparathyroidism** is caused due to the adenoma of the parathyroid gland.
- **Secondary hyperparathyroidism** is caused due to hypocalcemia in renal failure.
- **Oral manifestations**:
  - Hyperparathyroidism: It is a giant cell lesion due to the presence of multinucleated giant cells (osteoclasts). It causes:
  - Mobility and drifting of teeth
  - Osteitis fibrosa cystica (bone inflammation with cystic cavities due to bone destruction)
  - Brown tumor (granulation tissue overgrowth in response to bone destruction,brown, color is due to hemolysis causing release of hemosiderin).

Radiographic Features

Intraoral periapical radiographs reveal: Partial or complete loss of lamina dura and may be generalized in severe cases.

Tapered appearance of roots is due to loss of lamina dura.

Ground glass appearance is given by the numerous, small, randomly oriented trabeculations.

Orthopantomogram reveals osteitis fibrosa cystice as a localized cystic cavity as a result of bone destruction caused by excess osteoclastic activity.

Pathological fracture in severe cases.

Thinning of the cortical boundaries inferior border and mandibular canal in mandible and cortical outlines of maxillary sinus in maxilla.

3. Enumerate the radiographic appearance of jaw lesions.

Radiographic appearance	Lesions
Moth-eaten appearence	Chronic suppurative osteomyelitis
Punched-out appearance	Multiple myeloma Metastatic carcinoma Eosinophilic granuloma
Honeycomb appearance	Ameloblastoma Central hemangioma Central giant cell granuloma Central mucoepidermoid carcinoma
Soap-bubble appearance	Ameloblastoma Aneurysmal bone cyst Cherubism Hyperparathyroidism Central giant cell granuloma Odontogenic fibromyxoma
Tennis-racket appearance	Odontogenic fibromyxoma
Thumbprint/digital Copper beat appearance	Hypophosphatasia Crouzon syndrome
Heart shaped radiolucency	Nasopalatine cyst
Inverted pear-shaped radiolucency	Globulomaxillary cyst
Brandywine radiolucency	Type III dentinogenesis imperfecta
Teeth floating in airspace	Malignant diseases of jaw like osteosarcoma, Ewing's sarcoma, metastatic carcinoma, etc.
Teeth floating in cyst-like radiolucencies	Cherubism

4. Differential diagnosis of inter-radicular radiolucencies.

Radiolucencies present between the roots.

Anatomic Interradicular Radiolucencies

- Incisive foramen
- Intermaxillary suture
- Nutrient canals
- Radiolucent crypts of permanent teeth seen between the roots of the primary molars
- Radiolucent shadow of maxillary sinus extending down between the molars and premolars
- Mental foramen.

Pathological Inter-radicular Radioloucencies

- **Vertical bone loss:** Inter-radicular radiolucency closer to the involved tooth, contacting the mesial and distal aspects of the teeth.
- **Horizontal bone loss:** Bone loss occurs in a plane parallel to the cementoenamel junction of teeth.
- **Furcation involvement:** Bone destruction in the furcation area seen as radiolucency.
- **Globulomaxillary cyst:** Developmental nonodontogenic cyst along the fusion line between the maxillary process and the globular process of the frontonasal process in the embryonic life.
- **Inverted pear** or **tear-shaped** radiolucency between the roots of lateral incisor and canine.
- **Nasopalatine cyst:** Fissural cyst originates from the nests of epithelium that remains after disintegration of nasopalatine duct. Radiographically appears as a heart shaped radiolucency between the roots of maxillary central incisors
- **Lateral periodontal cyst:** Unusual inflammatory odontogenic cyst occurs in the periodontal ligament near the alveolar crest. It appears as inter-rradicular radiolucency between the mandibular canine and first premolar.

- **Median mandibular cyst:** True fissural cyst, originating from the epithelial inclusions during the fusion process or from the merging of a paired mandibular process at the fourth week of embryonic life. It is sees as a radiolucent line in the symphyseal region.

5. Differential diagnosis of pericoronal radiolucencies.

- **Anatomic radiolucencies:** Follicular space (soft tissue remnant of enamel organ) around the crown of erupting tooth which then merges with periodontal ligament space. Homogenous radiolucent halo with thin outer radiopaque border (compact bone becomes continuous with lamina dura).
- **Dentigerous cyst:** It is an odontogenic cyst around the crown of unerupted teeth seen as pericoronal radiolucency usually starting from the cementoenamel junction with the crown projecting into the radiolucency.
- **Unicystic ameloblastoma or mural ameloblastoma:** It is an odontogenic tumor arising from the wall of the dentigerous cyst and is commonly seen in the mandibular third molar region and is seen as pericoronal radiolucency with hyperostotic radiopaque border due to localized thinning of bone.
- **Adenomatoid odontogenic tumor or adenoameloblastoma:** It is an uncommon, benign, noninvasive odontogenic tumor that develops from the residual periodontal ligament and is usually associated with unerupted teeth (canine). The pericoronal radiolucency mimics a dentigerous cyst.
- **Ameloblastic fibroma:** Mixed odontogenic tumor is seen as unilocular or pericoronal radiolucency with a cortical expansion and root displacement.

VIVA VOCE

1. What are the different multilocular radiolucencies of the jaw?

- Soap-bubble appearance
- Honeycomb appearance
- Tennis-racket appearance.

2. Differential diagnosis of multiple separate radiolucencies.

- Multiple myeloma
- Basal cell nevus syndrome
- Hyperparathyroidism
- Metastatic carcinoma
- Langerhans cell histiocytosis.

3. Conditions associated with Codman's triangle.

This occurs when periosteum is elevated and maintains its osteogenic potential but is breached in the center and it is a feature of:

- Osteosarcoma
- Ewing's sarcoma
- Fibrosarcoma.

4. Name the primary sites from which malignant tumors commonly metastasize to jaw bones.

From breast, adrenal gland, colorectal, genital and thyroid in women and from lung, prostate, kidney, bone and adrenal gland in men.

5. Conditions associated with alveolar bone loss.

- Periodontal diseases
- Diabetes
- Histiocytosis X
- Leukemia
- Malignant neoplasm.

6. Name few radiolucent lesions associated with edentulous region.

- Residual cyst
- Primordial cyst
- Static bone cyst
- Central giant cell granuloma.

BIBLIOGRAPHY

1. Hisatomi M, Asaumi J, Konouchi H, et al. Comparison of radiographic and MRI features of a root-diverging odontogenic myxoma, with discussion of the differential diagnosis of lesions likely to move roots. Oral dis. 2003;9(3):152-7.
2. Hisyam Amirul Nik, Hishamuddin Nik, Ahmad A, et al. Adenomatoid odontogenic tumour: A clinical note. International Medical Journal. 2013;20(1):47-9.
3. Langland OE, Langlais RP, Preece JW. Principles of dental imaging. Lippincott Williams & Wilkins; 2002.
4. Öğütcen-Toller M, Metin M, Yıldız L. Metastatic breast carcinoma mimicking periodontal disease on radiographs. Journal of clinical periodontology. 2002.29(3):269-71.
5 White SC, Pharoah MJ, Goaz PW. Oral radiology: principles and interpretation. 4th edition. St Louis Mosby; 2009. pp. 448-52.

CHAPTER 39

Radiopaque Lesions

HIGHLIGHTS

Radiopacity refers to the portion of the image that appears white or light. Dense structures or structures with high atomic numbers absorb the X-rays and hence reduce the amount of radiation reaching the receptor resulting in a radiopaque image. Bone, enamel, dentin, cementum, and lamina dura are few examples of radiopaque structures. Dental restorative materials like amalgam, root canal obturating materials, metal and ceramic crowns, posts and acrylic resins appear radiopaque.

Learners are expected to study:

- Anatomical radiopacities of maxilla and mandible
- Periapical radiopaque lesions
- Generalized radiopaque conditions of jaws.
- Ground glass radiopacities
- Soft tissue radopacities.

ESSAY QUESTIONS

1. Discuss in detail the differential diagnosis of radiopaque lesions of the jaw.

True Periapical Radiopacities

Lesions present in the periapical region.

- Condensing osteitis
- Periapical idiopathic osteosclerosis
- Periapical cementosseous dysplasia
- Hypercementosis
- Odontome
- Foreign bodies.

Condensing osteitis (Focal sclerosing osteomyelitis):

- Sclerosis of bone induced by inflammation or infection that most occurs as a pulpo-periapical lesion.
- Mandibular first molar is commonly involved.
- Dense diffuse radiopacity is seen near the periapical region of a nonvital tooth.

Periapical idiopathic osteosclerosis (Enostosis):

- Localized growth of compact bone extending from inner surface of cortical bone
- Few mm-2 cm in diameter.
- Dense small isolated well-defined radiopacity is usually not contacting the teeth.
- Trabeculae blend with those of adjacent bone.

Periapical cementosseous dysplasia:

- Reactive fibro-osseous lesion derived from the periodontal ligament.
- Mature stage: Dense radiopacity surrounded by a radiolucent halo.
- Affinity to occur in the mandibular anterior region.
- The associated teeth are vital.

Hypercementosis:

- Excessive deposition of cementum on all portions of the roots or at the root apex.
- Occur due to periapical inflammation.
- Systemic diseases like Paget's disease are associated with the hypercementosis.
- Bulbous root surrounded by an intact periodontal ligament space and the lamina dura.

Odontome: It is a developmental hamartoma.

- ***Compound composite odontoma:*** A radiolucent halo surrounds a radiopaque mass containing many denticles or small radiopacities resembling teeth. It is frequently seen in the maxillary anterior region.
- ***Complex composite odontoma:*** Irregular calcified mass seen as dense radiopacity surrounded by a radiolucent halo. Its occurrence is common in the mandibular posterior region.

Foreign bodies: Extruded radiopaque restorative materials from the root canal treated teeth.

False Periapical Radiopacities

Structures not present in the periapical region, but the image is projected in the periapical region.

- ***Unerupted, impacted, supernumerary teeth:*** Radiopaque structure with central radiolucency representing the pulp chamber.
- ***Exostosis:*** Osseous hyperplasia of cortical and cancellous bone on the surface of the alveolar process.
- Torus palatinus is seen in the midline of the posterior hard palate as a dense radiopaque shadow superimposed over the periapical area of maxillary molar teeth.
- Torus mandibularis is seen bilaterally on the lingual aspect of the mandibular premolars as a dense radiopaque shadow.

Ectopic Calcifications (or) Soft Tissue Calcifications

- ***Sialolith*** is a calcareous deposit in the major or minor salivary gland and seen as small radiopacities (Fig. 1).
- ***A calcified lymph node*** is a linear radiopaque mass, well contoured, and well-defined.
- ***Phlebolith is a*** calcified thrombus occurring in the venules or veins due to vascular stasis. It is seen as small, well-defined radiopacity (Fig. 2).

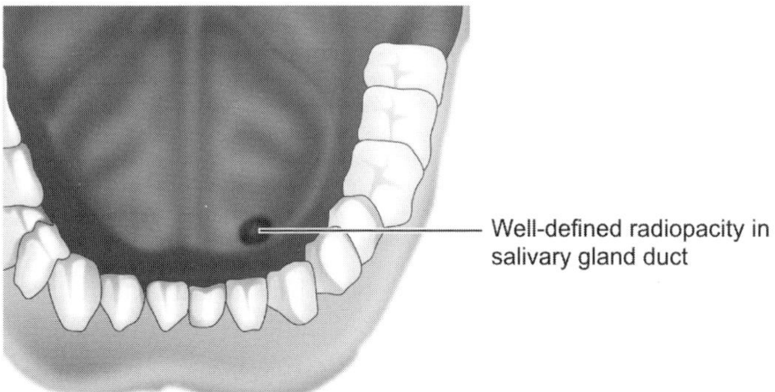

Fig. 1: Sialolith.

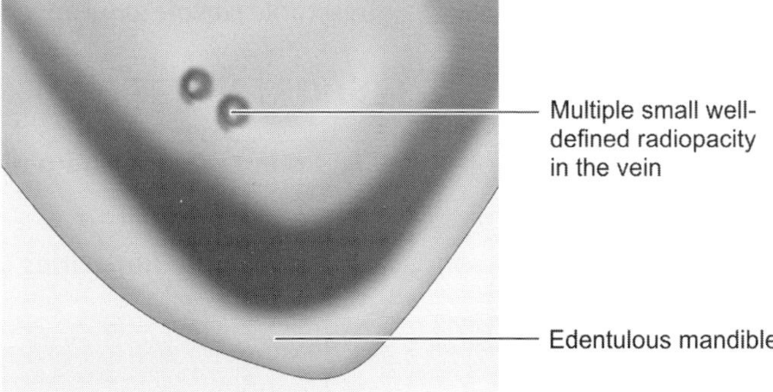

Fig. 2: Phlebolith appearing as multiple small radiolucencies in the vein.

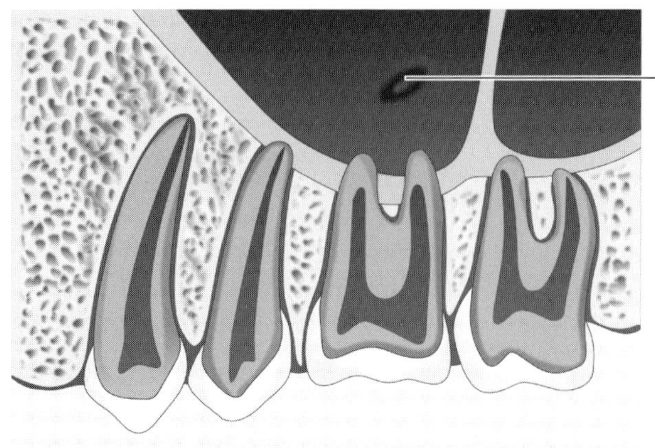

Fig. 3: Antrolith.

- ***Antrolith*** is calcareous deposits in the maxillary antrum (Fig. 3)
- ***Rhinolith*** is calcareous deposits in the nasal cavity seen as concentric rings of radiopacity.

Generalized Radiopacities of the Jaw

- Paget's disease
- Osteopetrosis
- Florid cement osseous dysplasia
- Diffuse sclerosing osteomyelitis.

Paget's Disease

- It is an osteodystrophy where physiological bone remodeling is affected.
- In the advanced stage, excess bone deposition is seen as fluffy balls called cotton-wool appearance (Fig. 4).

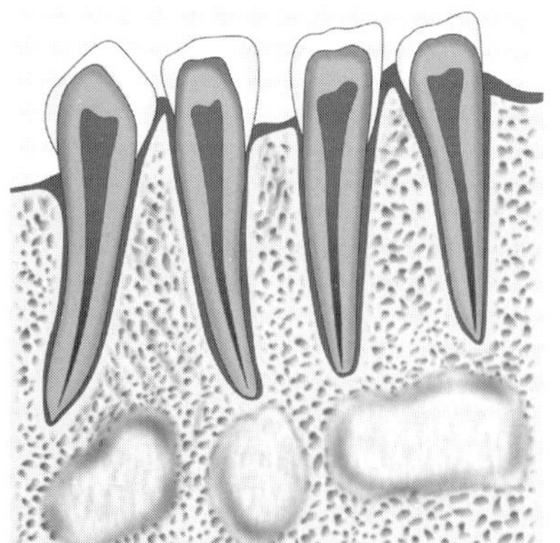

Fig. 4: Cotton wool appearence.

Osteopetrosis

- The bone disease occurs as a result of the failure of bone resorption due to non-functional osteoclasts. As a result of the increased bone density, and trabeculae the marrow spaces are obliterated.
- Multiple unerupted teeth are seen in the orthopantomograph, due to the presence of dense bone.

Florid Cement Osseous Dysplasia

- Reactive fibrosseous lesion
- Multiple lesions involving all four quadrants of tooth bearing regions of maxilla and mandible
- Diffuse radiopaque mass is seen in OPG called as cotton-wool appearance.

Diffuse Sclerosing Osteomyelitis

It is a reactive bone lesion. There is a proliferative response of bone to low grade infection and resemble ***cotton-wool*** appearance (Fig. 5).

SHORT NOTES

1. Enumerate the anatomical radiopacities of the jaw.

Anatomical Radiopacities Common to Both the Jaws

- Enamel
- Dentine

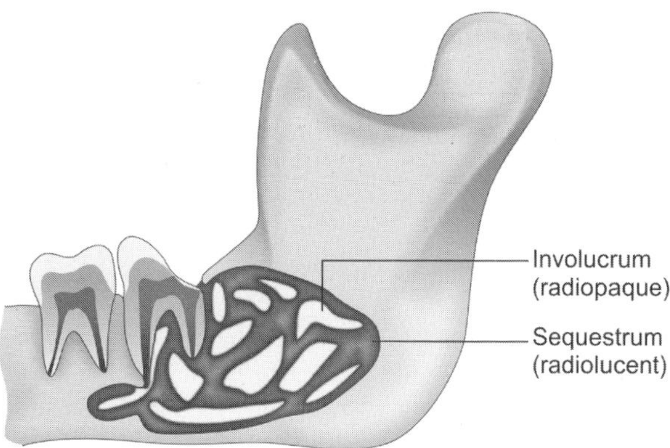

Fig. 5: Diffuse sclerosing osteomyelitis.

- Lamina dura
- Alveolar crest
- Trabeculations of alveolar bone.

Normal Anatomical Radiopaque Landmarks of the Maxilla

- Nasal septum
- Floor of nasal fossa
- Anterior nasal spine
- Nasolabial fold
- Floor of maxillary sinus
- Y line of Ennis
- Zygomatic process of maxilla
- Maxillary tuberosity
- Pterygoid hamulus
- Coronoid process of the mandible.

Normal Anatomical Radiopaque Landmarks of Mandible

- External oblique ridge
- Internal oblique ridge
- Mental ridge
- Genial tubercle
- Two thin radiopaque lines on either side of the inferior alveolar canal
- Inferior border of the mandible.

2. Enumerate the various conditions causing radiopacities in enamel, dentin, and pulp.

Restorative materials which appear radiopaque:

- Silver amalgam
- Gold
- Gutta-percha
- Stainless steel pins
- Silver points
- Calcium hydroxide
- Orthodontic appliance.

Talon's cusp: Hyperplasia of cingulum of maxillary or mandibular incisors.

The radiopaque image of talon's cusp is superimposed on the crown of the involved incisor.

Pulp stone: Foci of calcification in the pulp chamber seen a round or ovoid radiopacity occupying the pulp chamber.

3. Differential diagnosis of periapical radiopacities of jaw.

Refer Essay Question 1.

4. Discuss generalized radiopacities of jaw.

Refer Essay Question 1.

5. Radiographic features of Paget's disease.

Refer Essay Question 1.

6. Name the characteristic radiographic appearance of jaw lesions.

Radiographic appearance	Disease/conditions
Cottonwool appearance (Fig. 4)	Paget's disease Diffuse sclerosing osteomyelitis Florid osseous dysplasia
Orange peel/Peaud' orange appearance (Fig. 6)	Fibrous dysplasia
Ground glass appearance (Fig. 7)	Hyperparathyroidism Fibrous dysplasia Paget's disease Chondrosarcoma
Hair-on-end appearance/ sunray appearance (Fig. 8)	Sickle cell anemia Thalassemia Osteosarcoma Ewing's sarcoma
Driven snow appearance (Fig. 9)	Pindborg's tumor
Onion skin appearance (Fig. 10)	Garre's osteomyelitis
Sunray or sunburst appearance	Central hemangioma

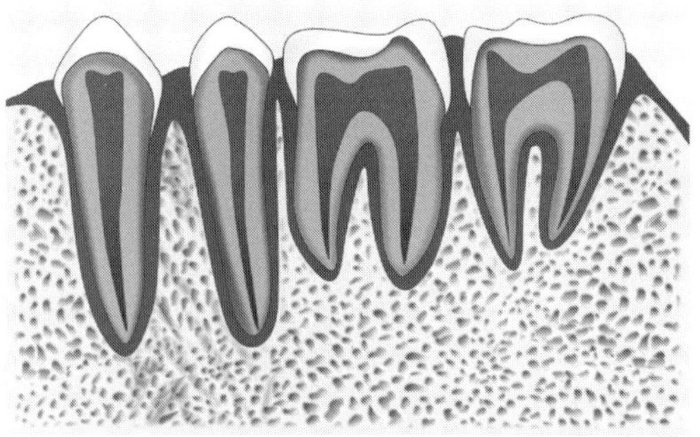

Fig. 6: Orange peel appearence.

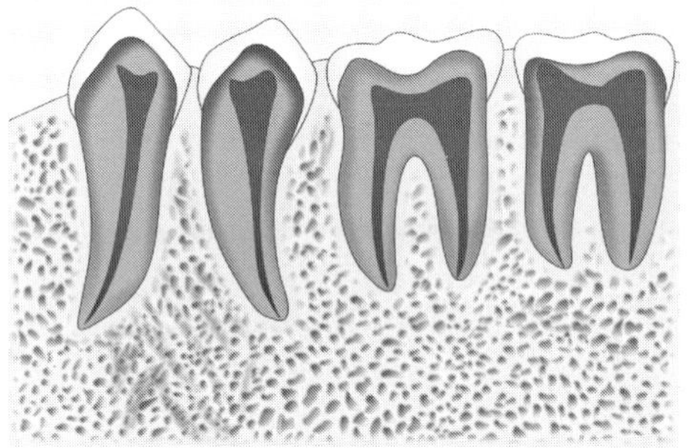

Fig. 7: Ground glass appearence.

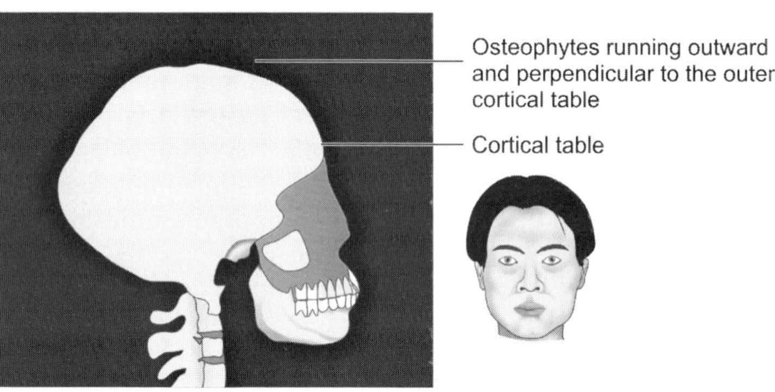

Fig. 8: Hair-on-end appearance.

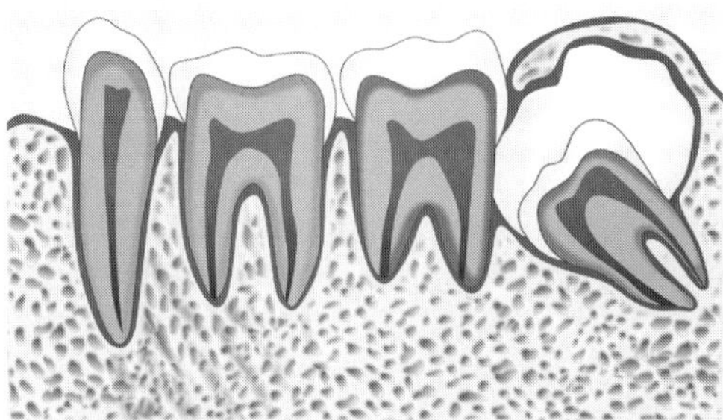

Fig. 9: Driven snow appearence.

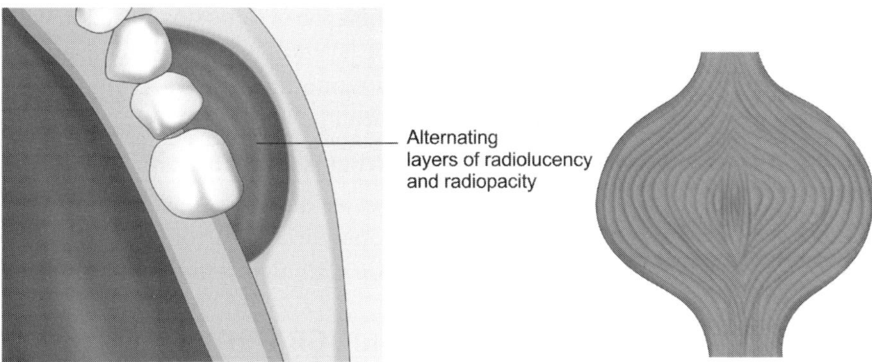

Fig. 10: Onion skin appearence.

7. Differential diagnosis of multiple separate radiopacities of jaws.

- Multiple impacted teeth/retained teeth:
  - Osteopetrosis—delayed eruption of teeth due to bone sclerosis.
- Multiple impacted supernumerary teeth are seen in:
  - Cleidocranial dysostosis
  - Gardner's syndrome
- Multiple exostoses: Multiple osseous hyperplasia in the buccal and lingual cortical bones of both the jaws seen as multiple separate radiopacities.
- Multiple hypercementosis: Club-shaped root apex due to excess cementum deposition is seen in many teeth in Paget's disease a hyperpituitarism.

MULTIPLE CHOICE QUESTIONS

1. Ground glass appearance in fibrous dysplasia is due to ***numerous small trabeculations***.
   a. Numerous small trabeculations
   b. Multiple bony islands
   c. Immature woven bones
   d. Wide marrow space
2. Club-shaped root with dense radiopacity seen within the periodontal ligament space is due to ***hypercementosis***.
   a. Hyperosteosis
   b. Hypercementosis
   c. Enostosis
   d. Cementicles
3. Generalized hypercementosis can occur in ***Paget's disease***.
   a. Fibrous dysplasia
   b. Hyperparathyroidism
   c. Rickets
   d. Paget's disease
   (**Note:** Generalized hypercementosis occur in Paget's disease and hyperpituitarism).
4. Focal hypercementosis can occur as a result of ***periapical infection***.
   a. Primary periodontal infection
   b. Secondary periodontal infection
   c. Periapical infection
   d. Root caries
5. Which of the following developmental anomaly resembles tooth like structure? ***Compound composite odontoma***.
   a. Complex composite odontoma
   b. Peg laterals
   c. Disto molar
   d. Compound composite odontome
   (**Note:** Compound composite odontome is common in the anterior maxillary region and complex composite odontome is common in the posterior mandibular region, appearing as an irregular dense radiopacity surrounded by radiolucent halo).
6. Well-defined radiopacity in the maxillary antrum is likely to be ***antrolith***.
   a. Phlebolith
   b. Antral septum
   c. Antrolith
   d. Roots of maxillary molars

VIVA VOCE

1. Differential diagnosis of cotton wool appearance.

- Paget's disease
- Diffuse sclerosing osteomyelitis
- Florid osseous dysplasia.

2. Radiographic appearance of fibrous dysplasia.

- Initially osteolytic stage—completely radiolucent
- Intermediate stage—radiopaque flecks in radiolucency (***salt and pepper appearance***)
- Advanced stage—dense radiopacity with many small closely arranged trabeculations seen as stippled or ***ground glass appearance*** or ***Peau d orange*** appearance.

3. Name the solitary radiopacities not necessarily contacting the teeth.

- Exostosis (palatine torus and torus mandibularis)
- Idiopathic osteosclerosis or enostosis
- Unerupted/impacted/supernumerary teeth.

4. What is onion skin appearance?

- It represents the laminar periosteal bone reaction commonly seen in malignant lesions of jaws
- Alternating layers of radiolucency and radiopacity seen as onion peel or onion skin appearance.
- This type of periosteal reaction with multiple layers of new bone on the buccal aspect of mandible is also seen in Garre's osteomyelitis.

5. What is target lesion?

Target lesion refers to well-defined, localized radiopaque area surrounded by a radiolucent halo, e.g. Benign cementoblastoma.

BIBLIOGRAPHY

1. Curé JK, Vattoth S, Shah R. Radiopaque jaw lesions: an approach to the differential diagnosis. Radiographics. 2012;32(7):1909-25.
2. Fowler CB. Benign and malignant neoplasms of the periodontium. Periodontology 2000. 1999;21(1):33-83.
3. Goaz PW, White SC. Oral radiology: principles and interpretation. Louis: Mosby; 1994.
4. Halstead CL, Hoard BC. Dental radiology and oral pathology. Curr probl Diagn Radiol. 1991;20(6):189-226.
5. Langland OE, Langlais RP, Preece JW. Principles of dental imaging. Lippincott Williams and Wilkins; 2002.
6. Yonetsu K, Yuasa K, Kanda S. Idiopathic osteosclerosis of the jaws: panoramic radiographic and computed tomographic findings. Oral Surg, Oral Med, Oral Pathol, Oral Radiol Endod. 1997;83(4):517-21.

3 PART

Part 3 Outline

CHAPTER 40

Forensic Dentistry

HIGHLIGHTS

Personal identification is a part of criminology investigation to identify the crimes and unknown deceased individuals. For establishing the details of the unidentified victims, dental findings can be used alone or in combination with other evidence. The art and science of applying dentistry in the detection or investigation of unknown person are evolved as a new branch named forensic odontology/dentistry. Keiser-Neilson in 1970 defined forensic odontology as a branch of forensic medicine that deals with the proper handling and examination of dental evidence and the proper evaluation and presentation of the dental findings to support the law and justice. Identification is made by comparing the known dental findings/records of an individual (*antemortem* data) with the identified characteristics of an unknown body (*postmortem* data). This chapter deals with the methods, interpretation and reporting system of dental and oral findings for personal identification.

Learners are expected to study about:

- Personal identification
- Antemortem records
- Dental age determination
- Lip print and palatal rugae
- Bite marks
- Deoxyribonucleic acid (DNA) analysis of dental samples.

ESSAY QUESTION

1. Enumerate the age determination in forensic dentistry or dental age determination.

Age estimation for an individual is requested for criminal investigations and civil purposes. Age estimation of unidentified bodies assists in narrowing the age group of the search and thereby focusing the antemortem data analysis.

Dental age estimations are based on age-related findings in teeth. Tooth development and eruption pattern are used in children and adolescent groups, whereas tooth morphology, regressive changes like attrition and abrasion are applied for the age estimation of adults and elderly individuals.

Gustafson's Method of Age Determination

Sectioning of teeth shows some characteristic signs at advancing ages and these signs are used in age estimation.

- Amount of secondary dentin deposition
- Plane of gingival attachment
- Sclerotic apical dentin—the apical translucency is absent or minimal at 20 years whereas it gradually increases with age and involves half of the root in around 70 years of age.
- Amount of secondary cementum at the apex.
- Extent of resorption at the apex.

By analyzing the root dentin transparency, the age of an individual from 20 years onward can be identified (Table 1).

Table 1: Analysis of root dentin transparency.

Age	Dentin transparency at the roots
Below 20 years	Transparent dentin is absent
21–30 years	Attempted formation of transparent dentin at the apical 3rd of roots
31–40 years	Transparent dentin involving full apical 3rd of roots
41–50 years	Transparent dentin beyond apical 3rd to middle 3rd of roots
51–60 years	Transparent dentin up to or beyond middle 3rd of roots toward the cervical region
61–70 years	Transparent dentin beyond middle 3rd to cervical 3rd of roots
Above 70 years	Transparent dentin on the entire root

Dental Radiographs in Age Determination

Dental radiographs are assessed for the following features:

- Morphology of jaw bones
- Appearance of tooth germs
- Evidence of mineralization in deciduous teeth during intrauterine life
- Beginning of mineralization in permanent teeth
- Amount of crown completion
- Level of root development in both erupted and unerupted teeth
- Amount of root resorption in deciduous teeth
- Presence of open apices in roots
- The dimension of the pulp chamber and root canals—secondary dentin deposition will reduce the pulp cavity size in advancing age group
- Tooth-to-pulp ratio
- Stage of third molar development.

Age estimation is grouped into three phases based on the above radiographic features:

1. Prenatal, neonatal and postnatal
2. Children and adolescents
3. Adults.

Age Determination from Mandible

Age determination from mandible is possible only for broad range of groupings like infancy, adult, and older age (Table 2).

Table 2: Age determination from mandible.

S. No.	Features	Infancy	Adult	Old age
1.	Body	Shallow and small	Thick and long	Shallow and long
2.	Mental foramen	At the lower margin of mandible	At the middle of mandible	Close to alveolar ridge
3.	Ramus	Oblique and short	Less obtuse angle with body	Oblique and long
4.	Condylar process	Placed at lower level than coronoid process	Placed above the level of coronoid process	Condylar neck bends backward
5.	Mediolateral angle (angle between the upper border of body and anterior border of ramus)	Obtuse	Right angled	Obtuse

SHORT NOTES

1. Describe the comparative dental identification.

The comparative dental identification is the process of comparing the dental findings in postmortem and antemortem dental records to determine similarities and exclude discrepancies.

The forensic dentist prepares the postmortem record by charting and written descriptions of the teeth, supported by the evidence of radiographs, photographs, and dental casts. This record is compared with an available antemortem dental record for personal identification.

This comparative analysis is helpful in the determination of sex, race, and age by analyzing the teeth, soft and hard tissue anatomical landmarks.

Forensic odontologists may obtain more information about the deceased based on tobacco habits, occupation, and other causes that bring about characteristic morphological changes in the teeth.

The comparative analysis may leads to four types of results:

1. *Positive identification*: There is adequate matching between antemortem and postmortem data in essential features without any significant discrepancies to prove that they belong to the same individual.
2. *Possible identification*: There will be sufficient matching between antemortem and postmortem data, but the insufficient details of either the postmortem remains or the antemortem evidence will make it impossible to establish the identity positively.
3. *Insufficient evidence*: The existing details are inadequate to validate the matching.
4. *Exclusion*: The antemortem and postmortem data are obviously mismatched. This finding has as equally significant as positive identification.

Advantages

- The comparative dental analysis is routinely used as a personal identification technique in criminal investigations, calamity, decayed or traumatized bodies, and in situations where visual identification is not possible.
- Dental identifications are rapid, more accurate and economically productive.

Disadvantages

- Poor quality of antemortem records.
- Inability to trace and obtain the antemortem data.
- Discrepancy between antemortem data and postmortem dental records.

2. Describe the dental records or dental charts or antemortem records in dentistry.

To identify a person, a forensic dentist must have a dental record received from the deceased person's dentist.

A dental record is the detailed documentation of the dental problems, a comprehensive medical history, oral examination findings, diagnosis, treatment, and follow-up details of a patient. The record also includes demographic information, diagnostic and treatment radiographs, study models, clinical photographs, laboratory reports, and drug prescriptions.

The dental team should be cautious and well organized in the record keeping tasks.

All information in the dental record should be legible, and when new entries are made, it should be certified with sign and date. The information should be clear and should not contain any short forms or acronym.

Retention and Storage

The dental clinic/hospital should have a record retention policy. Dental records may be stored with records storage service, preserved on microfilm, or scanned for electronic storage. The documentation and maintenance should be accurate. The release of the details for legal purpose if necessary is the part of the dentist's professional responsibility.

3. Describe the Gustafson's technique of age determination.

This method involves the removal of one or few teeth from the dead body and preparing longitudinal ground sections. The sections are assessed for the following:

- Level of attrition
- Amount of secondary dentin
- Periodontal attachment

- Secondary cementum deposition
- Evidence of sclerotic or translucent dentin.

All these features accessed from the deceased need to be compared with sections taken from teeth of known age to identify the age of deceased. By this technique, the age at death may be determined within about 7 years either way from the calendar age.

4. Describe the rugoscopy or palatal rugae in personal identification.

Rugae are the ridges formed by small folds of mucous membrane on the palate (Fig. 1). Rugoscopy is the study of rugae patterns and is used in the identification of an individual. There is an average of three to seven ridges for an individual, and the size, shape, and numbers of these ridges are considered unique to an individual. Hence rugoscopy is regarded as a reliable method in postmortem cases. Palatal rugae form an intrinsic and integral pattern for every single individual and can also help in sex determination. The ease of reproducibility and lower level of variation makes palatal rugae a potential tool in forensic odontology.

By determining the length of all rugae, Thomas et al. identified three categories:

1. Primary rugae (5–10 mm)
2. Secondary rugae (3–5 mm)
3. Fragmentary rugae (<3 mm).

The rugae are also classified into five types based on their shape:

1. *Straight:* Runs from origin to the ending in a straight line.

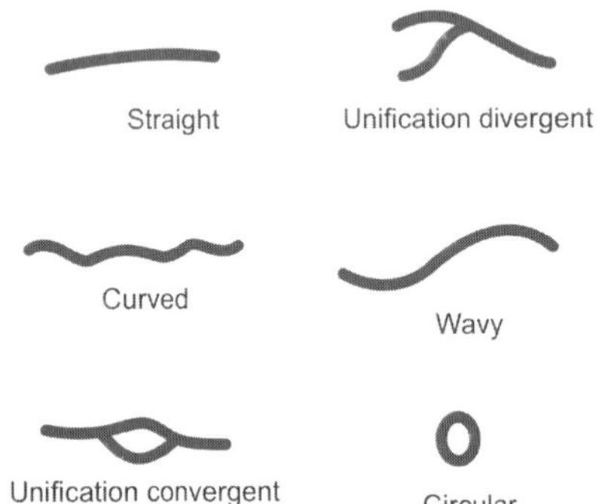

Fig. 1: Different shapes of palatal rugae.

2. *Curvy:* Crescent shape ridge with a gentle curve.
3. *Circular:* Continuous ring shape.
4. *Wavy:* Serpentine form.
5. *Unification pattern:* Two rugae that are united at a point.

Limitations of Rugoscopy

- Identification is not possible without the antemortem records. It is essential to keep the scanning record of rugae pattern, preservation of dental casts and computer records to apply rugoscopy as evidence.
- Worn-out dentures, misalignment of teeth, and palatal lesions can cause alterations in rugae patterns.
- Different patterns of rugae are genetically determined and can be used in population differentiation than individual identification.
- Palatal rugae are destroyed in fire accident cases and degeneration process, hence cannot be used in such incidents.

5. What is cheiloscopy or lip print?

Lip prints are the anatomical lines present on the lip between the labial mucosa and outer skin. The pattern is characteristic for each, and does not change during the life of a person. The study about the pattern of lip lines is known as cheiloscopy and useful in the personal identification.

Suzuki and Tsuchihashi, in 1970, devised a classification method of lip prints (Fig. 2):

- Type I: A clear-cut groove running vertically across the lip.
- Type II: Partial-length groove of type I.
- Type III: A branched groove.
- Type IV: An intersected groove.
- Type V: A reticular pattern.
- Type VI: Other patterns.

Recording the Lip Prints

The Magna brush method is frequently used to mark the lip prints. The lip impression is made against a glass or smooth, nonporous surface. After sometime the forensic white powder

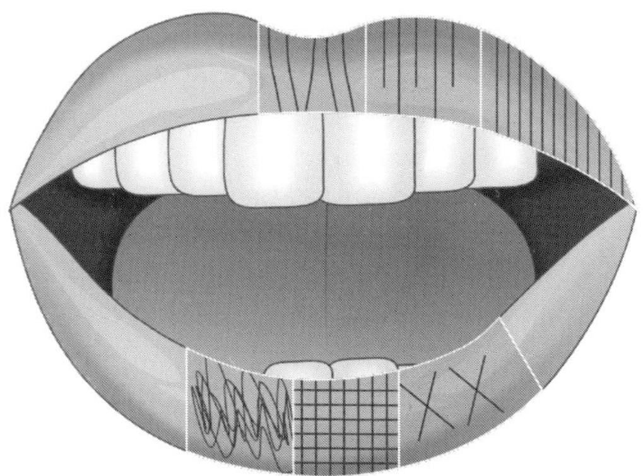

Type I: Complete straight
Type II: Partial straight
Type III: Branched
Type IV: Intersected
Type V: Reticular
Type VI: Undifferentiated

Fig. 2: Classification of lip prints.

sprinkled over the print Magna brush that will reveal the lip print in a definite pattern.

Lip Prints in Personal Identification

Lip print, being unique, can be used in the personal identification process. Lip prints are traced along with tooth marks on food products. It is possible to locate lip prints in the windows, painting, doors, plastic bags and cigarette end and frequently collected in incidents of murders, rapes and theft incidents. Record of clear lines permits the personal identification of human beings.

6. Describe the bite marks in personal identification.

Bite marks may be seen in nonaccidental injuries to the child and in a variety of crimes. Bite marks also left in the foodstuffs and other materials in the site of the crime.

Bite marks on the flesh: Bites are multifaceted injuries produced by crushing pressure from teeth. The typical human bite mark consists of a double arcade of marks corresponding to the upper and lower six anterior teeth and forming an oval or round shape impression. In the center of the oval, bruise due to tongue pressure or suction will be present.

Bite marks in foodstuff and other materials: Foods which tend to take the best impression of teeth are apple, cheese, and chocolate. Wooden materials are also used to identify the marks.

Collection of Evidence

- Recognition of mark as a human bite
- Preservation of evidence in a form suitable for analysis.

Processing Bite Mark Evidence

Morgue Procedure

- Photograph (black and white, color)
- Saliva washings
- Tissue specimens (for microscopic study)
- Impressions as needed.

Photographs should show the bite mark about the nearby anatomical landmarks, close-up exposure of the entire bite mark as well as the entire arch pattern.

Saliva washings for enzyme and blood group determination are obtained by swabbing the area with 10% cotton threads moistened with distilled water.

Interpretation of Bite Marks

- Incisors—rectangles
- Canines—triangles with some variation
- Premolars—single or dual triangles, diamond with some variation
- Molars—rarely leave marks, but when present, reflects the shape of the marking area.

Correlation of Evidence

Bite mark evidence is collected and interpreted to connect an individual with a crime during which the bite mark was made (Fig. 3). To explore the possibility of particular dentition as a cause for mark or not, an oral examination and accurate model of the dentition are needed.

The evidence collected is then interpreted and a comparison is made with the bite pattern in the tissue. The bite mark in the tissue usually exists as photograph record. In this

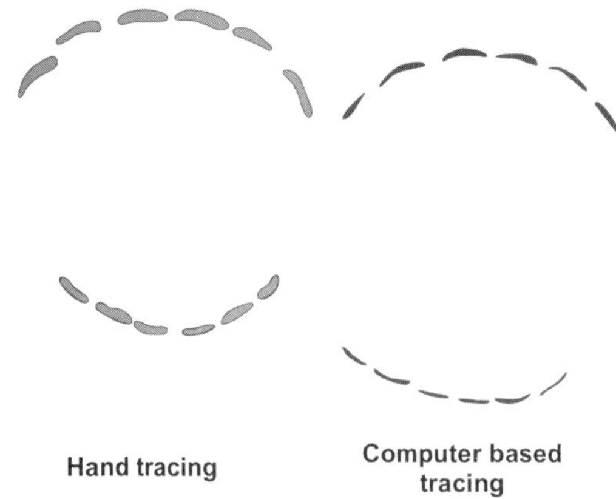

Fig. 3: Bite marks tracing.

comparison, it is necessary to decide whether the dentition in question is the common origin of the bite marks in the tissue.

Conclusion

There are three possibilities of bite mark analysis:

1. With reasonable dental certainty, the bite marks in the tissue and the exemplars have been left by the same teeth (high degree of possibility for two bite marks has common origin).
2. The bite mark in the tissue and exemplars are consistent (middle degree conclusion).
3. The bite mark in the tissue and exemplars are not constant (two bite marks do not have the same origin).

7. What are the various types of bite marks?

- *Amorous bite mark*:
  - This mark represents the areas where the tissues are stretched around the neck of the teeth and between the teeth.
  - The central area of the bite will be caused by tongue pressure pushing the tissues against the rugae on the palate.
- *Moderately aggressive bite marks*:
  - This mark usually found on the arms of the victim of attempted rape.
  - The bite has been made quickly and with moderate force.
  - It often leaves the biting edge of the teeth scraped across the tissue at central parts of the mark.
- *Aggressive bite marks*:
  - This wound cannot be positively identified as bite mark.
  - Not possible to identify which tooth has caused the bite.
  - Tissue scraping will be present.
- *Very aggressive bite marks*:
  - Most aggressive bites will result in tissue tear.
  - Usually involved sites are ears, nose, or nipples.
  - Very difficult to interpret because the tissue is removed by a combination of biting and tearing and there is only a rare possibility to relate individual parts of the mark to the individual teeth.

8. Describe the DNA analysis or DNA testing in forensic odontology or DNA analysis for personal identification from dental samples.

Dental source for DNA analysis includes components of tooth and tooth-supporting structures, jaw bones, oral fluids, biopsy specimen, and mucosal swabs.

The steps to be followed:

1. Collection method should be legible
2. Collected material should be verified for the quantity and quality
3. Authenticated methodology for DNA extraction and testing
4. Analysis of results.

After the sample collection, it should be preserved adequately and should not be subjected to temperature or moisture changes.

Teeth: Pulp, dentin, cementum and bony fragments provide DNA. It is obtained either by horizontal or vertical splitting, crushing/grinding, endodontic assess or ultrasonic wash.

Saliva or mucosal cells: Desquamated epithelial cells act as a source of DNA. Saliva is collected as a whole by using cotton swabs, filter papers, specialized tips or cytobrush.

Biopsy materials: They provide epithelial and connective tissue cells for DNA extraction.

DNA extraction is a three-step procedure that includes cell rupture, protein denaturation and inactivation, and DNA extraction.

The various DNA extraction techniques are:

- *Organic method* (phenol-chloroform)
- *Chelex 100* (rapid technique, minimal chance for contamination, expensive)
- *FTA paper* (absorbent cellulose paper with chemical substances)
- *Isopropyl alcohol method* (less expensive).

9. Describe the sex determination in forensic dentistry.

In forensic dentistry, sex determination of an individual is carried out based on the developmental pattern of teeth, eruption sequence, tooth morphology (size and shape).

Three methods are broadly applied to gender determination:

1. **Visual method or clinical identification**

This method of identification is carried out using gender differentiating dental records like tooth size and shape.

Tooth size: Buccolingual (BL) width of all maxillary teeth and mandibular lateral incisors and canines are larger in males than in females. The mesiodistal width of maxillary and mandibular canine and first molar are larger for men. The size of mandibular canine and intercanine distance is greater for males and helps in the sex differentiation with 74% accuracy.

Canine dimorphism: A distal accessory ridge of upper-and lower canines (present at the lingual surface between the mesial and distal marginal ridge) is frequently common in males and also more prominent in males than in females.

Dental index includes the incisor index, mandibular canine index, crown module, and crown index.

Incisor index is determined by using the formula: Ii = MDI2/MDI1 × 100 where MDI2 = Maximum mesiodistal diameter of the maxillary lateral incisor.

MDI1 = Maximum mesiodistal diameter of the central incisor.

The incisor index is commonly used, and the value is higher for males.

2. **Microscopic methods**

Barr bodies in sex determination: The study of X and Y chromosomes in the cells is utilized for sex determination. Buccal smears and tooth pulp are considered as a suitable sample for chromosome analysis, and quinacrine mustard stain is specific in the identification of Y chromosome. The pulp tissue is stained with 5% quinacrine hydrochloride and examined under fluorescent microscope. Cells that have Y chromatin display a blue-violet fluorescent spot and labeled as positive cells.

3. **Advanced methods**

Polymerase chain reaction (PCR): Dental pulp is subjected to ultrasonication to extract DNA followed by PCR for amplification of X and Y sequence in males and X sequence in females.

Sex determination using enamel protein: Amelogenin or AMEL is a protein matrix of enamel. The *AMEL* gene that encodes amelogenin is located on the X chromosome for females and the Y chromosome for males. The female has two identical *AMEL* genes, whereas the man has two different *AMEL* genes. This pattern of expression is used to find out the sex from DNA samples.

10. Dental jurisprudence.

Dental jurisprudence is a branch of law that deals with the dental practice. It includes legal requirements for patient safety, ethical boundaries, and related matters.

Risk Management

It describes the series of actions followed by dental practitioners to prevent legal complaints against them.

Legal Responsibilities of a Dental Practitioner

The dentist should avoid:

- Breach of contract
- Maligning a patient
- Permitting a hazard in the dental clinic
- Technical assault.

Dental malpractice:

Malpractices include the following:

- Professional misconduct
- Any unreasonable lack of skill execution:
  - Failure to diagnose
  - Improper diagnosis
  - Failure to inform the diagnosis or treatment of the patient
  - Wrong treatment (e.g. removal of wrong teeth)
  - Mortality and morbidity due to negligence.
- Lack of reliability in performance of professional duties
- Violating the rules and regulations of professional practice.

Dentist's Responsibilities

- Must be a registered practitioner
- Must execute a reasonable skill, care, and decision
- Must perform any procedure only getting consent from the patient
- Must refer cases to a specialist if the training/skill is insufficient
- Must use standard drugs, materials, and techniques
- Must give adequate instructions and information to the patient
- Must charge reasonably for the offered services
- Must respect the patient's privacy.

The dentist should obtain written consent from the patient when:

- Administering new drugs
- Carry out trial procedures or clinical trial
- Presenting or publishing the patient's photograph
- Administering general anesthesia
- Providing treatment for children in a public program
- Duration of treatment is more than 1 year.

11. Describe the recent advances in forensic dentistry.

Role of DNA

The use of DNA as a biological material for personal identification is the recent advance in forensic dentistry. Teeth are the excellent source of DNA material for deceased individuals because of their protected nature in the oral cavity.

DNA extracted from teeth of an unidentified individual is compared with a suspected known antemortem sample or to a parent or sibling.

Genomic DNA

Present in the cell nucleus and can be used as a source of DNA for forensic examination. Subjecting this DNA sample for PCR analysis will provide DNA profile that can be compared with known antemortem records.

Mitochondrial DNA

Cells contain a high number of mitochondria and mitochondrial DNA (mDNA). mDNA is maternally inherited.

For the forensic analysis, DNA from the teeth is obtained by either:

- Cryogenic grinding
- Restriction fragment length polymerization.

12. Enumerate the medicolegal importance of teeth.

- Teeth help to identify both living and deceased in the following:
  - Age estimation
  - Blood group detection
  - DNA sample extraction for comparison.
- Habit detection:
  - Blackish brown or reddish stains—habit of betel nut chewing
  - Dark brown stains on the inner aspect of incisors—habit of smoking.

- Racial identification :
  - In Chinese, Inuit, and Mongoloid, mandibular 1st premolar has three cusps
  - In Mongoloids, mandibular molars have three roots.
- Professional identification: Notched incisors suggest being the profession of tailor or cobbler.
- Identification of toxins on examination of teeth and gingiva:
  - Sulfuric acid causes chalky white appearance of teeth
  - Nitric acid causes yellow stain
  - Cocaine produces black stains on teeth
  - Lead poison causes bluish line along marginal gingiva
  - Copper sulfate causes bluish-green discoloration at the junction of tooth and gingiva.

13. Enumerate the work of forensic odontologists.

- Identification of unknown bodies from dental records
- Bite marks identification on the victim's body
- Tracing of bite marks from the materials, such as foodstuffs
- Match the identified bite marks with the teeth of the suspect and submitting this proof as an experts witness for the legal purpose
- Age estimation of skeletal remains
- Sex determination by microscopic examination of teeth.

MULTIPLE CHOICE QUESTIONS

1. The Demirjian system is used for ***dental age identification***.
   a. Sex determination
   b. Dental age identification
   c. Race identification
   d. Ethnic group identification
2. Whitehouse standards are useful for ***bone age determination***.
   a. Dental age identification
   b. Bone age identification
   c. Personal identification
   d. Comparative identification
3. Boyde's method of age determination is based on microscopic observation of ***dentin deposition***.
   a. Root development
   b. Root resorption
   c. Dentin deposition
   d. Cementum deposition
4. Biochemical method of age determination uses the ***collagen in dentin***.
   a. Collagen in pulp
   b. Collagen in dentin
   c. Undifferentiated cells in apex
   d. DNA extraction from gingiva
   [**Note:** Biochemical method of age determination uses the collagen (ascorbic acid) in dentin].
5. The half-formed roots of wisdom tooth denote the age of the individual as around ***17 years***.
   a. 21 years b. 13 years
   c. 30 years d. 17 years
6. The angle of the mandible is ***sharp in males and round in females***.
   a. Sharp in females and round in males
   b. Obtuse in males and females
   c. Sharp in males and round in females
   d. Oblique in males and females
7. Barr bodies in the nucleus are the indication for the ***female sex***.
   a. Male sex
   b. Female sex
   c. Jacob syndrome
   d. Jacobsen syndrome
   [**Note:** The absence of Barr bodies in nucleus denotes male sex, in male with Klinefelter's syndrome (genotype 47XXY), one Barr body is present].
8. Strangulation or victims of drowning may lead to ***pink discoloration of teeth***.
   a. Black discoloration of teeth
   b. Greenstick fracture of mandible
   c. Tongue protrusion
   d. Pink discoloration of teeth
   (**Note:** Strangulation or victims of drowning may lead to pink discoloration of teeth after 1.5–2 weeks).

9. In WINID tooth codes, the primary codes denote ***restored surfaces***.
   a. Modifiers
   b. Supernumerary teeth
   c. Restored surfaces
   d. Prosthetic replacement
10. In WINID tooth codes, the secondary codes are ***modifiers***.
   a. Modifiers
   b. Supernumerary teeth
   c. Restored surfaces
   d. Prosthetic replacement
   (**Note:** In WINID tooth codes, the primary codes denote *restored surfaces* and presence or absence of tooth. The secondary codes are *modifiers*, allowing for extra information but not for best match comparison).
11. Dorian method of bite mark analysis is applied when the bite is insufficiently defined to be a ***human bite***.
   a. Animal bite
   b. Human bite
   c. Teeth mark
   d. Postmortem evidence
   (**Note:** Dorian method of bite mark analysis involves removal of bitten tissue from assault victim for microscopic examination especially when the bite is insufficiently defined to be a human bite).
12. The study of biting marks made by teeth is known as ***odontoscopy***.
   a. Tooth sculpture
   b. Dental sculpture
   c. Odontoscopy
   d. Dentoscopy
13. In a population study, the intergroup marker is ***central incisor***.
   a. Molar
   b. Canine
   c. Premolar
   d. Central incisor
14. The study of the oral health status of an ancient population from the fossil or skeletal remnants is known as ***paleodontology***_
   a. Podiatry
   b. Paleodontology
   c. Trace evidence analysis
   d. Gerodontology

VIVA VOCE

1. What is odontobiography?

Identification of a deceased person using dental records and dentition from a legal perspective is known as odontobiography.

The dentition helps in the identification of individuals where other recognized methods like face recognition, moles, thumb or other fingerprints. They play a crucial role in facial reconstruction process for identification.

2. What is shovel tooth or blade shape tooth?

Upper and lower incisors are called as shovel-shaped teeth if they manifest a pronounced mesial and distal marginal ridge with a deep pit (palatal fossa) on the palatal surface (blade shape). This pattern is helpful in population analysis and is present 100% of Mongoloid origin population's central incisors.

FORENSIC RADIOLOGY

ESSAY QUESTIONS

1. Describe the intraoral radiographic techniques in forensic dentistry. (or) Briefly explain the radiographic techniques to obtain the intraoral image for a deceased.

Intraoral Radiographic Sources (for Intact Jaws)

To take intraoral radiographs of the dead body (morgue) with the entire jaw, the possibility of gaining access to place the film in the proper position is a difficult task. Mechanical mouth props are required if the jaws are in rigor mortis. To place the film in position, hemostats, taps, and gauze are used.

Intraoral Radiographic Sources (for Jaws Resected)

If the body is skeletonized, and jaws can be resected, the conventional radiographic techniques can be used. The specimen should be wrapped in multiple layers of plastic wrap. Radiographic film is then taped to the specimen and exposed. If the procedure can be delayed, then the sample should be stored in 10% formalin solution.

The postmortem radiograph should duplicate the antemortem film as closely as possible. If antemortem radiographs are not available then, conventional periapical and bitewing films should be obtained.

Exposure time should be reduced one-third for resected jaws and up to one-half for skeletonized jaws.

2. Describe the role of dental radiology in personal identification.

For identification purposes, properly exposed, mounted and labeled dental radiographs (both antemortem and postmortem) are as good as fingerprints.

In the case of "direct identification", the dentists compare the postmortem details with antemortem records and produce the evidence.

In the case of "unknown identification", no presumption of identification exists, and the dentist needs to provide a detailed description of the dentition and surrounding structures for comparison of missing person.

Personal identification of human remains is possible only when a specific dental finding on the corpse is matched with individual's data obtained during his life. The technique used for getting antemortem and postmortem radiographs should be as similar as possible to prevent the matching difficulties.

Two requirements are essential for positive radiographic identification in forensic dentistry:

1. The detail must be unique
2. The detail should be stable for long time.

Usually, one to four similarities and absence of disparity are taken for a positive identification.

Both extraoral-and intraoral radiographs, various anatomical landmarks, physical characteristics and disease status are used for identification purpose if antemortem data are available.

Missing and unerupted teeth, fillings, caries, root canal fillings, periapical and periodontal pathology are the common features useful for identification. The type of prosthetic restorations, the placement of retention pins and posts, the placement and type of implants can also be evaluated.

Accurate assessment of tooth development and age determination in a child and juvenile is also possible with dental radiographs.

Bone trabeculation pattern, anatomical landmarks like mental foramen and mandibular canal, nutrient canals are also served for identification.

3. What is the panoramic radiography in forensic identification?

The panoramic radiographic image reveals a wide range of anatomical, pathological and therapeutic details in both jaws and related structures on a single film. Hence the comparative analysis of antemortem and postmortem panoramic radiographs will reveal sufficient details in the oral and maxillofacial complex. In postmortem cases, dissection is not required for using the panoramic technique. The head portion of the body is introduced to the X-ray scanning area. A machine that can accommodate a patient in a prone position is preferred.

In a cadaver, the tube head travels 240° under the patient's head during exposure, and the radiograph is examined for the forensic purposes. Processing should be done with care by adopting technical recommendations to get an image of adequate quality and details.

SHORT NOTES

1. What is virtopsy?

"Virtopsy" refers to virtual autopsy—an imaging technique used to provide objective and permanent records of postmortem evidence. It is a blend of computed tomography (CT) and magnetic resonance imaging (MRI) to obtain the three-dimensional view. The benefit of this method is the avoidance of any sort of damage to the body by puncturing or resection and to "freeze" findings during the investigation. It is also possible to revisit the image on later periods either for submitting to court or for other purposes.

2. What is the role of dental radiology in age estimation?

- *Frontal sinus in age estimation*: Frontal sinus can be detected radiographically above the age of 6 years. It increases in size rapidly during puberty and stops increasing by 20 years of age.
- The formation and eruption stages of dentitions identified on the panoramic radiographs can be used for age estimation in children.
- In adults, pulp chamber volume is reduced by the increased secondary dentin deposition and is proportional to the age of an individual. This can be identified through dental radiographs and considered for age estimation.
- Chronology of third molar eruption also helps in age estimation.

BIBLIOGRAPHY

1. Aitchison J. Sex differences in teeth, jaws and skulls. Dent Pract. 1963;14:52-7.
2. Cottone JA, Standish SM. Outline of Forensic Dentistry. Chicago: Yearbook Medical Publishers; 1982.
3. Johnson LT, Cadle D. Bite mark evidence. Recognition, preservation, analysis and courtroom presentation. NY State Dent J. 1989;55(3):38-41.
4. Kahana T, Hiss J. Forensic radiology. Br J Radiol. 1999;72(854):129-33.
5. Luntz LL, Luntz P. Handbook for Dental Identification: Techniques in Forensic Dentistry. Philadelphia: JB Lippincott; 1973.
6. Marín L, Moreno F. Odontología forense: identificación odontológica de cadáveres quemados. Reporte de dos casos. Revista Estomatología. 2004;12(2):57-70.
7. Rawson RD, Ommen RK, Kinard G, et al. Statistical evidence for the individuality of the human dentition. J Forensic Sci. 1984;29(1):245-53.
8. Senn DR, Stimson PG.Bite marks. In Forensic Dentistry, 2nd edition. Boca Raton: CRC Press; 2010.
9. Thali MJ, Schweitzer W, Yen K, et al. New horizons in forensic radiology: the 60-second digital autopsy-full-body examination of a gunshot victim by multislice computed tomography. Am J Forensic Med Pathol. 2003;24:22-7.
10. Whittaker DK. Principles of forensic dentistry:1. Identification procedures. Dent Update. 1990;17(8):315-21.
11. Whittaker DK. Principles of forensic dentistry: 2. Non-accidental injury, bite marks and archaeology. Dent Update. 1990;17(9):386-90.

Appendix

Appendix Outline

RADIOGRAPHIC INTERPRETATION

- Image Nomenclatures
- Diagnostic Quality of Radiographs
- Anatomical Landmarks
- Normal Anatomical Structures

PATHOLOGICAL FEATURES

- Pulp and Periapical Diseases
- Periodontitis
- Restorative Materials
- Developmental Defects and Anomalies
- Fracture
- Impaction
- Imagined Caries—Misinterpretation

INTERPRETATIONS

APPENDIX

Milestone in Periapical Radiographic Interpretation

RADIOGRAPHIC INTERPRETATION OF DENTAL STRUCTURES (FIG. 1)

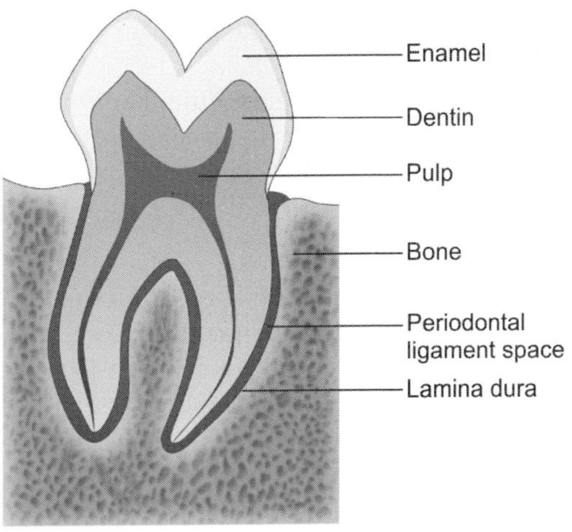

Fig. 1: Radiographic appearance of a tooth.

Image Nomenclatures

- ***Radiolucency:*** An area of darkness on a radiograph that indicates an object of low density which allows complete or partial penetration of X-rays (Fig. 2).
- ***Radiopacity:*** An area of lightness on a radiograph indicating the density of an object that prevents the penetration of X-rays (Fig. 2).
- ***Interpretation:*** Radiographic interpretation is the ability to assess and recognize the image revealed by a radiograph to diagnose a lesion, disease and condition revealed clinically.

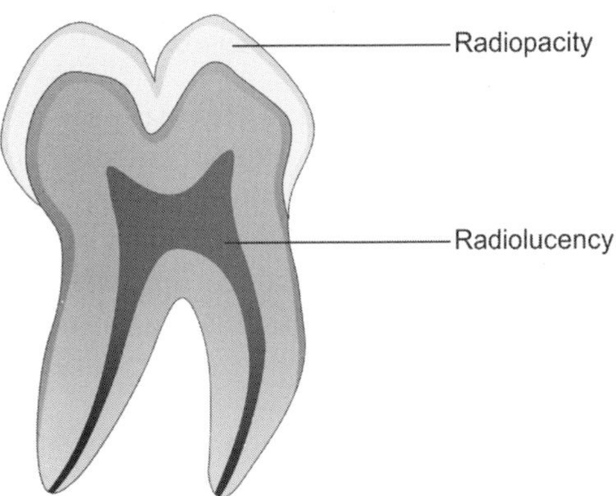

Fig. 2: Radiopque and radiolucent appearance.

Diagnostic Quality of Radiographs

Diagnostic Prichard criteria: To determine the adequate diagnostic accuracy of periapical radiographic angulation:

- The radiograph should show the tips of molar cusps without or little reveling the occlusal surface. Enamel caps, and pulp chambers should be clearly outlined.
- Open interproximal spaces.
- Proximal contacts should not overlap unless teeth are malpositioned.

Anatomical Landmarks

The following structures are more frequently seen in the intraoral periapical images.

Landmarks In Maxilla

Midpalatine suture: Vertical radiolucent line present in the midline between two maxillary central incisors (Fig. 3).

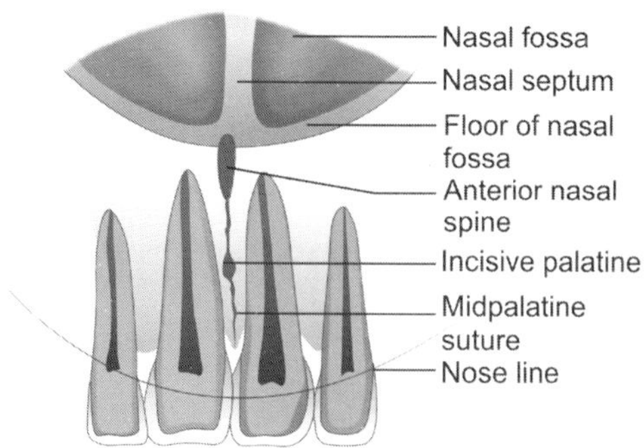

Fig. 3: Maxillary incisor region.

Incisive foramen or anterior palatine fossa: Round or ovoid radiolucent structure measuring less than 6 mm in diameter present between the roots of two maxillary central incisors, slightly above the root apices (Fig. 3).
Anterior nasal spine: Radiopaque structure in the midline above the incisive foramen (Fig. 3).
Nasal septum: Thick radiopaque line present in the midline and separates two nasal fossa.
Y line of ennis: Floor of nasal fossa and anterior wall of maxillary sinus intersect and form ***inverted "Y"*** (upside down – λ) line known as Y line of Ennis (Fig. 4).
Floor of maxillary sinus: Delicate, curvy, radiopaque line that overlaps the roots of maxillary premolars and molars or dipping between the roots of premolars and molars. It encircles a radiolucent maxillary sinus (Fig. 5).
Maxillary sinus: Well-defined radiolucent structure above the maxillary premolars and molars overlapping their root apices (Fig. 5).

Sometimes, fine radiopaque lines may run within the radiolucent space and compartmentalize the space indicating sinus septa.
Pneumatization: Expansion of the maxillary sinus floor and invading into the edentulous alveolor process.
Malar or zygomatic process: Thick, "U" shaped radiopaque structure that superimposes the roots of maxillary molars (Fig. 6).
Maxillary tuberosity: Round radiopaque projection representing the end of maxillary process. It is seen distal to maxillary 3rd molar (Fig. 6).
Coronoid process of mandible: Radiopaque structure resembling finger pad (proximal phalanx), present distal to and overlapping the crown of maxillary 3rd molar (Fig. 6).

Landmarks In Mandible

Lingual foramen: Small radiolucent dot surrounded by a radiopaque periphery, seen in the mandibular anterior alveolar process along the midline and well below the roots of central incisors. Nutrient vessels pass through this foramen (Fig. 7).
Genial tubercles: Round radiopaque structure that surrounds the lingual foramen (Fig. 7).

They are otherwise known as superior and inferior mental spines which are 4 in

Fig. 4: Maxillary canine region.

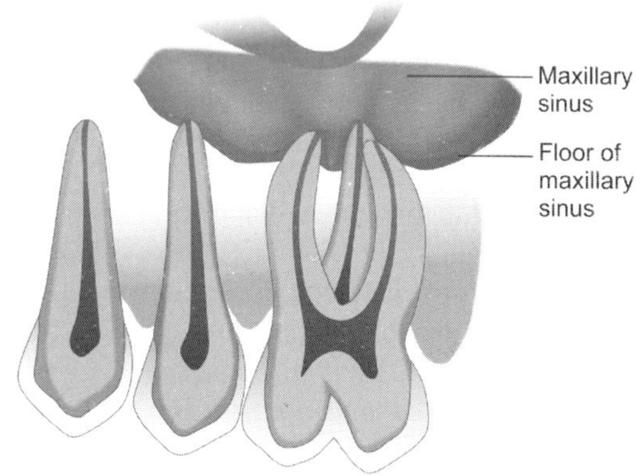

Fig. 5: Maxillary premolar region.

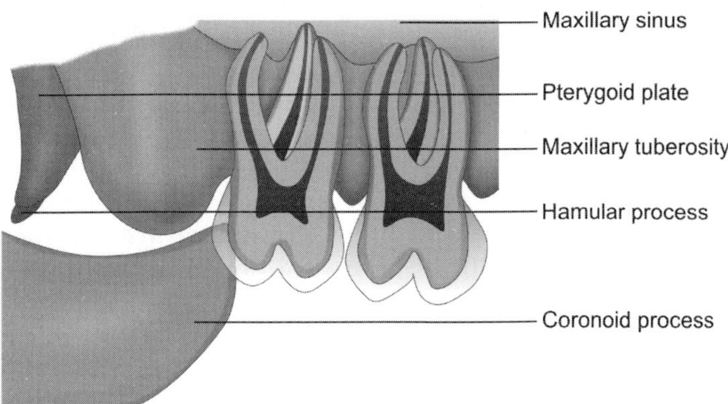

Fig. 6: Maxillary molar region.

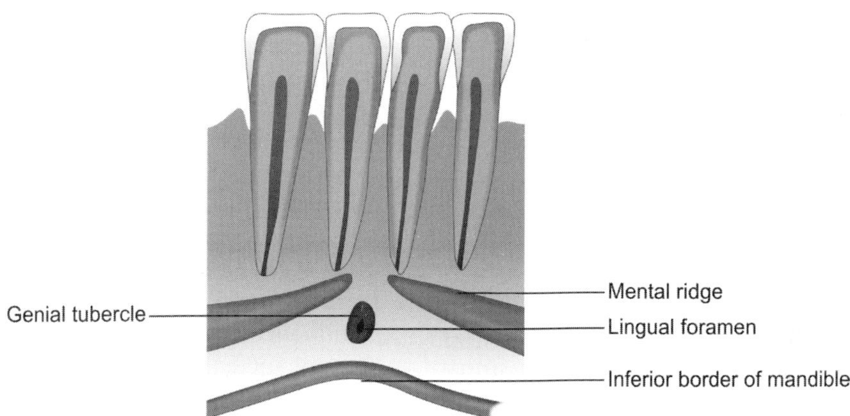

Fig. 7: Mandibular incisor region.

number and coalesced. On close observation of radiograph, we can see 2 on either side of lingual foramen. Along the superior mental spines, genioglossal muscle is attached and on inferior mental spines, geniohyoid muscle is attached.

Mandibular Canine

Mental ridge: Appears as an inverted 'v' shaped structure that extends between the premolars and crossing the midline at the inferior border of mandible and apices of anterior teeth (Fig. 7).

Mental fossa: Faint, diffused radiolucency overlying the apical 3rd of roots of mandibular incisors. Care should be taken to avoid misinterpretation as pathology.

Mental foramen: Round, radiolucent structure present between the roots of mandibular premolars (Fig. 8).

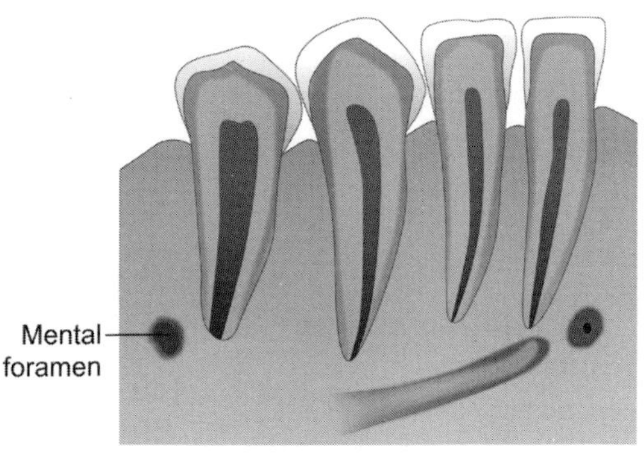

Fig. 8: Mandibular premolar region.

Mandibular Molar

External oblique ridge: A thin radiopaque line that extends from the anterior border of the ramus of mandible and sliding down to the cervical region of 3rd molar (Fig. 9).

Internal oblique ridge: A thin radiopaque line that runs below and in close approximation with the external oblique ridge (Fig. 9).

Mylohyoid ridge: Radiopaque line running posteroanteriorly from the 3rd molar to the premolar region along the root apices (Fig. 9).

Inferior alveolar canal or mandibular canal: Radiolucent line running postero-anteriorly from the lingual foramen on the ramus of mandible and ends at the mental foramen. Two thin radiopaque lines outline this radiolucent canal both superiorly and inferiorly representing cortical bone boundaries (Fig. 9).

Submandibular gland fossa: Occasionally seen as diffuse area of radiolucency below the root apices of mandibular molars.

Normal Anatomical Structures

Pulp cavity: The pulp cavity is the central part of the tooth known as pulp chamber which extends into the root as root canal, which opens into the periodontium via apical foramen and is enclosed all around by dentin (Fig. 1).

Healthy periapical tissues exhibit following important features:

- ***Lamina dura:*** A thin, continuous radiopaque line adjacent to the radiolucent line.
- ***Periodontal ligament space (PDL):*** A thin, continuous radiolucent line around the outline of the root.
- The trabecular pattern and density of the surrounding cancellous bone.

Lamina Dura

- It appears as radiopaque line that covers the alveolar socket and extends on the top of the interdental bone (Fig. 1).
- Because the facial and lingual bony plates are obscured by dense root structure, radiographic evaluation of bone changes in periodontal disease is based mainly on the interdental septa.
- With periodontal disease, the crestal lamina dura is indistinct, irregular, fuzzy, and radiolucent. Its appearance in radiograph is influenced by the shape and position of the root and angulation of the X-ray beam.

Periodontal ligament space: With disease, the periodontal ligament space may appear

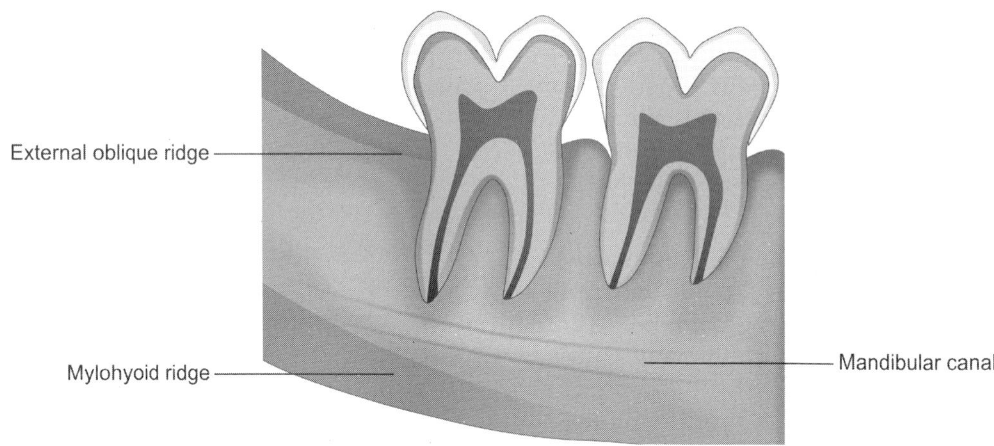

Fig. 9: Mandibular molar region.

at varying thicknesses that can show that the disease involvement is not consistent around the entire root (Fig. 1).

Alveolar bone and crest: Normal alveolar bone supporting dentition has a characteristic radiographic appearance. It exhibits a thin opaque cortical bone that covers the alveolar crest. The height of crest lies at a level approximately 0.5–2.0 mm below the level of cementoenamel junctions (CEJ) and is continuous with lamina dura of adjacent teeth. The distance considered as normal in young individuals would be from 1 to 2 mm between the cementoenamel junction and the bone crest.

- ***Crest*** is the most coronal portion of alveolar process.
- Between incisor teeth, the alveolar crest will usually appear **pointed.** In posterior teeth, it appears flat and will be **parallel** to a line between the adjacent CEJs where the enamel thins and disappears (Fig. 10).
- When viewing the lamina dura and the periodontal ligament, only the interproximal portions are visible. The buccal and lingual areas are not seen in the radiograph.
- It shows signs of apical recession with age or in periodontal diseases. Widening of the periodontal ligament space and loss of lamina dura can be interpreted as resorption of the alveolar bone.

Furcation

- The root complex is divided into two parts as root body and root cone. Furcation is the area at which the roots are separated.
- The part of the root before furcation is called as root body and part of root following the furcation area is known as root cone.
- Widening of PDL space at the apex of inter-radicular bony crest of the furcation is an indication of periodontal disease.

Trabecular bone: It is composed of thin radiopaque plates and rods surrounded by many small radiolucent marrow compartments (Fig. 11).

Blunder buss canal: Incompletely formed root with open apex in which the apical diameter of the pulp canal is greater than the coronal diameter. The canal walls are flared and diverged with funnel shaped apex (Fig. 12).

PATHOLOGICAL FEATURE

Pulp and Periapical Diseases

Dental caries: The carious process results in demineralization which is radiolucent because the carious lesion allows the beams to pass through easily than healthy tooth structure resulting in more remnant beam reaching the film to produce more interaction in the emulsion layer, thus producing more black metallic silver.

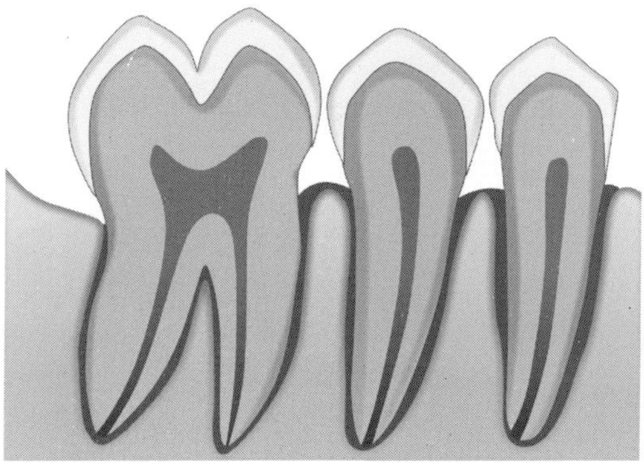

Fig. 10: Alveolar crest.

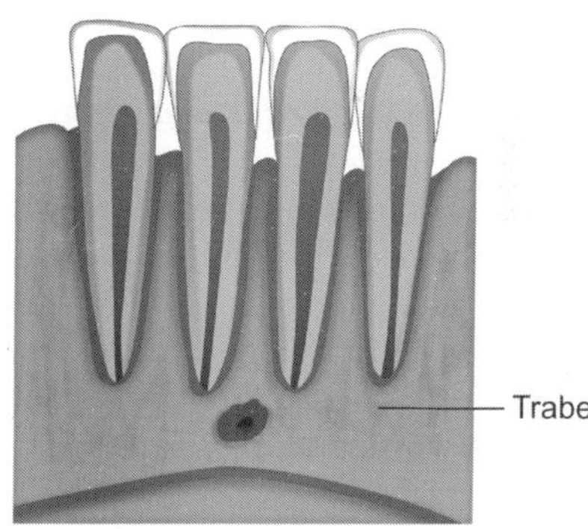

Fig. 11: Trabecular bone.

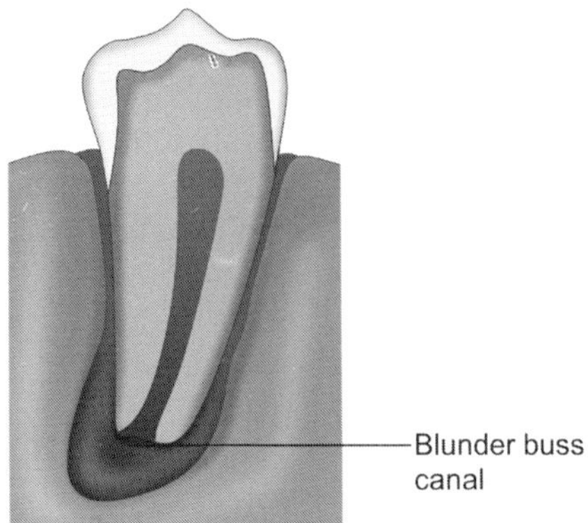

Fig. 12: Blunder buss canal.

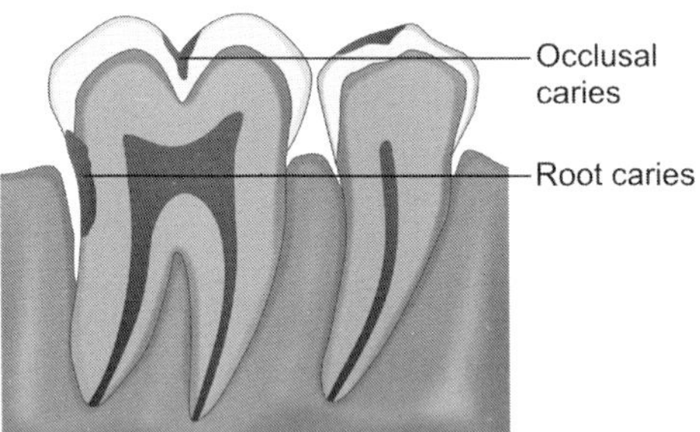

Fig. 13: Radiolucent appearance of caries.

Occlusal caries: Large carious lesions in the dentin give a diffuse appearance as they expand towards the pulp. The diffuse periphery of occlusal caries differentiates it from facial and lingual caries (Fig. 13).

Root Caries:

- On a radiograph, root caries produces a saucer shaped (scooped-out) appearance. The carious lesion has a ***diffuse periphery*** (Fig. 13).
- Frequently, root caries may be incorrectly interpreted as cervical burnout, especially when the radiolucency occurs under the proximal step of a metallic restoration.
- For root caries to occur ***there must be loss of crestal bone*** and exposure of the cementum.

Facial and Lingual (Palatal) Caries:

- Facial and lingual (palatal) caries originate in pits and grooves on the facial and lingual surfaces.
- The radiolucency is well-demarcated from the surrounding sound tooth structure. Its shape may be round, oval or semilunar, and depends on its location and degree of extension.
- Even after the carious lesion has penetrated the dentinoenamel junction and has spread along the junction, the undermined enamel tends to retain its integrity and provides a ***definite periphery to the lesion.*** This sharp demarcation differentiates facial and lingual caries from occlusal caries.

Pulpal pathosis: A pulpal condition usually caused by dental caries or deep restoration or exposed dentin due to cuspal fracture, severe attrition or cervical abrasion that causes pain precipitated by thermal or chemical stimulus and pain lasts for several seconds to minutes. Radiographic changes involve dentin and expanding towards pulp in Figure 14. Radiographically, radiolucent lesion extending into pulp chamber will be evident ***without periapical changes.***

Secondary caries (or) recurrent caries: Radiographic diagnosis of secondary or recurrent caries:

- Caries immediately next to restoration.
- Inadequate margins and excavation (Fig. 15).
- On a radiograph, calcium hydroxide produces a thin radiolucent line whereas recurrent caries produces a diffuse radiolucency.

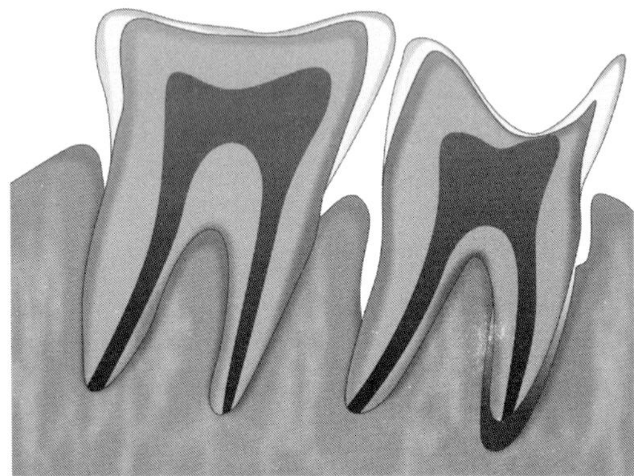

Fig. 14: Pulpal pathosis with and without periapical changes.

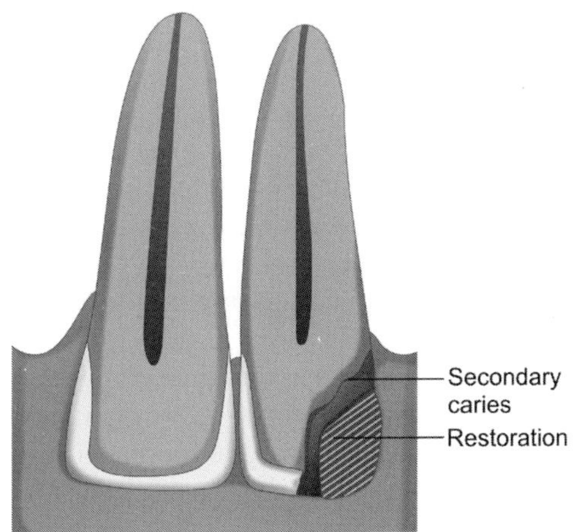

Fig. 15: Secondary caries.

Hidden Caries

- Hidden caries is a term used to describe occlusal dentin caries that is missed on a visual examination, but is large and demineralized enough to be detected by radiographs.
- They are found in pit or fissure lesions that develop through tiny enamel defects, progressing under seemingly intact tooth structure.
- The etiology of hidden caries is still unknown, although some authors believed to be related to the massive use of fluorides, which act in the remineralization of occlusal enamel lesions masking their evolution.
- It has been postulated that the incidence of hidden caries is increasing due to the use of fluoride which reduces or makes absent the demineralization characteristic of the carious lesion of enamel, hiding the caries progression into dentin.

Periapical Diseases

- Radiographically present as a periapical radiolucent lesion as a result of localized inflammatory reaction, infection in the root canal system and reducing the mineral density of the affected periapical bone. Advancing pulpal inflammation when exits, the apical foramen will exhibit radiographic signs, such as widened PDL and poorly demarcated periapical low density area due to demineralization.
  These changes are typically located at the apex of the tooth. Sometimes these lesions extend along the lateral surface of root due to the presence of the accessory canals. Widening of PDL is an early sign of periapical inflammation.
  Periapical lesions are confined to cancellous bone only. This is a result of periapical mineral loss in bone masked by denser, more mineralized cortical plate. Periapical lesion are seen immediately below the mesial root of first mandibular molar tooth, as it surrounded by more cancellous bone than normal counterpart, hence periapical radiolucent lesions are usually developed in mesial roots of mandibular 1st molar.
- Periapical radiolucent lesions are diagnosed only when there is a perforation of the overlying cortical plate.
- Radiolucent or low density presentations at periapical region are categorized as ***periapical rarefying osteitis*** including periapical periodontitis, periapical abscess, granuloma, and cyst/tumor while the radiopaque presentations are categorized as ***periapical sclerosing osteitis*** and ***idiopathic osteosclerosis.***
- Definitive diagnosis of periapical lesions is possible only with microscopic findings of the lesion. Radiographic findings are helpful in considering a provisional diagnosis.

The radiographic appearance of periapical lesions are not the exact replica when compared with the actual periapical lesion.

Reason

- **Anatomical note**—less contrast in the periapical lesion in cancellous bone and increased thickness of cortical bone.

- **Bisecting angle technique** causes geometric distortion that may increase or decrease the resolution or even inability to visualize.

Periapical Periodontitis

- Pulpal disease extends into surrounding periradicular tissues and cause inflammation.
- PDL space appears widened with distinct radiolucency.
- Discontinuity of lamina dura also seen at the apical region.

Periapical Granuloma

Circumscribed circular to ovoid radiolucent area at the periapical region that encloses the root end. The lesion shows a grayish appearance. It is the most common periapical radiolucent.

Periapical Abscess

- An inflammatory reaction to pulpal infection and necrosis characterized by slow ingress into periapical tissue and resultant inflammatory process cause periradicular bone resorption that manifest as a periradicular radiolucency on a radiograph (Fig. 16).
- This periapical condition may occur with a necrotic pulp of partially or definitely endodontically treated tooth with unfilled lateral or accessory canal in which continued bacterial contamination and leakage occurs.

Periapical Cyst

- Well-defined area of bone destruction seen as dark radiolucent lesion attached with root apex (Fig. 17).
- It is the second common periapical radiolucency.
- To differentiate cyst and granuloma radiographically, size of the lesion is usually considered. Periapical granuloma is usually less than 1 cm in size whereas cyst is more than 1cm in diameter.

Periapical Index

PAI 1: Normal periapical structure (Fig. 18).
PAI 2: Small changes in bone structure not pathognomic for apical periodontitis (Fig. 18).
PAI 3: Changes in bone structure with some mineral loss characteristic of apical periodontitis.
PAI 4: Periodontitis with well-defined radiolucent area (Fig. 18).
PAI 5: Severe periodontitis with exacerbating features and bone expansion (Fig. 18).

Periapical Rarefying Osteitis

- It occurs as a result of bone resorption in the periapical areas surrounded by a sclerotic periphery (Fig. 19).

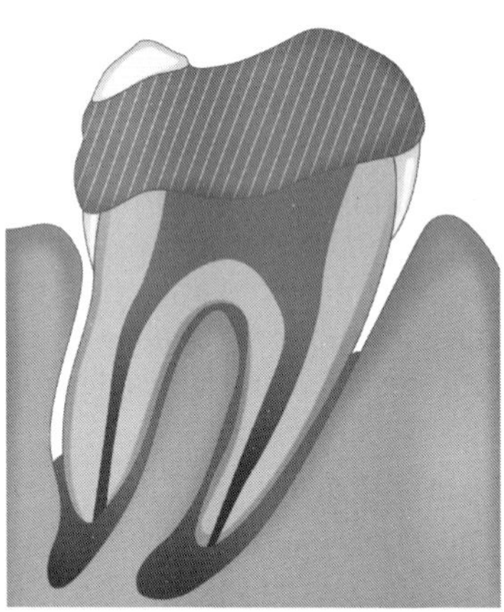

Fig. 16: Periapical abscess.

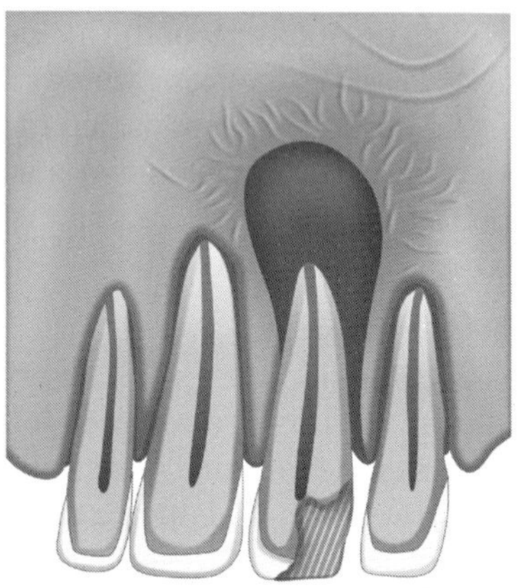

Fig. 17: Periapical cyst.

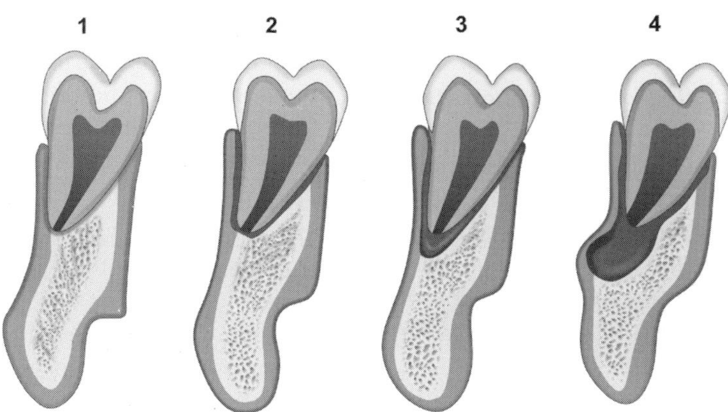

Fig. 18: Periapical index.

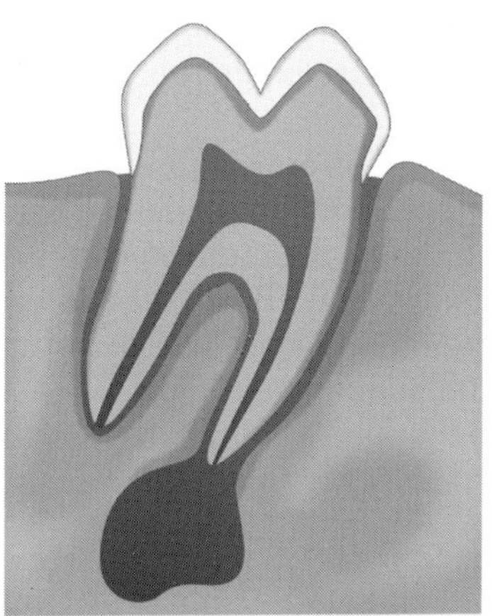

Fig. 19: Rarefying osteitis.

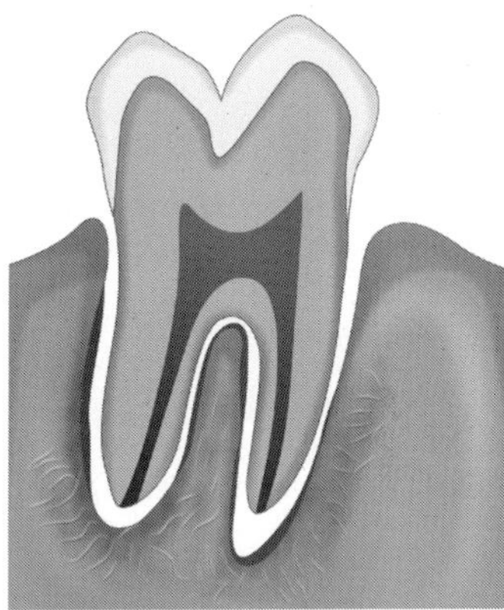

Fig. 20: Periapical sclerosing osteitis.

- Early lesions presents as a widening of the PDL space followed by a gradual loss of apical lamina dura.
- As the lesion grows with resorption, thinning of associated buccal and lingual cortices with possible expansion of the region.

Periapical Sclerosing Osteitis

- Also known as ***condensing osteitis or focal sclerosing osteitis*** occurs as a result of chronic low grade periapical infection in a tooth.
- Individual thickening of the trabeculae is noted within the marrow spaces surrounding the roots of the affected tooth with sclerosis of periapical bone (Fig. 20). This is a result of surrounding bone attempting to wall off the inflammation or repair the bone affected by the inflammatory process.

Idiopathic Osteosclerosis

- A dense bone island or enostosis are localized areas of increased radiopacities that occur due to unknown etiology. They occur in the periapical areas, extend beyond the apices of associated teeth and can also be found in the edentulous areas.
- Radiographically, these present as well-defined, densely homogeneous, non-expansile radiopacity with normal PDL

space and lamina dura when in close proximity to the apex of a tooth.

Condensing Osteitis (Focal Sclerosing Osteomyelitis)

The involved teeth will have an etiologic factor of low grade, chronic inflammation, such as necrotic pulp or extensive restorative material. Radiographically, the tooth shows increased radiopacity around one or more of the roots. This periradicular radiolucency resolves after endodontic therapy (Fig. 21).

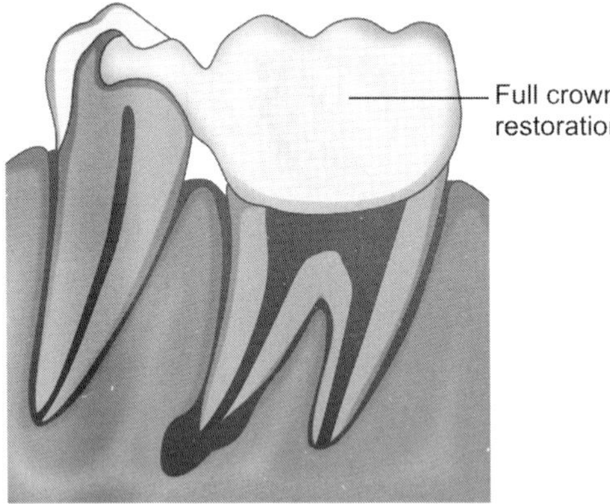

Fig. 21: Condensing osteomyelitis.

Root Resorption

- Root resorption is the loss of hard tissue of roots, i.e. dentin and cementum.
- Chronic infection or pressure will stimulate odontoclasts and then causes resorption.

Internal Resorption

- The pulp of only crown or both crown and root may be involved in the resorptive defect.
- Radiographically **internal root resorption** shows enlargement of pulp chamber or pulp canal or both. But the normal outline of the canal is maintained with thin layer of radiopaque dentin bordering the pulp chamber and canal.
- Enlargement of pulp canal characteristically appears as a ballooning out of the root canal (Fig. 22).
- The resorption appears as radiolucent with smooth well-defined margins and in oval or round shape, the outline of the root canal is usually distorted and the root canal and the radiolucent resorptive defect appear to be contiguous.
- More common in permanent dentition with high prevalence for maxillary incisors.

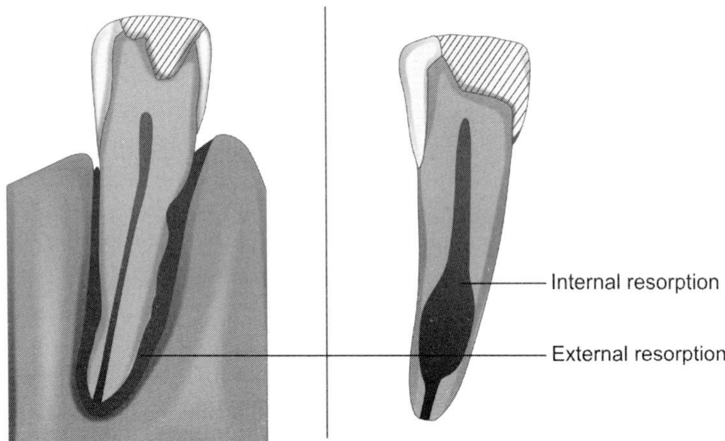

Fig. 22: Root resorption.

External Root Resorption

- Loss of root structure from the outer surface and localized at apical, middle or cervical third of roots.
- Radiographic appearance depends on severity of the process.
- External inflammatory root resorption is always accompanied by the resorption of the bone seen as a loss of lamina dura around the apex in addition to that of the root apex (Fig. 22).
- Early lesion ***appears cloudy radiolucent in the cervical region.***
- Of the teeth and borders appear poorly defined.
- The root canal outline appears normal and can usually be seen
- "Running through" the radiolucent defect indicating lamina or external structure.
- Superficial resorption appear as a shallow lesion with rounded contour, beginning at the apex and progressing towards coronal direction and seen as a slightly shortened root with blunt and square apex, whereas deep resorption begins at the cervical part of the root and appear as small narrow canals with scalloped margins.

Apical Scar

Apical scar results from endodontic treatment of periapical lesions which generally tend to resolve the lesion, but sometimes the granulation tissue produces excessive collagen fibers that results in a dense tissue scar.

This remains as a permanent, asymptomatic periapical lesion and appear as a well circumscribed radiolucency on the radiograph of endodontically treated tooth (Fig. 23).

Calcific Metamorphosis

A pulpal response to trauma by ***rapid deposition of hard tissue on the canal space.*** Entire space may appear obliterated radiographically due to extreme deposition (Fig. 24). Most common in anterior teeth.

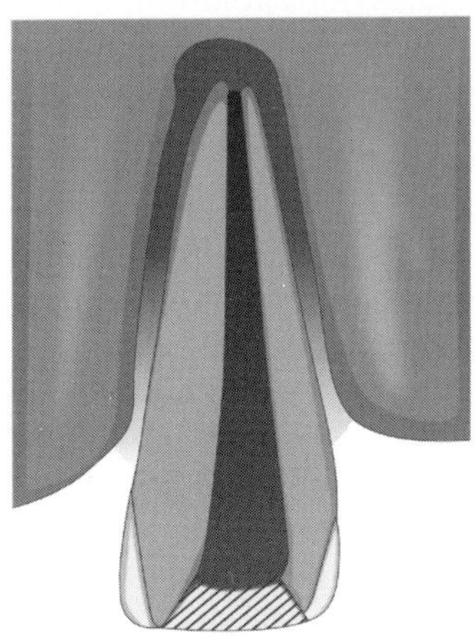

Fig. 23: Periapical scar.

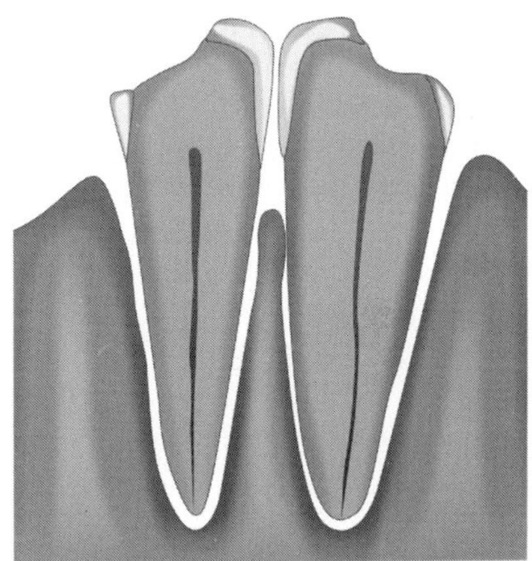

Fig. 24: Calcific metamorphosis.

Benign Fibro-Osseous Lesions

Noninflammatory periapical lesion are collectively called as **"Benign fibro-osseous lesions".** Normal bone is replaced by fibrous connective tissue containing abnormal cementum or bone. Cemento-osseous dysplasia (COD) is an example of fibro-osseous disease that occurs in jaws.

- Radiographically, these lesions exhibit early osteolytic, intermediate and mature stages.
- The osteolytic stage appears as well-defined radiolucencies at the apices of associated

teeth. These can be easily confused as pulpal disease; however, the affected teeth are vital and typically are asymptomatic.

- Intermediate stage lesions appear partly radiolucent and partly radiopaque with the initiation of hard tissue (bone or cementum) formation at the center of the lesion.
- Mature stage lesions appear completely radiopaque.

Endodontic/Periodontic Lesion (Pulpo-periodontal lesion)

A process involving diseases of the pulp and periodontium.

Classification of the Lesion Based on Etiology Diagnosis and Prognosis

- Primary pulpal lesion with extension into periradicular tissue (Fig. 25: Type 1).
- Primary pulpal lesion with extension to the periradicular tissue with secondary ***infection*** and inflammation of periodontal tissue (Fig. 25: Type 2).
- Primary periodontal lesion (Fig. 25: Type 3).
- Primary periodontal lesion with extension into pulpal tissue (Fig. 25: Type 4).
- Combined pulpal and periodontal lesion with independent disease process in both tissues are joined or coalesced in periradicular tissue.
- Concomitant pulpal-periodontal lesion in which the disease process exists independently in each tissue but are apparently not interlaced (Fig. 25: Type 5 and 6).

Periodontitis

A progressive destructive change in the supporting tissues that attaches the root of the teeth to alveolar bone leading to loss of bone.

In periodontal disease interpretation, we need to look for changes in the:

- Crestal bone
- Height and contour of alveolar bone
- Lamina dura
- Alteration in medullary bone pattern.

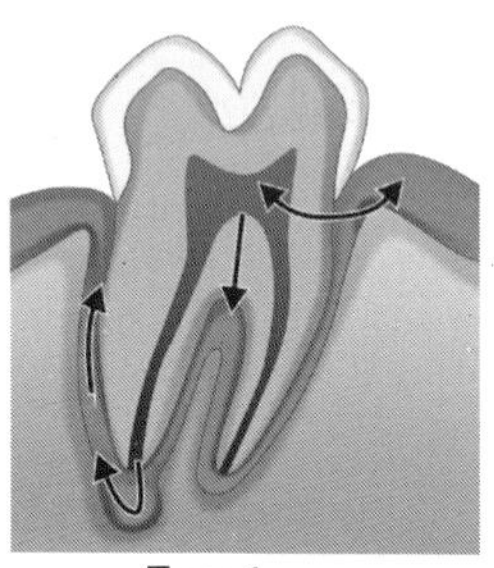

Type 1

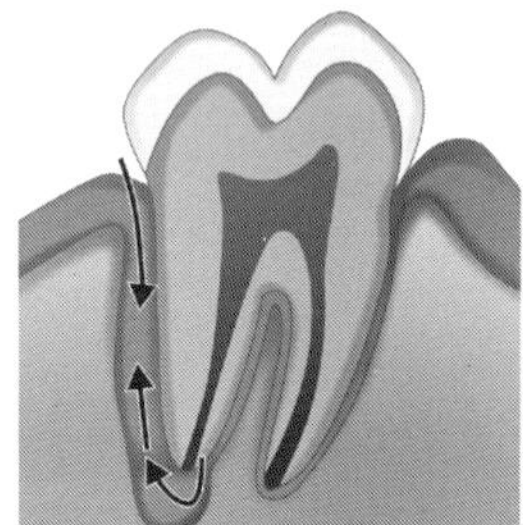

Type 2

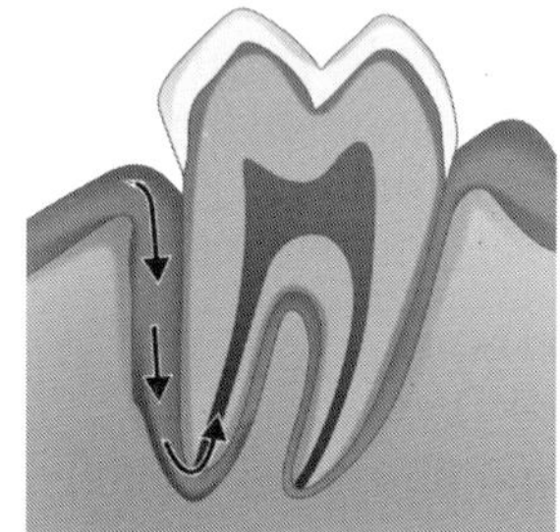

Type 3

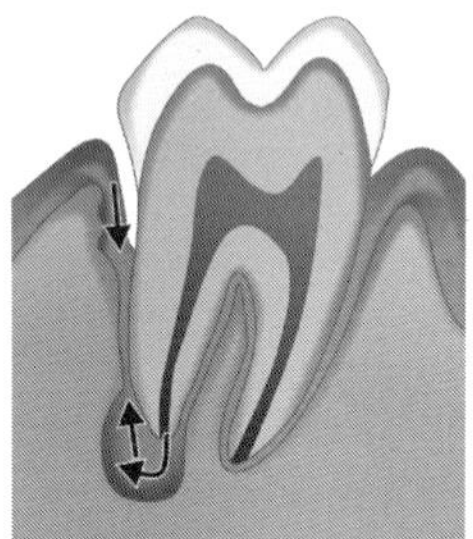

Type 4

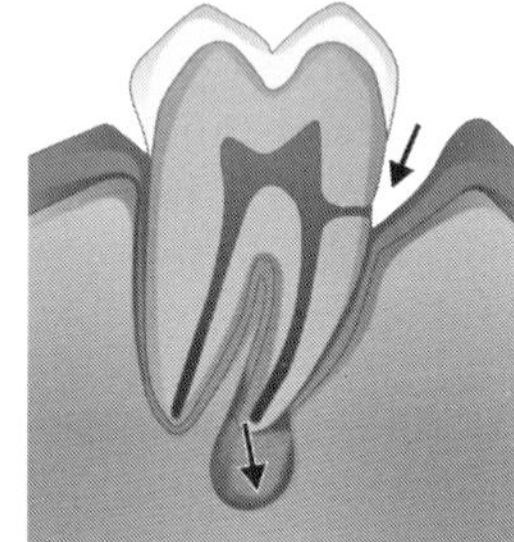

Type 5 and 6

Fig. 25: Types of pulpo-periodontal lesions.

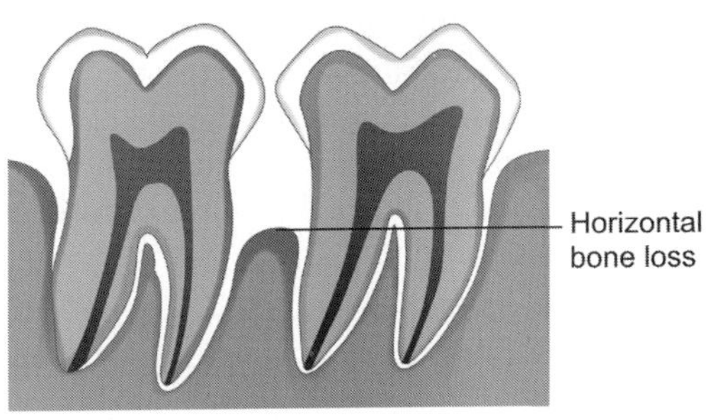

Fig. 26: Horizontal bone loss.

Horizontal Bone Loss

- When the remaining ***crest of the bone is parallel with a line between the cemento-enamel junctions of two adjacent teeth,*** it is called horizontal bone loss (Fig. 26).
- It is usually *caused by inflammation.*
- When the amount of remaining bone is fairly evenly distributed throughout the dentition, it is described as generalized horizontal bone loss. If confined to a specific area, localized horizontal bone loss is used.

Vertical Bone Loss (Angular Bone Loss)

- Irregular reduction in the height of crestal bone occuring in a plane that is at an angle to a line that is drawn from the CEJ of a tooth to an adjacent tooth (Fig. 27). These defects develop when bone loss progresses down the root of the tooth.
- With vertical bone loss, there will be ***greater bone loss on the mesial surface*** on one tooth in comparison to the adjacent tooth.
- Usually, ***inflammation and trauma from occlusion*** are combined in causing the destruction and irregular shape of the bone.

Radiographic Assessment of Periodontal Status

- Receding bone height related to CEJ.
- Loss of bone at interproximal space or at furcation.
- Widening of periodontal space.
- Loss of integrity of lamina dura.

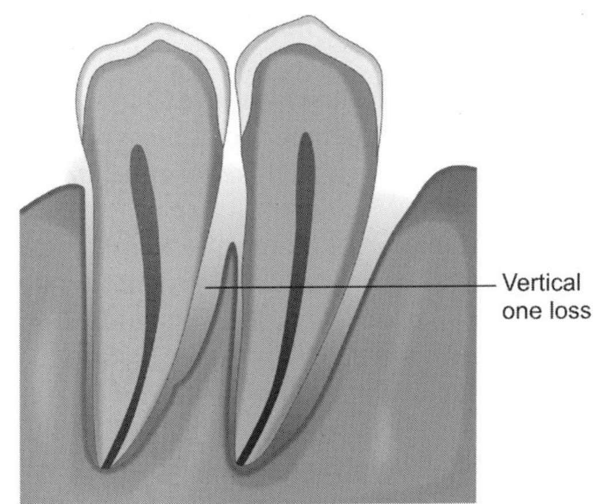

Fig. 27: Angular bone loss.

Stages of Periodontal Disease

Periodontal disease is also classified from stages 1 to 4 based on the severity of radiographic and clinical signs.

Stage 1: Gingivitis

- Clinically, the gingiva appears swollen and inflammed.
- In stage 1 disease, *no bone loss has occurred,* and ***dental radiographs appear normal.***

Stage 2: Early periodontitis

- Signifies the first appearance of radiographic abnormalities. The earliest radiographic signs of periodontitis are the ***loss of definition of the crestal bone.*** The alveolar crest loses its distinct sharp appearance and becomes ***blunted.***
- The bony margin becomes diffuse and irregular, and may show areas of localized erosion.
- In the incisor regions, there will be a blunting of the alveolar crests. In the premolar- and molar regions, there may also be loss of the normally sharp angle between the lamina dura and the alveolar crest.

Stage 3: Established periodontitis

- Clinically seen as pocket formation.
- Radiographically, the bony destruction usually extends to the buccal or lingual alveolar bony plate or both.

- There may also ***be horizontal or vertical defects***.
- Horizontal bone loss is used to describe the radiographic appearance of the loss of bone height in the region of ***several adjacent teeth***.
- Horizontal bone loss may be classified as mild (less than 10% bone loss), moderate (10–30%), or severe (>30%) depending on the extent of bone loss.
- In horizontal bone loss, both the buccal and lingual plates of bone as well as the interdental bone have been resorbed.
- Vertical bone defects also called as proximal ***intrabony defects.*** Radiographically, the vertical bone defect is generally "V shaped" and sharply outlined.
- ***Inconsistent bony margin*** is result of an uneven resorption of the alveolar cortical plate on lingual or facial surfaces, a feature of established periodontitis.

Stage 4: Advanced periodontal lesions

- Its a periodontal disease, bone loss is extensive.
- Furcation exposure (radiolucent area at the region of the furcation) starts from bone loss at the furcation of multirooted teeth.
- Furcation involvement is indicated ***by triangular radiolucency in the bifurcation area of mandibular first and second molars.***

Periodontal Abscess

It appears as *distinct radiolucency along the lateral aspect of the root.* However radiograph alone should not be considered for diagnosing periodontal abscess because the findings are often atypical due to:

- In early stage, it does not reveal any change.
- Abscess in the soft tissue wall of the periodontal pocket are less likely to demonstrate changes.
- Abscess on the facial and lingual aspect of the root are often obscured by the density of roots. Only interproximal location can be appreciated.
- The morphological changes on the bone may also give a false positive result.
- If sinus orifice is seen in the associated tooth a gutta percha point is placed through the sinus might locate the source of abscess in the radiograph.

Trauma from Occlusion

- Evidence of loss of lamina dura in the apices, furcations and marginal areas with thickening of PDL space (Fig. 28).
- Angular bone loss is characteristic feature.
- Cervical V shaped (angular bone loss), thickening of lamina dura, increase in density or apical bone sclerosis signs reflect an attempt by the periodontal tissues adapt by the new functional demand.

Alveolar Dehiscence

- Alveolar dehiscence exists when the alveolar cortical bone is resorbed along the entire length of the root (Fig. 29).
- Radiographically, there will be a radiolucency surrounding the affected root.

Furcation Involvement

Extension of bone loss between the roots of mutirooted teeth and eliminating the bone covering the root in that region. It is visible as radiolucency at the point of division.

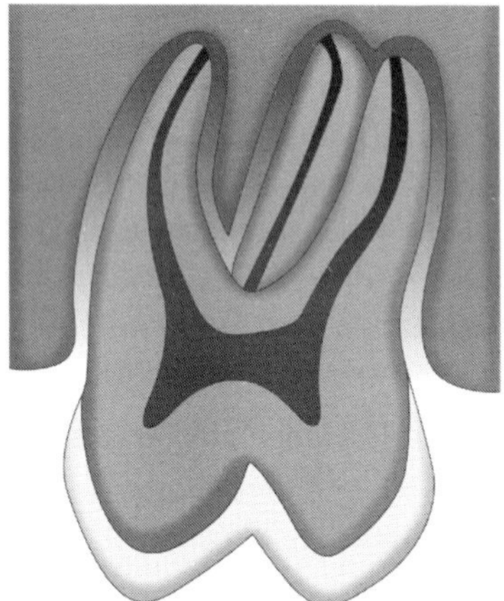

Fig. 28: Loss of lamina dura and widening of periodontal ligament space around the entire root structure.

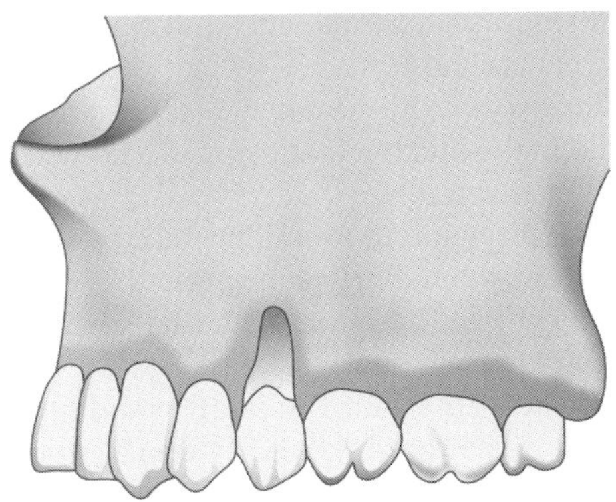

Fig. 29: Alveolar dehiscence.

Restorative Materials

According to Radiographic Density (Beginning with Most Radiopaque)

Group 1: Gold alloys, amalgam, silver.
Group 2: Gutta percha, zinc phosphate, or other base materials, composite with opacifier, rubber base impression material, calcium hydroxide group with opacifier.
Group 3: Porcelain.
Group 4: **Radiolucent**—calcium hydroxide, composite, resin.

Base Materials

Zinc phosphate cement and zinc oxide-eugenol paste, are used as cavity liners to protect the pulp of the tooth and appear as radiopaque. (If compared with amalgam, base material appears less radiodense).

Gutta Percha Cone

A radiopaque cone used for restoring pulp canal.

RC Filling

Radiopaque material placed into the root canal for obturation and sealing the canal space.

Post and Core Restoration

Seen in endodontically treated teeth. Cast metal appears radiopaque as amalgam or gold. The core portion of the restoration resembles the prepped portion of a tooth crown, and the post portion extends into the pulp canal (Fig. 30).

Acrylic Restoration

Often used as an interim or temporary crown or filling. Of all nonmetallic restorations, acrylic is the least dense and appears radiolucent or barely visible on a dental radiograph.

Splint

A stainless steel wire used for immobilization to support weak teeth which appears to the radiopaque (Fig. 31).

Pontic

Artificial tooth suspended from the retainer casting, occupies the space formerly filled by the crown of a natural tooth.

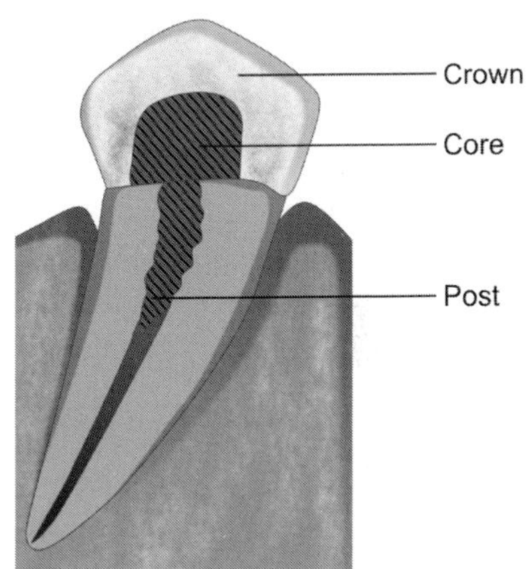

Fig. 30: Post and core restoration.

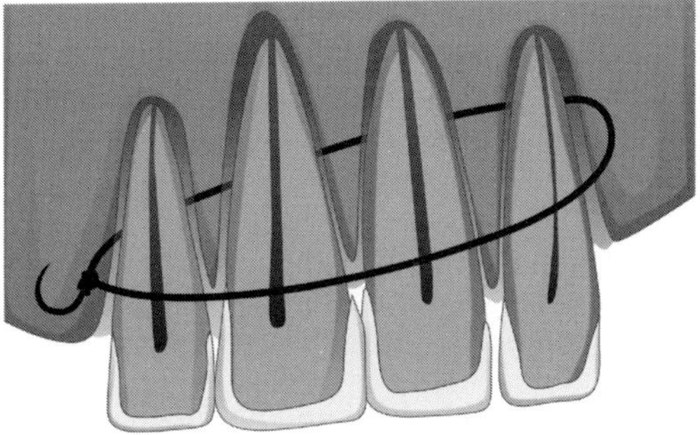

Fig. 31: Splint.

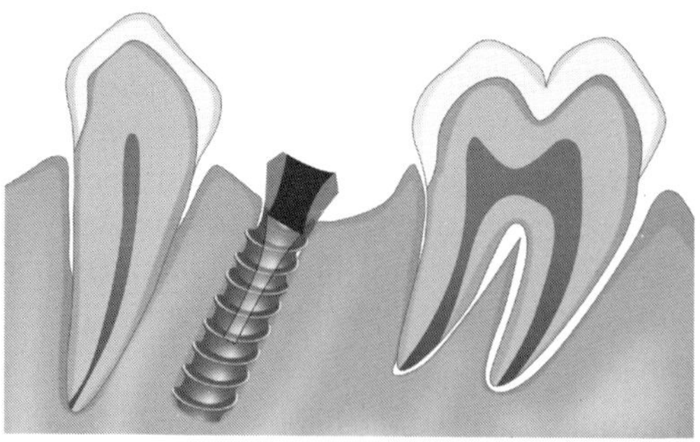

Fig. 32: Fixture and abutment.

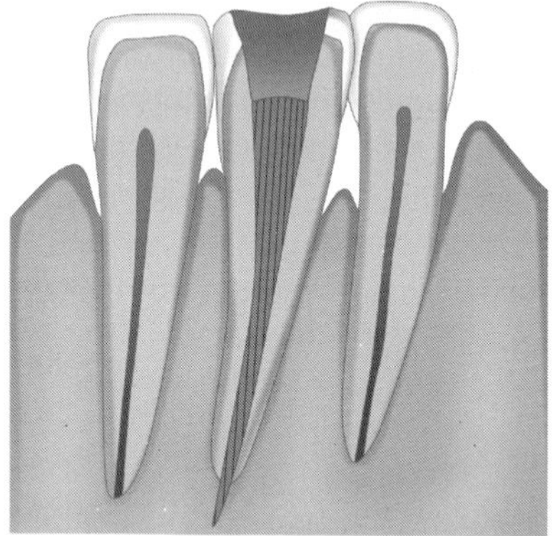

Fig. 33: Overfilled root canal.

Implant

A flat screw shaped device that pierces in alveolar process (that supports prosthesis) (Fig. 32).

Overfilling

Radiopaque root canal filling extending beyond the apical foramen. Inference: The root canal space completely obturated.

Overextension

Root canal filling extending beyond the apical foramen often result in failure to create an apical stop during instrumentation indicates that the root canal space is not completely obturated (Fig. 33).

Developmental Defects and Anomalies

Supernumerary teeth: These can cause crowding problems and are often associated with unerupted permanent tooth or malposed permanent tooth.

Dilaceration: It is defined as a deviation or bend in the linear relationship of a crown of a tooth to its root.

- The direction of root dilacerations should be considered in 2 planes, and they can be categorized as mesial, distal, labial/buccal, or palatal/lingual.
- If the roots bend mesially or distally, the dilaceration is clearly apparent on a periapical radiograph. However, when the dilaceration is toward the labial/buccal or palatal/lingual, the X-ray beam passes through the deflected portion of the root in an approximately parallel direction.
- The dilacerated portion then appears at the apical end of the unaltered root as a rounded opaque area with a dark "spot" in its center that is caused by the apical foramen of the root canal (this appearance is similar to a bull's eye or a target) (Fig. 34).
- The periodontal ligament space around the dilacerated portion of the root might be seen as a radiolucent halo, and the radiopacity of this segment of the root is usually greater than the rest of the root as a result of the increased thickness of tooth structure that the X-rays have to pass through. In some cases, especially in the maxilla, the geometry of the projections may stop the recognition of a dilaceration.

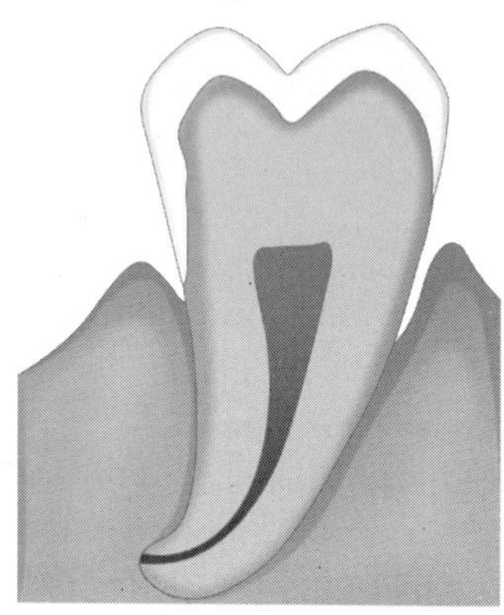

Fig. 34: Dilacerated root.

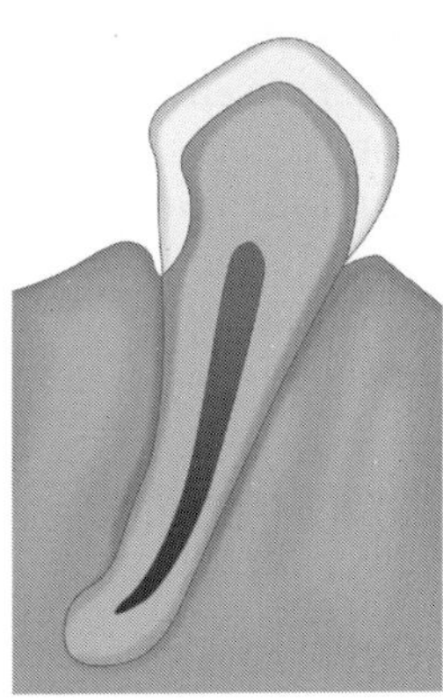

Fig. 35: Ankylosed tooth.

Ankylosis

Ankylosis of teeth is the fusion of the tooth to the bone, preventing the tooth from erupting. Radiographically, there is obliteration of periodontal ligament space suggestive of fusion between root, cementum and the alveolar bone (Fig. 35). Conventional radiographic diagnosis is however limited when ankylosis occurs in the lingual, labial and interradicular areas.

Enamel Hypoplasia

It appears as radiolucent area with radiopaque margins.

Amelogenesis Impefecta

Hypoplastic form: The crowns of the teeth either have very thin enamel or lack enamel completely.
Hypocalcified form: Enamel is less radiopaque than dentin on radiographs.
Hypomaturative form: Radiodensity of enamel is approximately the same as that of dentin.

Dentinogenesis Imperfecta

Radiographically, the teeth have bulbous crowns with constricted short roots. Initially, pulp chambers may be abnormally wide and resemble "shell teeth," but they will progressively obliterate.

Odontome

Radiological features manifest as a dense radioopaque lesion surrounded by a thin radiolucent halo corresponding to the connective tissue capsule.

Three developmental stages can be identified based on the radiological features and degree of calcification of the lesion at the time of diagnosis.

1. The first stage is characterized by radiotransparency due to the absence of dental tissue calcification.
2. The second or intermediate stage presents partial calcification.
3. The third or classically radiopaque stage exhibits significant calcification surrounded by a radiolucent halo.

Compound odontomas: Show an irregular radiopaque image with variations in contour and size, composed of multiple radiopacities corresponding to the so-called denticles (mini teeth).
Complex odontoma: Shows radiopacity which is not specific for tooth structure but resembling a disorganized, irregular single or multiple mass.

Fracture

Radiographic Features

Sharp radiolucent line within the anatomic boundaries. Deviation from normal anatomic outline.

- Discontinuity in the cortical border or step formation.
- In few situations increased density.
- A crown fracture that exposes the pulp chamber will result in endodontic disease.
- When this occurs the extent of pathology should be evaluated with a dental radiograph, blunt trauma may result in damage to the pulp without fracturing the tooth.
- A dental radiograph should be made of any tooth that is discolored from pulp hemorrhage.

Root Fracture

- **Vertical root fractures** (VRF) are longitudinal fractures that begin at the roots of teeth; these fractures occur primarily in the buccolingual plane (Fig. 36).

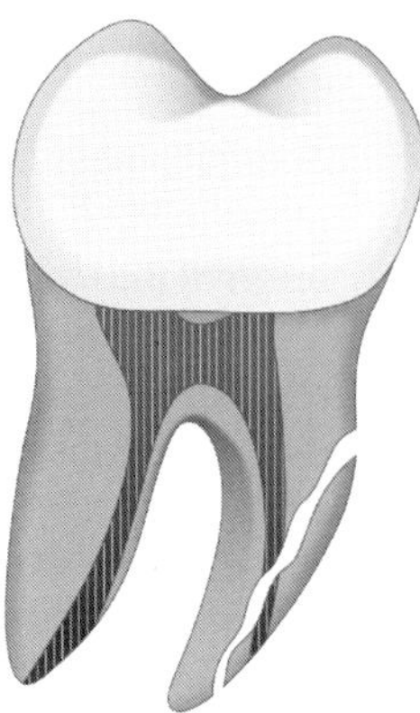

Fig. 36: Root fracture.

- VRFs in teeth without endodontic treatment are relatively common; they are more common in the posterior teeth of people over 40 years of age and may be caused by excessive forces from mastication or occlusion.
- Symptoms are usually minimal or absent in the early stages. With time, dull pain on mastication may develop as a result of the separation of the fractured root segments. Hence, careful radiographic evaluation is necessary when a patient reports with symptom of pain in a clinically sound tooth.
- *One limitation of the intraoral radiographs is the absence of radiographic signs when the X-ray beam is not parallel to the plane of the fracture.*
- *The images taken from three different angulations could increase detection ability in the intraoral images as vertical translucent line.*

Luxation

Total displacement of a tooth from its original position in the alveolus as a result of trauma.

Extrusive Luxation

A partial axial displacement of the tooth out of its socket.

Impaction

Partially or completely unerupted tooth is known as impacted tooth.

Complete impaction: Crown and root structures of 3rd molar are entirely below the level of alveolar crest.

Partial impaction: Portion of 3rd molar crown is above the alveolar crest.

An impacted tooth should be radiographically evaluated for position:

- Angulation
- Relation with adjacent vital structures like mandibular canal
- Root curvature
- Pathological changes

Pell and Gregory classification for mandibular third molar position in relation to ramus:

- **Class I:** Sufficient amount of space between distal aspect of second molar crown and ramus of mandible to accommodate the mesiodistal diameter of the third molar crown (Fig. 37).
- **Class II:** The space between distal aspect of second molar crown and ramus of mandible is insufficient to accommodate the mesiodistal diameter of the third molar crown (Fig. 37).
- **Class III:** All or most root of the third molar is on the ramus (Fig. 37).

Angulation of impacted teeth may be (Fig. 38):

- **Mesioangular:** Long axix of the crown 3rd molar is tilted mesial to the long axis of 2nd molar and below the level of occlusal plane.
- **Distoangular:** Long axix of the crown 3rd molar is tilted distal to the long axis of 2nd molar and below the level of occlusal plane.
- **Vertical:** Long axix of the crown 3rd molar is parallel to the long axis of 2nd molar and below the level of occlusal plane
- **Horizontal:** Long axix of the crown 3rd molar is perpendicular to the long axis of 2nd molar and below the level of occlusal plane.

Pell and Gregory classification for impacted maxillary third molar (Based on the relative depth of the impacted maxillary third molar in bone)

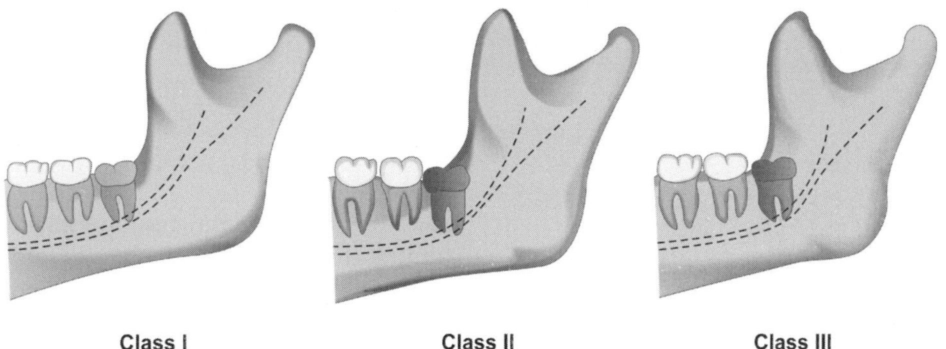

Fig. 37: Pell and Gregory classification of impaction in relation to ramus.

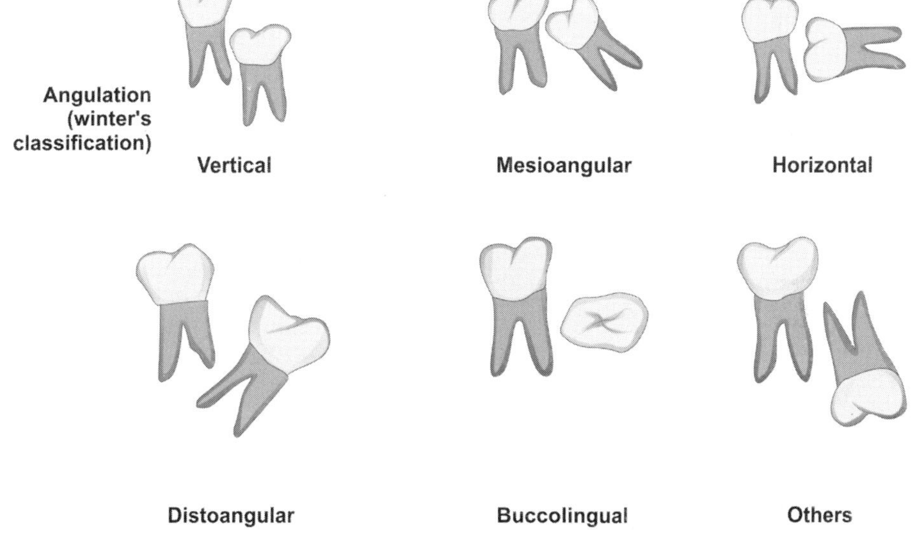

Fig. 38: Classification of impaction based on the crown angulation.

Class A: The lowest portion of the crown of the impacted maxillary third molar is on a line with the occlusal plane of the second molar.

Class B: The lowest portion of the crown of the impacted maxillary third molar is between the occlusal plane of the second molar and the cervical line.

Class C: The lowest portion of the crown of the impacted maxillary third molar is at or above the cervical line of the second molar.

Classification for maxillary canine impaction (Fig. 39)

- Horizontal
- Vertical
- Semivertical

Imagined Caries-Misinterpretation

Cervical Burnout

- A sharply defined radiolucent wedge at the alveolar bone crest may resemble

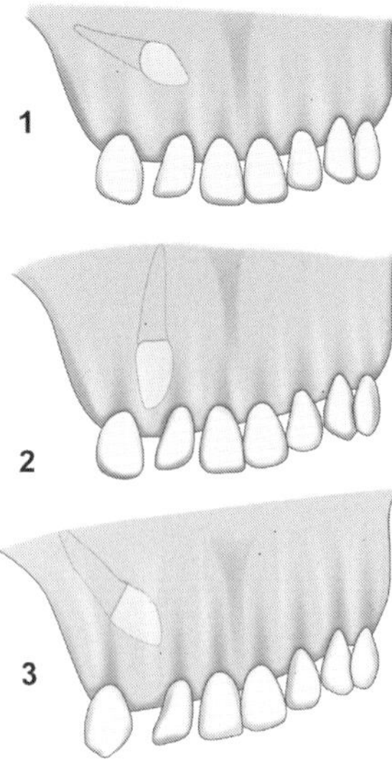

Fig. 39: Maxillary canine impaction.

interproximal or cemental caries burnout due to excessive exposure is called ***peripheral or cervical burnout.***

- Cervical burnout should not be mistaken for root caries or with caries under the proximal step of a Class II restoration.
- ***The final confirmation*** must be done clinically with the use of an explorer.
- A second radiograph made with a slightly different X-ray beam angulation and a change in exposure factors will enable the clinician to differentiate a cervical burnout from root caries.

Mach Band Effect

An optical illusion which produces artificial radiolucent areas in dentinal peaks bounded by occlusal and proximal enamel seen especially in premolar but also in molar teeth.

- Radiolucent restorations and linings may be mistaken for caries but these usually have clearly demarcated outlines and can be confirmed clinically.
- Developmental defects in enamel hypoplasia may appear as radiolucent dots outline of all visible changes on a radiograph should be carefully visualized to mark it as either.
  - Anatomical landmark
  - Pathological finding
  - Superimposed or overlapped structures
  - Artifact due to processing or technical error.

Aunty Minnie

The term **"Aunt Minnie"** describes an imaging finding that is ***both perfectly obvious and pathognomonic of a disease***. In other word if it looks like your aunt Minnie then it is your aunt Minnie, e.g. recurrent pericoronitis.

Uncle Fred: Represents a ***dull and unexciting abnormality*** that is frequently seen in a radiograph, e.g. attrition.

Cousin harry represents a ***rare abnormality which is uncommon*** to be noticed by a physician but like to see it, e.g. dentigerous cyst.

Why cannot you depend on radiographs alone to determine pulpal exposure to caries?

- Overangulation can create the appearance of pulpal exposure.
- "Burnout" of dentin between pulp and the carious lesion enlarges the lesion.
- Superimposition of caries over the pulp gives the illusion of pulpal invasion.

What are some developmental-acquired defects that might appear as caries?

- Defects in tooth structure often appear radiolucent.
- Hypoplastic defects in the enamel will mimic caries.
- Abrasion, especially toothbrush abrasion will mimic cervical caries.
- Severe attrition may mimic occlusal caries.

INTERPRETATION AND REPORTING

Periapical Abscess (Fig. 40)

Teeth seen: 45,46,47 and partial image of 48.

Anatomical landmarks: Nil.

Anatomical structures: Crown, root, pulp chamber, pulp canal and periapical region, crestal bone, trabecular pattern are normal in 45 and 47.

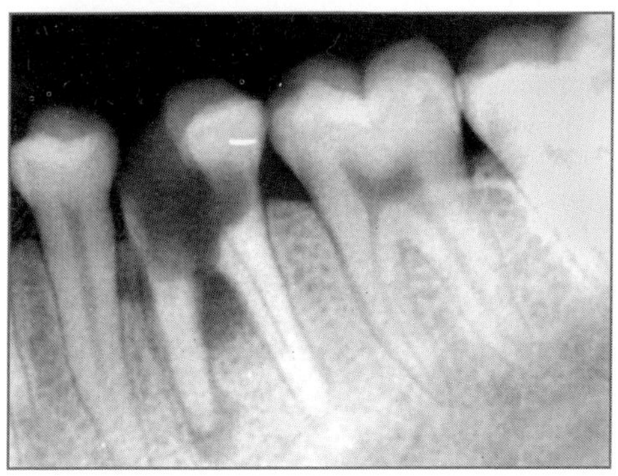
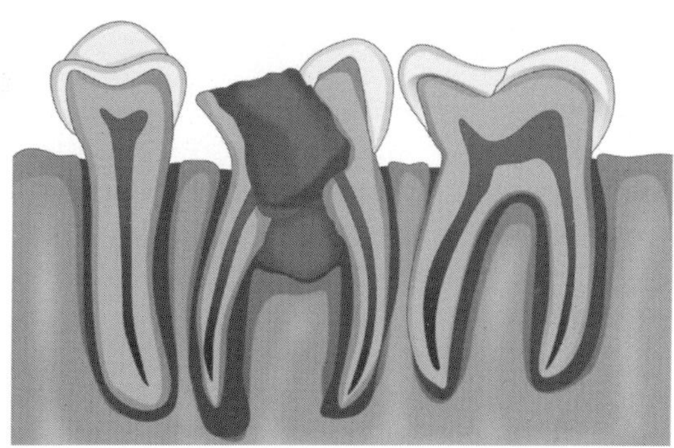

Fig. 40: Periapical abscess.

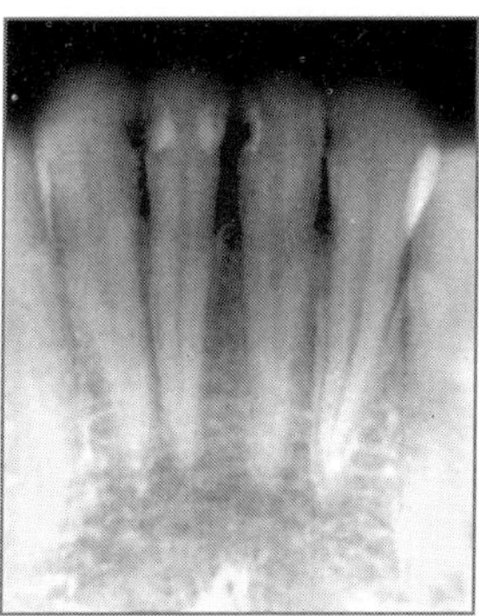
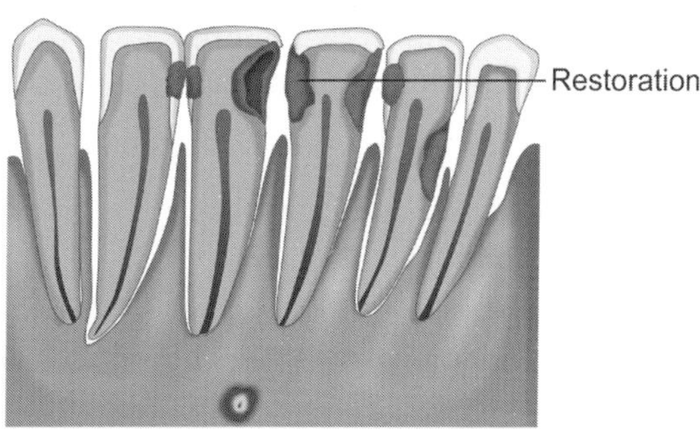

Fig. 41: Secondary caries.

Pathological Interpretation

- Radiolucency evident on coronal structure of 46 with loss of mesiolingual and mesio-buccal cusp architecture involving enamel, dentin and pulp.
- Periphery of the radiolucency is diffused extending towards pulp chamber of 46.
- Pulp canal is partially obliterated in mesial and distal root of 46.
- Loss of lamina dura is evident on the mesial and distal root of 46.
- PDL space is widened with distinct radiolucency in 46.
- A triangular radiolucency evident on the bifurcation area of 46 suggestive of furcation involvement.

Radiodiagnosis

Dental caries in 46 with periapical abscess.

Secondary Caries (Fig. 41)

Teeth seen: 31, 32, 41, 42 and partial image of 33 and 43.

Anatomical landmarks: Nutrient canal, genial tubercle, lingual foramen.

Pathological Interpretation

- Radiolucency evident on the mesial aspect of the coronal structure of 31 with thin group 2 radiopaque restorative boundary suggesting dislodged restorative material.
- Diffused radiolucency evident immediately next to the radiopaque restorative material involving pulp of 31.
- Lamina dura intact with normal PDL space, no periapical changes evident in 31.
- Group 2 restorative material evident on the mesial and distal surface of the coronal

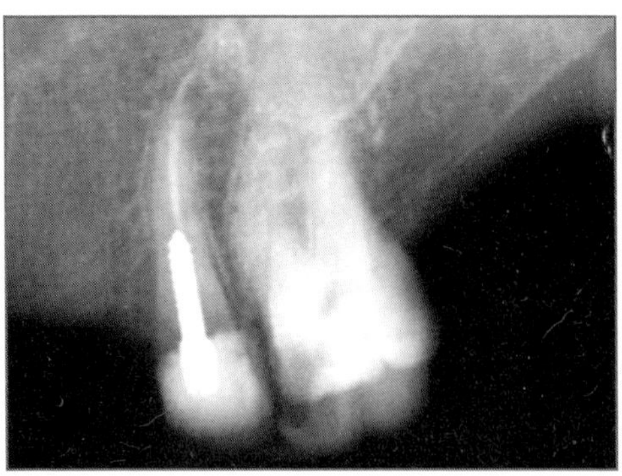

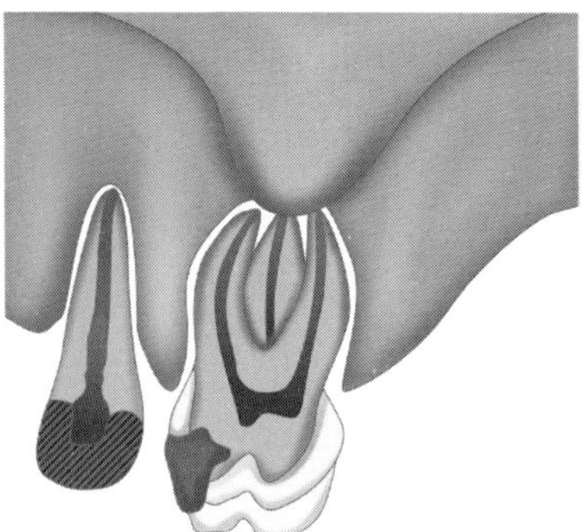

Fig. 42: Post and core restoration in premolar.

structure with restorative boundaries close to pulp in 41.

- ❖ Pulp canal is normal with intact lamina dura and PDL space, no periapical changes evident in 41.
- ❖ Radiolucency evident on the mesial surface of the coronal portion of 32 and 42 involving enamel.

Radiodiagnosis

- ❖ Secondary caries with pulpal involvement in 31.
- ❖ Restored crown in 41 without pulpal involvement.
- ❖ Enamel caries in 32 and 42.

Post and Core (Fig. 42)

Teeth seen: 25, 26

Anatomical structures: Edentulous region mesial to 25 and distal to 26 with normal alveolar bone pattern.

Anatomical landmarks: Zygoma

Pathological Interpretation

- ❖ Prefabricated metal post fitted and cemented into the pulp chamber and pulp canal of 25 which is continued with group 2 radiodense restorative material, probably gutta pecha on the apical third of 25, extending a bit beyond the apical foramen indicating complete obturation.
- ❖ Group 2 radiodense restorative material evident on the entire coronal structure indicating poor resteration.
- ❖ No periapical bone resorption evident in 25.
- ❖ Diffused radiolucency evident in mesio-proximal aspect of 26 involving both buccal-and palatal cusp. The radiolucency expanding from enamel towards dentin and mesial pulp horn. Lamina dura is intact with normal PDL space, no periapical bone resorption evident.

Radiodiagnosis

- ❖ Post and core restoration in 25.
- ❖ Proximal caries 26 with pulpal involvement.

Chronic Periodontitis (Fig. 43)

Teeth seen: 13,14,15

Anatomical structure: Crest of alveolar ridge distal to 15 in line parallel to apical third of root structure.

Anatomical landmarks: Zygoma, floor of maxillary sinus, maxillary sinus with septum.

Pathological Interpretation

- ❖ Radiolucent area evident on the occlusal surface of 14, 15 bounded by occlusal and proximal radiolucency of enamel.
- ❖ Radiolucency evident in the inter-radicular region between 13-14 and 14-15 indicating receeding crestal bone height. The bone recession extents from CEJ to apical third of root in distal aspect of 13 and mesial and distal aspect of 14 and 15.
- ❖ Loss of lamina dura evident in 14, 15 with irregular widening of PDL space along the entire root.

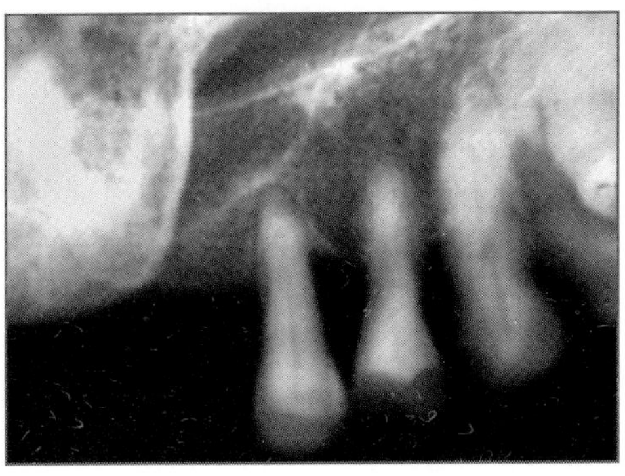

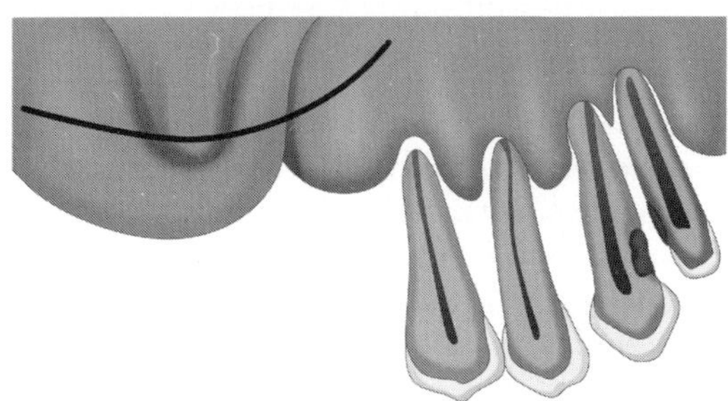

Fig. 43: Chronic periodontitis—established stage.

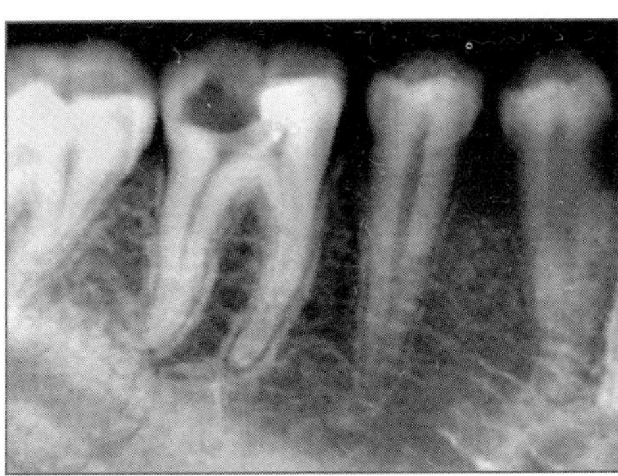

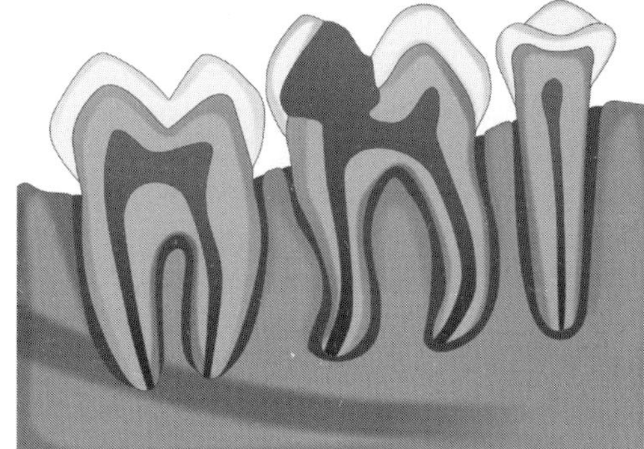

Fig. 44: Apical periodontitis.

- Cortical bone resorption in uneven suggesting inconsistent bony margin in 13, 14, 15 region.

Radiodiagnosis

- Mach band effect 14,15
- Chronic periodontitis (Stage 2: Established periodontitis).

Dental Caries with Apical Periodontitis (Fig. 44)

Teeth seen: 44, 45, 46 and partial image of 47
Anatomical landmarks: NIL
Anatomical structures: Crown, root, pulp chamber, pulp canal and periapical region, crestal bone, trabecular pattern are normal in 45 and 44.

Pathological Interpretation

- A well-defined radiolucency evident on the occlusal and distobuccal of 46 which is sharply demarcated from the surrounding tooth structure with a loss of distobuccal cuspal morphology evident.
- The radiolucency extends to involve the pulp chamber. Lamina dura is intact on mesial root with discontinuity evident on apical region of distal root of 46. PDL space is thickened in the apical region of mesial root of 46.
- Furcal area is normal with no evidence of resorption.

Radiodiagnosis

DC in 46 with apical periodontitis.

Root Stump (Fig. 45)

Teeth seen: 44, 45 ,47 and partial image of 48.
Anatomical landmarks: NIL
Anatomical structures: Crown, root, pulp chamber, pulp canal and periapical region, crestal bone, trabecular pattern are normal in 44, 45 and 47.

Pathological Interpretation

- Radiolucency evident in between 45 and 47 along the alveolar region suggesting a loss of coronal structure of 46, two distal root structures evident with the partial obliteration of the pulp canal and complete loss of lamina dura evident at the alveolar bone level suggesting the mesial and distal root structure of 46.
- The cervical end of root structures shows an irregular outline with hazy radiolucency indicating a sign of resorption.

Radiodiagnosis

Root stump 46.

Impaction (Fig. 46)

Teeth seen: 37, 38, partial image of 36.
Anatomical landmarks: Inferior alveolar canal, external oblique ridge.

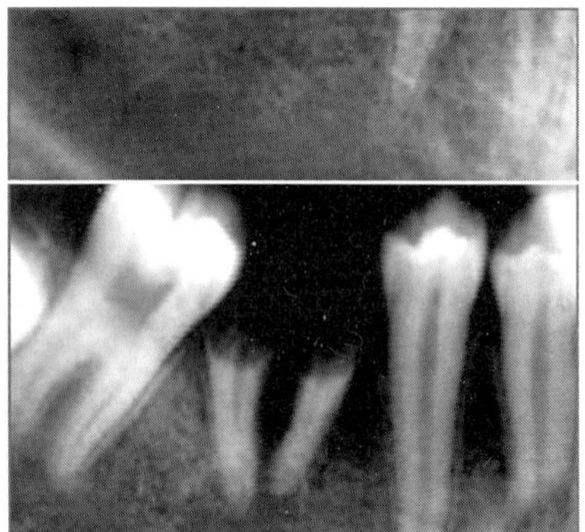

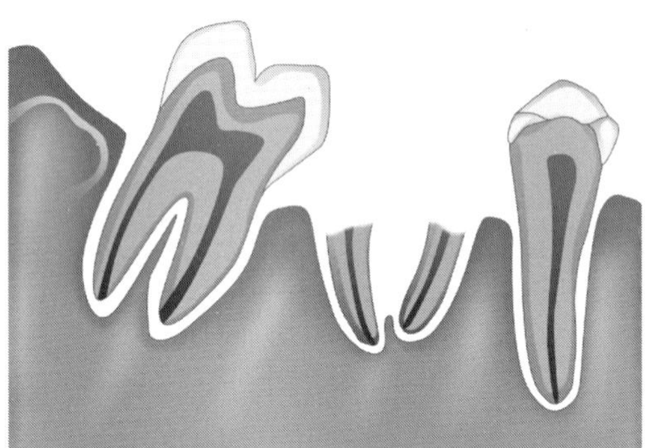

Fig. 45: Root stump.

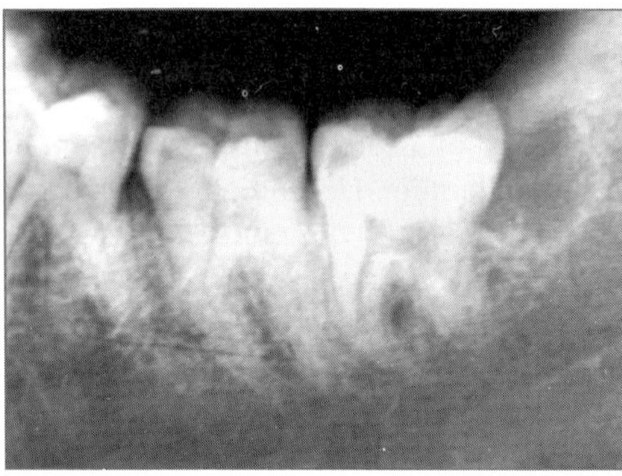

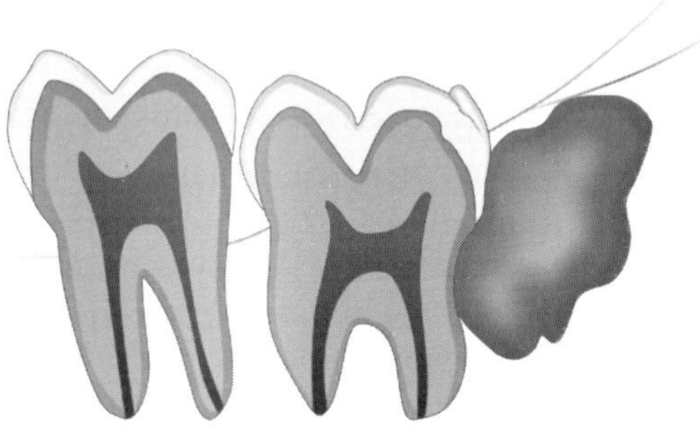

Fig. 46: Impacted 3rd molar.

Anatomical structures: Crown, root, pulp chamber, pulp canal and periapical region, crestal bone, trabecular pattern are normal in 45 and 47.

Pathological Interpretation

- Distal aspect of the crown of 38 is engorging on the ramus and is covered by alveolar crest.
- The distal aspect of coronal portion of 48 is impinging on the ascending ramus.
- No pulpal changes evident.
- Distal root apexogenesis is incomplete.

Radiodiagnosis

Pell and Geogrey Class II, Distoangular Impaction.

Canine Impaction (Fig. 47)

Teeth seen: 63, 24, partial image of 22.
Anatomical landmarks: Nil
Anatomical structures: Crown, root, pulp chamber, pulp canal and periapical region, crestal bone, trabecular pattern are normal in 45 and 47.

Pathological Interpretation

- Radiopaque orthodontic band is evident at the cuspal surface of 24.
- Tiny tooth structure revealing enamel, dentin and pulp chamber suggesting crown of 63, loss of root structure evident in 63 with blunted cervical 3rd.
- A tooth structure with complete formation of crown and root morphology is evident at the alveolar bone level, positioned horizontally in relation roots of 24 and 22.
- No bony changes evident in the region.

Radiodiagnosis

- Retained 63 with resorbed roots.
- Impacted 23.

Odontome (Fig. 48)

Teeth seen: 21, 22, partial image of 24, 25.
Anatomical landmarks: Nil
Anatomical structures: Crown, root, pulp chamber, pulp canal and periapical region, crestal bone, trabecular pattern are normal in 21 and 22.

Pathological Interpretation

- Multiple tiny radiopaque structures evident on the alveolar crest.
- A tooth structure resembling the morphology of crown evident at the alveolar bone level along the roots of 21, 22 and the

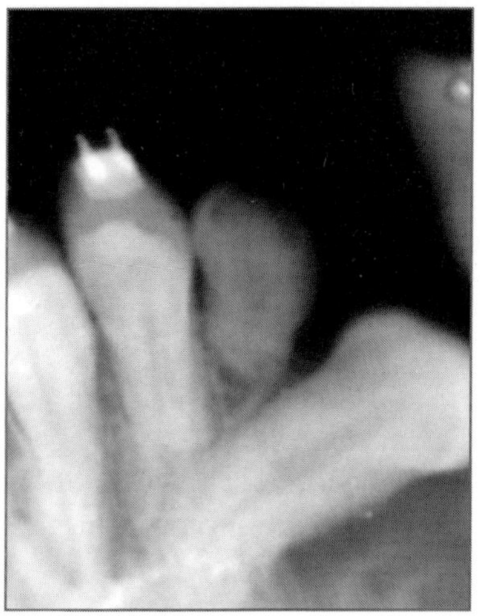

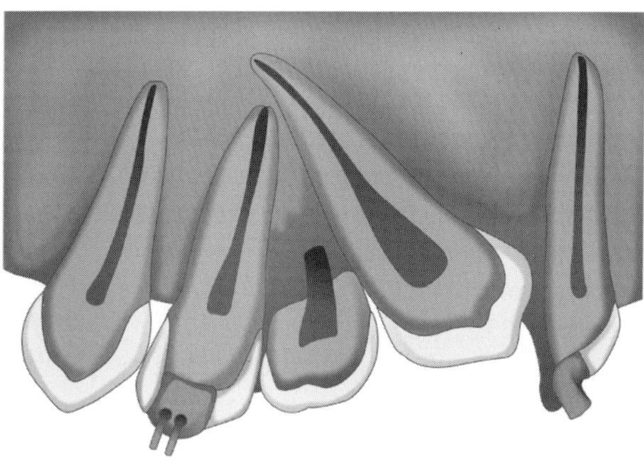

Fig. 47: Semivertical Impaction of maxillary canine.

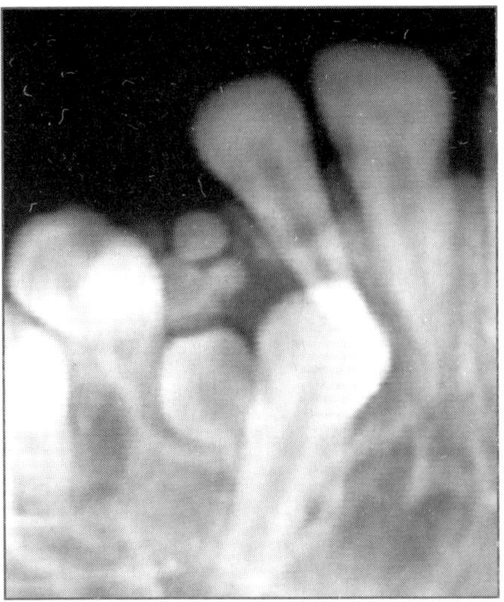
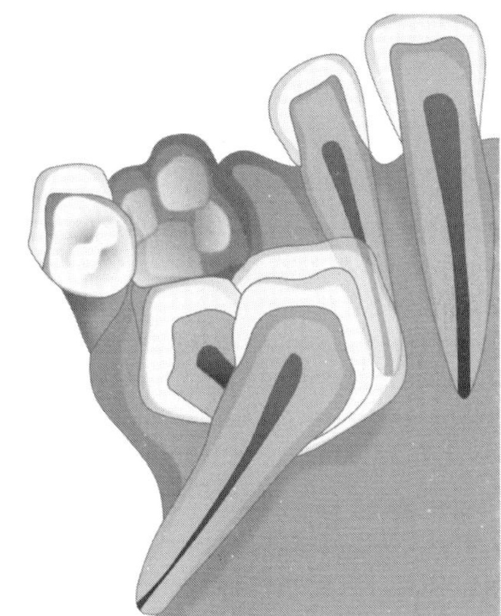

Fig. 48: Odontome.

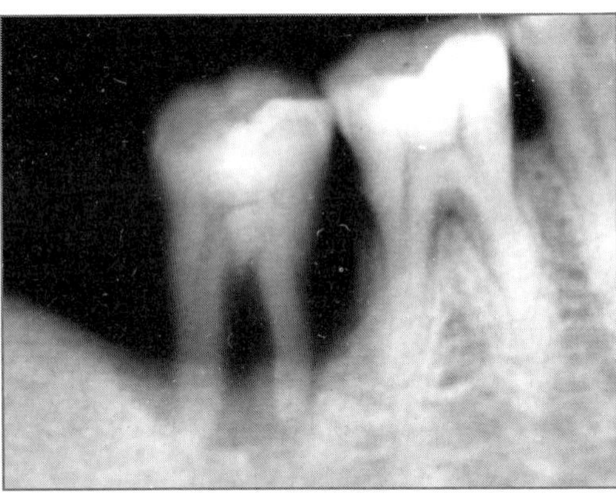
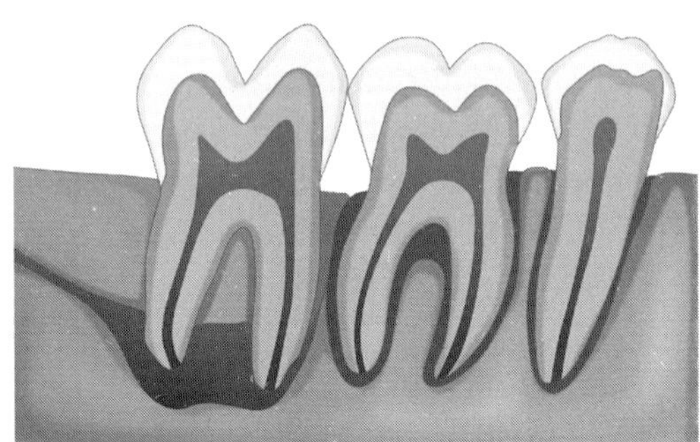

Fig. 49: Established chronic periodontitis.

incisal 3rd of the root apex of 22 suggesting impacted 23 positioned semivertically.

- A tiny radiopaque structure resembling the enamel, dentin and pulp of a crown structure evident overlapping the proximal surface of cervical 3rd of root of the impacted 23.
- Well-defined radiolucency surrounded by a radiopaque cortication is seen encircling impacted 23 and the adjacent crown like structure of multiple tiny radiopaque structures suggesting follicular space.

Radiodiagnosis

Odontome with impacted 23 with supernumerary teeth.

Established Chronic Periodontits (Fig. 49)

Teeth seen: 46, 47 and partial image of 45.
Anatomical landmarks: NIL
Anatomical structures: Crown, root, pulp chamber, pulp canal are normal in 45.

Pathological Interpretation

- Extensive crestal bone loss is evident between 46 and 47 in obtuse angle suggesting

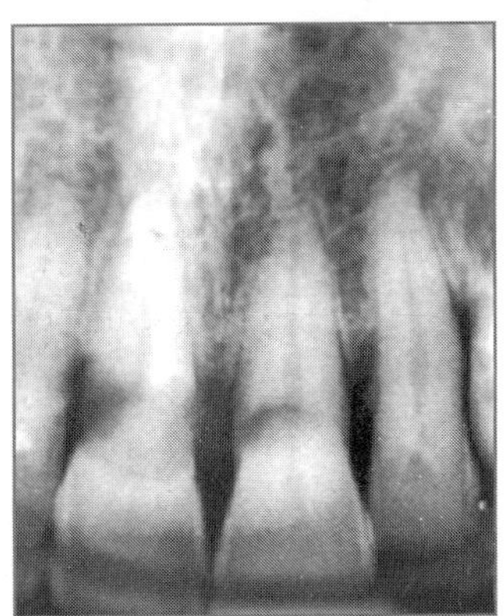
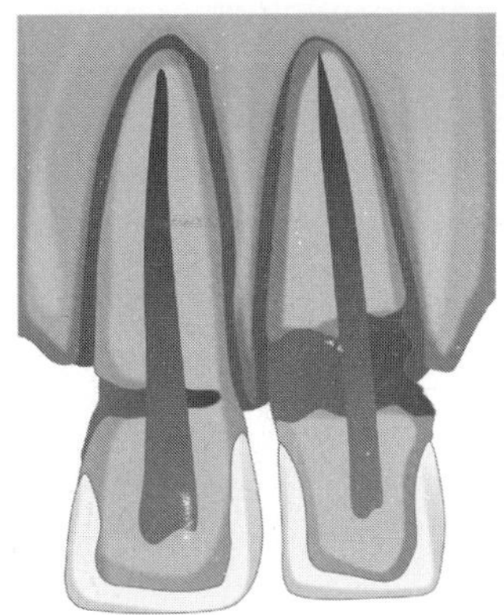

Fig. 50: Internal resorption.

vertical bone defect with distal aspect of 47 extending into root apex.

- Triangular radiolucency evident in the bifurcation area of 47.
- Resorption changes also evident in the bifurcation area of 46.
- No pulpal changes evident.
- Thickening of PDL space evident at the mesial and distal roots of 46, 47.

Radiodiagnosis

Chronic periodontitis: 46,47 (established stage or Stage IV).

Internal Resorption (Fig. 50)

Teeth seen: 11, 12 and partial image of 22.
Anatomical landmarks: Floor of nasal fossa, intermaxillary suture, nasal septum, shadow of upper lip.
Anatomical structures: Crown, root, pulp chamber, pulp canal and trabecular pattern are normal in 22.

Pathological Interpretation

- Radiolucency evident at the incisal edge of 11, 21 with evidence of loss of normal enamel structure in the incisal and middle 3rd region of 11, 21.
- Diffuse semicircular radiolucency evident in the cervial 3rd root of 11 involving pulp canal.
- Diffuse scooped out radiolucency evident on distoproximal aspect of cervical root portion of 21.
- Radiolucency expanding towards pulp. Incomplete oblieteraion of pulp canal evident in cervical and apical 3rd root of 21.
- Discontinuity of lamina dura and widening of PDL space in 21.
- Crestal bone loss evident between 21 and 22 extending upto the middle 3rd of roots of 21 and 22.

Radiodiagnosis

- Internal resortption in 11.
- Root caries in 21 with apical periodontitis.

Incomplete Obturation with Periapical Abcess (Fig. 51)

Teeth seen: 45,46, 47 and partial image of 48.
Anatomical landmarks: NIL

Pathological Interpretation

- Radiolucency evident on the occlusal surface of 46. Group I radiopaque restorative material evient on pulp chamber of 46 and Group II restorative material evident in the mesial-and distal canal of 46.
- Lateral adaptation of restorative material is incomplete in the distal root of 46.
- Well-defined radiolucency evident in the periapical region of distal root of 46 suggesting bone resorption.

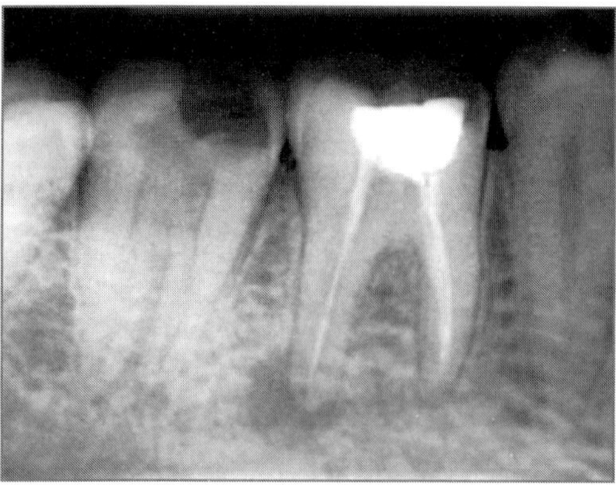
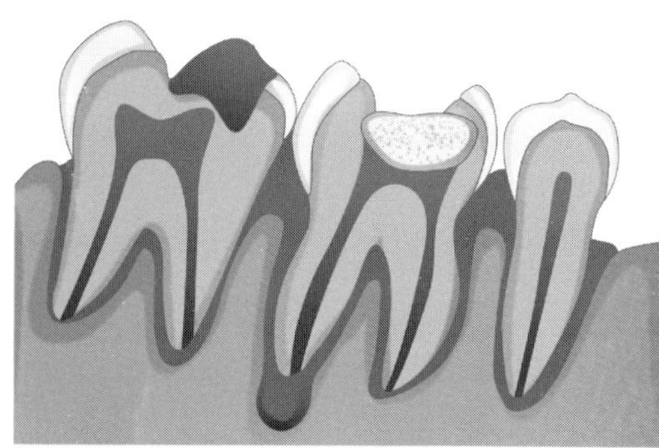

Fig. 51: Incomplete obturation with periapical abscess.

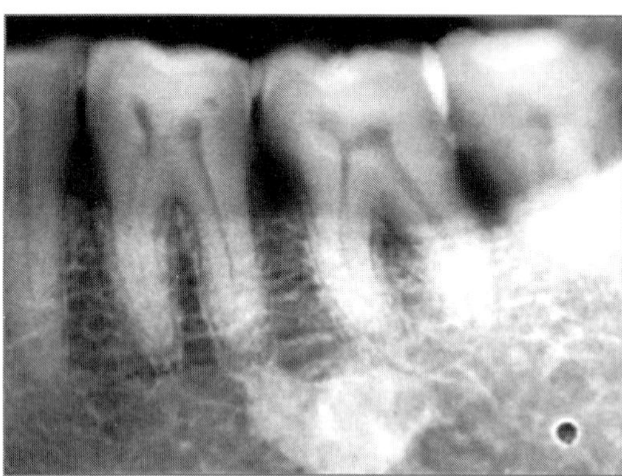
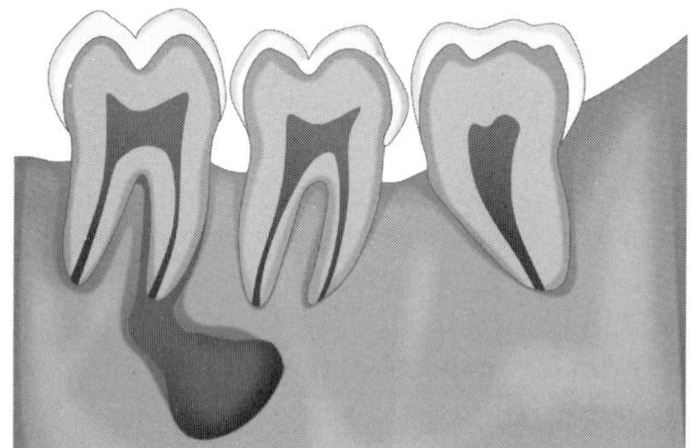

Fig. 52: Idiopathic osteosclerosis.

- Well-defined radiolucency evident on the crown structure of 47 involving enamel, dentin and pulp. The radiolucency is well demarcated from surrounding enamel and dentin.
- Irregular thickening of PDL space evident in apical region and furcal area of 47.

Radiodiagnosis

- Incompeletely obturated distal canal in 46 with periapical abscess.
- Facial/lingual caries in 47 with apical periodontitis.

Idiopathic Osteosclerosis (Fig. 52)

Teeth seen: 36, 37, and partial image of 35, 34.
Anatomical landmarks: NIL
Anatomical structures: Crown, root, pulp chamber, pulp canal and periapical region, trabecular pattern are normal in 36 and 35.

Pathological Interpretation

- Crestal bone loss evident between the roots of 35–36, and 36–37, bone reduction is perpendicular to CEJ of 35, 36 and 37. No pulpal or periapical changes evident in 35-37 region.
- Lamina dura intact with normal appearance of PDL space.
- Well-defined high, dense, homogenous radiopaque structure evident at the alveolar bone level adjacent and apical to roots of 36 and 37.

Radiodiagnosis

Idiopathic osteosclerosis.

Odontome (Fig. 53)

Teeth seen: 71, 32, 41, 42 and partial image of 33, 43.

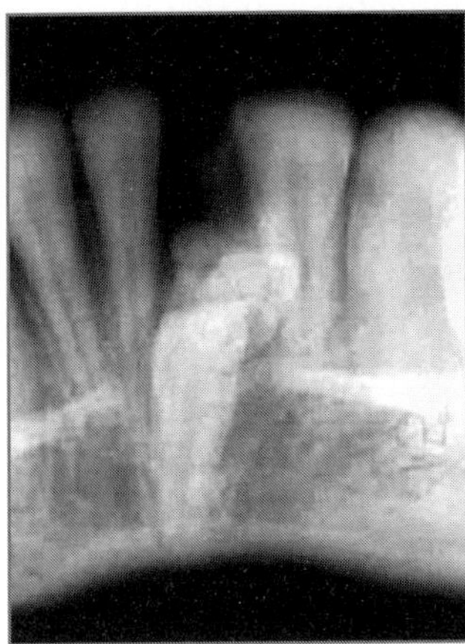
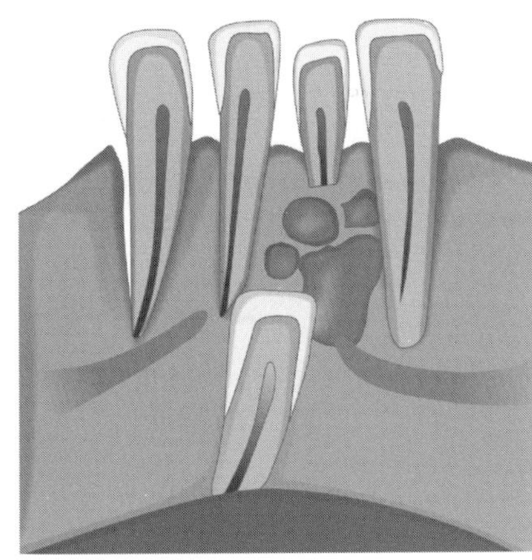

Fig. 53: Odontome and impacted tooth.

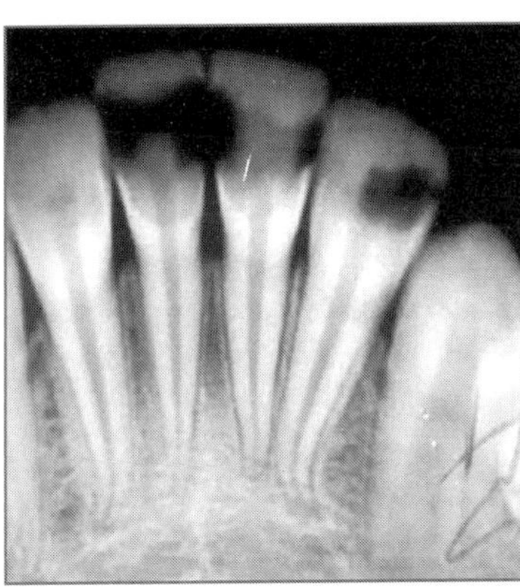
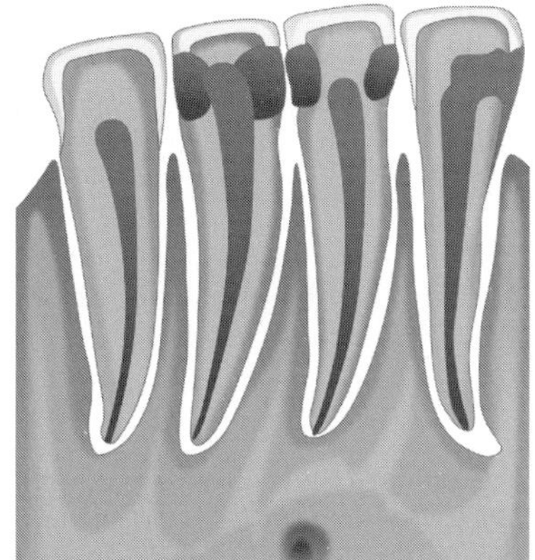

Fig. 54: Apical periodontitis.

Anatomical landmarks: Inferior border of mandible and mental ridge.

Anatomical structures: Crown, root, pulp chamber, pulp canal, periapical region and trabecular pattern are normal in 32, 41, 42, 33 and 43.

Pathological Interpretation

- Loss of apical root structure evident in 31.
- A tooth structure resembling the morphology of an incisor at the alveolar bone level between the root apices of 32 and 41 with normal enamel, dentin and pulp cavity.
- Multiple discrete radiopaque structures evident at the alveolar crest level between 32 and 41, overlapping the root of 41 and crown of impacted 31.
- The radiopaque mass is surrounded by a radiolucent rim.

Radiodiagnosis

- Impacted—31
- Retained—71
- Odontome

Dental Caries with Apical Periodontitis (Fig. 54)

Teeth seen: 32, 31, 41, 42 and partial image of 33, 43.

Anatomical landmarks: NIL

Pathological Interpretation

- Diffuse radiolucency evident on the coronal aspect of 41, involving enamel, dentin and pulp.

- Discontinuity of lamina dura evident in the apical region of 41.
- Mild cortical bone resortpion evident in the periapical region of 41.
- Radiolucency evident on the mesial-and distal proximal surface of crown of 31. On mesial aspect radiolucency is extending towards pulp. On distal aspect it is involving enamel and dentin.
- Discontinuity of lamina dura evident with uniform widening of PDL space along the root of 31.
- Well-defined radiolucency evident on the coronal structure of 32, which is sharply demarcated from the surroundin dentin and expanding to involve pulp.
- Discontinuity of the lamina dura evident at the root apex of PDL space is evident along the distal surface of the root.
- Well-defined radiolucency at the apical region of 32.

Radiodiagnosis

- Dental caries in 41 with apical periodontitis (PAI-4).
- Dental caries in 31 with apical periodontitis (PAI-3).
- Facial/Lingual caries in 32 with periapical abscess (PAI-5).

Restored Tooth with Periapical Abcess (Fig. 55)

Teeth seen: 34, 35, 36, 37.

Anatomical landmarks: NIL

Anatomical structures: Crown, root, pulp chamber, pulp canal and periapical region, crestal bone, trabecular pattern are normal in 34, 35 and 37.

Pathological Interpretation

- Group I restorative material evident on the coronal aspect of 36 involving enamel, dentin and pulp.
- Diffuse radiolucency evident encircling the mesial-and distal roots of 36 indicating bone resorption, discontinuity of lamina dura and thickening of PDL space evident.
- Radiolucency evident at the furcal region of 36.

Radiodiagnosis

Restored 36 with periapical abscess. (PAI-5).

Extrusion (Fig. 56)

Teeth seen: 21, 22, 11 and partial image of 12,23.

Anatomical landmarks: Intermaxillary sutures, floor of nasal fossa, nasal septum, nasal spine.

Anatomical structures: Partial axial displacement of tooth out of socket.

Pathological Interpretation

- Uniform widening of the pulp canal evident as radiolucency with smooth well-defined

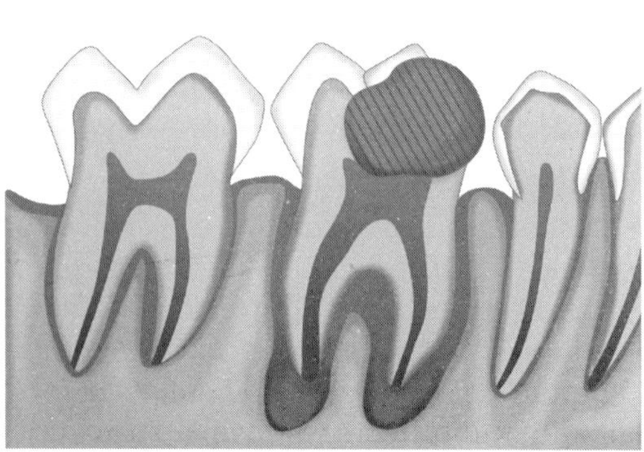

Fig. 55: Restored tooth with periapical abscess.

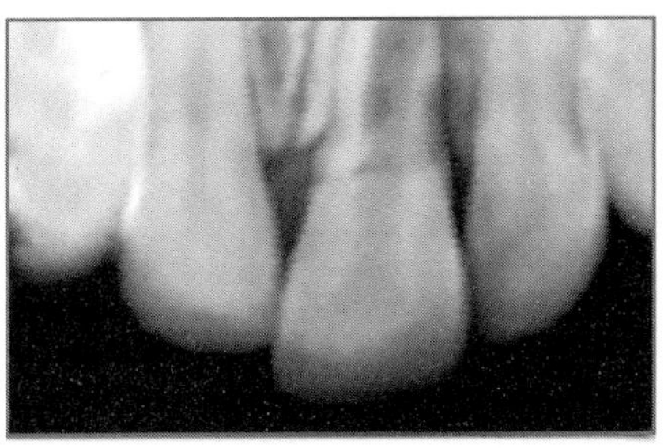

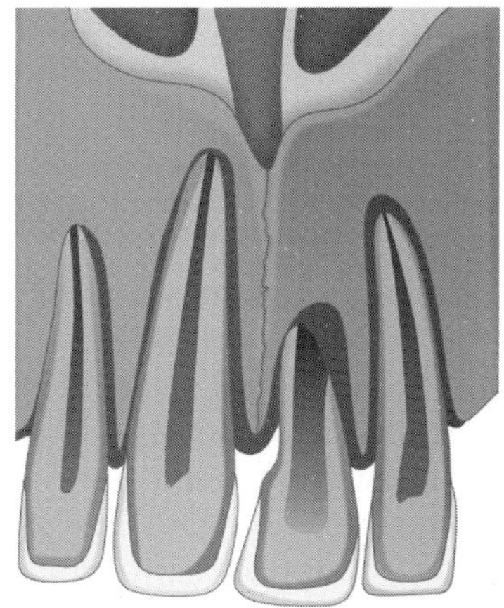

Fig. 56: Extrusion.

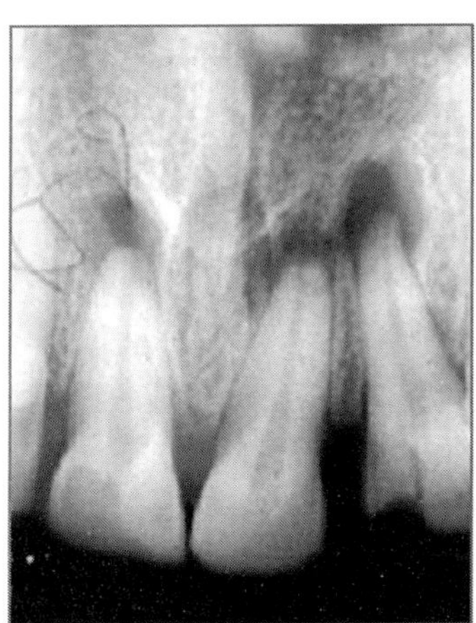
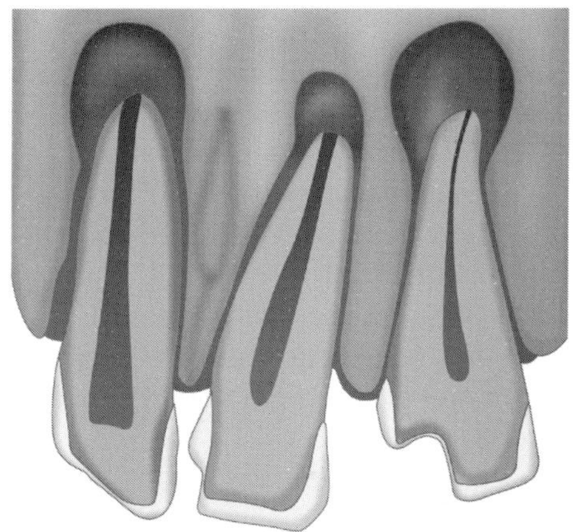

Fig. 57: Crown fracture with periapical cyst.

margin with distorted morphology of pulp canal.

- Bone rarefaction evident at the periapical region of 11.
- The apex of 21 is below the level of apices of 11 and 22.
- Root of 21 is partially displaced out of its socket as indicated by generalized thickening of PDL space and radiolucency at the lateral aspect of 21.

Radiodiagnosis

Extruded 21.

Coronal Fracture with Periapical Cyst (Fig. 57)

Teeth seen: 11, 21, 22, partial image of 12.

Anatomical landmarks: Intermaxillary suture, nasal septum, floor of nasal fossa.

Pathological Interpretation

- Partial loss of coronal tooth structure evident as radiolucent structure on the mesial side of coronal portion of 22 involving pulp.
- A thin radiolucent line running vertically on the midline, continuation with the

remaining crown structure suggestive of vertical fracture of the crown.

- A well-defined radiolucency encircling the apex of 22 with well-defined cortical boundary. The size of the radiolucency is approximately above 1 × 1 cm in size.
- Discontinuity of lamina dura with thickening of PDL space is evident.
- A step formation evident as radiolucency with clear radiopaque boundary evident on the mesioproximal angle of 21, and discontinuity of the incisal third of coronal structure is evident as shap radiolucent line in 11 and 21.
- Uniform widening of pulp canal is evident in the coronal third of roots of 11 and 21.
- Discontinuity of the lamina dura with widening of PDL space evident with diffuse radioluceny measuring less than 1 cm approximately, evident at the periapical region of 21 indicating bone resorption.
- Widening of PDL space with loss of lamina dura evident in 11 with diffused radiolucency measuring 1 × 1 cm in diameter approximately at the periapical region of 11.
- Loss of typical constriction of apical third of root structures evident in 11 and 21 appear as flattened surface.

Radiodiagnosis

- Coronal fracture 22 with periapical cyst. (PAI-5)
- Coronal fracture 11, 21 with periapical abscess and external root resorption.

Advanced Periodontitis (Stage 4) (Fig. 58)

Teeth seen: 32, 31, 41, 42 and partial image of 33, 43.

Anatomical landmarks: Lingual foramen, Genial tubercle, nutrient canal

Pathological Interpretation

- Reduction of crestal bone height is evident between 32–31, 31–41, the bone recession extends from CEJ to the apical third of 31, 32, 41 and perpendicular to the direction to CEJ.
- Thickening of PDL space evident along the root with loss of lamina dura.
- Nonhomogeneous radiopaque spike are evident at the middle third of root structure suggesting of subgingival calculus.

Radiodiagnosis

Advanced periodontitis (stage 4).

Incomplete Root Canal Obturation with Periapical Abscess (Fig. 59)

Teeth seen: 23, 24, 25, 26.

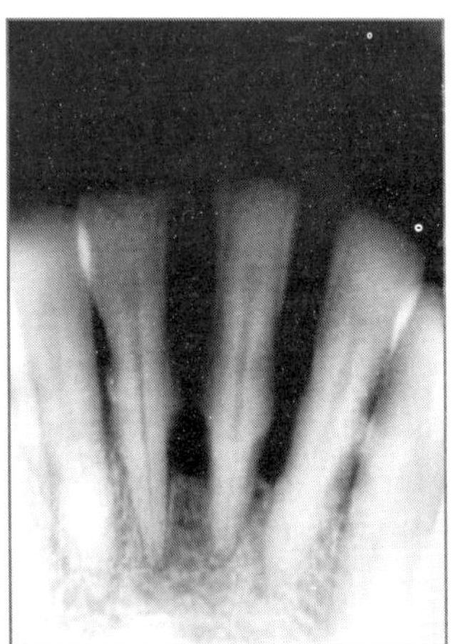

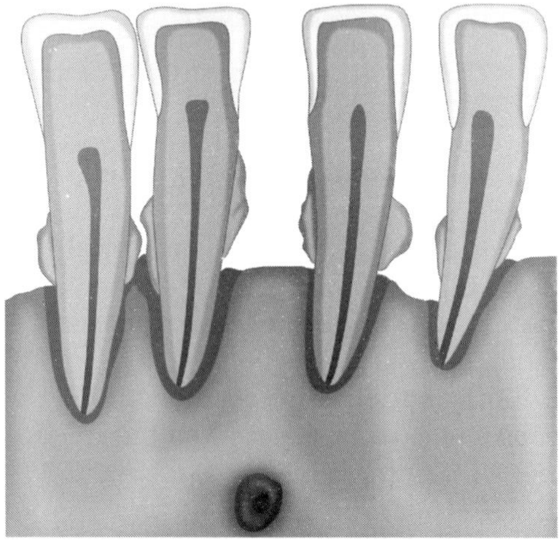

Fig. 58: Chronic periodontitis—advanced stage.

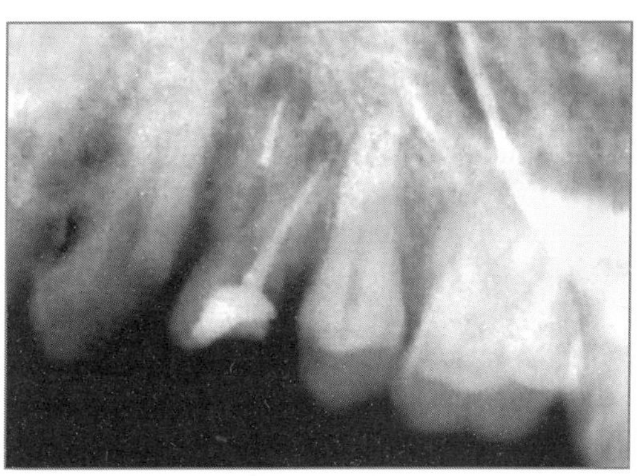
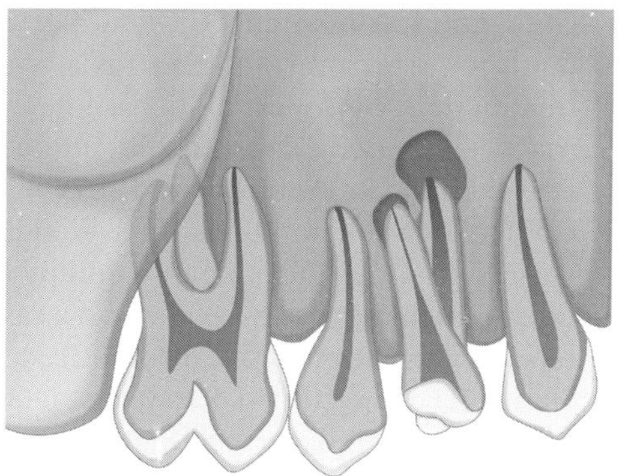

Fig. 59: Incomplete obturation with periapical abscess.

Anatomical landmarks: Zygoma, maxillary sinus.

Anatomical structures: Crown, root, pulp chamber, pulp canal and periapical region, crestal bone, trabecular pattern are normal in 26 and 25.

Pathological Interpretation

- Partial loss of coronal structure of 24 evident with loss of distal cusp morphology.
- Group I radiopaque restorative material evident on the coronal structure involving enamel, dentin and pulp chamber.
- Group II radiopaque restorative material evident on pulp canal of buccal root and incomplete obturation of pulp canal is evident on the palatal root with obturation material evident only the apical 3rd of palatal root.

Radiodiagnosis

- Well-defined radiolucency evident in the apical region of buccal and palatal root suggesting bone resorption.
- Incomplete root canal obturation of 24 with periapical abscess (PAI-4).

BIBLIOGRAPHY

1. American Association of Endodontists. Case Difficulty Assessment Form and Guidelines.
2. Andersson L, Blomlöf L, Lindskog S, et al. Tooth ankylosis: clinical, radiographic and histological assessments. Int J Oral Surg. 1984;13(5):423-31.
3. Berry JH. Cervical burnout and mach band: two shadows of doubt in radiologic interpretation of carious lesions. J Am Dent Assoc. 1983;106(5):622-5.
4. Cohen S, Burns RC. Pathways of the pulp. St. Louis: Mosby Inc.; 2006.
5. Cunningham AS, Blatt SD, Fuller PG, et al. The art of precepting: Socrates or Aunt Minnie?. Archives of pediatrics and adolescent medicine. 1999;153(2):114-6.
6. Dukić W, Filipović-Zore I, Bago I. Condensing osteitis-case report. Acta stomatologica Croatica. 2006;40(2): 182-8.
7. de Toledo BE, Barroso EM, Martins AT, et al. Prevalence of periodontal bone loss in Brazilian adolescents through interproximal radiography. Int J Dent. 2012;2012
8 Fuhrmann RA. Three-dimensional evaluation of periodontalremodeling during orthodontic treatment. Seminars in Orthodontics. 2002;8(1):23-28).
9. Fuss Z, Tsesis I, Lin S. Root resorption–diagnosis, classification and treatment choices based on stimulation factors. Dent Traumatol. 2003;19(4):175-82.
10. Guinta JL, Kaplan MA. Peripheral, soft tissue odontomas. Oral surgery, oral medicine, oral pathology. 1990;69(3):406-11.

11. Glickman I. Glickman's Clinical periodontology: prevention, diagnosis, and treatment of periodontal disease in the practice of general dentistry. 5th edition. Philadelphia. Saunder, Limited.1972
12. Gopikrishna V, Parameswaran A, Kandaswamy D. Criteria for management of calcific metamorphosis: review with a case report. Indian J Dental Res. 2004;15(2):54-7.
13. Haring JH, Howerton LJ. Paralleling technique. Haring JI, Iannucci JM, Howerton LJ, Jansen L. Dental Radiography: Principles and Techniques. 2nd edition. Philadelphia, PA: Saunders. 2000:pp.211-48.
14. Herrera D, Roldan S. O'Connor, A Sanz M The periodontal abscess (II). Short-term clinical and microbiological efficacy of 2 systemic antibiotic regimes. J Clin Periodontol. 2000;27(6):395-404.
15. Langlais RP, Langland OE, Nortje CJ. In: Diagnostic imaging of the jaws. 1st edition. Malvern: Williams and Wikins; 1995. pp. 87-102.
16. Langland OE, Langlais RP, Preece JW. Principles of dental imaging. Lippincott Williams & Wilkins; 2002.
17. McDonnell D. Dense bone island. A review of 107 patients. Oral Surg, Oral Med, Oral Pathol.1993;76(1):124-8.
18. Neelakantan P, John S, Subbarao CV. Restoring function and esthetics in a pair of twins with amelogenesis imperfecta. The Journal of Indian Prosthodontic Society. 2009;9(2):105.
19. Newman MG, Takei H, Klokkevold PR, et al. Carranza's clinical periodontology. Elsevier health sciences; 2011.
20. Owens BM, Schuman NJ, Mincer HH, et al. Dental odontomas: a retrospective study of 104 cases. J Clin Pediatr Dent. 1997;21(3):261-4.
21. Pell GJ, Gregory GT. Report on a ten-year study of a tooth division technique for the removal of impacted teeth. American Journal of Orthodontics and Oral Surgery. 1942;28(11):B660-6.
22. Peterson LJ, Ellis E, Hupp JR, Tucker MR, editors. Contemporary oral and maxillofacial surgery. St. Louis: Mosby; 1988.
23. Prichard JF. Interpretation of radiographs in periodontics. Int J Periodontics Restorative dentistry. 1983;3(1):8-39.
24. Ramfjord SP, Ash MM Jr. Significance of occlusion in the etiology and treatment of early, moderate and advanced periodontitis. J Periodontol. 1981;52(9): 511-7.
25. Riminucci M, Collins MT, Corsi A, et al. Gnathodiaphyseal dysplasia: a syndrome of fibro-osseous lesions of jawbones, bone fragility, and long bone bowing. J Bone Miner Res. 2001;16(9):1710-8.
26. Shields ED, Bixler D, el-Kafrawy AM. A proposed classification for heritable human dentine defects with a description of a new entity. Arch Oral Biol. 1973;18(4): 543-3.
27. Simon JH, Glick DH, Frank AL. The relationship of endodontic-periodontic lesions. J Periodontol. 1972;43(4):202-8.
28. Takagi Y, Fujita H, Katano H, et al. Immunochemical and biochemical characteristics of enamel proteins in hypocalcified amelogenesis imperfecta. Oral Surgery, Oral Medicine, Oral Pathology, Oral Radiology and Endodontology. 1998;85(4):424-30.
29. Thali MJ, Brogdon BG, Viner MD. Brogdon's forensic radiology. CRC Press; 2010.
30. Thomas MB, Hayes SJ, Gilmour AS. Radiographic evidence of postoperative healing 12 years following root canal treatment–a case report. Br Dent J. 2007; 203(11):635-39.
31. Tronstad L. Root resorption—etiology, terminology and clinical manifestations. Endod Dent Traumatol. 1988;4(6):241-52.
32. Williams TP, Brooks SL. A longitudinal study of idiopathic osteosclerosis and condensing osteitis. Dentomaxillofacial Radiol. 1998 ;27(5):275-8.

Index

Page numbers followed by *f* refer to figure, *fc* refer to flowchart, and *t* refer to table

D

I